FRRLS-FY ADULT
31022006499583
R 616.994 TURKINGTON
Turkington, Carol
The encyclopedia of cancer

10/05

REFERENCE

DISCARDED

D0023230

DISCHARGED

THE ENCYCLOPEDIA OF

CANCER

Carol Turkington
William LiPera, M.D.

DISCARDED

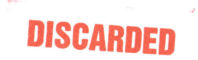

Facts On File, Inc.

The Encyclopedia of Cancer

Copyright © 2005 by Carol A. Turkington

All rights reserved. No part of this book may be reproduced or utilized in any form or by any means, electronic or mechanical, including photocopying, recording, or by any information storage or retrieval systems, without permission in writing from the publisher. For information contact:

Facts On File, Inc.
132 West 31st Street
New York NY 10001

Library of Congress Cataloging-in-Publication Data

Turkington, Carol.
The encyclopedia of cancer / Carol Turkington, William LiPera.
p. ; cm.
ISBN 0-8160-5029-5 (hc: alk. paper)
1. Cancer—Encyclopedias. I. LiPera, William J. II. Title.
[DNLM: 1. Neoplasms—Encyclopedias—English. QZ 13 T939e 2004]
RC262.T86 2004
616.99′4′003—dc22   2004043444

Facts On File books are available at special discounts when purchased in bulk quantities for businesses, associations, institutions, or sales promotions. Please call our Special Sales Department in New York at (212) 967-8800 or (800) 322-8755.

You can find Facts On File on the World Wide Web at http://www.factsonfile.com

Text and cover design by Cathy Rincon

Printed in the United States of America

VB Hermitage 10 9 8 7 6 5 4 3 2

This book is printed on acid-free paper.

CONTENTS

FOREWORD

In 2004 an estimated 1.4 million people in the United States will have been diagnosed with cancer, and 563,700 of these will die of their disease. Good news, however, is on the horizon. Death rates from the four most common cancers—lung, breast, prostate, and colorectal cancers—are on the decline. For all cancers combined, the death rate has begun to destabilize.

The steep decline in lung cancer rates in men and the recent slowing of the increased rates in women demonstrate the value of eduction and the impact of the antismoking campaign. Death rates from breast cancer continue to fall despite a gradual long-term increase in the rate of new diagnoses. Both these observations may be due in part to the increased use of mammographic screening, but other factors may be responsible as well.

Many advances in oncology (the study of tumors) have resulted from close interaction between the basic scientist and the clinical researcher. Biomedical research has dramatically enhanced our understanding of cancer and has provided a new branch of biological cancer treatment that has moved from the scientist's lab to the patient's bedside.

Biological therapy is an exciting and expanding field, tailored specifically to fighting individual cancers as well as alleviating many of the complications typically associated with chemotherapy and radiation. These treatments include monoclonal antibodies, cellular growth factors, anti-angiogenesis agents, and targeted receptor and enzyme inhibitors.

The field of oncology is growing at an unprecedented pace. The information and jargon that patients and their families are subjected to often heightens the fear that naturally accompanies a cancer diagnosis.

The purpose of this reference book is to detail, in a clear and distinct manner, commonly used terminology, the major cancers, their stages and complications, and cancer-screening and -prevention measures of which everyone should be aware.

All too often, when a patient is faced with a newly diagnosed cancer, fear, frustration, and anger take their toll. Although certainly justified, the stress that accompanies the confusion is often associated with natural misconceptions and should be quickly alleviated. Health-care givers are there to provide the answers to the questions that often plague the patient. Clarification and reinforcement of the multitude of new concepts the patient now faces will, we hope, relieve some of that anxiety.

That is the goal and purpose of this book: with increasing knowledge comes a positive attitude, which perhaps is the most critical factor in fighting a disease that in so many cases is now curable.

—William LiPera, M.D.

ACKNOWLEDGMENTS

The creation of a detailed encyclopedia involves the help and guidance of a wide range of experts. Without them, this book would not have been possible.

First of all, thanks to all the staff at Fox Chase Cancer Center in Philadelphia, and to Drs. William LiPera, Charles Pound, Mitchell Edelson, and Karen Krag. Also thanks to the staffs of the National Institute of Mental Health, the American Medical Association, the National Institutes of Health, American Heart Association, American Psychiatric Association, American Psychological Association, American Society of Hematology, the Cancer Information Service, the Food and Drug Administration, the National Cancer Institute, and the American Board of Plastic and Reconstructive Surgeons.

Thanks also to the National Prostate Cancer Coalition (NPCC); the National Institute of Nursing Research; American College of Obstetricians and Gynecologists; Complementary and Alternative Medicine; Exceptional Cancer Patient, Inc.; Well Spouse Foundation; Chemotherapy Foundation; American Society of Hematology; Cancer Liaison Program; Coalition of National Cancer Cooperative Groups; Widowed Persons Service; National Society of Genetic Counselors; Centers for Disease Control and Prevention, Division of Cancer Prevention and Control; Fertile Hope; Klinefelter Syndrome and Associates; American Urological Association Alliance for Prostate Cancer Prevention; American Foundation for Urologic Disease; American Prostate Society; CaP CURE; National Prostate Cancer Coalition; the Look Good . . . Feel Better program; Man to Man, Men's Cancer Resource Group; Patient Advocates for Advanced Cancer Treatments; Us Too International; American Brachytherapy Society; Cancer Hope Network; Cancer Information and Counseling Line; Cancer Information Service; Cancer Net; Cancer Research Institute; Cancer Survivors Network; CanSurmount; I Can Cope; International Union Against Cancer; CHEMOcare; Chemotherapy Foundation; National Association of Hospital Hospitality; Hereditary Cancer Institute; National Cancer Institute; Hospice Education Institute; HospiceLink; and the National Hospice and Palliative Care Organization.

Also, thanks to the National Hospice Foundation, Cancer Legal Resource Center, American College of Radiology, American Society of Clinical Oncology, Association of Community Cancer Centers, American College of Radiology, American Institute for Cancer Research, Cancer Research Foundation of America, Cancer Research Institute, European Organisation for Research and Treatment of Cancer.

Thanks also to ENCOREplus, National Alliance of Breast Cancer Associations, National Breast Cancer Coalition, National Lymphedema Network, Susan G. Komen Breast Cancer Foundation, Y-Me, Society of Gynecologic Oncologists, Breast Cancer Fund, Gilda's Club Worldwide, Make Today Count, National Asian Women's Health Organization, National Women's Health Information Center.

Thanks also to the librarians at the Hershey Medical Center medical library, the National Library of Medicine, the Reading Public Library, and the Pennsylvania State Library.

Finally, thanks to my agent, Gene Brissie of James Peter Associates, to Bert Holtje, to my editor James Chambers, to Vanessa Nittoli at Facts On File, and to Kara and Michael.

INTRODUCTION

Many people believe that their risk for cancer is much higher than it was 10, 20, or 30 years ago. It is true that the actual number of people who are diagnosed and who die of cancer each year has indeed grown, but the number has increased not because we are more at risk, but because the United States population is growing larger, and its biggest segment is entering old age.

Because cancer is more common among the elderly, it is not surprising that more cases are diagnosed as the average age of the U.S. population increases. A closer inspection of the numbers by age group shows the cancer risk for Americans is actually dropping. Only a few decades ago, fewer than one in 10 children with leukemia survived 10 years after diagnosis. With modern chemotherapy, the cure rate for these children is now almost 80 percent. Similar progress has been made fighting Hodgkin's lymphoma, bone and kidney cancers in children, and testicular cancer.

The fact is, a person's risk of being diagnosed with cancer and the risk of dying of cancer both have decreased since the early 1990s. Fewer than half the people diagnosed with cancer today will die of the disease. Some will be completely cured, and many more people survive for years with a good quality of life, thanks to treatments that control many types of cancer.

It's important to remember that "cancer" is not one disease but many different diseases with different causes. For that reason, one breakthrough cure for cancer that will solve the problem for everyone is unlikely. Instead, every year will bring new methods and treatments to cure different types of cancer.

There is no single treatment that is effective for all individuals. New treatments are available today that were not even imagined a few years ago, and medical researchers continue to find better ways to treat all types of cancer. Patients who have any doubts should feel comfortable in asking more than one doctor about their diagnosis and treatment plan. In fact, a patient's doctor can help arrange an appointment with another specialist—many health insurance companies pay for other opinions and some even require it.

Still, for all that is known today about cancer, many Americans have a lot of misconceptions about the disease. For example:

Myth: What you do when you are young does not have an impact on your chance of getting cancer later in life.

The truth is that poor lifestyle choices young people make can increase their risk of developing cancer—especially smoking, poor diet, lack of activity, sun exposure, and multiple sex partners (increasing the risk of human papillomavirus, a risk factor for cervical cancer). More than two-thirds of all fatal cancer cases can be prevented with simple lifestyle changes.

Myth: The medical industry will not tell the public about a cure for cancer because they make too much money treating cancer patients.

First of all, it is unlikely that there will ever be one all-encompassing cure for cancer, because cancer is actually many different diseases, and for several forms of cancer, cures are already available for most patients. It is also important to remember that scientists and doctors have family members and loved ones who die of cancer just as often as the rest of us do. All medical breakthroughs are quickly announced and applied, such as in the case of antibiotics and vaccines.

Myth: Electronic devices such as cell phones can cause cancer in the people who use them.

A few studies suggested a link between cell phones and certain rare types of brain tumors, but the consensus among well-designed population studies is that there is no consistent association between cell phone use and brain cancer.

Likewise, research has found no clear association between any other electronic consumer products and cancer. Cell phones, microwave ovens, and similar appliances emit low-frequency radiation—the part of the electromagnetic spectrum that includes radio waves and radar.

Ionizing radiation such as gamma rays and X-rays can increase cancer risk by damaging DNA in the body's cells, but low frequency, non-ionizing radiation does not cause these changes in DNA.

Myth: Living in a polluted city is a greater risk for lung cancer than smoking a pack of cigarettes a day.

Air pollution is much less likely to cause lung cancer than smoking cigarettes. Smoking or being frequently exposed to secondhand smoke is more dangerous than the level of air pollution encountered in U.S. cities. Air pollution does contribute to lung cancer risk, but it has a greater impact on heart disease, asthma, and chronic bronchitis.

Myth: Household pesticides can cause cancer.

Research does not support a link between cancer and using pesticides around the house. However, these products can be dangerous if consumers do not follow precautions regarding breathing and direct contact. Consumers should not avoid eating vegetables and fruit because of contamination fears, even though fruits and vegetables sold in groceries may contain trace amounts of pesticides, because these foods clearly help lower cancer risks.

Myth: Treating cancer with surgery causes it to spread throughout the body.

Surgical oncologists know how to safely take biopsy samples and remove tumors without spreading cancer. For a few types of cancer, surgeons take extra precautions to prevent any chance of the cancer spreading. For example, in testicular cancer the entire testicle is removed, so no cancer cells escape.

The Encyclopedia of Cancer is designed to answer questions just like these about all types of cancer, and includes the most up-to-date information on all major forms of this disease. It serves as a guide and reference to a wide range of subjects important to the understanding of cancer and includes a wide variety of contact information for organizations and governmental agencies affiliated with cancer issues, including current Web site addresses and phone numbers.

However, the book is not a substitute for prompt assessment and treatment by oncologic experts in the diagnosis and treatment of these diseases.

In this encyclopedia, we have tried to present the latest information in the field, based on the newest research. Although information in this book comes from the most recent medical journals and research sources, readers should keep in mind that changes occur very quickly in the field of oncology. A bibliography has been included for those who seek additional sources of information.

ENTRIES A–Z

ABCD   The abbreviation for a set of symptoms to watch out for that could indicate malignant MELANOMA. Any of the following symptoms should be brought to the attention of a dermatologist:

- **A** stands for asymmetry: One half of the mole does not match the other half. Melanomas tend to be irregular.
- **B** stands for border irregularity: Benign moles have nice smooth edges whereas melanomas are busily invading neighboring cells and tend to have irregular edges.
- **C** stands for color: If the color is intensely black or blue, or the color is uneven across the mole, this suggests a melanoma.
- **D** stands for diameter: If the mole is bigger than the size of a pea, then there is a greater chance that it is malignant.

abdominal cancer   A term that includes a number of different cancers that affect structures in the abdomen, including BLADDER CANCER, COLORECTAL CANCER, KIDNEY CANCER, LIVER CANCER, PANCREATIC CANCER, small intestine cancer, and STOMACH CANCER.

abdominoperineal resection   The surgical removal of the anus and the lower part of the rectum to treat cancer of the rectum and anus. Although this operation was once a common treatment for ANAL CANCER, it is not used as much today because RADIATION THERAPY with or without CHEMOTHERAPY is an equally effective treatment option but does not require a COLOSTOMY.

To perform an abdominoperineal resection, the doctor removes the anus and the lower part of the rectum by cutting into the abdomen and the perineum (the space between the anus and the scrotum in men, or the anus and the vulva in women). LYMPH NODES may also be taken out at the same time or in a separate operation (LYMPH NODE DISSECTION).

A doctor then creates a COLOSTOMY, which is an opening (stoma) on the outside of the body for waste to be eliminated. Patients with a colostomy must wear a special bag, to collect body wastes, which sticks to the skin around the stoma with a special glue and is thrown away after it is used. The bags are not visible under clothing, and most people can take care of the bags themselves.

achlorhydria   Also known as hypochlorhydria, this term describes a reduced ability to produce hydrochloric acid in the stomach, which places a patient at higher risk for STOMACH CANCER. Since hydrochloric acid is necessary to digest protein and is also required to stimulate the next stage of digestion, achlorhydria can cause significant problems with digestion and absorption.

acinar cell carcinoma   See PANCREATIC CANCER.

acral-lentiginous melanoma   See MELANOMA.

acrylamide   This substance is found in certain high-carbohydrate foods, such as french fries and potato chips, that may cause cancer, according to a study by Sweden's National Food Administration. Testing done in Sweden and several other countries found high levels of acrylamide in french fries, some brands of potato chips, some types of breakfast cereal, and some types of bread fried or baked at high temperatures. Regular bread and boiled foods did not contain significant levels of the substance.

The higher the heat at which the starches are cooked, the greater the level of acrylamide in the food. How acrylamide, previously known as an industrial chemical, forms in the cooking process remains a mystery.

According to Swedish tests conducted for the U.S. Center for Science in the Public Interest, a large order of fast-food french fries contains 39 to 82 micrograms of acrylamide, several hundred times the amount that the Environmental Protection Agency (EPA) says is allowable in an 8-ounce glass of water (0.12 micrograms).

In the original Swedish research, a kilogram (2.2 pounds) of potato chips was shown to contain an average of 1,212 micrograms of acrylamide. The equivalent weight in boiled potatoes held fewer than 3 micrograms, while a kilogram of soft bread held an average of 50, and breakfast cereals had 298. Unexplained differences in acrylamide levels were found between brands and types of products. For instance, breakfast cereals that were coated in sugar and then processed seemed to contain higher levels of acrylamide. French fries cooked until they were brown rather than just lightly done also contained higher levels.

Acrylamide, sometimes used in water-treatment facilities, is a known carcinogen in rats, but there is no conclusive proof that it causes cancer in humans. However, scientists are worried that because it can cause cancer in animals, it is probable that it also causes cancer in human beings; the EPA considers acrylamide a probable human carcinogen. In addition to being a carcinogen in rats, acrylamide is also a known neurotoxin, which can cause nerve damage resulting in weakness in the hands and feet.

Experts did not warn consumers against eating foods with the potentially cancer-causing substance but noted that further study is necessary to determine the extent of the risk—and how to reduce it. The findings of the Swedish study were greeted with some skepticism, in part because they were announced at a government news conference rather than in a peer-reviewed scientific publication. However, subsequent studies in Norway, Britain, Switzerland, Germany, and the United

States drew similar conclusions. Health experts were concerned enough to call a special meeting in Geneva of 23 scientists from universities and national food authorities, including the U.S. Food and Drug Administration.

Instead of warning consumers with specific advice, these scientists suggested people should eat a balanced and varied diet with plenty of fruits and vegetables and limit consumption of fried and fatty foods. Scientists already had warned consumers about various cancer risks posed by food: for instance, grilling or barbecuing meat can form carcinogenic substances.

The Swedish National Food Administration, which first discovered acrylamide in food, advises consumers to avoid burning food during frying, deep-frying, broiling, and grilling. (The agency also noted that cigarettes are a source of acrylamide.)

So far 200 analyses have been completed in North America and Europe. The UN health groups intend to set up a network to channel data from governments, universities, and industry into one central database and to include research from Africa, Asia, and South America.

Critics of the acrylamide studies complain that the claim that acrylamide poses a human cancer risk is based exclusively on high-dose studies in laboratory animals and say that there is no evidence that humans who eat the observed levels of acrylamide are exposed to any risk of any type of cancer.

Whenever a substance has been shown to cause cancer in test animals, the food industry, including the American Council on Science and Health, has argued that high-dose studies in animals do not predict risk of human cancer. This argument first appeared 30 years ago when animal testing showed the presence of potent carcinogens called nitrosamines in cured meats. However, regulations governing carcinogens in food are not based on human experiments, because it is impossible to conduct human epidemiological studies in this area for ethical reasons.

actinic keratosis A precancerous condition of thick, scaly patches of skin, also called solar keratosis, that can lead to malignant skin tumors (SQUAMOUS CELL CARCINOMA OF THE SKIN). Caused by long-term overexposure to the sun, it is usually found in older people but is appearing more and more often among younger patients. This common skin lesion affects one out of every six people. Untreated, it can invade the surrounding tissue or internal organs. Lesions occur most often on the face, back of hands and forearms, neck, and exposed scalp. The lesions develop slowly, eventually growing to about a quarter of an inch, sometimes fading and reappearing. There are usually several keratoses at one time on areas of the body exposed to sunlight.

Actinic damage of the lips is called "actinic cheilitis"; if it becomes squamous cell carcinoma, about a fifth of these lesions will spread.

Those at greatest risk for these lesions have fair skin, blond or red hair, and blue, green, or gray eyes. People with dark skin can develop keratoses if they are exposed to the sun without protection, although those with black skin rarely have these lesions. Individuals with compromised immune systems, as a result of chemotherapy, AIDS, or organ transplants, are at higher risk. One recent survey found keratoses in more than half of the men and a third of the women aged 65 to 74. Some experts believe that most people who live to be 80 or more will develop actinic keratoses.

Since more than half a person's lifetime sun exposure occurs before age 20, keratoses can appear in young people who have not been protected from sun damage.

While not all keratoses need to be removed, there are a number of treatments for those that do. The most common method is CRYOSURGERY, in which the lesion is frozen with liquid nitrogen. Two medicated creams (5-FU or masoprocol) are also effective in removing keratoses, especially when there are many lesions. Treatments cause the skin to become intensely red, causing some pain and skin breakdown.

acupressure   A noninvasive treatment, based on the same principles as ACUPUNCTURE, in which therapists press on acupuncture points with their fingers instead of using needles. (Other therapists use electrical impulses, heat, laser beams, sound waves, friction, suction, or magnets instead of their fingers at the acupressure points, but the goal is still the same.)

While acupressure cannot cure cancer, numerous studies have shown it is effective in relieving the NAUSEA associated with CHEMOTHERAPY treatment or surgery. The technique can be used by itself or as part of other systems of manual healing such as shiatsu massage.

acupuncture   A technique in which very thin needles of varying lengths are inserted through the skin to treat a variety of conditions. Although there is no evidence that acupuncture is effective as a treatment for cancer, clinical studies have found it to be effective in treating NAUSEA caused by CHEMOTHERAPY drugs and surgical anesthesia. This finding was supported by a National Institutes of Health expert panel consisting of scientists, researchers, and health-care providers. There is also some evidence that acupuncture may lessen the need for conventional pain-relieving drugs. A small clinical trial recently found acupuncture was effective in reducing the number of hot flashes men experienced after hormonal therapy for PROSTATE CANCER.

Acupuncture has been practiced for the past 2,000 years and is an important component of traditional Chinese medicine, still practiced today. Traditional Chinese practitioners believe that health depends on a vital energy called *qi* (pronounced "chee"), which they believe flows through pathways in the body called meridians. They believe that an obstruction along a meridian blocks the natural flow of energy, creating pain and disease. Also important to Chinese physicians is the idea of the opposing forces of yin and yang, which, when balanced, are said to work together with *qi* to promote physical and mental wellness. The insertion of needles into precise points on the skin is believed to unblock energy flow, balance yin and yang, and restore health. Originally, 365 acupuncture points were identified, corresponding to the number of days in a year, but gradually the number grew to more than 2,000.

Some practitioners in the West reject the traditional philosophies of Chinese medicine and claim that acupuncture works by stimulating the production of natural painkilling substances in the body called endorphins. Because Western scientists have found it hard to study meridians (they do not exactly correspond to nerve or blood circulation pathways), some do not believe that meridians exist at all. Nevertheless, several studies have found that acupuncture used along with mainstream medicine can have real benefits, such as helping to relieve pain and reduce the nausea and vomiting caused by chemotherapy. There is no evidence that acupuncture alone is effective for treating or preventing cancer.

Traditional acupuncture needles were made of bone, stone, or metal (including silver and gold), but modern disposable acupuncture needles are made of very thin stainless steel. In 1996 the U.S. Food and Drug Administration approved the use of acupuncture needles by licensed practitioners; by law, needles must be labeled for one-time use only.

The procedure should cause little or no discomfort because the needles are as thin as a strand of hair. They are usually left in place for less than half an hour. Some acupuncturists twirl the needles or apply low-voltage electricity to them as a way to enhance the results. When conducted by a trained professional, acupuncture is generally considered safe. Relatively few complications have been reported, but there is a risk that a patient may be harmed if the acupuncturist is not well trained.

There are more than 10,000 acupuncturists in the United States, and about 32 states have established training standards for licensing the practice of acupuncture. Medicare does not cover acupuncture, but it is covered by some private health insurance plans and HMOs. Consumers should consult an experienced, qualified practitioner who is state licensed or board certified. The American Academy of Medical Acupuncture (http://www. medicalacupuncture.org) can refer patients to physicians (M.D.s or D.O.s) who practice acupuncture.

acute lymphocytic leukemia   See LEUKEMIA.

adenocarcinoma   Cancer that begins in cells that line certain internal organs and that have glandular properties (*adeno* means "gland"). Adenocarcinoma can develop in almost any part of the body, including the breast, esophagus, lung, pancreas, prostate, small intestines, stomach, urethra, or vagina.

adenoid cystic carcinoma (ACC)   A relatively rare cancer usually first appearing in the minor salivary glands of the head and neck. It tends to grow slowly, often spreading to the lungs, liver, breast, bone, and other organs, although it can also be primary to these sites. It is often highly resistant to CHEMOTHERAPY.

Salivary gland cancers account for about 3 percent of all malignant HEAD AND NECK CANCER in North America, and of that 3 percent, about 25 percent are ACC. Of all salivary gland tumors, only about 10 percent to 15 percent originate in minor salivary glands.

Typically, patients are about 45 when first diagnosed. The disease affects men and women equally. It is quite typical for this cancer to recur at the original site many years after its initial treatment.

There appears to be some evidence that there are two kinds of ACC: most cases seem to be slow-growing, but the second type is a much faster, more aggressive form. There are also three distinct types of ACC cells: cribriform, tubular, and solid, a combination of which may appear in one tumor. There is some evidence that the solid type is a more aggressive form of ACC, leading to an earlier death. A tumor needs to consist of at least 30 percent solid pattern to be considered a solid tumor.

Cause

No one knows for sure what causes ACC, although research suggests that there appear to be abnormal characteristics of DNA on chromosomes 6, 12, 13, and 19 for ACC cells.

Treatment

Because of ACC's reputation for being unpredictable, aggressive treatment is generally recommended. The most common and effective treatments for ACC are surgery and radiation, with one or both used depending upon the location of the tumor. Because of the high propensity for spread and the difficulty in achieving clean surgical margins, many doctors recommend surgical removal followed by radiation treatment to the tumor region. Because ACC can spread microscopically through a region, it can be difficult to detect. Radiation is an effective way to treat the area all around the original tumor bed, including the lymph nodes and major nerves in the head and neck.

No type of chemotherapy has shown to be effective in a significant number of ACC patients or over an extended period of time. There has been limited success in using chemotherapy for slowing or stopping ACC tumor growth, but in most cases the cancer begins to grow again within a year or two. There has also been limited success using ANTI-ANGIOGENESIS INHIBITORS.

Prognosis

Because ACC is usually slow growing, most people live a long time after diagnosis, even in cases of more advanced tumor involvement. In many of the longer-term studies, 60 percent to 70 percent of study participants are still alive 10 years after their initial diagnosis. With newer treatments, earlier diagnosis, and more sophisticated techniques and equipment, it is expected that ACC cancer patients will continue to experience longer life spans with better quality of life than before.

adenoma   A noncancerous tumor that appears in the lining or inner surface of an organ, most often in the colon or rectum. Occasionally, adenomas also appear in the breast, adrenal glands, or elsewhere.

Because cancerous cells may one day appear within an adenoma, these benign growths should be removed. In fact, experts suspect that COLORECTAL CANCER may begin from adenomas.

adenomatoid tumor   A very rare, benign tumor of the epididymis. On ultrasound it appears as a well-defined mass separate from the testicle. See also TESTICULAR CANCER.

adenomatous hyperplasia   A type of abnormal or heavy bleeding during menopause (ENDOMETRIAL HYPERPLASIA) that may be triggered by excessive growth of the uterine lining. It may be the first sign of ENDOMETRIAL CANCER (a type of UTERINE CANCER).

adenomatous polyps   Small benign growths in the intestines that can be found in up to 15 percent of American adults. Although they do not usually cause symptoms, they can obstruct the passage of feces if they become large enough and can lead to occasional bleeding. Invasive cancer develops in about 5 percent of adenomatous polyps.

adenovirus   A group of viruses used in gene therapy that are altered so they can carry a specific tumor-fighting gene.

adjuvant therapy   Treatment given after the primary treatment of cancer to increase the chances of a cure. Adjuvant therapy may include CHEMOTHERAPY, RADIATION THERAPY, or HORMONAL THERAPY.

adrenal cancer   Cancer of the adrenal glands, a pair of small organs located above the kidneys that produce corticosteroid hormones. These hormones help to control the metabolism of protein, fat, and carbohydrates, and regulate sodium and potassium levels in the body. The adrenal glands also secrete epinephrine and norepinephrine, two hormones that help regulate the part of the nervous system that is responsible for heartbeat, digestion, and breathing. While most abnormal growths in the adrenals are not malignant, there are two very rare types of cancerous tumors that may occur in this area.

Adrenocortical Cancer

This cancer begins in the outer layer of the adrenals. It is rare and usually appears in adults between 40 and 50; only 75 to 115 new cases are diagnosed in the United States each year.

Symptoms   Stomach pain, weakness, weight loss, high blood pressure. Men may experience loss of sex drive, impotence, or breast enlargement; women may notice a deepening of the voice, oily skin, hairiness, or an enlarged clitoris. All of these gender-related symptoms are due to the excessive production of hormones as a result of the tumor. Adrenocortical tumors that do not produce hormones are called "nonfunctioning tumors."

Diagnosis   Blood and urine tests can evaluate hormone levels; endocrine studies, imaging tests, angiography, and contrast X-rays of the veins are all used to diagnose this condition.

Stages   *Stage I* indicates a tumor less than 5 cm, with no spread into the lymph nodes, local tissue, or distant metastases. *Stage II* indicates a tumor bigger than 5 cm, with no spread of cancer into lymph nodes, local tissue, or distant sites. *Stage III* indicates a tumor that has spread into local tissue and/or lymph nodes but has not spread to distant sites. *Stage IV* refers to a tumor that has spread to other parts of the body. *Recurrent* cancer has returned to the original site or has spread to a different part of the body after treatment.

Treatment   This depends on the health of the patient and the stage of the disease but usually includes surgery to remove the adrenal glands, lymph nodes, and any other tissue that contains cancer. This may be followed by CHEMOTHERAPY and/or RADIATION THERAPY. Additional treatment may be given to alleviate symptoms resulting from the excess hormones produced by the cancer.

Pheochromocytoma

This rare type of cancer appears in the inner core of the adrenals and may be genetic. Patients often have high blood pressure due to the release of large amounts of catecholamine.

Symptoms   Headaches, sweating, palpitations, anxiety, and constipation.

Diagnosis   Blood tests, urinalysis, and imaging tests can be used to diagnose this type of cancer.

Staging   The least serious is *localized benign pheochromocytoma,* in which a tumor is localized in one area and has not spread. *A regional pheochromocytoma* has spread to local lymph nodes or to other tissue surrounding the original tumor. *Metastatic pheochromocytoma* indicates that the malignancy has spread to other parts of the body. *Recurrent pheochromocytoma* indicates that the cancer has returned after being treated, either in the original area or in another part of the body.

Treatment   Typically, this type of cancer is treated with surgery; radiation therapy or chemotherapy also may be used.

adrenal medullary tumors   See THYROID CANCER.

adrenocortical cancer   Cancer of the adrenal gland is a rare cancer characterized by malignant cells in the outside layer of the adrenal gland (the adrenal cortex). The adrenal glands are located one above each kidney in the back of the upper abdomen; the inside layer of the adrenal gland is called the adrenal medulla. Cancer that starts in the adrenal medulla is called pheochromocytoma.

Symptoms

The cells in the adrenal cortex produce hormones that help the body work properly. When these cells become cancerous, they may produce many hormones, which can cause symptoms such as high blood pressure, weakening of the bones, or diabetes. If male or female hormones are affected, the body may go through changes such as a deepening of the voice, facial hair, swelling of the sex organs, or swelling of the breasts.

Cancers that make hormones are called functioning tumors. However, many adrenal cortex cancers do not make extra hormones and are called nonfunctioning tumors. Other symptoms of these tumors include abdominal pain, unexplained weight loss, or weakness.

Diagnosis

Blood and urine tests can assess hormone levels; a computed tomography (CT) scan of the abdomen and other special X-rays may be done to assess the tumor.

Stages of Cancer

Once cancer of the adrenal cortex has been found, a doctor will order tests to see how far the cancer has spread; this is called staging. The following stages are used for cancer of the adrenal cortex.

Stage I: The cancer is less than 5 centimeters (less than 2 inches) and has not spread into tissues around the adrenal gland.
Stage II: The cancer is more than 5 centimeters (bigger than 2 inches) and has not spread into tissues around the adrenal gland.
Stage III: The cancer has spread into tissues around the adrenal gland or has spread to the lymph nodes around the adrenal gland. Lymph nodes are part of the lymph system and are small, bean-shaped organs that make and store infection-fighting cells.
Stage IV: The cancer has spread to tissues or organs in the area and to lymph nodes around the adrenal cortex, or the cancer has spread to other parts of the body.
Recurrent: The cancer has returned after it has been treated. It may recur in the adrenal cortex or in another part of the body.

Treatment

There are treatments for all patients with cancer of the adrenal cortex, including surgery, CHEMOTHERAPY, and RADIATION THERAPY. The chance of recovery depends on how far the cancer has spread and on whether a doctor was able to surgically remove all of the cancer.

Surgery The adrenal gland may be removed (an adrenalectomy), in addition to tissues around the adrenal glands that contain cancer. LYMPH NODES in the area also may be removed in a procedure called a LYMPH NODE DISSECTION.

Chemotherapy The cancer drug mitotane may be used if the cancer is not operable or has spread to other parts of the body.

Radiation therapy Radiation for cancer of the adrenal cortex usually comes from a machine outside the body (external radiation therapy).

Symptom management In addition to chemotherapy, radiation therapy, and/or surgery, a patient may receive therapy to prevent or treat symptoms caused by the extra hormones that are produced.

advance directives A written document, completed and signed when a person is legally competent, that explains what the person would or would not want if unable to make decisions about medical care. Common advance directives include:

- health-care proxy (or health-care power of attorney), which gives another person the authority to make decisions for the patient when the patient is unable to do so.
- living will, which directs a doctor whether to use, not start, or stop treatment that is keeping a dying patient alive when the patient cannot make those wishes known.
- non-hospital (do not resuscitate) DNR ORDER, which directs emergency staff to not resuscitate a person when not in a hospital or other health-care facility.

Advance directives are an important part of any patient's personal affairs, since such a document allows someone else to make treatment decisions on a patient's behalf when the person is no longer capable of making those decisions.

Patients should prepare and sign advance directives that comply with state law and give copies to family, friends, and doctors. The document should reflect the patient's wishes and appoint someone to make decisions who is willing to carry out those wishes.

aflatoxins Toxic substances made by certain types of mold (*Aspergillus flavus* and *A. parasiticus*) found in peanuts, corn, wheat, rice, cottonseeds, barley, soybeans, Brazil nuts, and pistachios. Eating food contaminated with aflatoxins has been linked to LIVER CANCER.

The molds that produce aflatoxin grow in warm, humid climates in the southeastern United States; the mold can also be produced in the field when rain falls on crops such as corn and wheat that are left in the field to dry. Aflatoxin-producing mold can even grow on plants damaged by insects, drought, poor nutrition, or unseasonable temperatures.

Aflatoxin has been called the most potent natural carcinogen known to humans; rat studies suggest males are especially susceptible to cancer after aflatoxin exposure. Poor diet also seems to predispose animals to cancer after eating aflatoxins.

Still, scientists know very little about why or how the aflatoxins are produced by the mold, and because it is sometimes difficult to see, all susceptible crops are subject to routine testing in the United States. Unfortunately, it is not possible to detect the mold with 100 percent accuracy.

While the way agricultural products are stored can affect the mold's growth, the length of time of such storage is also important. The longer the products are stored in bins, the greater the chance that environmental conditions favorable to aflatoxin production will be created. Aflatoxins are more common in poor-quality cereals and nuts; while most of these low-grade products do not enter the human food market, they are sold as animal feed, which can go on to contaminate animal products such as meat and milk. For this reason, cottonseed meal (a product often contaminated with high levels of aflatoxin) is banned as an animal feed. Cottonseed oil, however, rarely contains aflatoxin.

Milk is commonly contaminated, and powdered nonfat milk can contain eight times more than the liquid product. Measurable levels can be found in some baby foods that use dry milk to boost the protein content of the product.

Pasteurization, sterilization, and spray-dry processing techniques can substantially reduce aflatoxin contamination of dried milk. Meat products are less often contaminated because little aflatoxin is carried over into the meat, except for pig's liver and kidneys.

In humans, aflatoxin consumption is believed to cause liver cancer, according to some east African studies that seem to show a correlation between the two. Data from the African studies were strong enough to prompt the U.S. Food and Drug Administration and the Environmental Protection Agency to develop strict regulations to control levels in human food and animal feed sold in the United States.

For these reasons, consumers should not eat moldy food, especially grains or peanuts, and should be cautious about eating unroasted peanuts sold in bulk.

AFP   See ALPHA-FETOPROTEIN.

African Americans and cancer   African Americans have the highest overall cancer incidence and death rates of all racial groups in the United States, as well as the highest rates for certain cancers. Although overall cancer rates have been inching down for African Americans in the last 10 years, there is a long way to go. Since 1992 cancer incidence and death rates for African-American men have been dropping by up to 2.7 percent each year, yet the death rate for all cancers combined is still about 30 percent higher for African Americans than for Caucasians. About 132,700 new cancer cases and 63,100 deaths are expected among African Americans in 2003, according to the American Cancer Society. Prostate cancer and BREAST CANCER rates in African Americans provide the most dramatic evidence of the cancer gap.

Continued higher incidence and death rates among some racial and ethnic groups suggest that not all populations have benefited equally from cancer prevention and treatment control efforts.

Such disparities may be due to multiple factors, such as late stage of disease at diagnosis, barriers to health-care access, history of other diseases, biological and genetic differences in tumors, health behaviors, and the presence of risk factors. Once diagnosed, African Americans with cancer, at all stages, survive for shorter periods than Caucasian Americans.

Causes

One way to bring down high cancer death rates among African Americans is early detection. Regular cancer-related checkups, mammograms, and blood tests find cancer early, when treatment is more successful. About half of all cancers can now be discovered early by such screening methods, but African Americans do not seem to be getting these tests regularly. Most cancers detectable by screening are diagnosed at a later stage in African Americans than in Caucasians.

Recently a landmark report, "Unequal Treatment: Confronting Racial and Ethnic Disparities in Health Care," concluded that racial discrimination within health-care settings contributes to poor medical care for many African Americans and other minorities. Time pressures on medical professionals and low-end health insurance plans were also cited as reasons why minorities were more likely to get substandard medical care. In this study, lower quality medical care was found even when minority patients' income, age, medical condition, and insurance coverage were similar to those of Caucasian patients.

African-American Men

African-American men have the highest death rates and highest incidence rates for lung, prostate, and colorectal cancers. Between 1995 and 1999, African-American men had the highest cancer incidence and death rates of all racial groups in each age group, except for African-American men under 20.

The 10 most common cancers in African-American men are (in order beginning with the most common) PROSTATE CANCER, LUNG CANCER, COLORECTAL CANCER, MOUTH CANCER, STOMACH CANCER, ESOPHAGEAL CANCER, LYMPHOMA, PANCREATIC CANCER, BLADDER CANCER, and KIDNEY CANCER. African-American men have the highest rate of prostate cancer and death in the world—more than twice the rates for Caucasian men in the United States.

African-American Women

Among women, African Americans have the highest incidence of colorectal cancer and lung cancer. While African-American women are less likely than Caucasian women to develop breast cancer, they are more likely to die from the disease.

The 10 most common types of cancer in African-American women (beginning with the most common) are breast cancer, colorectal cancer, lung cancer, UTERINE CANCER, CERVICAL CANCER, pancreatic cancer, OVARIAN CANCER, lymphomas, stomach cancer, and MULTIPLE MYELOMA.

Lung Cancer and African Americans

Despite a reduced rate across all races, lung cancer is still much more prevalent among African Americans than in the general population. Each year 73 out of 100,000 African Americans get lung cancer, compared with 54 out of 100,000 Caucasians. In addition, African Americans develop the disease at a much younger age than their Caucasian counterparts. For example, among men ages 40 to 54 African Americans are two to four times more likely to develop lung cancer than Caucasians. Studies also show African Americans with early-stage disease are less likely to undergo surgery, the primary curative option for early lung cancer. The five-year survival rate for African Americans is 35 percent, compared to 46 percent for Caucasians. The reasons for this disparity are unclear. The percentage of African Americans who smoke is higher than the percentage of smokers in the general U.S. population, but African Americans smoke fewer cigarettes than do Caucasians.

The type of cigarettes could be a factor, since between 75 percent and 90 percent of African-American smokers prefer menthol cigarettes, compared with 20 percent to 30 percent of Caucasian smokers, and research has found that menthol cigarettes are higher in tar and other carcinogens. Other factors that may account for the disparity between African Americans and Caucasians could include exposure to cancer-causing materials in the workplace and access to health care.

Erasing Disparity

The AMERICAN CANCER SOCIETY (ACS) has been working to eliminate the higher minority cancer burden for several years, providing funding for research into cancer prevalence, prevention, and treatment in low-income communities, and culturally appropriate programs and services for different populations. The ACS also works to secure insurance coverage for screening tests and treatment.

"Let's Talk about It" is a prostate health education program for African Americans cosponsored by the group 100 Black Men of America, Inc. The Man to Man Program of the American Cancer Society enlists survivors and others concerned about prostate cancer to help people newly diagnosed with the disease and to develop local support groups, screenings, and educational events.

after loading   A technique in which radiation is directed to a specific site in the body as part of RADIATION THERAPY. In this method, a tube or needle is placed near the cancer area and loaded with radioactive material. After a certain prescribed period of time, the tube is removed from the patient's body.

age and cancer   There is a definite link between age and onset of certain cancers; some are more typical in childhood, some in early adulthood, others in middle age, and some in old age. In general, however, patients become more likely to get cancer as they get older, even if no one in their family has had cancer at all. The average age for all cancers combined is 68 years old; the median ages for the top four cancers are

- LUNG CANCER, age 70
- COLORECTAL CANCER, age 72
- BREAST CANCER, age 63
- PROSTATE CANCER, age 69

According to the latest government studies, published in 2002, breast, prostate, lung, and colorectal cancers are the most frequently occurring cancers in the age group of 50 to 64. These cancers continued to rank highest in even older populations, although their relative ranking varies among older age groups. Even if cancer incidence remains steady, the number of people diagnosed with cancer in the next 50 years is expected to double, barring any major breakthroughs in prevention. The aging of the population alone will increase the number of people who are diagnosed and treated for cancer. Advances in cancer prevention, detection, and treatment should continue to reduce cancer death rates.

Researchers have found that age does not affect relative survival rates, but type of cancer and extent of the disease do play important roles. An estimated 8.9 million cancer survivors were alive as of January 1, 1999; of these survivors, 60 percent were 65 years and older, and 32 percent were 75 years and older.

During the period 1987 to 1999, lung, colorectal, breast, and prostate cancers represented more than half of all cancer cases. For men under 50 years, prostate cancer incidence increased while lung and colorectal cancer rates decreased. For men 50 and over, lung and colorectal cancer incidence decreased in most age groups while prostate cancer increased for men 50 to 64.

During the same period, breast cancer incidence increased for women aged 50 to 64. Lung cancer decreased for many age groups but continued to increase for older women. Colorectal cancer increased for women under 50 but decreased for women aged 50 to 64 and age 75 and older.

Death rates for these four cancers continued to decline. Lung cancer death rates decreased during the 1990s in men of all ages and in women under age 65, but lung cancer accounted for almost one-third of cancer deaths in men and one-fourth of cancer deaths in women. Most age groups showed declines, but lung cancer death rates for women aged 65 to 74 continued to rise.

Agent Orange A toxic herbicide containing DIOXIN used by U.S. soldiers during the Vietnam War. Shortly after their military service in Vietnam, some veterans reported a variety of health problems (including cancer) that many attributed to exposure to Agent Orange or other herbicides.

According to the U.S. Veterans' Administration, the following cancers are believed to be linked to exposure to Agent Orange: HODGKIN'S DISEASE, MULTIPLE MYELOMA, NON-HODGKIN'S LYMPHOMA, PROSTATE CANCER, respiratory cancers (LUNG CANCER and cancers of the larynx or trachea), soft tissue sarcoma (other than osteosarcoma, chondrosar-

coma, KAPOSI'S SARCOMA, and MESOTHELIOMA), and possibly at least one type of childhood LEUKEMIA (acute myelogenous leukemia) related to a parent's service in Vietnam.

Agent Orange was the code name for a herbicide developed in the 1940s for military use in tropical climates; serious testing for military applications did not begin until the early 1960s. The purpose of the product was to destroy enemy cover in dense terrain by defoliating trees and shrubbery. Agent Orange (named for the orange band that was used to mark the drums in which the herbicide was stored) was tested in Vietnam in the early 1960s and used more heavily during the height of the war (1967–68). It was eventually phased out of use and discontinued in 1971.

Agent Orange was a mixture of two chemicals (2,4-D and 2,4,5-T) that was combined with kerosene or diesel fuel and dispersed by aircraft, vehicle, and hand spraying. An estimated 19 million gallons of Agent Orange were used in South Vietnam during the war.

The earliest health concerns about Agent Orange focused on the product's contamination with TCDD, one of a family of dioxins that are cousins of cancer-causing compounds called polychlorinated biphenyls (PCBs). The TCDD found in Agent Orange is believed to be harmful to humans; in animal tests, TCDD has caused a wide variety of fatal diseases. TCDD is a man-made and always unwanted by-product of the chemical manufacturing process. The Agent Orange used in Vietnam was later found to be extremely contaminated with TCDD.

The Agent Orange Settlement Fund was created in response to class action lawsuits by Vietnam veterans and their families over injuries allegedly incurred as a result of their exposure to chemical herbicides used during the Vietnam War. The suit was brought against the major manufacturers of these herbicides and was settled out of court in 1984 for $180 million dollars—reportedly the largest settlement of its kind at that time. The Settlement Fund was distributed to class members according to a distribution plan established by the courts. Because the class involved an estimated 10 million people, the fund was distributed to Vietnam vets and their families in the United States through two separate programs designed to provide benefits to those most in need of assistance.

A payment program provided cash to totally disabled veterans and survivors of deceased veterans, and an assistance program provided money for social services organizations to establish programs to benefit all the affected veterans. The payment program distributed a total of $197 million to about 52,000 veterans, beginning in 1988 and ending in 1994. The assistance program functioned as a foundation, distributing $74 million to 83 organizations between 1989 and 1996. These agencies, which ranged from disability and veterans service organizations to community-based not-for-profits, provided counseling, advocacy, medical, and case-management services. During this period, these organizations helped more than 239,000 Vietnam veterans and their families.

The Department of Veterans Affairs has developed a comprehensive program to respond to vets' medical problems, including health-care services, disability compensation for veterans with service-connected illnesses, scientific research, and outreach and education.

agranulocytosis   See NEUTROPENIA.

AIDS (acquired immunodeficiency syndrome) An acquired defect in immune system function, caused by the human immunodeficiency virus (HIV), that is associated with a higher risk for certain cancers, such as KAPOSI'S SARCOMA, NON-HODGKIN'S LYMPHOMA, and a multitude of life-threatening opportunistic infections.

alcohol   An estimated 2 to 4 percent of all cancer cases are thought to be caused either directly or indirectly by alcohol. There is a strong association between heavy alcohol use and cancers of the esophagus, pharynx, and mouth, (oral cancers) and a more controversial association linking alcohol with liver, breast, and colorectal cancers. Together, these cancers kill more than 125,000 people each year in the United States. The oral and esophageal cancer risk from drinking alcohol is especially pronounced if a person smokes or eats a high-fat diet.

Alcohol can promote several types of cancer by damaging cells in the oral cavity and larynx. When a person drinks excessively the sensitive tissues of the upper respiratory tract are directly exposed to alcohol in beverages, damaging cells and possibly triggering cancer. Cancer of the liver is probably preceded by alcoholic liver cirrhosis, which develops after years of drinking.

Alcohol is also believed to indirectly affect cancer of the liver, colon, and breast, but experts do not know quite so much about how drinking alcohol affects the development of these other cancers. Experts do know that the risk for developing BREAST CANCER, the second most common cancer in American women, rises with increased alcohol consumption, which is why experts recommend that women at a high risk for breast cancer consider not drinking.

Prevention
To guard against developing alcohol-related cancers, experts suggest men should drink no more than two one-ounce drinks a day; women should have no more than one one-ounce drink a day. Different limits are recommended for men and women because alcohol affects the sexes differently. A woman's body has more fat and less muscle than a man's, so alcohol cannot be diluted as quickly in a woman's body, nor can a woman metabolize alcohol as quickly. The result is that alcohol stays in a woman's blood longer.

aleukemia   A lack of a certain type of white blood cell. Usually, LEUKEMIA triggers an overwhelming number of immature white blood cells; a person with aleukemia will have a normal-to-low white blood cell count, but the BONE MARROW (the normal source of blood cell production) will usually be packed with leukemic cells. Aleukemia occurs in about 30 percent of all leukemia cases. The condition will not alter the eventual outcome of the disease.

alkaline phosphatase test (ALP)   A test that measures the amount of an enzyme called alkaline phosphatase in the blood. This enzyme is found in all tissues, especially in the liver, bile ducts, placenta, and bone. Since damaged or diseased tissue releases enzymes into the blood, ALP measurements can be abnormal in many conditions, including cancer. (Serum ALP is also high in some normal circumstances, such as during normal bone growth, pregnancy, or in response to a variety of drugs.) The ALP test is one of several that may be used to help diagnose cancers that typically spread to the bone (such as PROSTATE CANCER, KIDNEY CANCER, LIVER CANCER or BREAST CANCER). The normal range is 44 to 147 IU/L. Higher-than-normal levels may indicate LEUKEMIA, liver cancer or bone cancer or noncancerous diseases of the liver and bile system. The ALP test can be further analyzed to detect if a high level is originating from bone or liver.

alkaloid A member of a large group of nitrogen-containing chemicals that are produced by plants. Some alkaloids have been shown to be effective against cancer and have been developed into anticancer drugs, including vinblastine and vincristine, a product of the periwinkle plant family, and VP-16 (from the mandrake family). Alkaloid drugs are used to treat a variety of cancers, including BREAST CANCER, LUNG CANCER, HODGKIN'S DISEASE, LYMPHOMA, and LEUKEMIA.

alkylating agents A family of CHEMOTHERAPY drugs that inhibits cancer cell growth by interfering with a cell's DNA. Alkylating agents cause the most damage to cells in the active phase of the cell cycle; in high doses, they can also kill cells in the "resting" phase.

Alkylating agents are used to treat BREAST CANCER, LUNG CANCER, LEUKEMIA, and LYMPHOMA. Examples of these drugs include mustargen, leukeran, Cytoxan (cyclophosphamide), thiotepa, streptozicin, and busulfan.

Side Effects

Alkylating drugs may cause sterility if used for a long period of time, and they slightly increase the risk of leukemia after a long latent period.

ALL See LEUKEMIA.

Alliance for Lung Cancer Advocacy, Support, and Education (ALCASE) The only nonprofit organization dedicated solely to helping people with LUNG CANCER and those at risk for the disease improve the quality of their lives through advocacy, support, and education. ALCASE provides services to patients, family members, and healthcare providers throughout the United States. ALCASE tries to

- advocate for better awareness of prevention, diagnosis, treatment, and living with lung cancer.
- provide psychosocial support.
- provide education about the disease and how best to live with it. For contact information, see Appendix I.

allicin A phytochemical found in onions and GARLIC that experts suspect may help protect against cancer. Allicin is most widely recognized for its action as an antiviral, antifungal, and antibacterial agent with the ability to block the toxins produced by bacteria and viruses. It is also an ANTIOXIDANT and helps to eliminate toxins from the body.

allogeneic bone marrow transplant See BONE MARROW TRANSPLANTS.

alopecia See HAIR LOSS.

alpha-fetoprotein (AFP) A protein produced by a developing fetus that also serves as a marker for cancer in adults. A high level of AFP suggests the presence of LIVER CANCER or TESTICULAR CANCER. Typically, the AFP level rises when the cancer is growing and falls when the cancer is shrinking or has been surgically removed. AFP levels should usually return to normal within a month of surgery if all of the tumor has been removed. However, the higher the initial AFP level, the longer it will take to return to normal. A blood test of AFP may measure the progress of the disease and the success of treatment. Only rarely do patients with other types of cancer (such as STOMACH CANCER) have high AFP levels.

AFP is normally less than about 5 ng/ml, but cancer cannot be assumed until the level surpasses 25 ng/ml. A very small number of healthy people have a naturally high level of this protein in their blood, although even among these individuals, the level is still less than 25 ng/ml.

Nonmalignant conditions that also can cause high AFP levels include ataxia telangiectasia, Wiscott-Aldrich syndrome, pregnancy, or liver conditions such as cirrhosis or hepatitis.

alveolar ridge cancer See HEAD AND NECK CANCER.

alveolar soft part sarcoma A rare soft tissue tumor that commonly affects the thigh in adults, and the head and neck in children. Five-year survival is more than 60 percent.

See also SARCOMAS, SOFT TISSUE.

American Brachytherapy Society (ABS) A nonprofit professional organization founded in 1978 that seeks to provide insight and research into the use of BRACHYTHERAPY (internal RADIATION THERAPY) in malignant and benign conditions. Members include physicists, physicians, and other health-care providers interested in brachytherapy. The mission of the ABS is to provide information directly to the consumer, promote the highest standards of practice of brachytherapy, and help health-care professionals by encouraging improved and continuing education for radiation ONCOLOGISTS and other health-care professionals involved in the treatment of cancer. In addition, the ABS promotes clinical and laboratory research into the practice of brachytherapy. For contact information, see Appendix I.

American Brain Tumor Association A nonprofit association that funds brain tumor research and provides information to help patients make educated decisions about their health care, including online support services, links, bibliographies, and personal patient stories. The group also offers a pen-pal service; a variety of volunteer opportunities; printed materials concerning research into and treatment of brain tumors; and listings of physicians, treatment facilities, and support groups throughout the country. A limited selection of Spanish-language publications is available. For contact information, see Appendix I.

See also BRAIN CANCER.

American Cancer Society (ACS) A voluntary organization that supports research, and offers a variety of services to patients and their families. It provides printed materials in English and Spanish, and conducts educational programs. The society also sponsors a number of related support groups, including CANCER SURVIVORS NETWORK, I CAN COPE PROGRAM, INTERNATIONAL ASSOCIATION OF LARYNGECTOMEES, LOOK GOOD . . . FEEL BETTER PROGRAM, and REACH TO RECOVERY. A local ACS group may be listed in the white pages of the telephone directory. For contact information, see Appendix I.

American Foundation for Urologic Disease A nonprofit organization founded in 1987 that supports research; provides education to patients, the general public, and health professionals; and offers patient support services for those who have or may be at risk for a urologic disease or disorder. The staff provides information on urologic disease and dysfunctions, including PROSTATE CANCER treatment options, bladder health, and sexual dysfunction. It also offers prostate cancer support groups (Prostate Cancer Network). Some Spanish-language publications are available.

The group publishes *Family Urology,* the official magazine of the foundation, which reaches more than 100,000 individuals each quarter. It also offers a membership program to help support the foundation's mission and to keep medical professionals, patients, family members, and friends informed about urologic disorders, the latest treatment options, and up-to-date research findings. The foundation's education councils have distributed more than six million brochures nationwide to patients, grassroots organizations, physicians, medical specialty groups, allied health-care workers and corporations. For contact information, see Appendix I.

American Indians/Alaska Natives and cancer While American Indians/Alaska Natives experience some of the lowest cancer rates among all groups, they do experience higher death rates and incidences for certain cancers. The Indian Health Service reports a large variability in cancer rates among this population, especially in areas such as the Northern plains and Alaska.

Among American Indians/Alaska Natives, men have the lowest PROSTATE CANCER incidence among all groups, and women from these groups have the lowest BREAST CANCER incidence. However, American Indian/Alaska Native women have the third highest rate of death from LUNG CANCER after Caucasians and African Americans.

American Institute for Cancer Research (AICR)
A nonprofit group that provides information about cancer prevention, particularly through diet and nutrition, and supports research at sites throughout the country. The institute offers a toll-free nutrition hotline, pen-pal support network, a wide array of brochures for consumers and health professionals, and materials with information about diet and nutrition and their link to cancer and cancer prevention.

The AICR also supports the CancerResource, an information and resource program for cancer patients. A limited selection of Spanish-language publications is available.

Since its founding in 1982, the American Institute for Cancer Research has grown into the nation's leading charity in the field of diet, nutrition, and cancer. AICR also offers a wide range of cancer prevention education programs and publications for health professionals and the public. Through these pioneering efforts, AICR has helped focus attention on the link between cancer and lifestyle choices. Over the past several years, the Institute has spent between 66 percent and 72 percent of its funds on research and education. For contact information, see Appendix I.

American Prostate Society (APS)   A nonprofit organization that provides information on the latest treatments for PROSTATE CANCER, prostatitis, prostate growth (BPH), and impotence. In addition to a Web site featuring FAQs and other information, the APS provides a free newsletter on request. For contact information, see Appendix I.

American Society of Clinical Oncology (ASCO)
A nonprofit organization dedicated to supporting all types of cancer research, but especially patient-oriented clinical research. ASCO's mission is to facilitate the delivery of high-quality health care, foster the exchange of information, further the training of researchers, and encourage communication among the various cancer specialties.

ASCO has more than 16,000 professional members worldwide, including clinical ONCOLOGISTS specializing in medical ONCOLOGY, therapeutic radiology, surgical oncology, pediatric oncology, gynecologic oncology, urologic oncology, and hematology; students; oncology nurses; and other health-care practitioners. International members make up 20 percent of the total membership and represent 75 countries worldwide. For contact information, see Appendix I.

American Society of Plastic and Reconstructive Surgeons   A professional organization founded in 1931 to promote quality care for plastic surgery patients, to provide educational programs, and to support the activities of its members. To become a member, each plastic surgeon must be certified by the American Board of Plastic Surgery. In addition to its professional activities, the society maintains a speakers' bureau and a patient referral service to help patients choose a plastic surgeon. Material describing procedures and results is also available. For contact information, see Appendix I.

AML   See LEUKEMIA.

amyloidosis   A condition affecting about 15 percent of patients with MULTIPLE MYELOMA. There is also a less-common type called primary amyloidosis. In both conditions, deposits of protein fragments called light chains that appear in different parts of the body, such as the tongue, heart, nerves, and muscles. This can lead to carpal tunnel syndrome, weakness, weight loss, low blood pressure, shortness of breath, light-headedness, and renal and heart failure.

anal cancer   A fairly rare cancer of the anus that is often curable and begins in the end of the large intestine. The anus is about an inch and a half long and opens to allow the passage of stool during a bowel movement. Cancer can start either in the part of the anus that is inside the body, or the outside part. The seriousness of the cancer depends to some extent on where it starts. Many kinds of tumors can develop in the anus. Some are benign at first but later develop into cancer.

SQUAMOUS CELL CARCINOMA (affecting the outer anus) is the most common type of anal cancer and is more likely to occur in men. If the anal cancer is found only in the surface cells where it started, it is called squamous cell carcinoma in situ (CIS); it may also be called BOWEN'S DISEASE.

Sometimes a tumor can grow in an area between the anus and the rectum; this area is called the cloaca and these types of cancers are known as cloacogenic carcinomas.

About 15 percent of anal cancers begin in the anal area glands and are known as adenocarcinomas. Paget's disease is a type of adenocarcinoma that spreads through the surface layer of the skin and can occur in the anal area. (Paget's disease of the bone and of the breast are entirely different diseases.)

A few anal cancers are basal cell carcinomas; another 1 to 2 percent are malignant melanomas, another type of skin cancer. Melanomas are far more common on parts of the body that get exposed to the sun than around the anus. Unfortunately, most anal melanomas are found at a late stage because they cannot easily be seen.

The risk of anal cancer is rising, with homosexual men most at risk. In 2002, 3,900 new cases were diagnosed, affecting more women than men. Although fairly rare, anal cancer is serious; about 500 Americans died of this disease in 2002.

Cause

Anal cancer has been linked to infection with the human papilloma virus, which is why many experts consider anal cancer to be a type of sexually transmitted disease.

Stages

Stage 0 (CARCINOMA IN SITU): Very early cancer found only in the top layer of anal tissue.

Stage I: Cancer has spread beyond the top layer of anal tissue and is smaller than 2 cm (less than 1 inch).

Stage II: Cancer has spread beyond the top layer of anal tissue and is larger than 2 cm (about 1 inch), but it has not spread to nearby organs or lymph nodes.

Stage IIIA: Cancer has spread to the LYMPH NODES around the rectum or to nearby organs such as the vagina or bladder.

Stage IIIB: Cancer has spread to the lymph nodes in the middle of the abdomen or in the groin or has spread to both nearby organs and the lymph nodes around the rectum.

Stage IV: Cancer has spread to distant lymph nodes within the abdomen or to organs in other parts of the body.

Recurrent: The cancer has returned after treatment, either in the anus or in another part of the body.

Treatment

Treatment for anal cancer depends on the type of disease, stage, and patient's age and general health and may include surgery, RADIATION THERAPY, and/or CHEMOTHERAPY.

Surgery In a local resection, only the cancer is removed, and the sphincter muscle around the anus can be saved so that the patient can continue to pass body wastes as before. ABDOMINOPERINEAL RESECTION is an operation in which the anus and the lower part of the rectum are removed by cutting into the abdomen and the perineum (the space between the anus and the scrotum or the anus and the vulva). An opening (stoma) is made on the outside of the body for waste to pass; this is called a COLOSTOMY. Although this operation was once commonly used for anal cancer, it is not used as much today because radiation therapy with chemotherapy is an equally effective treatment option but does not require surgery. Patients who do need surgery and a colostomy must wear a special bag to collect body wastes. Lymph nodes may also be removed at the same time or in a separate operation.

Radiation therapy and chemotherapy These are usually combined to shrink tumors and make an abdominoperineal resection unnecessary.

Patients with Stage 0 anal cancer usually have local resection. Stages I and II may call for either local resection for some small tumors or external radiation therapy with chemotherapy. Some patients may also receive internal radiation therapy. If cancer cells remain after therapy, patients may then need surgery of the anal canal to remove the cancer.

Stage IIIA patients usually have radiation therapy with chemotherapy; depending on how much cancer remains after chemotherapy and radiation, local resection or surgery to remove cancer in the anal canal may be done.

Stage IIIB patients will probably have radiation therapy and chemotherapy followed by surgery. Depending on how much cancer remains after chemotherapy and radiation, local resection or surgery to remove the anus and the lower part of the rectum (abdominoperineal resection) may be done. During surgery, the lymph nodes in the groin may be removed.

To relieve symptoms only, Stage IV patients may have either surgery, radiation, or a combination of chemotherapy and radiation. For those whose cancer has recurred, choice of treatment will be based on what treatment was given initially. Patients who had been given surgery may receive radiation and chemotherapy if the cancer recurs. Those treated with radiation and chemotherapy may have surgery the next time.

analgesia See PAIN CONTROL.

anaplasia Cells in a malignant tumor that have reversed to a primitive state and have no organized structure; this type of tumor is usually more aggressive.

anaplastic astrocytoma See BRAIN CANCER.

anaplastic oligodendroglioma See BRAIN CANCER.

anaplastic thyroid See THYROID CANCER.

androgens Male hormones (such as testosterone) that are also used to treat cancer. Androgens appear to change the hormonal environment in the cancer cell, removing the stimulus to grow so that the cancer cell does not divide. The exact mechanism is unknown. They are rarely used to treat advanced BREAST CANCER, and they are not recommended in PROSTATE CANCER.

Androgens may cause patients to retain salt and water. Women receiving androgens will notice a deepening of their voice after a period of time. Patients who take androgens for more than three months may have decreased sexual interest, increased body hair, and acne.

Androgen medications include

- calusterone (Methosarb)
- dromostanolone propionate (Drolban, Macleron, Permastril)
- fluoxymesteron (Halotestin, Ora-Testryl)
- nandrolone decanoate (Deca-Durabolin)
- testosterone propionate (Neohombreol, Oraton)

anemia A common side effect in patients with cancer that may cause debilitating FATIGUE. It is caused by a decline in hemoglobin, the part of the blood that carries oxygen to the body's tissues. The decline in hemoglobin is caused by a reduction in the number of red blood cells. About three in four cancer patients will experience fatigue caused by anemia that may be secondary to the cancer itself or be caused by treatment.

The causes of anemia are decreased bone marrow production (from CHEMOTHERAPY or the cancer itself), bleeding, or shorter lifespan of the red cells.

Several forms of anemia may occur in patients with cancer. *Hemolytic anemia* occurs when red blood cells get destroyed too soon, rarely as a result of chemotherapy. More commonly, it is a result of an autoimmune response or an enlarged spleen. *Hypoplastic anemia* occurs when the BONE MARROW makes too few red blood cells, either as a result of chemotherapy or radiation. Levels of white blood cells and platelets also decline. *Iron-deficiency anemia* occurs when there is too little iron in the blood, which leads to a lack of hemoglobin, which in turn causes anemia. In those with cancer, iron deficiency may be a result of bleeding (such as from a tumor in the colon). *Pernicious anemia* occurs when there is a lack of vitamin B_{12} absorption. People with some types of intestinal cancer may have trouble absorbing enough B_{12}. In addition, many cancer patients often are malnourished.

angiogenesis The formation of a network of blood vessels that penetrates into cancerous growths, supplying nutrients and oxygen and removing waste products, helping cancer grow and spread.

The walls of blood vessels are formed by cells that divide only about once every three years. However, when the situation requires it, angiogenesis can stimulate them to divide. Angiogenesis is regulated by both activator and inhibitor molecules. Normally the inhibitors predominate, blocking growth. Should a need for new blood vessels arise (such as to repair a wound), angiogenesis activators increase in number and inhibitors decrease. This prompts the formation of new blood vessels.

In cancer, malignant tumor cells release molecules that send signals to surrounding normal host tissue, activating certain genes to produce proteins that encourage growth of new blood vessels. Other chemicals, called angiogenesis inhibitors, signal the process to stop.

Scientists have recently discovered a gene (Id1) that stimulates angiogenesis in certain cancers by turning off the production of a naturally occurring angiogenesis suppressor.

The Id1 gene is highly expressed in MELANOMA, breast, head and neck, brain, cervical, prostate, pancreatic, and TESTICULAR CANCER, resulting in lower numbers of suppressors and increased tumor blood vessel formation.

Because cancer cannot grow or spread without the formation of new blood vessels, scientists are trying to find ways to stop angiogenesis. Efforts to find a way to use the angiogenesis suppressor called TSP-1 as an anticancer agent are under way in animal studies. Because the suppressor occurs naturally throughout the body, it cannot be used as a drug, but it could potentially be paired with another molecule and programmed to be released only in tumors. In animal studies, angiogenesis inhibitors have successfully stopped the formation of new blood vessels, causing the cancer to shrink and die.

If the results of clinical trials show that angiogenesis inhibitors are both safe and effective in treating cancer in humans, these agents may be approved by the U.S. Food and Drug Administration and made available for widespread use. Detailed information about ongoing clinical trials evaluating angiogenesis inhibitors and other promising new treatments is available from the CANCER INFORMATION SERVICE.

Researchers have been studying angiogenesis ever since they realized that cancer cells can release molecules to activate the process. From such studies more than a dozen different proteins, as well as several smaller molecules, have been identified as "angiogenic," meaning that they are released by tumors as signals for angiogenesis. Among these molecules, two proteins appear to be the most important for sustaining tumor growth: vascular endothelial growth factor (VEGF) and basic fibroblast growth factor (bFGF). VEGF and bFGF are produced by many kinds of cancer cells and by certain types of normal cells as well.

Although many tumors produce angiogenic molecules such as VEGF and bFGF, their presence is not enough to begin blood vessel growth. For angiogenesis to begin, these activator molecules must overcome a variety of angiogenesis inhibitors that normally restrain blood vessel growth. Almost a dozen naturally occurring proteins can inhibit angiogenesis, including proteins called angiostatin, endostatin, and thrombospondin. A finely tuned balance between the concentration of angiogenesis inhibitors and activators determines whether a tumor can induce the growth of new blood vessels. To trigger angiogenesis, the production of activators must increase as the production of inhibitors decreases.

It has been known for many years that cancer cells originating in a primary tumor can spread to another organ and form tiny, microscopic tumor masses that can remain dormant for years. A likely explanation for this tumor dormancy is that no angiogenesis occurred, so the small tumor lacked the new blood vessels needed for continued growth. One possible reason that angiogenesis did not occur may be that some primary tumors secrete the inhibitor angiostatin into the bloodstream, which then circulates throughout the body and inhibits blood vessel growth at other sites.

angiogenesis inhibitor Substance (also called "anti-angiogenesis agent") that may prevent the growth of blood vessels from surrounding tissue to a solid tumor.

See also ANGIOGENESIS.

angiosarcoma See SARCOMA.

ANLL See LEUKEMIA.

anorexia See APPETITE LOSS.

anoscopy A procedure that enables a doctor to see the anus and anal canal using a tube called an anoscope. The procedure allows visualization of tears in the canal's lining and also of tissue that may be cancerous.

First the doctor performs a digital rectal exam, and then inserts a lubricated anoscope a few inches to enlarge the rectum so that the doctor can see the entire anal canal using a light. A specimen for biopsy can be taken if needed. During the test, the doctor might ask the patient to bear down and relax as the tube is inserted, because this will help to guide it in the easiest direction and also can help the doctor to identify bulges along the lining of the rectum.

Patients can feel the pressure of the anoscope inside, but most do not feel pain. There are no significant risks from this test, although if patients have hemorrhoids, they may experience a small amount of bleeding after the anoscope is removed.

anthocyanins A group of plant chemicals within the larger category of PHYTOCHEMICALS called PHE-NOLICS that give intense color to certain red and blue fruits and vegetables. (Blueberries are especially rich in anthocyanins.) These plant pigments are very powerful ANTIOXIDANTS and are being studied extensively for their ability to fight cancer and to delay several diseases associated with the aging process.

anthraquinones A family of drugs that some experts believe may be effective as CHEMOTHERAPY against cancer.

anthrax An infectious and deadly bacterium that causes a fatal disease, but that has also been studied as an experimental cancer treatment. In mice a modified anthrax toxin killed tumor cells. Tumor cells in humans contain high levels of a protein known as urokinase, which is the target for the new anthrax cancer treatment. Senior researchers at the National Institutes of Health genetically altered the structure of the anthrax toxin so that it invades only cells that express the urokinase protein.

In the lab the new treatment worked well on fibrosarcoma (a tumor of the connective tissue), MELANOMA, and LUNG CANCER. After one anthrax treatment, the toxin reduced tumor size by 65 percent to 92 percent, depending on the type of tumor; two treatments eliminated 88 percent of the fibrosarcomas and 17 percent of the melanomas.

The tumor cells began to die just 12 hours after the first treatment. Even more encouraging, the toxin accomplished this without damaging nearby healthy cells.

The treatment is an advance in the field known as toxin fusion protein therapy, which involves taking two different, normally separate proteins and fusing them into a single protein. Protein fusion therapy has almost exclusively targeted tumor cells by binding the fused protein to their surface.

Human trials using the anthrax toxin may begin by 2005, but it might be eight to 10 years before anthrax treatments are generally available.

antiandrogen A class of drugs that blocks the function of male hormones, used in the treatment of PROSTATE CANCER. Antiandrogens interfere with the action of testosterone on prostate cancer cells that are stimulated by androgen. Antiandrogens include Casodex (bicalutamide) and flutamide (Eulexin).

anti-angiogenesis agents See ANGIOGENESIS INHIBITORS.

antibody-dependent cell-mediated cytotoxicity The killing of antibody-coated target cells by effector cells (lymphocytes, macrophages, and natural killer cells).

anticancer antibiotics A group of CHEMOTHERAPY drugs that block cell growth by interfering with a cell's DNA. Anticancer antibiotics are also called antitumor antibiotics or antineoplastic antibiotics; (examples include bleomycin or Adriamycin).

anti-CEA antibody An antibody against CARCINOEMBRYONIC ANTIGEN (CEA), a protein present on certain types of cancer cells. It is used in a radiologic scan to detect hidden types of cancer, especially when the CEA is elevated in cancers such as colon cancer.

antiemetics See ANTINAUSEA MEDICATION.

anti-estrogen A substance (such as tamoxifen) that blocks the activity of estrogens, the family of hormones that promote the development and maintenance of female sex characteristics.

anti-idiotype vaccine A vaccine made of antibodies that see other antibodies as the antigen (target) and bind to them. Anti-idiotype vaccines can stimulate the body to produce antibodies against tumor cells.

antimetabolite A type of CHEMOTHERAPY drug that interferes with the normal metabolic processes within cells. Because the antimetabolite is similar to a nutrient, it fools the cancer cell into ingesting it. The chemotherapy drugs fluorouracil, methotrexate, and mercaptopurine are all antimetabolites that prevent growth of a cell at a short, specific time in its reproduction cycle by interfering with important enzyme reactions within the cell.

Antimetabolites may sometimes need to be administered over hours, days, or weeks. Side effects of antimetabolites can be severe, including blood cell disorders or gastrointestinal problems such as diarrhea; sometimes cancer cells can become resistant to a particular antimetabolite.

antinausea medication A type of drug that can prevent or reduce NAUSEA and vomiting, common side effects of CHEMOTHERAPY and RADIATION THERAPY. Popular antinausea drugs include Decadron, Compazine, Thorazine, metoclopramide, Ativan, Valium, Marinol, dronabinol, Kytrel, Anzemet, Zofran, Aloxi, and Emmend. Often a combination of these drugs is prescribed; if the first combination does not work, others may work better. Quite often antinausea medication is given along with chemotherapy drugs to head off nausea.

antineoplastic antibiotics See ANTICANCER ANTIBIOTICS.

antioxidants Compounds that fight cell damage caused by FREE RADICALS, a rogue type of oxygen molecule that can attack cells throughout the body. Although free radicals serve important functions, such as helping the immune system fight off disease, at excessive levels they can cause problems.

Free radicals are formed both during normal metabolism and in response to infection and some chemicals. They cause damage to fatty acids in cell membranes, and the products of this damage can then damage important proteins and DNA. The most widely accepted theory of the biochemical basis of many types of cancer is that they are triggered by free radical damage to tissues.

A number of different mechanisms are involved in protection against, or repair after, free radical damage, including a number of nutrients—especially vitamin E, beta carotene, vitamin C, and selenium. Collectively these are known as antioxidant nutrients, and they limit the cell and tissue damage caused by toxins and pollutants.

Side effects Supplements containing high doses of antioxidants can cause severe side effects, including internal bleeding, and may be toxic in patients taking anticoagulant medication (blood thinners). No one should take these or any supplements without consulting a doctor. In addition, high doses of vitamin E are potentially harmful if combined with blood-thinning drugs. It is safer to consume antioxidants as part of a healthy diet. Antioxidants are found in:

- fruits and vegetables (especially blueberries and yellow fruits and vegetables)
- brown rice and other whole grains
- meats
- eggs
- dairy products

antiperspirants and breast cancer Despite persistent rumors in the media and on the Internet about a link between antiperspirants or deodorants and BREAST CANCER, scientists at the NATIONAL CANCER INSTITUTE say they are not aware of any research to support a link between the use of these products and the subsequent development of breast cancer.

The U.S. Food and Drug Administration, which regulates food, cosmetics, medicines, and medical devices, also does not have any evidence or research data to support the theory that ingredients in underarm antiperspirants or deodorants cause cancer.

antitumor antibiotics See ANTICANCER ANTIBIOTICS.

aplastic anemia Not a single disease, but a rare group of closely related disorders characterized by the failure of the BONE MARROW to produce all three types of blood cells: red blood cells, white blood cells, and platelets. Aplastic ANEMIA affects fewer than 1,000 Americans each year.

Cause

The exact cause of aplastic anemia is unknown, although it has been linked to exposure to certain drugs, chemicals, and radiation. It is also believed that some cases of aplastic anemia are inherited and that some cases are due to a viral infection.

Symptoms

Patients with aplastic anemia have much lower quantities of each of the three blood cell types, which triggers symptoms. Fewer white blood cells leads to unexplained infections; fewer platelets causes unexpected bleeding; and fewer red blood cells causes FATIGUE.

Diagnosis

Blood samples can reveal the number of each type of blood cell circulating in the blood. When two or three of the cell counts are extremely low, doctors will suspect aplastic anemia. A definitive diagnosis is made if a bone marrow biopsy shows a great reduction in the number of cells in the marrow itself.

Treatment

Patients with severe aplastic anemia require immediate treatment to stabilize their disease until a BONE MARROW TRANSPLANT can be performed. Patients with mild or moderate symptoms often receive red blood cell transfusions, platelet transfusions, and/or drug therapy, although STEM CELL transplantation is also an option for some of these patients.

apoptosis Programmed cell death that naturally occurs during the development of a person's tissues and organs. During fetal development, apoptosis plays a vital role in determining the final size and form of tissues and organs. As more cells are created than are required to produce tissues and organs, the body programs unwanted cells to die, either by suppressing the chemical signals that direct them to go on living or by sending the unwanted cells a specific signal to die. Experts believe that the suppression of apoptosis is associated with the uncontrolled cell growth in LEUKEMIA and other cancers. Apoptosis also occurs when viruses infect cells. Apoptosis differs from cell necrosis, in which cell death may be triggered by a toxic substance.

apoptotic enhancers A class of proteins named for their ability to stimulate programmed cell death.
See also APOPTOSIS.

appetite loss A frequent problem experienced by cancer patients, either as a result of the disease itself or due to side effects of treatment. People may lose their appetite while struggling with cancer because of mouth sores that make eating painful, because the taste of food changes, because CHEMOTHERAPY-related NAUSEA or stomach pain alters appetite, or because pain itself can trigger appetite loss.

Appetite loss is a serious problem among cancer patients because it can lead to poor nutrition, which can interfere with recovery.

Treatment

Drugs such as megace or MARINOL (derived from MARIJUANA) may be used to improve appetite. Patients also should eat

- small, frequent meals
- nutritious snacks

- skim milk
- new foods or spices
- high-calorie, high-protein food
- attractive, appetizing meals

In addition, patients should eat during the times when they feel most comfortable, stimulate appetite with light exercise, take medications with high-calorie drinks, and eat at a friend's home or a good restaurant. Patients should also try using lemon-flavored drinks, rinse their mouths before eating, and try cold, white food (ice cream, milk shakes, boiled chicken). Many patients find that meat becomes unpleasant to eat at this time; patients should try to substitute other high-protein meals they find more palatable.

aromatase inhibition   A type of HORMONAL THER-APY used in postmenopausal women with hor-mone-dependent BREAST CANCER in which production of the female hormone estradiol is blocked in the adrenal gland. Examples include Femara, Aromasin, and Arimidex.

aromatase inhibitors   A group of drugs used in ANTI-ESTROGEN therapy that lower the amount of estrogen being produced by the body. Limiting the amount of estrogen produced means there is less estrogen available to reach cancer cells and make them grow.

In postmenopausal women, estrogen is no longer produced by the ovaries, but it is converted from androgen, another hormone. Aromatase inhibitors keep androgen from being converted to estrogen, so that less estrogen enters the blood-stream and reaches estrogen receptors.

Anastrozole (Arimidex), letrozole (Femara), and exemestane (Aromasin) are the aromatase inhibitors currently being used for postmenopausal women with BREAST CANCER that has spread beyond the breast. Each of these drugs is adminis-tered in pill form.

In the past, these drugs were used primarily by women who had already tried other anti-estrogen therapies (such as tamoxifen) and whose cancer was no longer controlled by those drugs. However, today many doctors recommend an aromatase

inhibitor *before* tamoxifen for postmenopausal women whose disease has spread.

An ongoing study is assessing the usefulness of giving Arimidex to postmenopausal women with earlier-stage disease after they have completed five years of tamoxifen. When the results become known, standard treatment recommendations may change.

Results of the ATAC (Arimidex and Tamoxifen Alone or in Combination) study, announced in December 2002, showed that Arimidex is better than tamoxifen (Nolvadex) in postmenopausal women diagnosed with early-stage estrogen-receptor-posi-tive breast cancer and/or progesterone-receptor-pos-itive breast cancer. Arimidex reduced the risk of breast cancer recurrence by 17 percent more than tamoxifen alone. Arimidex also decreased the chances of breast cancer developing in the other breast by almost 80 percent (60 percent better than tamoxifen). In addition, Arimidex was able to deliver these benefits with fewer side effects than tamoxifen, including fewer cases of ENDOMETRIAL CANCER, fewer blood clots, and fewer hot flashes.

However, the combination of tamoxifen and Arimidex did not work any better than either tamoxifen or Arimidex alone. The ATAC study was the largest breast cancer trial ever conducted, with more than 9,000 women participating in more than 20 countries.

See also SELECTIVE ESTROGEN-RECEPTOR MODU-LATORS.

arsenic   A naturally occurring element widely distributed in the Earth's crust that is considered to be carcinogenic, although it is also sometimes used to treat cancer. Although arsenic has been known as a poison since ancient times, people in many regions of the world consume small amounts of arsenic every day in their drinking water. Exposure to these relatively small doses of arsenic has been linked to several kinds of cancer.

In the environment, arsenic combines with oxy-gen, chlorine, and sulfur to form inorganic arsenic compounds, which are used primarily to preserve wood. Arsenic in animals and plants combines with carbon and hydrogen to form organic arsenic compounds, which are used as pesticides, primarily on cotton plants.

As a Carcinogen

Inorganic arsenic compounds are more toxic than organic arsenic. Several studies have shown that inorganic arsenic increases the risk of LUNG CANCER, SKIN CANCER, BLADDER CANCER, LIVER CANCER, KIDNEY CANCER, and PROSTATE CANCER. The World Health Organization, the U.S. Department of Health and Human Services, and the U.S. Environmental Protection Agency (EPA) each has determined that inorganic arsenic is a human carcinogen. Arsenic cannot be destroyed in the environment, it can only change its form.

People can be exposed to arsenic by

- eating or drinking tainted substances
- breathing air containing arsenic
- breathing sawdust from wood treated with arsenic, or breathing smoke from burning arsenic-treated wood
- living near uncontrolled hazardous waste sites containing arsenic
- living in areas with unusually high natural levels of arsenic in rock
- drinking water from wells contaminated with arsenic

The EPA has set limits on the amount of arsenic that industrial sources can release to the environment and has restricted many uses of arsenic in pesticides. The EPA has set a limit of 0.05 parts per million for arsenic in drinking water.

Recent research has found that exposure to small amounts of arsenic in drinking water may interfere with the expression of genes involved in helping cells repair damaged DNA. The process, known as DNA repair, is considered a major part of the body's ability to fight cancer. Initial findings suggest that arsenic may act as a cocarcinogen—not directly causing cancer, but allowing other substances, such as cigarette smoke or ultraviolet light, to cause mutations in DNA more effectively.

Tests can measure the level of arsenic in blood, urine, hair, toenails, or fingernails. The urine test is the most reliable for arsenic exposure within the previous few days, but tests on hair and nails can measure exposure to high levels of arsenic over the previous six to 12 months. Although these tests can determine if a person has been exposed to above-average levels of arsenic, they cannot predict how the arsenic levels in the body will affect health.

As Chemotherapy

Although arsenic is normally considered a deadly poison and carcinogen, some research suggests it can help save the lives of cancer patients with a severe form of LEUKEMIA. Based on preliminary Chinese studies, researchers at the Memorial Sloan-Kettering Cancer Center in New York treated 12 patients, none of whom had responded to conventional therapy, with arsenic trioxide, or Trisenox. The patients all had relapsed acute promyelocytic leukemia (APL), a subtype of acute myelogenous leukemia (AML), the most common form of acute leukemia in adults.

With the new treatment, 11 achieved remission lasting between 12 and 39 days and suffered only mild side effects. After two cycles of therapy, highly sensitive tests were performed on the patients to see if there were any molecular signs of leukemia left. Three patients tested positive and later relapsed, while eight patients tested negative and remained in remission as long as 10 months.

Researchers explained that their findings proved that arsenic kills the cancerous cells causing APL, including those cells that have become resistant to the most successful conventional form of treatment (a drug called all-trans retinoic acid).

Arsenic-containing preparations have been used as medicines for more than 2000 years. Arsenic-based treatment was first used in the United States and Europe more than 100 years ago for leukemia therapy as well as for treatment of infections, but these treatments were replaced by modern chemotherapy and antibiotics. More recently, interest in arsenic-based therapy was revived by reports of the antileukemic activity of some traditional Chinese preparations. It is also used to treat MYELOMA and MYELODYSPLASTIC SYNDROME.

arterial embolization   The blocking of an artery by a clot of foreign material (usually gel foam) performed by physicians as a type of cancer treatment that blocks the flow of blood to a tumor. It is usually used to treat LIVER CANCER.

artificial sweeteners   Research studies have not provided clear evidence of an association between artificial sweeteners and cancer, nor do they conclusively rule out such a possibility, according to scientists. The link between sweeteners and cancer began when early studies showed that cyclamate, one of several types of artificial sweeteners, caused BLADDER CANCER in laboratory animals, suggesting that cyclamate also may increase the risk of bladder cancer in humans. For this reason, the U.S. Food and Drug Administration (FDA) banned the use of cyclamate in 1969.

Results of animal studies conducted since then have not found proof that cyclamate is a carcinogen. Nevertheless, other issues must be resolved before cyclamate can be approved for commercial use, such as whether cyclamate enhances the effect of a cancer-causing substance, or whether large amounts of cyclamate could be dangerous.

Saccharin, another artificial sweetener, was also banned by the FDA when other animal studies linked the sweetener with the development of bladder cancer.

The FDA consequently proposed a ban on saccharin in April 1977, but the Saccharin Study and Labeling Act passed seven months later placed an 18-month moratorium on any action against saccharin by the FDA. The act also required that all food containing saccharin bear a label warning that "Use of this product may be hazardous to your health. This product contains saccharin, which has been determined to cause cancer in laboratory animals." The moratorium was subsequently extended to May 1997. During 1978 and 1979, the National Cancer Institute (NCI) and FDA conducted a population-based study on the possible role of saccharin in causing bladder cancer in humans and found that in general, people in the study who used an artificial sweetener had no greater risk of bladder cancer than anyone else. However, when only the data for heavy users were examined, there was some suggestive evidence of an increased risk, particularly in people who consumed both diet drinks and sugar substitutes and who used at least one of these heavily. In the study, which included a large number of elderly people, "heavy use" was defined as six or more servings of sugar substitute, or two or more 8-ounce servings of diet drinks daily.

The results of the NCI-FDA study, together with findings of additional research with laboratory animals, suggested that consumption of saccharin was not a strong risk factor for bladder cancer in humans. More recent animal studies also suggest that saccharin is unlikely to be a risk factor for cancer in humans. Two government scientific panels found that any link between saccharin and cancer was weak, although a third scientific panel of nongovernment experts voted 4-3 against ruling that saccharin was not a carcinogen.

In May 2000 officials at the National Institute of Environmental Health Sciences and its subdivision, the National Toxicology Program, announced that saccharin would no longer appear on their list of "cancer threats." In December 2000 Congress passed the Saccharin Warning Elimination via Environmental Testing Employing Science and Technology Act ("SWEETEST Act") after a National Toxicology Program review concluded that saccharin poses no health hazard to humans. The report concluded that the observed bladder tumors in rats were caused by mechanisms not relevant to humans, and no data in humans suggest that a carcinogenic hazard exists. The legislation allowed manufacturers to remove the warning labels from saccharin packages.

Aspartame, a third type of artificial sweetener, was approved in 1981 by the FDA after tests showed that it did not cause cancer in laboratory animals, although not all the laboratory experiments agreed. At present, aspartame is a common artificial sweetener and is distributed under the trade name of Nutrasweet or Equal. Interest in aspartame was renewed by a 1996 publication which suggested that an increase in the number of persons with BRAIN CANCER between 1975 and 1992 may be associated with the introduction and use of this sweetener in the United States. However, a recent analysis of NCI statistics on cancer incidence in the United States does not support an association between the use of aspartame and an increased incidence of brain tumors. These data show that the overall incidence of brain and central nervous system cancers began to rise in 1973, eight years before the approval of aspartame, and continued to rise until 1985. Increases in overall brain cancer incidence have occurred primarily in the 70 and older age group, a group that has not been exposed to the highest doses of aspartame since its 1981 introduction. Since 1985 the incidence of these cancers has stabilized, and in the last three years for which data are available (1991–93), the incidence has decreased slightly. Thus, at this time, there is no clear link, based on animal or human studies, between the use of aspartame and the development of brain tumors.

Sunett and Splenda

Acesulfame potassium (Sunett) is a calorie-free sweetener contained in hundreds of sugar-free products ranging from puddings to chewing gum. First approved in 1988, it was approved for liquid beverages 10 years later. It is 200 times sweeter than table sugar, and blending Sunett with other low-calorie sweeteners can create a beverage with a more sugarlike taste than one sweetened with any single low-calorie sweetener. However, the Center for Science in the Public Interest has raised questions about Sunett's safety, saying a few tests on rats indicated a possibility of a link with cancer, although not proof that the sweetener could cause cancer. The Calorie Control Council counters that the safety of acesulfame potassium has been confirmed by more than 90 studies and endorsed by a committee of the World Health Organization.

The FDA approved a new "high intensity" artificial sweetener called sucralose (Splenda) in April 1998. Splenda, a white crystalline powder that dissolves in water, is 600 times sweeter than sugar. In the lab, parts of the sugar molecule are replaced with chlorine atoms, and only a small portion of the resulting compound is absorbed by the body. Unlike other sweeteners, most of it passes straight through the body without being digested—somewhat like the artificial fat product made with olestra called Olean. The FDA has approved Splenda for use in almost every kind of processed food, including soda, ice cream, baked goods, jellies, chewing gum, puddings, and fillings. It also can be used by consumers as a tabletop sweetener to add directly to foods. The new sweetener also is safe for diabetics, the FDA says. The agency spent more than a decade deciding whether to approve the new sweetener. It reviewed 110 studies in animals and people to verify Splenda's safety and reported that long-term studies of extremely high doses found no evidence of cancer, birth defects, or immune system problems.

Splenda is sold in more than 25 countries, including Canada; millions of consumers around the world have been using the product since 1991.

asbestos A group of six different minerals that have been used in a variety of building materials because of their heat-resistant properties. Asbestos minerals have long fibers that are strong and flexible enough to be spun and woven. Because of these characteristics, asbestos has been used for a wide range of manufactured goods, such as roofing shingles, ceiling and floor tiles, paper products, asbestos cement products, friction products (automobile clutch, brake, and transmission parts), heat-resistant fabrics, packaging, gaskets, and coatings.

Asbestos fibers may be released into the air during demolition work, building or home maintenance, repair, and remodeling. When products containing asbestos break down, fibers can enter the air or water. Asbestos fibers are generally not broken down to other compounds and will remain virtually unchanged over long periods. Everyone is exposed to low levels of asbestos in the air, ranging from 0.00001 to 0.0001 fibers per milliliter of air; levels are highest in cities and industrial areas. People working in industries that make or use asbestos products or who are involved in asbestos mining may be exposed to high levels of asbestos, as can those who live near these industries. Drinking water may contain asbestos from natural sources or from asbestos-containing cement pipes.

Breathing high levels of asbestos fibers for a long time may result in scar-like tissue in the lungs and in the lining of the lungs. Breathing lower levels of asbestos may cause plaques in the lungs, which can occur in workers and sometimes in people living in areas with high environmental levels of asbestos. Effects on breathing from pleural plaques alone are not usually serious, but higher exposure can lead to a thickening of the pleural membrane that may restrict breathing. The U.S. Department of Health and Human Services, the World Health Organization, and the U.S. Environmental Protection Agency (EPA) have determined that asbestos can cause two types of cancer: LUNG CANCER and

MESOTHELIOMA (cancer of the lining surrounding the lung or abdominal cavity). Studies also suggest that breathing asbestos can increase a person's chances of getting cancer in other parts of the body, such as the stomach, intestines, esophagus, pancreas, and kidneys, but this is less certain. People who smoke and are exposed to asbestos have a significantly higher risk of getting lung cancer.

Diagnosis

Low levels of asbestos fibers can be measured in urine, feces, mucus, or lung washings. Higher-than-average levels of asbestos fibers in tissue can confirm exposure but not determine whether the person will get cancer. A thorough history, physical exam, and diagnostic tests are needed to evaluate asbestos-related disease. Chest X-rays are the best screening tool to identify lung changes resulting from asbestos exposure. Lung function tests and CAT scans also can help diagnose asbestos-related disease.

Prevention

Materials containing asbestos that are not disturbed or deteriorated do not usually pose a health risk. People who think they may have been exposed to asbestos at home should contact their state or local health department or the regional offices of the EPA to find out how to test the home and find a company trained to remove or contain the fibers.

In 1989 the EPA banned all new uses of asbestos, although asbestos used before this date is still allowed. The EPA requires school systems to inspect for damaged asbestos and to eliminate or reduce the exposure by removing the asbestos or by covering it up. The EPA regulates the release of asbestos from factories and during building demolition or renovation to prevent asbestos from getting into the environment. The EPA has proposed a concentration limit of 7 million fibers per liter of drinking water for long fibers. The Occupational Safety and Health Administration has set limits for exposure to asbestos in workplace air.

ascites The presence of excess fluid in the abdomen, usually caused by liver disease but also a symptom of many types of cancer. The types of cancer that are more likely to cause ascites are: breast, lung, colon, stomach, pancreatic, ovarian, and endometrial.

If cancer cells have spread to the lining of the abdomen (peritoneum), they can cause irritation that leads to fluid buildup. Cancer in the liver can block the circulation of blood through the liver, triggering a buildup of fluid in the abdomen. Liver damage also can result in less blood protein being produced, which may upset the body's fluid balance, causing fluid to build up in the body tissues, including the abdomen.

It is also possible for cancer cells to block the lymphatic system, which is responsible for draining off excess tissue fluid. If some of these channels are blocked, fluid can build up.

Symptoms

Ascites may cause the abdomen to become painfully swollen, making it hard to feel comfortable. It can make patients feel very tired and breathless or cause NAUSEA, indigestion, and a reduced appetite.

Treatment

Ascites can be treated by removing the excess fluid with a drain, which is inserted by a doctor. The length of the time the drain needs to stay in place depends on the amount of fluid that needs to be drained off. A large amount of fluid requires hospitalization for two or three days. Because ascites may recur, drainage may need to be performed more than once. Alternatively, the doctor may prescribe a diuretic to help the patient pass more urine than normal so as to slow the buildup of the ascitic fluid. In some cases, a permanent shunt may be inserted to drain the fluid directly into a large vein.

Ashkenazi Jews and cancer Mutations in two BREAST CANCER genes (*BRCA1* and *BRCA2*) appear more often among Ashkenazi Jews than in the general population.

Researchers have long known that some inherited diseases occur more commonly in certain ethnic groups than they do in the general population because of the "founder effect," which occurs in groups that have been isolated for religious, cultural, or geographical reasons and that descend from a small group of common ancestors. In such groups, disease-associated mutations get passed down with greater frequency because any mutations present in the founders become common in their offspring.

Researchers believe the *BRCA1* and *BRCA2* mutations that today occur with a relatively high degree of frequency in Ashkenazi Jews originated in common ancestors approximately 600 hundred years ago. The word *Ashkenazi* is derived from the Hebrew word for "Germany." Today the term is used to refer to Jews who have ancestors from Eastern or Central Europe, such as Germany, Poland, Lithuania, Ukraine, and Russia. Today there are Ashkenazi Jews all over the world and many are intermarrying. For centuries, political and religious factors ensured their genetic isolation from the population at large.

In addition, recent studies have shown that people of Ashkenazi Jewish descent may be at greater risk for breast and ovarian cancer than the general population. In 1995 scientists from the National Institutes of Health discovered that a particular mutation in the breast cancer gene called *BRCA1* was present in one percent of the general Jewish population. In comparison, the percentage of people in the general U.S. population who have any mutation in *BRCA1* has been estimated to be between 0.1 and 0.6 percent. A second study the next year found two additional mutations (one in the *BRCA1* gene and one in *BRCA2*) to have a greater prevalence in the Ashkenazi Jewish population, bringing the overall risk for carrying one of these three mutations to 2.3 percent.

About one in 40 Ashkenazi Jews carries one of three *BRCA1* or *BRCA2* mutations, while approximately one in 500 members of the general population carry any *BRCA1* or *BRCA2* mutation. Moreover,

- Twenty percent of Ashkenazi Jews who have been diagnosed with breast cancer before the age of 40 have a *BRCA1* mutation.

- Twenty-nine percent of Ashkenazi Jews with a family history of two or more breast cancers carry one of these mutations.

- Seventy-three percent of Ashkenazi Jews with a family history that includes two or more cases of breast cancer and at least one case of OVARIAN CANCER carry one of these mutations.

Asian-American women and cancer   Cancer is the leading cause of death among Asian-American women, a subgroup of Asian/Pacific Islanders. When Asian women migrate to the United States, their risk of BREAST CANCER rises sixfold compared to the women in their native countries; those Asian-American women who immigrated to the United States at least a decade ago have a risk of breast cancer that is 80 percent higher than that of new immigrants. For those born in the United States, the breast cancer risk is similar to that of U.S. Caucasian women. Exposure to Western lifestyles (especially diet and nutrition) has been the most popular explanation for the dramatic differences between breast cancer incidence in Asian women living in the United States and those living in Asia.

Asian-American women have the lowest rates of early detection screening for breast and CERVICAL CANCER, and the lowest breast cancer mortality rate of all ethnic groups in America. Among ethnic populations in this country, Asian-American women are also the least likely to have ever had a mammogram, probably because of barriers due to cultural beliefs and practices, mistrust of Western medicine, and socioeconomic factors.

The most recent breakdown among Asian-American women for the incidence of breast cancer per 100,000 women (from 1988 to 1992) is

- Korean women: 29
- Vietnamese women: 38
- Chinese women: 55
- Filipino women: 73
- Japanese women: 82
- Native Hawaiian women: 106

(In comparison, Caucasian women had a reported incidence of 112 per 100,000 women.)

The death rate from breast cancer among Asian-American women (1988–1992) is the lowest of the main ethnic populations in the United States. Asian-American women have a combined mortality rate of 13 deaths for every 100,000 women, compared to a rate of 27 out of every 100,000 Caucasian women, and 15 out of every 100,000 Latina women. Among Asian-Americans, the mortality rate was 7 per 100,000 for Korean and Southeast

Asian women, 12 per 100,000 for Filipino women, 13 per 100,000 for Japanese women, and 11 per 100,000 for Chinese women. The lower number of Asian-American women who die of breast cancer reflects the lower incidence of the disease.

The National Asian Women's Health Organization created the Asian American Women's Breast and Cervical Cancer Program as a way to address the problem of breast cancer in this community. This program is a unique intervention whose goals are to improve screening outreach and cancer education and eliminate the threat of these diseases in Asian-American communities nationwide.

Asian/Pacific Islanders and cancer While Asian/Pacific Islanders experience lower incidence of cancer in general and lower death rates compared with other minority groups, they do experience higher death and incidence for certain specific types of cancers. (Of course, Asian/Pacific Islanders are not a homogenous population and contain subgroups that have different cancer rates.)

Both men and women in this group experience the highest incidence of LIVER CANCER and STOMACH CANCER of any group. While the liver cancer incidence for American Indian/Alaska Natives is much lower, Asian/Pacific Islanders and American Indian/Alaska Natives are the only populations in which the liver is among the top ten cancer sites.

Asian/Pacific Islander women have the third highest breast cancer incidence, but Asian/Pacific Islander women have the lowest breast cancer death rates. They also have the third lowest COLORECTAL CANCER death rates. Asian/Pacific Islander men have the third highest rate for LUNG CANCER and colorectal cancer, and high death rates for liver cancer and stomach cancer.

aspartame See ARTIFICIAL SWEETENERS.

aspiration biopsy See BIOPSY.

aspirin This common painkiller helps decrease the risk for a number of diseases, including several cancers. According to research, daily use of aspirin may help reduce the risk of several types of cancer, including COLORECTAL CANCER and cancers of the

esophagus, stomach, rectum, prostate, and pancreas. In particular, studies have found that people who took aspirin daily were about half as likely to develop colon cancer and may also experience modest reductions in the polyps that can lead to colon cancer.

A daily aspirin may also help decrease PANCREATIC CANCER risk by as much as 43 percent, according to University of Minnesota researchers. The researchers studied the use of aspirin and other nonsteroidal anti-inflammatory drugs by 28,283 postmenopausal women who responded to health questionnaires in the Iowa Women's Health Study from 1992 to 1999. Women who took aspirin had a 43 percent lower rate of pancreatic cancer than nonusers, and the risk of the cancer declined with increasing frequency of aspirin use, the team reported. Of 80 people in the study who developed pancreatic cancer, 33 were women who never used aspirin and 27 used it less than once a week. There were 10 cases among women who took aspirin two to five times a week and 10 among those using it six times or more weekly.

Scientists are not sure exactly how aspirin may prevent cancer. They theorize that it limits the production of prostaglandins, a hormone-like substance that may be involved in tumor growth.

Consumers should ask their doctor if an aspirin a day is right for them; it is generally recommended to prevent heart disease for men over age 40 and women past menopause. For some people, a daily dose of aspirin is not recommended because of potential side effects or other medical conditions.

Association for the Cure of Cancer of the Prostate See CAP CURE.

Association of Community Cancer Centers (ACCC) The nation's leading ONCOLOGY policy organization for the cancer care team, dedicated to helping cancer professionals adapt to the complex challenges of program management, reimbursement, legislation, and regulations. In the 1970s the ACCC presented the first U.S. meeting on hospital oncology units and hospice care; throughout the 1990s, association support resulted in passage of ACCC's off-label drug legislation in 39 states. The association helps to ensure that cancer programs are adequately funded. ACCC priorities also include cancer patient advocacy and the development of guidelines for standard patient care.

ACCC members include medical and radiation ONCOLOGISTS, surgeons, cancer program administrators, hospital executives, practice managers, oncology nurses and social workers, and cancer program data managers. ACCC Institution/Group Practice members include more than 650 medical centers, hospitals, oncology practices, and cancer programs across the United States. For contact information, see Appendix I.

astrocytoma   See BRAIN CANCER.

ataxia telangiectasia (AT)   A progressive degenerative disease that affects several body systems and leads to a higher risk of several types of cancer. Children with AT tend to develop malignancies of the blood system almost a thousand times more often than do children in the general population. LYMPHOMA and LEUKEMIA are common types of cancer although the risk of most types of cancer is higher. Unfortunately, these patients are also unusually sensitive to radiation, which means that they cannot tolerate the RADIATION THERAPY usually given to cancer patients.

The condition affects boys and girls equally in about one out of 40,000 births, but experts suspect that many children with the condition, particularly those who die at a young age, are never properly diagnosed. Therefore, this disease may actually be much more common.

Cause
AT is a hereditary disease; in 1988 the gene responsible for AT was mapped to chromosome 11.

Symptoms
Children with AT appear normal at birth. The first signs of the disease usually appear after age 2, when balance becomes uncertain and speech is slurred as a result of a lack of muscle control (ataxia). The onset of this muscle problem marks the beginning of progressive degeneration of the cerebellum that gradually leads to a general lack of muscle control. As muscle control worsens, chil-

dren lose their ability to read and write and eventually must be confined to a wheelchair.

Soon after the onset of the ataxia, tiny red spidery veins (telangiectasias) begin to appear at the corners of the eyes or on the surface of the ears and cheeks exposed to sunlight. These harmless veins, together with ataxia, characterize the disease.

Treatment
There is currently no way to slow the progression of the disease or prevent cancer, so treatment is aimed at easing symptoms as they appear. Because AT is a rare disease, very little research is available about what drugs might help these children. Physical, occupational, and speech therapy can help children maintain flexibility, gamma-globulin injections help supplement the immune systems of AT patients, and high-dose vitamins may be of some help.

Prognosis
There is no cure for AT. If they do not develop cancer, most children with AT are confined to wheelchairs by the age of 10 because they cannot control their muscles. Patients usually die from respiratory failure or cancer by their teens or early twenties. A few live into their forties, but they are extremely rare.

Ataxia Telangiectasia Children's Project   A nonprofit organization founded in 1993 by a family in Florida with two young sons who have ATAXIA TELANGIECTASIA (AT). The AT Children's Project was formed to raise funds for scientific research aimed at finding a cure and improving the lives of all children with ataxia telangiectasia. The organization also seeks to improve the accurate diagnosis of AT patients by increasing public awareness and by educating physicians. It is developing an international registry of AT patients. For contact information, see Appendix I.

autoclave-resistant factor   A substance found in soybeans that may slow down or stop the spread of cancer. This substance does not break down in an autoclave (a device that uses high-pressure steam to kill microorganisms and clean medical equipment).

autologous blood transfusion The use of a patient's own blood for a blood transfusion. Typically, a patient's blood is removed, stored, and then transfused back when needed.

An autologous blood transfusion with STEM CELL transplant involves the intravenous infusion of the patient's own BONE MARROW or circulating stem cells after high dose CHEMOTHERAPY and/or radiation. Without the transplant and restoration of the bone marrow, high dose treatment would be lethal.

autologous bone marrow transplant See BONE MARROW TRANSPLANTS.

axillary dissection Removal of the LYMPH NODES located in the armpit, usually during BREAST CANCER surgery such as a LUMPECTOMY. The lymph nodes are removed to determine whether breast cancer has spread. The standard breast cancer operations call for removal of these nodes to determine further treatment and prognosis, depending on whether the nodes are "positive" (with malignant cells) or "negative" (containing no cancer cells).

See also SENTINEL NODE BIOPSY.

bacteria and viruses   A number of cancers have been linked to infectious agents, including parasites, viruses (such as the HUMAN PAPILLOMAVIRUS and some of the viruses that cause hepatitis), and the *Helicobacter* bacterium that causes ulcers. Prevention could be as simple as getting hepatitis vaccinations, practicing safe sex by using a latex condom, and discussing with a doctor the possibility of antibiotic treatment of ulcers.

B3 antigen   A protein found on some tumor cells.

barbecued meat   Several recent reports suggest that eating barbecued meat may promote cancer due to ingestion of cancer-causing substances (POLYCYCLIC AROMATIC HYDROCARBONS) that are produced when fat from the meat drips onto the flames. The substances rise up in the smoke and settle back on the meat.

Experts recommend that consumers limit the amount of barbecued meat they eat. If consumers insist on barbecuing, the meat should be precooked in an oven or microwave before being transferred to the barbecue. This will result in shorter open-flame cooking time and fewer polycyclic aromatic hydrocarbons.

barium enema   A barium enema (lower gastrointestinal series) is an X-ray procedure that uses barium sulfate and air to outline the lining of the colon and rectum.

barium swallow   A series of X-rays of the esophagus taken after a patient drinks a barium-containing solution. The barium coats and outlines the esophagus on the X-ray for better viewing. Barium swallow is used to help diagnose cancers of the throat and ESOPHAGEAL CANCER.

basal cell carcinoma   The most common form of SKIN CANCER, affecting more than 750,000 Americans each year. One out of every three new cancers is a skin cancer, and 83.5 percent of skin cancers are basal cell carcinomas.

Basal cells are small, round skin cells that are found in the lower portion of the outermost skin layer. When these cells become malignant, they typically develop into small skin tumors that grow locally, sometimes destroying skin and nearby tissues. This can be especially troublesome if the tumor grows on the face, where it can be disfiguring in addition to interfering with function of facial structures, such as the eyelids or mouth. Basal-cell tumors rarely spread and are almost never fatal. However, an untreated tumor can grow deeper into surrounding tissues. Although about 90 percent of basal cell cancers occur on the face, this cancer may grow on any unprotected portion of the body exposed to sunlight.

Incidence

Until recently, those most likely to get basal cell carcinoma were older people (especially men) who spent a great deal of time outdoors. The incidence increases significantly in those with outdoor occupations and those who live in sunny climates; in Queensland, Australia, more than half the local white population has had a basal cell carcinoma by age 75. The number of new cases has risen sharply in the last decade because of the thinning ozone layer and extensive sunbathing.

In addition, younger people are being diagnosed with the disease. Today almost as many women as men are getting basal cell cancer.

Causes

Chronic overexposure to sunlight is the cause of 95 percent of all basal cell carcinomas. In a few cases, contact with ARSENIC, exposure to radiation, and complications of burns, scars, or vaccinations are contributing factors.

Symptoms

A basal cell tumor often occurs on the side of the eye or the nose, although it can appear in any location. These tumors are usually very slow-growing, although if untreated they can eventually get quite large. The five most typical characteristics of basal cell carcinoma are very different from each other, and often two or more features are found in one tumor. Basal cell carcinoma may be

- a sore that bleeds or oozes, remaining open for three or more weeks
- a reddish patch or irritated area (often on the shoulder, chest, arms, or legs) that may itch or hurt, or cause no sensation at all
- a smooth growth with an elevated, rolled border and indented center, developing tiny blood vessels on its surface as it grows
- a shiny bump that is pearly or translucent, often pink, red, white, tan, black, or brown
- a scar (white, yellow, or waxy) with poorly defined borders; the skin itself looks shiny and taut. This last sign is less frequent but may indicate an aggressive tumor. This rare type of basal cell cancer is called a morpheaform basal-cell carcinoma

As the cancer slowly grows, the center of the nodule may form an ulcer, producing a crater that bleeds, crusts, or forms a scab.

Diagnosis

A diagnosis of basal cell carcinoma is made after physical examination and biopsy (removal and examination of a piece of tissue). During a biopsy, a doctor may shave away only a small piece of abnormal skin; in other cases, the doctor will simply remove the entire abnormal area and send it to the laboratory for examination.

Treatment

If tumor cells are found, the growth can be removed by surgery or destroyed by radiation. The treatment is based on type, size, and location of the tumor, whether it has recurred, and on the patient's age and health. It can almost always be performed on an outpatient basis. Local anesthetics are used, and not much pain is felt during removal.

Once treatment is finished and the cancer is gone, the doctor will schedule regular follow-up skin examinations.

Surgical removal The most common way to remove a basal cell carcinoma is to have the doctor remove the entire growth and an additional border of normal skin as a safety margin. The site is then stitched closed, and the tissue is sent to the lab to determine if all malignant cells have been removed.

Electrosurgery In this procedure, (also called curettage and electrodesiccation), the doctor scrapes cancerous tissue from the skin with a curette. Next, the doctor uses an electric needle to burn a safety margin of normal skin around the tumor at the base of the scraped area. This technique is repeated twice to make sure the tumor has been completely removed.

Cryosurgery With this technique, the doctor does not cut the growth but instead freezes the lesion by applying liquid nitrogen with a special spray or a cotton-tipped applicator; this method does not require anesthesia and produces no bleeding. It is easy to administer and is the treatment of choice for those who have bleeding disorders or are intolerant of anesthesia.

Laser surgery This method focuses a beam of light on the lesion either to excise it or destroy it by vaporization. The major advantage of this technique is that it seals blood vessels as it cuts. In removing skin cancer, incisional laser surgery offers no real advantage over scalpel surgery.

Mohs surgery Microscopically controlled surgery that involves removing very thin layers of the malignant tumor and checking each layer thoroughly under a microscope. This is repeated until the tissue is free of tumor. This method saves the most healthy tissue and has the highest cure rate. It is often used for tumors that recur and for tumors in areas where basal cell carcinomas are known to recur after other treatment techniques (such as the nose, ears, and around the eyes).

Radiation therapy In this method, X-rays are directed at the malignant cells; it usually takes several treatments several times a week for a few weeks to totally destroy a tumor. Radiation therapy may be used with older patients or with those in poor health, or with tumors that are deep and recurrent.

Other treatments Researchers are studying the possible use of INTERFERON, a genetically engineered product of the human immune system, as a possible treatment of some basal cell carcinomas. Interferon interferes with viral multiplication and increases the activity of natural killer cells (a type of white blood cell and part of the body's immune system). Less common or experimental therapies include topical fluorouracil (an anticancer drug applied directly to the skin), CHEMOTHERAPY with systemic retinoids, or photodynamic therapy (killing cancer with a combination of special sensitizing chemicals and light).

Prognosis

When removed early, basal cell carcinomas are easily treated, but the larger the growth, the more extensive the treatment. While this type of skin cancer almost never spreads, it can destroy surrounding tissue. Since removal of a tumor scars the skin, large tumors may require reconstructive surgery and skin grafts.

The outlook for this type of cancer is excellent; 95 percent can be cured if treated early. However, 36 percent of patients who have been treated for one basal-cell cancer develop a second basal-cell cancer within the next five years—usually near the same place and within the first two years. Therefore, it is important to examine the surgical site from time to time to check for recurrences. Especially problematic are basal cell carcinomas on the scalp, nose and sides of the nose, and around the ears. If the cancer recurs, the doctor may recommend a different type of treatment the second time (most likely Mohs surgery).

Prevention

Because basal-cell cancer results from unprotected exposure to sunlight, protecting skin from the sun can help prevent these tumors. This includes

- Using sunscreen with an SPF of 15 or above, with a broad spectrum of protection against both ultraviolet-A and ultraviolet-B rays.

- Avoiding sun exposure during peak intensity (in most parts of the United States, from about 10 A.M. to 3 P.M.).

- Using sunglasses with ultraviolet light protection.

- Wearing long pants, a shirt with long sleeves, and a hat with a wide brim.

- Limiting sun exposure when taking certain drugs, including some antibiotics and certain drugs used to treat psychiatric illness, high blood pressure, heart failure, acne, or allergies.

- Limiting sun exposure when using some nonprescription skin-care products containing alpha hydroxy acids, which can make skin more vulnerable to damage from sunlight.

- Performing skin self-examinations every one to two months. Use a mirror to check for skin abnormalities on less visible areas (back, shoulders, upper arms, buttocks, and the soles of the feet).

B43-BAP immunotoxin A toxic substance linked to an antibody that attaches to and kills tumor cells.

B cell acute lymphocytic leukemia See LEUKEMIA.

BCG solution A form of BIOLOGICAL THERAPY for BLADDER CANCER in which a catheter is used to introduce a solution into the bladder. The solution contains live, weakened bacteria (bacille Calmette-Guérin), which activate the immune system. The BCG solution used for bladder cancer is not the same thing as BCG vaccine, which is used for tuberculosis in countries outside the United States.

Beckwith-Wiedemann syndrome (BWS) A rare overgrowth syndrome that occurs in about one out of every 15,000 births. About 10 percent of infants and children with the syndrome develop cancer, and the period of highest risk for developing cancer is before the age of four. In general, children outgrow the visible signs of BWS by adolescence.

The most common types of cancer that occur in children with the syndrome are KIDNEY CANCER and LIVER CANCER. Other types of cancer, which occur more rarely, include ADRENAL CANCER, neuroblastoma, and RHABDOMYOSARCOMA. Children with BWS who have uneven growth of limbs have an increased risk of developing cancer, and children with large kidneys appear to be at greater risk for WILMS' TUMOR.

Symptoms

Most children have only a few of the many distinct characteristics of the syndrome. The most common characteristics, which can range from mild to severe, are a large tongue, large body size and weight, abdominal wall defects, uneven growth of limbs or organs, ear lobe creases or pits, low blood sugar, swallowing/eating problems, hearing loss, speech defects, and behavior problems.

Cancer Screening

Infants and small children with BWS need to be frequently screened for cancer, including an abdominal ultrasound at least every three months until age seven or eight to check for early-stage Wilms' tumor. Blood levels of ALPHA-FETOPROTEIN (AFP) should be checked every six to 12 weeks until children are three or four years old. (An elevated level of AFP can suggest the presence of liver cancer.)

The risk of cancer decreases with time, particularly beyond the age of eight years. Screening beyond that age is of uncertain value and is thus not routinely recommended. Nonetheless, for some parents, continued screening may be reassuring.

Bence-Jones protein A protein that is excreted in the urine of most patients with MULTIPLE MYELOMA and sometimes in the urine of patients with other types of cancer. This protein is part of the antibodies abnormally produced because of the cancer.

The malignant plasma cells in most patients with myeloma produce complete proteins known as immunoglobulins, which normally consist of both long and short chains (otherwise known as heavy and light chains). However, in 15 percent to 20 percent of patients, the plasma cells produce only light-chain proteins, which are called Bence-Jones proteins after the person who discovered them. Patients who have this type of protein in their urine are said to have "Bence-Jones myeloma," or, more often, "light-chain myeloma."

benign prostatic hyperplasia (BPH) Abnormal growth of benign prostate cells that triggers benign growth of the prostate. In the past, it was commonly used to refer to an enlarged prostate. Although this condition is not cancer, it can cause many of the same symptoms as PROSTATE CANCER. Benign prostatic hyperplasia does not usually affect sexual function, but it causes problems because as the prostate enlarges, it presses against the bladder and the urethra, blocking the flow of urine.

Once the prostate begins to enlarge, it can grow in one of two ways. Cells can multiply around the urine passageway through the prostate, squeezing it closed. The second type of growth is more likely to cause symptoms and involves enlargement of the middle lobe: cells grow into the urine tube and even up and into the bladder. This type of growth most often needs to be treated with surgery.

Cause

BPH is the result of small noncancerous growths inside the prostate that may be related to hormone changes that occur with aging. By age 60, more than half of all American men have microscopic signs of BPH, and by age 70, more than 40 percent have enlargement that can be felt on physical examination.

The prostate normally starts out about the size of a walnut, and begins to enlarge in all men by the time they reach 40, growing to the size of an apricot; by age 60, it may be as big as a lemon. Prostate growth generally continues throughout a man's lifetime. Effects of this growth vary from minor annoyance to almost unbearable discomfort. By age 60, one in four men are so severely affected by symptoms that treatment is required.

Symptoms

This condition is normally diagnosed by its symptoms. A man who has BPH may find it difficult to urinate or maintain more than a dribble of urine. He also may need to urinate frequently, or he may have a sudden, powerful urge to urinate. Many men are forced to get up several times a night; others have an annoying feeling that the bladder is never completely empty. Straining to empty the bladder can make the condition worse; the bladder stretches, the bladder wall thickens and losses its elasticity, and the bladder muscles become less efficient.

The pool of urine that collects in the bladder can foster urinary tract infections, and trying tc force a urine stream can produce pressure that eventually damages the kidneys.

Complications

BPH can lead to a number of problems. For instance, a completely blocked urethra is a medical emergency that requires immediate catheterization, a procedure in which a tube called a catheter is inserted through the penis into the bladder to allow urine to escape. Other serious potential complications of BPH include bladder stones, urinary infection, kidney damage, and bleeding.

Self Test

The AMERICAN UROLOGICAL ASSOCIATION has developed a seven-question self-test to help patients assess the severity of BPH symptoms. The test asks men to rate how often over the past month they have

- had a sensation of not emptying the bladder completely after urinating
- had to urinate again less than two hours after urinating
- stopped and started again several times during urination
- found it difficult to postpone urination
- had a weak urinary stream
- had to push or strain to begin urination
- had to get up several times at night to urinate (how many times)

Scoring

For the first six questions:

- 1 point for having problems less than one time in five
- 2 points for having problems less than half the time
- 3 points for having problems about half the time
- 4 points for having problems more than half the time
- 5 points for having problems almost all the time

For the seventh question:

- 1 point for each time a man gets up at night
- 5 points for getting up five times or more

MILD: 1 to 7 points
MODERATE: 8 to 19 points
SEVERE: 20 to 35 points

Diagnosis

BPH is diagnosed with a detailed medical history focusing on the urinary tract (kidneys, ureters [the pair of tubes that carry urine from the kidneys to the bladder], the bladder, and the urethra).

The initial medical evaluation typically includes a physical exam called a DIGITAL RECTAL EXAM (DRE), a urinalysis to check for infection or bleeding, and a blood test to measure kidney function. Some physicians may also check the level of PROSTATE-SPECIFIC ANTIGEN (PSA), using a PSA test to help rule out the likelihood of cancer. PSA is a protein that is produced by the cells of the prostate gland.

In addition, other tests may help a urologist determine whether BPH has affected the bladder or kidneys. These include tests that measure the speed of urine flow, pressure in the bladder during urination, and the amount of urine that remains in the bladder after urination.

Some other tests that are widely used are expensive, sometimes risky, and unnecessary for most men, according to an expert panel sponsored by the U.S. Public Health Service practice guidelines. These include

- CYSTOSCOPY, in which the doctor inserts a viewing tube up the urethra to get a direct look at the bladder
- UROGRAM, an X-ray in which urine is made visible after dye is injected into a vein
- ULTRASOUND, a test that obtains images of the kidneys and bladder after a probe is placed on the abdomen

Treatment

There is no cure for prostate growth, but there also is no connection between BPH and prostate cancer. Although BPH may not be a threat to life, if not properly treated it can lead to extremely serious consequences, including kidney damage and failure. Some men may require treatment with medicine or surgery to relieve symptoms. Although BPH cannot be cured, its symptoms often can be relieved by surgery or by drugs. According to some experts, mild to moderate symptoms worsened in only about 20 percent of the cases, improved (without any specific treatment) in another 20 percent, and remained about the same in the rest.

If a man has no serious complications, such as the inability to urinate, kidney damage, frequent urinary tract infections, major bleeding through the urethra, or bladder stones, the best approach for treating BPH is not clear. The practice guidelines advise doctors to leave treatment decisions to the patient after discussing the benefits and side effects of each treatment option.

The options selected by an individual man are tied to his own preferences. For instance, some men with significant symptoms or complications want immediate relief and are willing to undergo surgery or begin a drug regimen. Others are reluctant or unwilling to undergo surgery or to take pills daily for an extended period.

Watchful waiting Men whose symptoms are mild often opt for "watchful waiting," having regular checkups and getting further treatment only if their symptoms become bothersome. The USPHS Clinical Practice Guidelines call watchful waiting "an appropriate treatment strategy for the majority of patients." Men who choose watchful waiting should have regular, perhaps annual, checkups, including DREs and laboratory tests.

For those who choose watchful waiting, a number of simple steps may help to reduce bothersome symptoms. These include limiting fluid intake in the evening, especially alcohol or caffeinated beverages, which can trigger the urge to urinate and can interfere with sleep; taking time to empty the bladder completely; and not allowing long intervals to pass without urinating. Men monitoring prostate conditions should also be aware that certain medications prescribed for other conditions may make their symptoms worse. These include some over-the-counter cough and cold remedies, prescribed tranquilizers, antidepressants, and drugs to control high blood pressure. Switching to a different prescription may help. Watchful waiting, of course, is not always enough for BPH, and surgery or drug therapy may be required. Here is a close look at both options:

Surgery Several types of surgery can relieve the symptoms of an enlarged prostate, including the following:

Transurethral resection of the prostate (TURP). Trans-urethral resection of the prostate is considered to be the best way to treat prostate enlargement, and accounts for a majority of all prostate surgery. However, its use is beginning to decline as alternatives have become more widely available. This procedure relieves symptoms quickly, generally improving the urinary flow within weeks. By inserting a slim fiber optic scope through the penis and up the urethra as far as the prostate, the surgeon pares away the lining of the prostate and excess prostate tissue, expanding the passageway for the urine flow. The TURP procedure ordinarily does not cause incontinence or impotence.

Transurethral incision of the prostate (TUIP). This procedure is used on small prostate glands and is far less common than TURP. As in TURP, TUIP is performed by passing an instrument through the penis to reach the prostate; however, the surgeon makes only one or two small incisions to relieve pressure in the prostate rather than trimming away tissue. As the TURP, the procedure considerably increases the urine flow. TUIP is an outpatient procedure with a low risk of side effects. Men interested in having children may want to consider this procedure, because it usually does not affect ejaculation or fertility.

Laser surgery. Using a laser, a doctor can vaporize prostate tissue directly. In laser-induced and laser-assisted surgery, high-energy instruments heat prostate tissue to the boiling point, thereby killing the tissue.

Indigo laser. In this minimally invasive procedure, a urologist threads a special indigo fiber into a tube through the urethra and into the prostate. The fiber optic tip is carefully placed in the area targeted for treatment; laser energy through the tip is then used to precisely destroy the enlarged part of the prostate. The destroyed prostate tissue is then absorbed naturally into the body. As the prostate shrinks over a few weeks, pressure on the bladder and the urethra eases, decreasing the symptoms of BPH. Symptoms continue to improve over several months. The treatment is typically an outpatient procedure and can be completed in less than 30 minutes. There are several anesthesia options, including general, spinal, and local. Choice of anesthesia depends on the patient and the size of his prostate. Patients must use a catheter until the swelling subsides; this is usually removed within a week. This is a relatively recent therapy, which some have compared favorably to the "gold-standard" TURP.

Transurethral needle ablation (TUNA). This recently approved technique can be done with a local anesthetic on an outpatient basis. An instrument is inserted through the penis into the prostate's urine tube. Heat is applied to prostate tissues through needles, which removes excess tissue; that tissue later dies. Some clinical studies have reported that TUNA improves the urine flow with minimal side effects when compared with other procedures. TUNA is similar to lasers and other noninvasive techniques. The TUNA works best on moderately enlarged prostates, but is not very effective on very large prostates or those that have a median lobe.

Targis. This type of microwave treatment was approved by the U.S. Food and Drug Administration in late 1997. As other new therapies, this has appeared to be effective in the short term, but has yet to demonstrate long-term benefits.

Prostatectomy. This generalized term is used to describe any procedure that surgically removes prostate tissue. A radical prostatectomy is performed for cancer and involves removal of the entire prostate. Only the inner part of the prostate is removed during an open prostatectomy (also called a suprapubic prostatectomy), which is done for men with BPH with very large prostates (about 5 percent of all cases) that are too big to remove using a scope.

Drug Therapy

Millions of American men have chosen drugs rather than surgery since drug therapy for BPH was first tried in the early 1990s. Although regarded as less effective than surgery, drugs are also less invasive and usually free of major side effects. There are two major classes of drugs:

Alpha adrenergic blockers originally were used to treat high blood pressure by relaxing smooth muscles in blood vessel walls. In BPH, they relax the muscular portion of the prostate and the bladder neck, allowing urine to flow more freely. In the average patient, these drugs increase the rate of urine flow and reduce symptoms, often within days. Side effects include dizziness, fatigue, and headache.

Finasteride shrinks the prostate by blocking an enzyme that converts the male hormone testosterone into a stronger, growth-stimulating form. Some studies show that use of finasteride for at least six months can increase urinary flow rate and reduce symptoms. It seems to work best for men who have greatly enlarged prostates.

In a small percentage of men, the drug can affect sexual activity, decreasing a man's interest in sex, diminishing his ability to have an erection, and causing problems with ejaculation. It sometimes also causes tenderness or swelling of the breasts and causes a drop in PSA levels. These side effects can be reversed by stopping the drug.

Some doctors think that combining the two types of drugs may produce better results. This is most often done in men with large prostates.

Other Treatments

Researchers are working to develop BPH treatments that are more effective and produce fewer side effects. These include using laser surgery, powerful electric currents, and microwaves. Doctors have also tried to enlarge the urethra by inserting a balloon into it and inflating it with fluid and by inserting a stent (a small metal coil) into the urethra to hold it open. This treatment has a significant risk of long-term complications and is generally done only in patients where other treatments are not an option.

benign uterine tumor   See FIBROID.

benzene   A flammable colorless liquid with a sweet odor that evaporates quickly and dissolves in water. Benzene is a human carcinogen, according to the Department of Health and Human Services; long-term exposure to high levels of benzene in the air can cause LEUKEMIA.

Benzene is widely used by U.S. industries to make other chemicals that are used to make plastics, resins, and nylon and synthetic fibers. Benzene is also used to make some types of rubbers, lubricants, dyes, detergents, drugs, and pesticides. Benzene can be produced naturally, as happens with volcanoes and forest fires, and it is a natural part of crude oil, gasoline, and cigarette smoke.

Outdoor air contains low levels of benzene from tobacco smoke, car exhaust, and industrial emissions. Indoor air generally contains higher levels of benzene from products that contain it such as glues, paints, paint thinners, furniture wax, and detergents. Air around hazardous waste sites or gas stations contains higher levels of benzene. Leakage from underground storage tanks or from hazardous waste sites containing benzene can result in benzene contamination of well water. People working in industries that make or use benzene may be exposed to the highest levels of it. Finally, a major source of benzene exposure is tobacco smoke.

Breathing very high levels of benzene can be fatal, while high levels can cause drowsiness, dizziness, rapid heart rate, headaches, tremors, confusion, and unconsciousness. Eating or drinking foods containing high levels of benzene can cause vomiting, irritation of the stomach, dizziness, sleepiness, convulsions, rapid heart rate, and death. Long-term exposure to benzene can affect the blood. It harms the bone marrow, can lower red blood cell count (leading to anemia) and can cause excessive bleeding. It can also damage the immune system, increasing the chance for infection.

Several tests, such as a breath test or blood test can reveal, whether a person has been exposed to benzene. This must be done shortly after exposure. Benzene metabolites can also be measured in the urine, but this test also must be performed soon after exposure. It is not a reliable indicator of how much benzene a patient has been exposed to, since the metabolites may be from other sources.

Safety Levels

The U.S. Environmental Protection Agency has set the maximum permissible level of benzene in drinking water at 0.005 mg/L (milligram per liter). The agency requires that spills or accidental releases into the environment of 10 pounds or more of benzene be reported to the government. The Occupational Safety and Health Administration has set a permissible exposure limit in the workplace of 1 part of benzene per million parts of air during a 40-hour workweek.

benzidine　A synthetic carcinogenic chemical that does not occur naturally in the environment. This crystalline solid may be grayish yellow, white, or reddish gray and will only evaporate slowly, especially from water and soil. Benzidine is also called 4,4'-diphenylenediamine or Fast Corinth Base B.

Benzidine causes cancer, most often BLADDER CANCER, according to studies of workers who were exposed for years to levels much higher than those experienced by the general public. Some evidence suggests that benzidine may cause cancer in the stomach, kidney, brain, mouth, esophagus, liver, gallbladder, bile duct, and pancreas. Most of the exposed workers studied did not develop cancer, even after such high exposures.

In the past, industry used large amounts of benzidine to produce dyes for cloth, paper, and leather, but it has not been manufactured for sale in the United States since the mid-1970s, and major U.S. dye companies no longer make benzidine-based dyes. Nor is benzidine used any longer in medical laboratories or in the rubber and plastics industries. However, small amounts of benzidine may still be manufactured or imported for scientific research in laboratories or for other specialized uses. Some benzidine-based dyes (or products colored with them) may also still be imported. Today, most benzidine still entering the environment probably comes from waste sites where it had been thrown away. Some may also come from the physical, chemical, or biological breakdown of benzidine-based dyes, or from other dyes where it may exist as an impurity. Only very small amounts of free benzidine will dissolve in water at moderate environmental temperatures. When discharged to waterways, it will sink and become part of the bottom sludge.

Benzidine exists in the air as very small particles, which may be brought back to the Earth's surface by rain or gravity. In soil, most benzidine is likely to be strongly attached to soil particles, so it does not easily pass into underground water. Benzidine can slowly be destroyed by certain other chemicals, light, and some microorganisms (for example, bacteria). Certain fish, snails, algae, and other forms of water life may take up and store very small amounts of benzidine, but accumulation in the food chain is unlikely.

Because benzidine is a synthetic chemical that does not occur naturally in the environment, most people are not likely to be exposed to it via contaminated air, water, soil, or food. Today no releases to air, water, or soil are reported on the Toxic Release Inventory. Only rarely has benzidine been detected in areas other than waste sites, and it has not been found in food. People living near a hazardous waste site could be exposed to benzidine by drinking contaminated water or by breathing or swallowing contaminated dust and soil. Benzidine can also enter the body by passing through the skin. Some dyes made from benzidine may still be imported for use in the United States. They may contain small amounts of benzidine as a contaminant or may be broken down in the body to benzidine. If consumers use such dyes to dye paper, cloth, leather, or other materials, they may be exposed through breathing or swallowing dust, or through skin contact with dust. Workers may be exposed in a similar way if they work at or near hazardous waste sites.

Because benzidine can cause cancer, the EPA has issued regulations listing it as a priority chemical, subject to inspection and control. The EPA allows 0.10 parts of benzidine per million parts of waste transported to waste disposal sites and requires that any release of a pound or more of benzidine or its salts to the environment be reported to the National Response Center. EPA's Office of Water also issues guidelines advising that benzidine concentration limits be less than 1 part benzidine in a trillion parts of water. Although zero benzidine is preferred, lifetime exposure to these concentrations is estimated to result in no more than one additional case of cancer in a million persons exposed.

The U.S. Occupational Safety and Health Administration considers benzidine to be a carcinogen and has issued regulations to reduce the risk of exposure in any workplace in which it might still be found. The National Institute for Occupational Safety and Health recommends that worker exposure to benzidine-based dyes be as low as feasible, since it considers benzidine to be

an occupational carcinogen. EPA's Office of Water has set a discharge limit for benzidine-based dye applicators.

beta-carotene   A carotenoid. A common plant chemical within a group of more than 600. Beta-carotene is converted by the body into vitamin A, which has many vital functions including the growth and repair of body tissues, formation of bones and teeth, resistance of the body to infection, and development of healthy eye tissues. Whereas vitamin A supplements can be toxic, excess beta-carotene is safely stored away and converted to vitamin A only when the body needs it. Epidemiological studies have linked high intake of foods rich in beta-carotene and high blood levels of the micronutrient to a lower risk of cancer (particularly LUNG CANCER).

Beta-carotene acts as an ANTIOXIDANT and immune system booster and is found in bright-orange-colored fruits and vegetables such as carrots, pumpkins, peaches, and sweet potatoes. Some experts suspect it may be possible to decrease cancer risk by supplementing the diet with beta-carotene.

Most, but not all, beta-carotene in supplements is synthetic, consisting of only one molecule (natural beta-carotene found in food is made of two molecules). Researchers originally saw no meaningful difference between natural and synthetic beta-carotene, but this view was questioned when the link between beta-carotene-containing foods and lung cancer prevention was not duplicated in studies using synthetic pills.

The most common beta-carotene supplement is 25,000 IU (15 mg) per day, though some people take as much as 100,000 IU (60 mg) per day. Excessive beta-carotene (more than 100,000 IU, or 60 mg, per day) sometimes tints the skin yellow-orange. Individuals taking beta-carotene for long periods of time should also supplement with vitamin E, as beta-carotene may reduce vitamin E levels.

bile duct cancer   This relatively rare cancer occurs in the system that drains bile from the liver to the intestine. Also known as cholangiocarcinoma, or biliary cancer, bile duct cancer is the most common cause of bile duct obstruction next to gallstones and true pancreatic cancer. It is often caused by cancer originating in the pancreas. Bile duct cancer is slightly more common in men and usually occurs in middle age.

Symptoms

The most common symptom of bile duct cancer is jaundice, in which the skin (and sometimes the whites of the eyes) turns yellow. Other symptoms include itching, abdominal pain, poor appetite and weight loss, fever, dark-red urine, and light-colored stools.

Diagnosis

Bile duct cancer can be diagnosed with X-rays, ultrasound, MRI and CT scans, cholangiography (X-rays taken after contrast dye has been injected), and endoscopic retrograde cholangiopancreatography (ERCP). A final diagnosis may not be conclusive without abdominal surgery. However, brushings taken during ERCP can often confirm the diagnosis.

Stages

Bile duct cancer has only two stages: localized or unresectable (inoperable). Localized bile duct cancer can be completely removed with surgery; unfortunately, this occurs in only a minority of cases. Most people have unresectable cancer, in which the malignancy cannot be completely removed. By the time the diagnosis is made, the cancer often has invaded the nearby liver or spread along the common bile duct and into adjacent lymph nodes. Spreading of this cancer throughout the body is common.

Risk Factors

Risk factors include

- *History of primary sclerosing cholangitis (PSC):* This condition scars and narrows the bile ducts, blocking bile from reaching the intestines. Many patients eventually develop liver failure and require a liver transplant; between 10 percent and 20 percent of patients develop bile duct cancer. Experts suspect that progressive injury and regeneration of the bile ducts predispose patients with PSC to cancer. More than half of patients with PSC have a history of inflammatory bowel disease (most often ulcerative colitis).

- *Congenital bile duct abnormalities:* These birth defects include dilation of the common bile duct and Caroli's disease (dilation of the intrahepatic bile ducts). It is thought that prolonged sludging of bile in these dilated spaces and subsequent infection predispose patients to carcinoma, again through progressive injury and repair. The overall lifetime risk of bile duct cancer in these patients is 10 percent.

- *Benign bile duct tumors*

- *Parasitic infection:* Bile duct infections are most often seen in the Far East. Parasites include *Clonorchis sinensis* (most common in Japan, Korea, Vietnam) and *Opisthorchis viverrini* (most common in Thailand, Laos, Malaysia). *Clonorchis* is acquired by eating freshwater fish harboring the *Clonorchis* cyst; infection with this worm increases the risk of developing biliary tract carcinoma by 25- to 50-fold.

- *Toxic exposures:* Thorium dioxide (Thorotrast), used as a contrast dye in radiologic procedures between 1930 and 1950, has been shown to promote cancers in the liver and bile ducts.

Treatment

Treatment depends on the stage of the disease and includes surgery, radiation, and CHEMOTHERAPY. Surgical removal is the only way to cure the disease. Bile duct cancers within the liver are treated by removing a portion of the liver. Occasionally, a liver transplant will be attempted. Bile duct cancers near the joining of the bile ducts are treated differently depending upon how extensive the tumor is. Tumors confined below the right and left hepatic ducts are treated with removal of the extrahepatic bile ducts, gallbladder, and LYMPH NODES. Tumors that extend above the duct confluence may require removal of a lobe of the liver.

If the tumor cannot be removed surgically, bypass procedures may be performed to prevent obstruction of the gastrointestinal and biliary tracts, and to relieve the patient's symptoms (either with surgery or with stents).

biliary cancer See BILE DUCT CANCER.

bilobectomy The removal of more than one of the five lobes of the lungs.

biochanin A An isoflavone found in SOY PRODUCTS currently being studied as a possible cancer preventive.

bioflavonoids Chemical compounds related to vitamin C that have demonstrated an ability to slow down cancer growth and even turn cancer cells back into normal, healthy cells. These naturally occurring compounds act primarily as plant pigments and ANTIOXIDANTS, which fight cell damage caused by FREE RADICALS, a rogue type of oxygen molecule that can attack cells throughout the body.

Lemons, grapes, plums, grapefruit, cherries, blackberries, and rosehips are some of the richest dietary sources of bioflavonoids. Additional sources include other citrus fruits, green peppers, broccoli, tomatoes, and herb tea (especially stinging nettle tea). Bioflavonoids belong to a large group of more than 2,000 phytochemicals called phenols that are known to be very powerful antioxidants. Many studies have identified their unique role in protecting vitamin C from oxidation in the body, thereby allowing the body to reap more benefits from vitamin C.

Different bioflavonoids tend to have different health effects on the body, but in general, a diet high in bioflavonoids is associated with a lower incidence of many diseases, including cancer. For example, green TEA extract, which contains these compounds, protects against the development of some types of cancer, and a recent Hawaiian study suggests that consumption of certain flavonoids cuts the risk of LUNG CANCER in half.

Side Effects

Anyone taking bioflavonoid supplements should inform a doctor before undergoing surgery; bioflavonoids may interfere with the results of some blood and urine tests.

biological response modifier (BRM) A substance that can improve the body's natural response to infection and disease. There are many types of these modifiers, some produced by the body and others created in the lab. Many ongoing studies are investigating the use of these substances in BIOLOGICAL THERAPY to treat a wide variety of cancers.

The primary biological response modifiers include antibodies, COLONY-STIMULATING FACTORS, CYTOKINES (including INTERFERON and INTERLEUKINS), MONOCLONAL ANTIBODIES, and vaccines. Researchers continue to discover new BRMs, learn more about how they function, and develop ways to use them in cancer therapy. All of these substances alter the interaction between cancer cells and the body's immune defenses, restoring the body's ability to fight cancer. Biological therapies may be used to stop or control processes that allow cancer cells to grow, make cancer cells more recognizable to the immune system, boost the killing power of immune system cells, and alter the malignant growth patterns to make them more like healthy cells. BRMs also block or reverse the process that turns a normal cell into a cancerous cell and enhance the body's ability to repair normal cells damaged by other forms of cancer treatment, such as CHEMOTHERAPY or radiation. BRMs also stop cancer cells from spreading to other parts of the body.

Some BRMs are a standard part of treatment for certain types of cancer, while others are being studied as prospective treatments, either alone or in combinations. They are also being used with other treatments, such as RADIATION THERAPY and chemotherapy.

biological therapy A relatively new type of cancer treatment, sometimes called immunotherapy, biotherapy, or BIOLOGICAL RESPONSE MODIFIER therapy. Biological therapies may be used to stop or suppress processes that allow cancer growth and make cancer cells more recognizable and therefore more susceptible to destruction by the immune system. Biological therapies also boost the killing power of immune system cells and alter cancer cells' growth patterns to promote healthy behavior. They can be used to block or reverse the process that changes a normal cell into a cancerous cell and to enhance the body's ability to repair normal cells damaged by other forms of cancer treatment, such as CHEMOTHERAPY or radiation. Biological therapy also can help prevent cancer cells from spreading to other parts of the body.

Nonspecific Immunomodulating Agents

These substances boost the immune system, targeting important immune system cells and triggering increased production of CYTOKINES and immunoglobulins. Two nonspecific immunomodulating agents used to fight cancer are bacille Calmette-Guérin (BCG) and levamisole. BCG is used to treat superficial BLADDER CANCER following surgery. Levamisole is used with fluorouracil (5-FU) after surgery to treat stage III COLORECTAL CANCER. Levamisole may act to restore depressed immune function.

Biological Response Modifiers (BRMs)

Antibodies, cytokines, and other immune system substances produced in the lab for use in cancer treatment that alter the interaction between the body's immune defenses and cancer cells to boost the body's ability to fight the disease. BRMs include interferon, interleukins, COLONY-STIMULATING FACTORS, MONOCLONAL ANTIBODIES, and vaccines.

Interferons

An interferon is a type of naturally occurring cytokine. There are three major types: interferon alpha, interferon beta, and interferon gamma; interferon alpha is the type most widely used in cancer treatment.

Interferons can improve the way a cancer patient's immune system fights cancer cells and may slow the growth of cancer cells or promote their transformation into cells with more normal behavior. Researchers believe that some interferons may also stimulate natural killer (NK) cells, T cells, and macrophages, boosting the immune system's anticancer function.

The U.S. Food and Drug Administration (FDA) has approved the use of interferon alpha for the treatment of certain types of cancer, including hairy cell LEUKEMIA, MELANOMA, chronic myeloid leukemia, and AIDS-related KAPOSI'S SARCOMA. Studies have shown that interferon alpha may also be effective in treating other cancers such as KIDNEY CANCER and NON-HODGKIN'S LYMPHOMA. Researchers are exploring combinations of interferon alpha and other BRMs or chemotherapy in clinical trials to treat a number of cancers.

Interleukins

Interleukins are also cytokines that occur naturally in the body and can be produced synthetically. There are many different kinds of interleukins, but interleukin-2 (IL-2 or aldesleukin) has been the most widely studied in cancer treatment. IL-2 stimulates the growth and action of cancer-killing immune cells such as lymphocytes. The FDA has approved IL-2 for the treatment of kidney cancer and melanoma. Interleukins are being studied as potential treatments for colorectal, ovarian, lung, brain, breast, and PROSTATE CANCER, some leukemias, and some LYMPHOMAS.

Colony-Stimulating Factors (CSFs)

CSFs (sometimes called hematopoietic growth factors) usually do not directly affect tumor cells; rather, they encourage BONE MARROW STEM CELLS, the source of all blood cells, to divide and develop into white blood cells, platelets, and red blood cells. The CSFs' stimulation of blood cell production may benefit patients undergoing cancer treatment, which can damage the body's ability to make blood cells, resulting in an increased risk of infections, anemia, and bleeding.

By using CSFs to stimulate blood cell production, doctors can increase the doses of anticancer drugs without increasing the risk of infection or the need for transfusion with blood products. As a result, researchers have found CSFs particularly useful when combined with high-dose chemotherapy.

Some examples of CSFs include

- *G-CSF (filgrastim) and GM-CSF (sargramostim)* can increase the number of white blood cells, thereby reducing the risk of infection in patients receiving chemotherapy. G-CSF and GM-CSF can also stimulate the production of stem cells in preparation for stem cell or bone marrow transplants.
- *Erythropoietin* can increase the number of red blood cells and reduce the need for red blood cell transfusions in patients receiving chemotherapy.
- *Oprelvekin* can reduce the need for platelet transfusions in patients receiving chemotherapy.

Researchers are studying CSFs in clinical trials to treat some types of leukemia, metastatic colorectal cancer, melanoma, LUNG CANCER, and other types of cancer.

Monoclonal Antibodies (MOABs)

Antibodies made in the laboratory that are produced by a single type of cell and are specific for a particular antigen. Researchers are trying to figure out how to create MOABs specific to the antigens found on the surface of the cancer cell being treated. MOABs that react with specific types of cancer may enhance a patient's immune response to the cancer. MOABs can be programmed to interfere with the growth of cancer cells. In addition, MOABs may be used with CHEMOTHERAPY drugs, radioactive substances, other biological response modifiers, or other toxins so that when the antibodies latch onto cancer cells, they deliver these poisons directly to the tumor, helping to destroy it.

MOABs may help destroy cancer cells in bone marrow that has been removed from a patient in preparation for a bone marrow transplant. MOABs carrying radioisotopes may also prove useful in diagnosing certain cancers, such as colorectal, ovarian, and prostate. Rituxan (rituximab) and Herceptin (trastuzumab) are examples of monoclonal antibodies that have been approved by the FDA. Rituxan is used for the treatment of B-cell non-Hodgkin's lymphoma with and without chemotherapy. Herceptin is used to treat metastatic BREAST CANCER in patients with tumors that produce large amounts of a receptor protein called HER-2. These tumors occur in about 25 percent of breast cancer cases.

Researchers are also testing MOABs in clinical trials to treat lymphomas, leukemias, colorectal cancer, lung cancer, BRAIN CANCER, prostate cancer, and other types of cancer.

Cancer Vaccines

Researchers are developing vaccines for cancer treatments that may encourage the patient's immune system to recognize and reject cancer cells, preventing cancer from recurring. In contrast to vaccines against infectious diseases, cancer vaccines are designed to be injected after the disease is diagnosed, rather than before it develops.

Cancer vaccines given when the tumor is small may be able to cure the cancer. Early cancer vaccine studies focused on patients with melanoma, but today vaccines are also being studied in the treatment of many other types of cancer, including lymphomas and cancers of the kidney, breast, ovary, prostate, colon, and rectum. Researchers are also investigating ways that cancer vaccines can be used in combination with other BRMs.

Side Effects

Biological therapies can cause a number of side effects, including rashes or swelling at the site where they are injected. Several biological response modifiers, including interferons and interleukins, may cause flulike symptoms including fever, chills, NAUSEA, vomiting, and APPETITE LOSS. FATIGUE is another common side effect, and blood pressure may be affected. The side effects of IL-2 can often be severe, depending on the dosage given. Patients need to be closely monitored during treatment. Side effects of CSFs may include bone pain, diarrhea, edema, fatigue, fever, and appetite loss. The side effects of MOABs vary, and serious allergic reactions may occur. Cancer vaccines can cause muscle aches and fever.

biomarker A substance that may indicate the presence of a type of cancer when present in high levels in blood, other body fluids, or tissues. Examples of biomarkers include CA 125 (marker for OVARIAN CANCER), CA 15-3 and CA 27-29 (BREAST CANCER), CEA (ovarian, lung, breast, pancreatic, and gastrointestinal tract cancers), and PSA (PROSTATE CANCER).

biopsy A procedure that samples a small amount of tissue or cells for microscopic examination to diagnose cancer and to estimate how far it has spread. There are different biopsy techniques, depending on which tissue or organ is being sampled.

In a *skin* or *muscle biopsy*, for example, a small incision is made in the skin using a scalpel, and a small portion of skin or muscle is removed.

In a *needle biopsy*, a sterile hollow needle is inserted through the skin to remove a small sample of a deeper organ such as the kidney or breast. In some cases, the biopsy needle will be guided with ultrasound scanning or CT scanning to more precisely locate the area being sampled.

Biopsies can also be done during endoscopy procedures (such as BRONCHOSCOPY or COLONOSCOPY) using a sampling instrument at the end of the endoscope.

While many biopsies are performed outside the hospital using only mild local pain medication, an *open biopsy* is part of a surgical operation that opens a major body cavity such as the chest or abdomen. This type of biopsy requires general anesthesia and hospital admission.

The time required for a biopsy varies according to the specific type of biopsy procedure. For example, a simple skin biopsy usually takes about one minute, while a needle biopsy of the kidney takes about 15 minutes. Open biopsies requiring general surgery can take much longer.

Once inside the lab, the biopsy sample is stained and examined under the microscope. Microscopic examination can tell whether the tissue sample is normal, part of a benign (not cancerous) tumor, or malignant (cancerous). Laboratory examination can also identify the type of cancer and may be used to evaluate the chance that cancer has spread to other parts of the body. Besides being used for cancer diagnosis, a biopsy procedure can also be done to identify the causes of inflammations and infections.

Preparation

The patient's preparation will depend on the specific biopsy procedure that is being done. For an open biopsy that requires general anesthesia, patients will need to stop eating and drinking hours before the procedure. For a colonoscopy and possible colon biopsy, laxatives and enemas will be prescribed in addition to diet changes.

The Procedure

In a *skin or muscle biopsy,* the area to be biopsied is first numbed with a local anesthetic and thoroughly cleaned. A small piece of tissue is removed with a scalpel, and the small wound is sutured.

In a *needle biopsy,* the biopsy area is numbed and cleaned, and a sterile hollow needle is inserted through the skin to take the sample.

In an *endoscopic biopsy,* a forceps attachment at the end of the endoscope is used to snip off a small tissue sample.

In an *open biopsy* under general anesthesia, a sample of tissue can be cut directly from an organ that has been exposed with a surgical incision.

While some biopsy results are available rather quickly, others may take several days.

Risks

Most small biopsy procedures are very safe and carry only a small risk of bleeding or infection at the biopsy site. For larger open biopsies, there are additional risks that accompany general anesthesia and larger surgical procedures.

When to Call the Doctor

Patients should consult a doctor after a biopsy in the event of a fever or pain, swelling, redness, pus, or bleeding at the biopsy site or at the site of the surgical wound.

biotherapy   Treatment to stimulate or restore the ability of the immune system to fight infection and disease, and to lessen side effects caused by some cancer treatments. Biotherapy is also known as IMMUNOTHERAPY, BIOLOGICAL THERAPY, or BIOLOGICAL RESPONSE MODIFIER (BRM) therapy.

birth control pills and cancer   There has been some concern in the past about the possible effect of oral contraceptive use on BREAST CANCER and CERVICAL CANCER risk. However, the National Institute of Child Health and Human Development Women's Contraceptive and Reproductive Experiences Study found that women who took oral contraceptives at some point in their lives are no more likely to develop breast cancer between the ages of 35 and 64 than are other women the same age. The study appeared in the June 27, 2002, issue of the *New England Journal of Medicine.* The women studied were members of the first generation of American women to use birth control pills. About 80 percent of U.S. women born since 1945 have used oral contraceptives.

In the study, researchers interviewed more than 9,200 Caucasian and African-American women between the ages of 35 and 64 living in Atlanta, Detroit, Philadelphia, Los Angeles, and Seattle. About half of the participants had recently been diagnosed with breast cancer, while the other half had not. The women were interviewed in person and asked a series of questions about their use of oral contraceptives and other hormones as well as their reproductive, health, and family issues.

Women who had used any type of oral contraceptive did not have a greater risk than other women of developing breast cancer. In addition, birth control pill use among women with a family history of breast cancer was not associated with a significantly increased breast cancer risk, nor was starting to use the pills at a young age. Results were generally similar across age and racial groups.

Studies of birth control pills and cancer were first started in the early 1970s, and a 1996 formal review of 54 smaller studies conducted over the past 25 years found a slightly increased risk of breast cancer in women who were current or recent users of oral contraceptives. Other previous studies had not found an increased risk of breast cancer among oral contraceptive users. Studies have consistently shown that using birth control pills reduces the risk of ovarian cancer, and there is some evidence that long-term use of birth control pills may increase the risk of cervical cancer. There is also some evidence that the pills may increase the risk of certain cancerous liver tumors.

Oral contraceptives first became available to American women in the early 1960s, when they quickly became the most popular form of birth control in the United States. However, experts were concerned about the role hormones play in a number of cancers, and how hormone-based birth control pills might contribute to their development.

Currently, two types of birth control pills are available in the United States. The most common contains two synthetic versions of natural female hormones (estrogen and progesterone) normally produced by the ovaries. The second type of pill available in the United States is called the minipill and contains only a progestogen. The minipill is less effective in preventing pregnancy than the combination pill, so it is prescribed less often.

bisphosphonates   A family of drugs (also called disphosphonates) used to treat dangerously high blood calcium levels caused by several cancers as well as to prevent bone fractures and pain when the cancer has spread to the bones.

See also BONE CANCER.

bladder cancer   The bladder is the hollow organ in the lower abdomen that stores urine, which passes from each kidney into the bladder through a tube called a ureter. Urine leaves the bladder through another tube, the urethra. Bladder cancer is the sixth most common cancer in the United States, excluding non-MELANOMA SKIN CANCERS. In 2002 there were about 56,500 new cases of bladder cancer diagnosed in the United States (about 41,500 in men and 15,000 in women). In 2002 there were also about 12,600 deaths from bladder cancer (about 8,600 men and 4,000 women).

The wall of the bladder is lined with cells called transitional cells and squamous cells. More than 90 percent of bladder cancers begin in the transitional cells, and this is called "transitional cell carcinoma." About 8 percent of bladder cancer patients have squamous cell carcinomas.

Cancer that occurs only in cells in the lining of the bladder is called superficial bladder cancer, or CARCINOMA IN SITU. After treatment, this type of bladder cancer often recurs as another superficial cancer in the bladder.

However, some cancer that begins as a superficial tumor may grow through the lining and into the muscular wall of the bladder, where it is known as *invasive* cancer. Invasive cancer may extend through the bladder wall and may grow into a nearby organ such as the uterus or vagina (in women) or the prostate gland (in men).

When bladder cancer spreads outside the bladder, cancer cells are often found in nearby lymph nodes. If the cancer has reached these nodes, cancer cells may have spread to other lymph nodes or other organs, such as the lungs, liver, or bones.

Cause

No one knows the exact causes of bladder cancer, but there are certain risk factors that increase a person's likelihood of developing this type of malignancy. The risk factors for bladder cancer include

- *Smoking.* The biggest risk factor for bladder cancer is smoking; cigarette smokers are two to three times more likely than nonsmokers to get bladder cancer. Pipe and cigar smokers are also at increased risk. Some of the carcinogens in tobacco smoke are absorbed from the lungs and get into the blood, where they are filtered by the kidneys and concentrated in the urine. These chemicals in the urine damage the cells that line the inside of the bladder, increasing the chance of cancer.

- *Age.* The chance of getting bladder cancer increases as people get older. People under 40 rarely get this disease.

- *Job.* Some types of jobs carry a higher risk of bladder cancer because of carcinogens in the workplace. Chemicals called aromatic amines (such as BENZIDINE and beta-naphthylamine), sometimes used in the dye industry, can cause bladder cancer. Workers in the rubber, chemical, and leather industries are at risk as well, as are hairdressers, machinists, metal workers, printers, painters, textile workers, and truck drivers.

- *Infections.* A parasitic worm called *Schistosoma hematobium,* which can migrate to the bladder, is linked to squamous cell carcinoma. Although this parasite is found mostly in Northern Africa, it does cause rare cases of bladder cancer in the United States among people who had the worm before moving to this country.

- *Chronic inflammation.* Urinary infections, kidney and bladder stones, and other causes of chronic bladder irritation have been linked with bladder cancer (especially squamous cell carcinoma of the bladder), but they do not necessarily cause bladder cancer.

- *Treatment with cyclophosphamide or arsenic.* These drugs, which are used to treat cancer and some other conditions, increase the risk of bladder cancer.

- *Race.* Caucasians get bladder cancer twice as often as African Americans and Hispanics; the lowest rates are among Asians.

- *Gender.* Men are two to three times more likely than women to get bladder cancer.

- *Family history.* People with family members who have bladder cancer are more likely to get the disease.

- *Personal history.* People who have had bladder cancer have an increased chance of getting the disease again.

- *Bladder birth defects.* In the fetus there is a connection between the navel and the bladder that normally disappears before birth. If part of this connection remains after birth, it could become cancerous and form an ADENOCARCINOMA. Cancer starting in this way is rare, causing less than one half of a percent of bladder cancers, but it represents about a third of the adenocarcinomas of the bladder. In another rare birth defect, called exstrophy, the skin, muscle, and connective tissue in front of the bladder fail to close completely, leaving a defect in the abdominal wall. This leaves the inside of the bladder exposed to chronic infection, which may eventually lead to formation of an adenocarcinoma of the bladder.

- *Aristocholia fangchi.* This Chinese herb is included in some dietary supplements and herbal remedies and was linked to bladder cancer (and kidney failure) among people who took it as part of an herbal weight-loss program. Experimental studies have shown that chemicals found in this herb can damage DNA and cause bladder cancer in rats.

While studies have found that the ARTIFICIAL SWEETENER saccharin causes bladder cancer in animals, research has not found that saccharin causes cancer in people.

Symptoms

Common symptoms of bladder cancer include bloody urine, painful urination, and frequent urination (or feeling the urge to urinate without results). These are not definite signs of bladder cancer, since infections, benign tumors, bladder stones, or other problems also can cause such symptoms. Anyone with these symptoms should see a doctor for diagnosis and treatment as early as possible.

Diagnosis

If a patient has symptoms that suggest bladder cancer, the doctor may check general signs of health, order lab tests, including blood and urine tests, and conduct a physical exam that may include a rectal or vaginal exam. Other tests may include an *intravenous pyelogram* (IVP, also known as an intravenous urography), in which the doctor injects dye into a blood vessel. The dye then collects in the urine, making the kidney, ureters, and bladder show up on X-rays. *Retrograde pyelography,* like the IVP, uses special dye to outline the lining of the bladder, ureters, and kidneys on X-rays. The difference is that in retrograde pyelography the dye is injected through a urinary catheter rather than into a vein.

In a *cystoscopy,* the doctor uses a thin, lighted tube called a cystoscope to look directly into the bladder and sometimes to remove samples of tissue. The patient may need anesthesia for this procedure. For a small number of patients, the doctor removes the entire cancerous area during the biopsy.

A *CT* or *MRI scan* of the pelvis provides information about whether the cancer has spread to tissues next to the bladder, to nearby lymph nodes in the pelvis, or to distant organs. These scans are used only if spread beyond the bladder is suspected.

An *ultrasound test* can be useful in determining the size of a bladder cancer and whether it has spread beyond the bladder.

Staging

If bladder cancer is diagnosed, the doctor needs to know the extent of the disease to plan the best treatment. "Staging" is a careful attempt to find out whether the cancer has invaded the bladder's muscle wall or spread to other parts of the body. The doctor may determine the stage of bladder cancer at the time of diagnosis, or the patient may need more tests, such as scans, ultrasound, intravenous pyelogram, BONE SCAN, or a chest X-ray. Sometimes staging is not complete until the patient has surgery.

The stages of the disease include

Stage 0: Cancer cells are found only on the surface of the inner lining of the bladder. This is called superficial cancer or carcinoma in situ.

Stage I: Cancer cells are found deep in the inner lining of the bladder but have not spread into the bladder muscle.

Stage II: Cancer cells have spread into the muscle of the bladder.

Stage III: The cancer cells have spread through the muscular wall of the bladder to the layer of tissue surrounding the bladder. The cancer cells may have spread to the prostate (in men) or to the uterus or vagina (in women).

Stage IV: The cancer extends to the wall of the abdomen or to the wall of the pelvis. The cancer cells may have spread to lymph nodes and other parts of the body far away from the bladder, such as the lungs. When cancer spreads to another part of the body, the new tumor has the same kind of abnormal cells and the same name as the primary tumor. For example, if bladder cancer spreads to the lungs, the cancer cells in the lungs are actually bladder cancer cells. The disease is metastatic bladder cancer, not lung cancer, and it is treated as bladder cancer, not as lung cancer.

Treatment

People with bladder cancer may have any combination of the following: surgery, RADIATION THERAPY, CHEMOTHERAPY, or BIOLOGICAL THERAPY. Surgery is a common treatment for bladder cancer, but the type of surgery depends on the tumor's stage and grade.

Transurethral resection (TUR) In this method, the doctor can treat early (superficial) bladder cancer by inserting a cystoscope into the bladder through the urethra and removing the cancer, burning away any remaining cancer cells with an electric current. The patient may need to be in the hospital and may need anesthesia. For a few days after TUR, patients may have some blood in their urine and difficulty or pain when urinating. After TUR, patients may also have chemotherapy or biological therapy.

Radical cystectomy This technique is used for invasive bladder cancer, or if a superficial cancer involves a large part of the bladder. Radical cystectomy involves the removal of the entire bladder, the nearby lymph nodes, part of the urethra, and any nearby organs that may contain cancer cells. In men, the nearby organs that are removed are the prostate, seminal vesicles, and part of the vas deferens. In women, the uterus, ovaries, fallopian tubes, and part of the vagina are removed.

When the entire bladder is removed, the patient needs a new way to store and pass urine. In one common method, the surgeon uses a piece of the person's small intestine to form a new tube through which urine can pass. The surgeon attaches one end of the tube to the ureters and connects the other end to a new opening in the wall of the abdomen, called a stoma. A flat bag, which is held in place with a special adhesive, fits over the stoma to collect urine. The operation to create the stoma is called a urostomy or an ostomy.

For some patients the doctor is able to use a part of the small intestine to make a storage pouch (called a continent reservoir) inside the body. Urine collects in the pouch instead of going into a bag; the pouch is connected to the urethra or to a stoma. If the surgeon connects the pouch to a stoma, the patient uses a catheter to drain the urine.

Because in a radical cystectomy the surgeon removes a woman's uterus and ovaries, menopause occurs at once. Hot flashes and other symptoms of menopause caused by surgery may be more severe than those caused by natural menopause.

In the past, nearly all men were impotent after radical cystectomy, but improvements in surgery have made it possible for some men to avoid this problem. Men who have had their prostate gland and seminal vesicles removed no longer produce semen, so they have dry orgasms. Men who wish to father children may consider sperm banking before surgery or sperm retrieval later on.

Segmental cystectomy   In this procedure, used when a patient has a low-grade cancer that has invaded the bladder wall in just one area, the doctor removes only part of the bladder.

Sometimes, when the cancer has spread outside the bladder and cannot be completely removed, the surgeon removes the bladder but does not try to get rid of all the cancer, or the surgeon does not remove the bladder but makes another way for urine to leave the body. The goal of the surgery may be to relieve urinary blockage or other symptoms caused by the cancer.

Radiation therapy   This technique uses high-energy rays to kill cancer cells. A small number of patients may have radiation therapy before surgery to shrink a tumor; others may have radiation after surgery to kill cancer cells that may remain in the area. Sometimes patients who cannot have surgery have radiation therapy instead.

Doctors use both internal and external types of radiation therapy to treat bladder cancer. In radiation administered from a machine outside the body (*external radiation*), most patients are treated five days a week for five to seven weeks. Treatment may be shorter when external radiation is given along with radiation implants (*internal radiation*).

Internal radiation requires hospitalization for several days. In this technique, the doctor places a small container of a radioactive substance into the bladder through the urethra or through an incision in the abdomen. To protect others from radiation exposure, patients may not be able to have visitors or may have visitors for only a short period of time while the implant is in place. Once the implant is removed, no radioactivity is left in the body. Some patients with bladder cancer receive both kinds of radiation therapy.

The side effects of radiation therapy depend on the treatment dose and the part of the body that is treated. Patients are likely to become very tired during therapy, especially in the later weeks of treatment. External radiation may permanently darken the skin in the treated area, or make it temporarily red, dry, tender, and itchy. Patients often temporarily lose hair in the treated area as well.

In addition, radiation therapy to the abdomen may cause nausea, vomiting, diarrhea, or urinary discomfort, and it may temporarily compromise the immune system.

Radiation treatment for bladder cancer can also temporarily affect sexuality. Women may experience vaginal dryness, and men may have difficulty with erections.

Chemotherapy   This method of treatment uses drugs to kill cancer cells. Patients with superficial bladder cancer may have *intravesical chemotherapy* after the cancer is removed with TUR. With this technique, the doctor inserts a catheter through the urethra, instilling liquid drugs into the bladder, where they remain for several hours. Usually, the patient has this treatment once a week for several weeks, although the treatments may continue once or several times a month for up to a year.

If the cancer has deeply invaded the bladder or spread to LYMPH NODES or other organs, the doctor may give drugs through a vein (*intravenous chemotherapy*) in cycles with a recovery period after each treatment period. The patient may have chemotherapy alone or combined with surgery, radiation therapy, or both. Although chemotherapy is usually given on an outpatient basis, depending on which drugs are used and the patient's general health, a short hospital stay may be required.

Biological therapy Biological therapy (also called immunotherapy) uses the body's immune system to help prevent cancer from recurring, usually after TUR for superficial bladder cancer. The doctor may use intravesical biological therapy with BCG solution that contains live, weakened bacteria to stimulate the immune system to kill cancer cells. The solution is placed through a catheter into the bladder, where it remains for about two hours. BCG treatment is usually given once a week for six weeks.

BCG therapy can irritate the bladder, so that patients may feel an urgent need to urinate. Patients also may have pain, especially when urinating, and may experience fatigue, nausea, a low-grade fever, or chills.

Follow-up Care

Bladder cancer can return in the bladder or elsewhere in the body. If the bladder was not removed, the doctor will perform cystoscopy and remove any new superficial tumors that are found. Patients also may have urine tests to check for signs of cancer. Follow-up care also may include blood tests, X-rays, or other tests.

blast crisis (blast phase)   The phase of chronic myelogenous LEUKEMIA in which the number of immature, abnormal white blood cells (blasts) in the BONE MARROW and blood is extremely high.

blast phase   See BLAST CRISIS.

blood cancers   Cancer of the blood includes three major types: LYMPHOMA, LEUKEMIA, and MULTIPLE MYELOMA. These cancers are formed either in the BONE MARROW or the lymphatic tissues of the body, affecting the way the body produces blood and provides immunity. The risk of developing blood cancers usually increases with age, and men are more susceptible than women.

Responses to treatment and survival rates for each of these cancers vary a great deal. Overall survival rates for people with blood cancer have doubled in the past 30 years because of more effective radiation and CHEMOTHERAPY treatments: In 1960, only 4 percent of children diagnosed with leukemia survived, but today, 79 percent are expected to live if they receive the best treatment available. Nevertheless, leukemia remains the leading cause of death by disease in children.

In general, adults are more likely than children to get blood cancer, because the risk increases with age; about 106,200 Americans are diagnosed with one of the blood cancers and about 57,500 die of the disease each year. Lymphomas are the most common blood cancers, accounting for about 55 percent of new cases, with leukemia having 28 percent, and myeloma about 14 percent. Less common forms of blood cancers account for about 3 percent of cases.

Cause

The actual causes of blood cancer are still unknown. Scientists are trying to identify when and why the body starts producing abnormal cells and how those cells begin invading the body's blood system. As these questions are answered, the information is used to improve prevention and treatment options.

The three types of blood cancers all involve an uncontrolled growth of abnormal cells within the blood and bone marrow. Blood carries oxygen and nutrients to all organs of the body, helps in healing, and fights viruses, bacteria and other foreign material in the body. It is made up of

- *plasma*, the watery, yellowish fluid in which the blood cells are suspended and move through veins and arteries of the body
- *red blood cells*, which contain hemoglobin, a body protein that carries oxygen to body tissues
- *platelets*, the smallest cells, which are responsible for clotting
- *white blood cells* (leukocytes), which protect the body from disease and infection

There are five main types of white blood cells, including lymphocytes, that are produced in the lymph tissue (including the lymph glands, spleen, thymus, tonsils and bone marrow). Lymphomas arise from lymphocytes, which make up about 25 percent of all white blood cells. The number of lymphocytes circulating in the blood varies and can increase or decrease as the body fights infection.

Lymph nodes are part of the lymphatic system, a network of thin tubes similar to blood vessels that branch into all parts of the body. The major external lymph node clusters are found in the neck, armpit and groin. Lymph nodes become enlarged during disease or infection; although swollen lymph nodes often are not a sign of a serious problem, they can be a symptom of lymphoma. Leukemia and multiple myeloma may not result in swollen lymph nodes. Leukemia usually starts in the bone marrow, and myeloma originates from plasma cells, which are formed in bone marrow.

Prevention

Because the exact cause of these cancers has not been discovered, there are no specific prevention recommendations. However, it is a good idea to limit exposure to excessive radiation and hazardous chemicals. Studies show that benzene (found in unleaded gasoline), asbestos, and pesticides may increase the risk of some blood cancers. When coming in close physical contact with benzene or other hazardous chemicals, consumers should take precautions by wearing protective clothing and gloves.

Treatment

The cure rate for leukemias and lymphomas today is remarkable, considering that the prognosis of most blood cancers 30 years ago was poor. Still, for many people, remission is the best hope, although recurrences are not uncommon. Chemotherapy is the standard therapy; radiation therapy is used for localized disease or to shrink tumor bulk that is compressing a vital body structure.

Bone-marrow transplants are being performed more often in many parts of the country to treat lymphoma and leukemia. In this procedure, very high doses of chemotherapy or irradiation are given to kill the cancer cells. But because healthy cells in the bone marrow also die, the patient is then given an infusion of STEM CELLS from the bone marrow or peripheral blood. Bone-marrow transplants have tremendous risks, including death, and tend to be more successful in younger patients and when the disease is in an early stage.

Since bone-marrow transplant for blood cancers is a specialized procedure, a transplant candidate should look for a hospital that performs bone-marrow transplants regularly.

Newer treatments, such as BIOLOGICAL THERAPIES, are already being used routinely in combination with other therapies. Biological therapy uses special immune system cells and proteins to stimulate the body's immune system to kill cancer cells. Biological agents such as INTERFERONS, INTERLEUKINS, MONOCLONAL ANTIBODIES, tumor-necrosis factors and COLONY-STIMULATING FACTORS are natural substances found in the body that help alter the way the immune system reacts to cancer. Researchers now are able to create reproductions of some of these biological agents in laboratories. These reproductions imitate the natural immune agents, and are used to augment the anti-tumor immune response of the patient.

blood vessel cancer   See SARCOMA.

bone cancer   Tumors in the bone may be either malignant or (more commonly) benign. Both types of tumors may grow and compress healthy bone tissue and absorb or replace it with abnormal tissue, but benign tumors do not spread and are rarely life threatening.

Cancer that appears first in the bone is rare, affecting about 2,500 new patients each year in the United States. More commonly, the bones are the site of tumors that have spread from another organ, such as the breast, lung, or prostate.

There are several types of cancer that do begin in the bone: osteosarcoma, Ewing's sarcoma, and chondrosarcoma. Osteosarcoma is the most common type of bone cancer, which develops in new tissue in growing bones. Chondrosarcoma begins first in cartilage, and Ewing's sarcoma begins in immature nerve tissue in bone marrow. Osteosarcoma and Ewing's sarcoma tend to occur more frequently in children and adolescents, while chondrosarcoma occurs more often in adults.

Risk Factors

A number of factors may put a person at increased risk for getting bone cancer, which occurs more often in children and young adults (especially those who have had radiation or chemotherapy for other conditions). Adults with Paget's disease, a noncancerous condition characterized by abnormal development of new bone cells, may be at higher risk for osteosarcoma. A small number of bone cancers have genetic origins. Children with an inherited cancer of the eye are at a higher risk of developing osteosarcoma.

Symptoms

Pain is the most common symptom of bone cancer, but symptoms may vary depending on the location and size of the cancer. Tumors that occur in or near joints may cause swelling or tenderness in the affected area. Bone cancer can interfere with normal movements and can weaken the bones, occasionally leading to a fracture. Other symptoms may include fatigue, fever, weight loss, and anemia.

Diagnosis

In addition to a personal and family medical history and a complete medical exam, the doctor may suggest a blood test to determine the level of an enzyme called ALKALINE PHOSPHATASE. A large amount of alkaline phosphatase can be found in the blood when the cells that form bone tissue are very active, which occurs when children are growing, when a broken bone is mending, or when a tumor triggers the production of abnormal bone tissue. Because high levels of this enzyme can normally be found in growing children and adolescents, this test is not a completely reliable indicator of bone cancer.

X-rays can show the location, size, and shape of a bone tumor. If X-rays suggest that a tumor may be cancerous, the doctor may recommend special imaging tests such as a bone scan, a CT (or CAT) scan, an MRI, or an angiogram.

Either a needle or incisional BIOPSY can detect bone cancer. During a needle biopsy, the surgeon makes a small hole in the bone and removes a sample of tissue from the tumor with a needle-like instrument. In an incisional biopsy, the surgeon cuts into the tumor and removes a sample of tissue.

Treatment

Treatment options depend on the type, size, location, and stage of the cancer, as well as the person's age and general health. Surgery is often the primary treatment. Although amputation is sometimes necessary, pre- or post-operative CHEMOTHERAPY has often made it possible to spare the limb. When possible, surgeons avoid amputation by removing only the cancerous section of the bone and replacing it with a prosthesis.

Chemotherapy and radiation, alone or in combination, may also be used. Because of the tendency for Ewing's sarcoma to spread rapidly, multidrug chemotherapy is often used, in addition to RADIATION THERAPY or surgery on the primary tumor.

bone marrow   The soft, spongy material found inside bones that contains immature cells called STEM CELLS, which produce all of the body's red blood cells and platelets, and most of the white blood cells. Stem cells produce

- white blood cells (leukocytes), which fight infection;
- red blood cells (erythrocytes), which carry oxygen to organs and tissues;
- platelets (thrombocytes), which enable the blood to clot.

Bone marrow plays an important part in the development, diagnosis, and treatment of cancer. In LEUKEMIA, a type of cancer in which the production of white blood cells in bone marrow spirals out of control, these cells infiltrate vital organs and glands, making them enlarge or malfunction. The cells can also crowd out healthy cells, preventing the bone marrow from producing enough normal cells.

In addition to leukemia, many other kinds of cancer can be diagnosed by checking the bone marrow for malignant cells in a test called a BONE MARROW ASPIRATION and BIOPSY.

bone marrow aspiration   A test in which a needle is inserted into the bone to obtain a sample of BONE MARROW, the spongy substance on the inside of the bone in which blood cells are manufactured. During the test, a hollow needle is inserted through the subcutaneous tissue and bone to withdraw about a half teaspoon of marrow with a syringe. After the test, there will be some pain or soreness at the site. The sample will be analyzed for iron stores, red blood cell and white blood cell production and maturation, and number of megakary-ocytes (cells that produce platelets).

A bone marrow aspiration is used to determine the cause of an abnormal blood test, to confirm the diagnosis of anemia, LEUKEMIA, leukocytosis (an increase in white blood cells), MULTIPLE MYELOMA, LEUKOPENIA (a reduction of white blood cells), or THROMBOCYTOPENIA (a reduction of platelets in the blood), or to evaluate response to cancer treatments.

bone marrow biopsy   This procedure is similar to BONE MARROW ASPIRATION but uses a larger-bore needle to take a core of bone and marrow to be analyzed. This type of BIOPSY adds additional information to a standard bone marrow aspiration, including the architecture of the bone and the presence of cancer cells that have spread from other parts of the body.

bone marrow metastases   Cancer that has spread from the original tumor to the BONE MARROW.

bone marrow transplants   Procedures in which the patient's cancerous bone marrow is replaced with normal marrow. In a similar fashion, doctors also can transplant a patient's STEM CELLS. Bone marrow transplants are used as part of CHEMOTHERAPY or RADIATION THERAPY treatments; in this procedure, a patient's marrow is removed and stored so that a much higher dose of drugs or radiation can be given, which would otherwise have damaged the bone marrow. After the treatment is finished, the healthy marrow is then transplanted back by IV infusion. The bone marrow cells circulate through the bloodstream and find the way to the bone marrow.

Transplants may be autologous (an individual's own marrow, saved before treatment, is reintroduced), allogeneic (marrow donated by someone else is used), or syngeneic (marrow donated by an identical twin).

Bone marrow transplants are used to treat several types of cancer, including LEUKEMIA and LYMPHOMA, MULTIPLE MYELOMA, and childhood BRAIN CANCER and neuroblastoma. In addition, researchers are evaluating the effectiveness of bone marrow transplants for the treatment of various other types of cancer, including KIDNEY CANCER and cancers of the breast and ovary.

bone scan   An imaging technique that uses radiation to create images of the entire skeleton (or a portion of it) on a computer screen or film, identifying areas of bone (called "hot spots") where the cells are unusually active, either breaking down or repairing tissue. Having hot spots does not necessarily mean that there is cancer in a bone; bone can break down and repair itself for other reasons, such as in infections or arthritis.

A bone scan can be done to look at a particular joint or bone. In cancer diagnosis, it is more usual to scan the whole body. During the test, a small amount of radioactive material is injected into a blood vessel and travels through the bloodstream; it collects in the bones and is detected by a scanner.

boron neutron capture therapy   A type of RADIATION THERAPY in which the patient is given an intravenous infusion containing the element boron, which concentrates in the tumor cells. The person then receives radiation therapy with atomic particles called neutrons from a small research nuclear reactor. The radiation is absorbed by the boron, killing the tumor cells without harming normal cells. This type of treatment was first proposed in 1936, and although results have not been promising, there is still some research interest in this method.

bowel cancer   See COLORECTAL CANCER.

Bowen's disease   A precancerous condition, also called squamous cell cancer in situ, characterized by a scaling, reddish-pink, slightly raised growth (usually on the face or hands). The disease is more often found among men with fair skin; chronic sun exposure is the primary cause. About a third of patients have many lesions.

Squamous cell cancers that occur as a result of Bowen's disease are usually more aggressive than those caused by ACTINIC KERATOSES. It is not unusual for a cancer that develops from Bowen's disease to spread to the LYMPH NODES.

Some studies suggest that patients with Bowen's disease may develop other premalignant and malignant tumors, not directly linked to the squamous cell carcinoma such as actinic keratoses, BASAL CELL CARCINOMA, adnexal carcinoma (OVARIAN CANCER), PROSTATE CANCER, LUNG CANCER, and ANAL CANCER.

Treatment

The condition is treated by surgically removing the diseased patch of skin, or destroying it by freezing or cauterization. Once removed, these skin conditions do not return.

brachytherapy A procedure in which radioactive material sealed in needles, seeds, wires, or catheters is placed directly into or near a malignant tumor. The procedure is also called internal radiation, implant radiation, or interstitial radiation therapy. In another version of this treatment, high-dose-rate remote brachytherapy (or high-dose-rate remote radiation therapy or remote brachytherapy), the radioactive source is removed between treatments.

The term *brachytherapy* is derived from the ancient Greek words for "short distance." Brachytherapy has been used for more than a century to treat CERVICAL CANCER, PROSTATE CANCER, ENDOMETRIAL CANCER, BREAST CANCER, and heart disease.

Henri Becquerel discovered natural radioactivity in 1896 when he noticed that uranium produced a black spot on photographic plates that had not been exposed to sunlight. Two years later, Marie and Pierre Curie, working in Becquerel's laboratory, extracted polonium from a ton of uranium ore. Later in the same year, they extracted radium. In 1901 Pierre Curie came up with the idea of inserting a small radium tube into a tumor, which signaled the birth of brachytherapy. Two years later, Alexander Graham Bell made a similar suggestion (completely independently) in a letter to the editor of *Archives Roentgen Ray*. With these early experiences, scientists found that inserting radioactive materials into tumors caused cancers to shrink.

In the early 20th century, major brachytherapy work was done at the Curie Institute in Paris and at Memorial Hospital in New York. The advent of high-voltage teletherapy for deeper tumors and the problems associated with radiation exposure from high-energy radionuclides led to a decline in the use of brachytherapy toward the middle of the last century. However, over the past 30 years, scientists have again become interested in the use of brachytherapy.

The discovery of man-made radioisotopes and remote AFTER LOADING techniques has reduced radiation exposure hazards. In addition, newer types of imaging scans (CT scan, MRI, ultrasound) and sophisticated computers have made it easier to position the radiation for the best doses.

Brachytherapy has been proven to be effective and safe, and it provides an alternative to surgical removal of the prostate, breast, or cervix—while reducing the risk of certain long-term side effects.

There are two different kinds of brachytherapy: permanent, in which the seeds remain inside of the body and gradually decay, and temporary, in which the seeds are placed inside of the body and are later removed. Prostate cancer is treated with permanent brachytherapy, while temporary implants are used with many gynecologic cancers.

There are several different types of seeds that are used in brachytherapy:

- *Palladium seeds* (Pd-103) produce radiation more rapidly and over a shorter period of time. Some researchers think that palladium seeds are best suited to treat faster growing, more aggressive tumors.
- *Iodine seeds* (I-125) are usually recommended for use in the treatment of slow-growing tumors.
- *Echogenic seeds* have a special feature that helps the doctor place them within cancerous tissue.

Even though very sensitive Geiger counters could detect radiation in the body of someone with radioactive seeds, the person would not be considered radioactive. Despite the very low risk, some doctors recommend that close contact with pregnant women and small children be avoided for some period of time after the initial procedure.

See also the AMERICAN BRACHYTHERAPY SOCIETY.

BRAF gene A gene popularly known as the "MELANOMA gene" that—when mutated—appears to cause many cases of malignant melanoma and several other types of cancer. The BRAF gene is one of a chain of genes that must all be switched on to enable a cell to grow and divide. A mutation in the BRAF gene causes it to remain in the "on" position all the time, causing cells to keep dividing and multiplying. The mutation is not inherited; rather, it appears to be a spontaneous event possibly caused by overexposure to ultraviolet rays from the Sun.

A recent study of BRAF mutations found the abnormal gene in 69 percent of papillary THYROID CANCER cases and in a small number of LUNG CANCER and HEAD AND NECK CANCER cases. In the past, other studies also have linked the abnormal gene with OVARIAN CANCER and SARCOMA.

brain cancer A complex group of diseases that strike more than 100,000 Americans annually either with a primary or metastatic brain tumor. A patient's symptoms, outlook for survival, and treatment depend on the precise location of the tumor. Brain cancer may cause severe symptoms, and the cure rate for many types of tumor is low.

The overall incidence of brain and central nervous system cancers began rising in 1973 and continued to increase until 1985, primarily among people over age 70. However, since 1985 the incidence of these cancers has stabilized, and in the last several years the incidence has decreased slightly.

Brain tumors are the second leading cause of cancer death in children under age 15 and in young adults up to age 34. Brain tumors are also the second fastest-growing cause of cancer death among those over age 65, and unlike the first and third fastest growing causes (LUNG CANCER and MELANOMA), there is no way to reduce the risk.

During 2002, 17,000 primary malignant tumors of the brain or spinal cord (9,600 in men and 7,400 in women) were diagnosed in the United States; about 13,100 people will die from these tumors. This type of cancer accounts for approximately 1.4 percent of all cancers and 2.4 percent of all cancer-related deaths.

Benign Tumors

A malignant tumor is life threatening because it consists of cancer cells growing out of control, but a benign tumor in the brain may also be life threatening because of its location. Although benign tumors are not particularly harmful in most parts of the body, the brain is housed within the rigid confines of the skull, so any abnormal growth can place pressure on sensitive tissues and impair functions.

Any tumor located near vital brain structures can seriously threaten health. For example, a benign tumor growing next to an important blood vessel in the brain does not have to grow very large before it can block blood flow. A benign tumor deep inside the brain may be hard to remove because of the risk of damaging vital brain centers. Because of their location, brain tumors are difficult to treat, and the cure rate for most is significantly lower than that for other types of cancer.

Primary vs. Metastatic Brain Tumors

Primary brain tumors originate within the brain, and about 44 percent of them are benign. Metastatic (secondary) brain tumors appear in the brain after spreading from other parts of the body. These secondary brain tumors are a common complication of cancer elsewhere in the body, and the incidence may be increasing. The most common sources of brain metastases are melanoma and lung, breast, colon, and kidney cancers.

An important difference between tumors that began in the brain and those that spread to the brain from other locations lies with their continuing potential to spread. While malignant tumors from elsewhere in the body often spread to many sites and keep on spreading, malignant brain tumors that originate in the brain rarely spread outside the central nervous system.

Risk Factors

Most brain tumors are not associated with any risk factors, and they seem to occur for no apparent reason. However, there are a few risk factors associated with brain tumors, including radiation, immune system problems, and family history of certain types of cancer. Environmental factors such as exposure to vinyl chloride (an odorless gas used in the manufacturing of plastics), aspartame, or electromagnetic fields from cellular telephones or high-tension wires have been suggested as risk factors. However, most researchers have not found conclusive evidence that clearly implicates any of these factors.

Radiation Most radiation-related brain tumors are caused by radiation to the head given for the treatment of other cancers.

Immune system disorders People with a weakened immune system have an increased risk of developing LYMPHOMAS of the brain. A weak immune system may occur as a congenital disorder, as a side effect of CHEMOTHERAPY treatment for other cancers or to prevent transplant rejections, or as a result of AIDS.

Family history Rarely, some types of brain tumors seem to occur over and over in some families. In general, patients with familial cancer syndromes have many tumors that appear during childhood. Some of these families have well-known tumor-causing disorders, such as

- *Neurofibromatosis type 2.* This inherited condition is associated with schwannomas of both hearing nerves, multiple meningiomas, or spinal cord ependymomas.

- *Tuberous sclerosis.* This inherited condition may cause noninfiltrating subependymal giant cell astrocytomas in addition to benign tumors of the skin, heart, or kidneys.

- *Von Hippel-Lindau disease.* This condition is associated with an inherited tendency to develop hemangioblastomas in the cerebellum as well as other cancers.

General Symptoms

Tumors in different parts of the brain will disrupt different functions and therefore cause different symptoms that are not unique to brain cancer—they would be caused by any disease involving that particular location within the brain.

The following symptoms immediately suggest the possibility of a brain tumor:

- a new seizure in an adult
- gradual loss of movement or sensation in an arm or leg
- unsteadiness or imbalance, especially if it is associated with headache
- loss of vision in one or both eyes, especially if it is more peripheral vision loss
- double vision, especially if it is associated with headache

- hearing loss with or without dizziness
- speech difficulty of gradual onset

While a headache is probably the most common symptom of a brain tumor, most people with headache (even persistent or severe headache) do not have a tumor. However, some kinds of headache do suggest a tumor:

- steady headache that is worse in the morning
- persistent headache with nausea or vomiting
- headache accompanied by double vision, weakness, or numbness

Cerebral hemisphere tumors Common symptoms of these tumors include seizures, difficulty with speech or language, a change of mood (such as depression or sadness), personality change, or changes in hearing, sight, or sensations. There may be weakness or paralysis on the side of the body opposite from where the tumor is located in the brain (because the left side of the brain controls the right side of the body and vice versa).

Basal ganglia Because this part of the brain controls muscle movements, a tumor here typically causes abnormal movements or abnormal body positioning.

Cerebellum The cerebellum controls coordination of movement, so tumors in this area may cause lack of coordination in walking, problems with fine motor coordination, and changes in speech rhythm.

Brain stem This part of the brain controls some of the most basic and vital operations in the body, including breathing and heartbeat. This area also controls muscles and sensations and is where most of the cranial nerves begin. Tumors in this part of the brain may cause weakness, stiff muscles, or problems with sensation, hearing, facial movement, and swallowing. Double vision and poor coordination are common early symptoms of brain-stem tumors. Because the brain stem is such an essential part of life, it is impossible to surgically remove tumors from it.

Cranial nerves Tumors that begin in the cranial nerves can affect vision, hearing, or facial sensations. The most common brain tumor in this category is the acoustic neuroma, which grows on the acoustic, or hearing, nerve and causes loss of hearing in one ear. Tumors may cause visual loss if they affect the optic nerve, facial paralysis if they affect the facial nerve, or facial pain if they affect the trigeminal nerve.

Diagnosis

An early diagnosis is critical for the successful treatment of a brain tumor. When a doctor suspects a brain tumor because of a patient's medical history and symptoms, there are a number of specialized tests and techniques that can confirm the diagnosis.

The first test is often a traditional neurological exam, which checks the eyes, reflexes, hearing, sensation, movement, balance, and coordination.

Next a doctor will use special imaging techniques and lab tests to detect a tumor and pinpoint its location and type. Scans include CT or MRI scan. Positron emission tomography (PET) scans provide a picture of brain activity rather than structure. Some scientists believe that PET scans offer important diagnostic clues, especially for recurrent brain tumors. Scientists are also examining whether PET can help physicians tell the difference between benign and malignant tumors before performing a biopsy or surgery. Similar results can be obtained with SPECT (single photon emission computed tomography) or functional MRI.

The final step in confirming the diagnosis of a brain tumor is a biopsy, in which a small sample of tissue is taken from the suspected tumor and is examined in a lab.

Tumor Grade

Tumor grade indicates the degree of malignancy and is based on the appearance of the tumor cells under the microscope. Grading a tumor is an attempt to predict a tumor's growth rate and tendency to spread, which can help doctors determine both the prognosis and treatment.

Types of Brain Tumor

Brain tumors of adults and children often form in different areas and from different cell types, and may have a different prognosis and treatments. There are many different kinds of tumors that can be found in brain tissue, including:

- chordomas
- choroid plexus papillomas
- craniopharyngiomas
- ependymoma
- pineal tumors, including the gliomas (astrocytomas, ependymomas, oligodendrogliomas, ganglioneuromas, mixed gliomas, brain-stem gliomas, and optic nerve gliomas), germ cell tumors, and neuroectodermal tumors (including medulloblastomas, neuroblastomas, pineoblastomas, medulloepitheliomas, ependymoblastomas, and polar spongioblastomas)
- meningiomas
- pituitary adenomas
- schwannomas
- vascular tumors (including hemangiosarcomas)

Chordomas Chordomas, which are more common in people in their 20s and 30s, develop from remnants of the flexible spine-like structure that forms and dissolves early in fetal development and is later replaced by the spinal cord. The tumors start in the bone at the back of the skull or at the lower end of the spinal cord. Although these tumors are often slow growing, they can recur after treatment many times over 10 to 20 years. They usually do not spread or metastasize to other organs and are usually treated with a combination of surgery and radiation.

Choroid plexus papilloma This rare, benign tumor appears most often in children before age 12. It makes up about 4 percent of all primary brain tumors in this age group. Choroid plexus tissue is located within the ventricles and produces cerebrospinal fluid. Choroid plexus papillomas grow slowly and eventually block the flow of cerebrospinal fluid, leading to hydrocephalus and increased pressure within the skull. The treatment of choice is surgery; tumor removal cures hydrocephalus in half of the patients. The remaining patients require a shunt in addition to tumor removal.

Choroid plexus carcinoma, the rare malignant and inoperable form of this tumor, may be treated with radiation.

Craniopharyngiomas These brain tumors usually affect infants and children. Although generally categorized as benign, they may be considered malignant because they can damage the hypothalamus, the area of the brain that controls body temperature, hunger, and thirst. Like chordomas, these tumors develop from cells left over from early fetal development. Craniopharyngiomas are often located near the brain's pituitary gland.

Treatment for these tumors usually includes surgery; sometimes radiation therapy is used.

Pineal Region Tumors

The pineal gland is a small structure located deep within the brain between the cerebral hemispheres. It produces hormones, including melatonin, which responds to changes in light. Tumors in the pineal gland itself account for about 1 percent of all brain tumors.

When possible, doctors will begin treatment with surgery or perform a biopsy to confirm the tumor type, and may also recommend radiation or chemotherapy, or both. The three most common types of pineal gland tumors are gliomas, germ cell tumors, and primitive neuroectodermal tumors.

Gliomas About half of all primary brain tumors are gliomas (tumors that grow from glial cells). There are three types of glial cells (astrocytes, oligodendrocytes, and ependymal cells). Normal glial cells grow and divide very slowly; most brain and spinal cord tumors develop from these slow-growing cells.

Within the brain, gliomas usually are found in the cerebral hemispheres, but they also may strike other areas, especially the optic nerve, the brain stem, and (particularly among children) the cerebellum.

Gliomas are classified into several groups because there are different kinds of glial cells: astrocytomas, ependymomas, oligodendrogliomas, ganglioneuromas, mixed gliomas, brainstem gliomas, and optic nerve gliomas.

Astrocytoma is the most common type of glioma; it develops from star-shaped glial cells called astrocytes. Astrocytes help support and nourish neurons. When the brain is injured, astrocytes form scar tissue that helps repair the damage. Most astrocytomas cannot be cured because they spread throughout the surrounding normal brain tissue, and sometimes into the cerebrospinal fluid path-

ways. With only very rare exceptions, astrocytomas do not spread outside of the brain or spinal cord.

A few special types of astrocytoma have a particularly good prognosis, including noninfiltrating astrocytomas (juvenile pilocytic astrocytomas and subependymal giant cell astrocytomas).

Doctors will often assign grades to an astrocytoma after a biopsy, ranging from I to IV (the higher the grade, the more malignant). The grade is determined by how closely cells are packed together within the tumor, how abnormal the cells are, how many of the cells are dividing or proliferating, whether blood vessels are growing near the tumor, and whether some cancer cells have spontaneously degenerated.

Grade I and II (well-differentiated): These low-grade astrocytomas contain cells that are relatively normal and are less malignant than those in the other two grades. They grow relatively slowly and may sometimes be completely removed through surgery, but more often they spread into normal brain tissue and therefore cannot be surgically cured. After as much of the tumor as possible is removed surgically, radiation therapy is usually given. However, radiation is not as effective against low-grade astrocytomas as it is against more aggressive astrocytomas. In some cases radiation therapy may not be given or may be postponed until certain symptoms develop. Average survival time for patients with low-grade astrocytomas is approximately six to eight years. However, even very slow-growing astrocytomas are life threatening if they are inaccessible.

Grade III (anaplastic): These mid-grade tumors grow more rapidly than lower-grade astrocytomas and contain cells with some malignant traits. Surgery is used to treat anaplastic astrocytomas, but it is not a cure. After as much of the tumor as possible is removed surgically, radiation therapy is given, usually followed by chemotherapy (usually intravenous BCNU, the initials of the drugs most commonly used to treat tumors). Many other drugs and combinations of drugs have been studied, but none have been shown to produce better results. Various clinical trials offer promising but unproven new treatments. Average survival for patients with anaplastic astrocytomas is about three years.

Grade IV (glioblastoma multiforme): These tumors (sometimes called high-grade astrocytomas) grow rapidly, invade nearby tissue, and contain cells that are very malignant. After as much of the tumor as possible is surgically removed, radiation therapy is given, usually followed by chemotherapy (usually intravenous BCNU). Many other drugs and combinations of drugs have been studied, but none have been shown to produce better results. Various clinical trials offer promising but unproven new treatments. Chemotherapy may be used before, during, or after radiation. Glioblastoma multiforme are among the most common and devastating primary brain tumors in adults; average survival for patients with these tumors is about 12 to 18 months.

Ependymoma. This is a type of glioma that usually affects children and develops from cells that line the hollow cavities of the brain and the canal containing the spinal cord. Ependymal cells help form part of the pathway through which cerebrospinal fluid travels, so tumors in this area may block cerebrospinal fluid from leaving the ventricles, causing the ventricles to become very large (hydrocephalus). Unlike astrocytomas and oligodendrogliomas, ependymomas do not usually spread into normal brain tissue; about 85 percent are very slow growing. As a result, some ependymomas can be completely removed and cured by surgery and radiation therapy. Chemotherapy is sometimes used, especially for recurrent tumors.

Spinal cord ependymomas have the greatest chance of surgical cure. Ependymomas may spread along the cerebrospinal fluid pathways but do not spread outside the brain or spinal cord.

Oligodendrogliomas. These develop from glial cells called oligodendroglia that are responsible for producing myelin. Myelin surrounds and insulates axons of nerves in the brain and spinal cord. Cells of the oligodendroglia help neurons transmit electric signals through axons. Oligodendrogliomas develop within the brain's cerebral hemispheres and may spread along the cerebrospinal fluid pathways, but they rarely invade areas outside the brain or spinal cord. They represent about 5 percent of all gliomas and occur most often in young adults. A small number of patients with oligodendrogliomas, however, have survived for 30 or 40 years.

Doctors often treat these tumors with surgery followed by chemotherapy and radiation therapy, but the tumors spread much like astrocytomas and usually cannot be completely removed by surgery.

Ganglioneuromas. These are the rarest form of glioma and contain both glial cells and mature neurons. They grow relatively slowly and may occur in the brain or spinal cord. These tumors have a high cure rate with surgery alone, or surgery combined with radiation therapy.

Mixed gliomas. These contain more than one type of glial cell (usually astrocytes and other glial cell types). Treatment focuses on the most malignant cell type found within the tumor.

Brain-stem gliomas. These are named for their location at the base of the brain rather than the cells they contain and are most common in children and young adults. Surgery is not usually used to treat brain-stem gliomas because of their vulnerable location. Radiation therapy sometimes helps to reduce symptoms and improve survival by slowing tumor growth.

Optic nerve gliomas. These are found on the optic nerve and are particularly common in individuals who have neurofibromatosis. Treatment may include surgery, radiation, or chemotherapy.

Germ cell tumors These appear in the pineal area and develop from the cells normally found in the ovaries or testicles destined to become egg cells or sperm cells (germ cells). During embryonic and fetal development, germ cells may not migrate properly, so that they move into abnormal locations such as the brain. There they may develop into germ cell tumors, similar to those that can form in the ovaries or testicles.

The most common germ cell tumor in the brain is the GERMINOMA. Germ cell tumors of the nervous system are very rare in adults but occur more often during childhood.

Primitive neuroectodermal tumors (PNETs) These are extremely malignant brain tumors in the pineal area usually affecting children and young adults. Many scientists believe that these tumors grow from primitive cells left over from early development of the nervous system. PNETs usually grow rapidly and spread easily within the brain and spinal cord; rarely, they spread outside the central nervous system.

More than 25 percent of all childhood brain tumors are a type of PNET called a *medulloblastoma*. Other more rare PNETS include *neuroblastomas, pineoblastomas, medulloepitheliomas, ependymoblastomas,* and *polar spongioblastomas.* Because their malignant cells often spread in a scattered, patchy pattern, PNETs are difficult to remove completely through surgery. Doctors usually remove as much tumor as possible with surgery, then prescribe radiation and chemotherapy.

Meningiomas

These tumors are mostly benign and develop from the meninges—the thin membranes that cover the brain and the spinal cord. Meningiomas account for about 24 percent of all brain tumors and affect people of all ages, although they are most common in middle age. Meningiomas usually grow slowly, generally do not invade surrounding normal tissue, and rarely spread to other parts of the body. Still, they can cause symptoms and damage by pressing on the brain or spinal cord.

About 85 percent of these tumors are benign and can be cured with surgery, which is the preferred treatment for accessible meningiomas; this treatment is more successful for these tumors than for most tumor types.

However, some meningiomas grow dangerously close to vital structures within the brain and cannot be cured by surgery alone. Other meningiomas are malignant and may recur many times after surgery or occasionally even spread to other parts of the body.

Radiation therapy may control regrowth of meningiomas that cannot be completely removed, or those that recur after surgery. Chemotherapy or hormonal drugs are being studied in clinical trials, but they have no proven benefit. Because of their slow growth, small meningiomas that cause no symptoms can usually be watched rather than treated (especially in the elderly).

Pituitary Adenomas

Benign tumors that affect the pituitary gland account for about 10 percent of all brain tumors. There are two types of these adenomas—secreting and nonsecreting. Secreting tumors release unusu-

ally high levels of pituitary hormones that trigger a group of symptoms, depending on which hormone is involved, including impotence, lack of menstrual periods, galactorrhea, abnormal body growth, Cushing's syndrome (excess cortisol production), or hyperthyroidism. Surgery or the drug bromocriptine is used to treat prolactin-secreting pituitary adenomas, while larger, nonsecreting adenomas are treated with surgery and radiation therapy, if needed.

Schwannomas

These usually benign tumors grow from the Schwann cells that form a protective sheath around nerve fibers. One of the more common forms of schwannoma affects the eighth cranial nerve, which contains nerve cells important for balance and hearing. Facial paralysis may occur if the tumor involves the adjacent seventh nerve. Also known as vestibular schwannomas or acoustic neuromas, these tumors may grow on one or both sides of the brain and are potentially curable with stereotactic radiosurgery. For malignant schwannomas, radiation therapy is often given after surgery.

Vascular Tumors

These rare, benign tumors are found in the blood vessels of the brain and the spinal cord. The most common vascular tumor is the *hemangioblastoma,* which is linked in a small number of people to a genetic disorder called VON HIPPEL-LINDAU'S DISEASE. Hemangioblastomas do not usually spread, and surgery can cure the problem.

Lymphomas

These tumors tend to spread throughout the brain and may be found in many different areas. Brain lymphomas occur in 2 to 6 percent of people with advanced AIDS.

Because they are so invasive, they cannot be cured by surgery. Instead, radiation therapy to the entire brain followed by chemotherapy may help, particularly in people without AIDS. Brain lymphomas respond better to chemotherapy than do other brain tumors, and many different combinations of drugs appear to be effective. Corticosteroids also may help shrink the tumor. In people without AIDS, treatment with radiation and chemotherapy can produce long-lasting remissions, but the success rate for those with a weakened immune system is not as good. Although people with AIDS may respond to the treatment, (particularly radiation), their disease may be so advanced that they do not live long in any case.

Childhood Brain Tumors

Tumors that have spread to the brain from other locations are less common in children than are tumors that appear first in the brain (primary brain tumors). Children can get most of the same tumors as adults, but there are some special types of childhood astrocytomas that tend to have a particularly good prognosis, including noninfiltrating astrocytomas (juvenile pilocytic astrocytomas and subependymal giant cell astrocytomas). Juvenile pilocytic astrocytomas most commonly appear in the cerebellum, but they also may be found in the optic nerve or the hypothalamus. Subependymal giant cell astrocytomas occur in the brain's ventricles and are almost always associated with tuberous sclerosis (an inherited condition that may also cause epilepsy, mental retardation, and tumors of the skin and kidneys).

Certain tumors possibly of mixed glial and neuronal origin that occur in children and young adults (and rarely in older adults) also have a good prognosis. These include the pleomorphic xanthoastrocytoma and the dysembryoplastic neuroepithelial tumor. Although they appear malignant under the microscope, these tumors are relatively benign and most are cured by surgery alone.

The most common childhood tumor is the supratentorial astrocytoma (not involving the cerebellum, brain stem, or spinal cord); this makes up between 25 percent and 40 percent of all tumors that occur in childhood. Other childhood tumors between 10 percent and 20 percent include cerebellar astrocytomas, brain-stem glioma, and medulloblastoma. Ependymomas occur between five percent and 10 percent; craniopharyngiomas occur between six percent and nine percent, and pineal tumors occur between .5 percent and 2 percent. All other kinds of tumors make up between 12 percent and 14 percent.

Treatment

Brain tumors are difficult to treat. Although survival may be prolonged by treatment, most malignant brain tumors are not cured by surgery, radiation, or chemotherapy.

Surgery   Tumor removal is usually the first step in treating brain cancer. Some tumors may be cured by surgery or a combination of surgery and radiation therapy. These tumors include meningiomas, some ependymomas, ganglioglioneuromas, and cerebellar astrocytomas.

Tumors such as anaplastic astrocytomas and glioblastomas cannot be cured surgically because cells from the tumor spread too quickly into normal surrounding brain tissue. However, surgery can reduce the size of a tumor, increasing the effectiveness of radiation or chemotherapy. In addition, surgery may ease some symptoms caused by brain tumors, particularly those caused by mounting pressure within the skull.

Surgery is not very effective against some types of brain tumor, such as lymphomas.

Radiation therapy   Combining surgery and radiation therapy against brain tumors can be effective; most brain tumors that cannot be completely removed by surgery are treated with radiation to try to kill any remaining cancer cells. However, each treatment risks damaging surrounding normal brain tissue. Radiation may be given either from an external source or internally by placing radioactive material directly within the tumor (interstitial radiotherapy or BRACHYTHERAPY). Because high doses of radiation can damage normal brain tissue, the goal is to deliver the highest dose of radiation to the tumor with the lowest possible dose to normal surrounding brain areas. Techniques such as three-dimensional treatment planning (conformal radiation) and STEREOTACTIC RADIOSURGERY (with a GAMMA KNIFE or a linear accelerator) have been developed to spare normal tissue. At present, there is no evidence to indicate that these techniques are superior to standard external beam radiation therapy.

Because radiation is most effective against rapidly growing cells, high-grade (very aggressive) tumors tend to be more responsive to radiation than low-grade tumors. For example, glioblastomas and anaplastic astrocytomas respond well, and up to half of all medulloblastomas and almost all germinomas can be cured by radiation therapy. Unfortunately, this is the exception. Most brain tumors, including low-grade astrocytomas, oligo-dendrogliomas, and ependymomas, are not cured by radiation therapy.

Although radiation is more damaging to cancer cells than to normal cells, healthy brain tissue can be damaged by radiation. In a condition called "radiation necrosis," a large amount of dead tissue may accumulate where the irradiated tumor had been, months to many years after radiation is given. In most cases, the dead tissue includes both malignant and benign tissue. Although patients with radiation necrosis usually do better than patients whose tumor has recurred, radiation necrosis can occasionally be fatal. Even those patients who do not develop radiation necrosis may experience significant changes in brain function if large portions of the brain were treated. Symptoms, which include memory loss, diminished libido, or poor tolerance to cold, are usually much less severe than those caused by the tumor, but they can still have a negative affect on a patient's quality of life.

Chemotherapy　Chemotherapy treatment of brain tumors is only minimally successful, which is why these drugs are usually used only for very aggressive tumors. A "good" surgical result can still leave the patient with severe physical incapacity, and successful radiation therapy to the brain can have harmful long-term side effects. The drugs are often given together with, or after, radiation therapy. However, some types of brain cancer, such as lymphomas, respond very well to chemotherapy.

The oral chemotherapy drug Temodar (temozolomide), is an effective oral chemotherapy drug to be able to cross the blood-brain barrier. Unlike other organs, the brain has a barrier between the blood and the brain that prevents the entry of many drugs, including some chemotherapy drugs. This protects the brain from toxins but also interferes with beneficial substances aimed at killing tumors or other brain diseases. Malignant tumors usually disrupt the blood-brain barrier, but the disruption may not be complete. Consequently the amount of a chemotherapy drug given by mouth or by IV that reaches a brain tumor may be less than ideal. A drug that can cross the blood-brain barrier, thus, is much more effective in killing tumor cells.

In the Future

There are a variety of experimental treatment techniques that scientists are currently studying that could be used to treat brain tumors. These include boron neutron capture therapy, gene therapy, immune therapy, and unconventional chemotherapy.

Boron neutron capture therapy　In this experimental type of radiation therapy, a compound containing the element boron is injected into the patient's blood. This chemical compound concentrates selectively in the brain tumor, and the brain is then irradiated with neutrons. When a neutron hits a boron atom, a type of high-energy radiation is released that does not extend far into the surrounding normal brain tissue. The value of this approach remains to be determined.

Gene therapy　Some scientists are trying to manipulate genes to treat very aggressive gliomas. In this approach, a genetically modified virus that cannot reproduce or spread is injected into a brain tumor. The virus has been altered with a special gene that makes tumor cells susceptible to an antivirus drug. The antivirus drug is harmless to normal brain cells, but it kills any cancer cells that have been infected with the genetically altered virus. This treatment is still in the earliest stages of evaluation.

Immunotherapy　This technique uses monoclonal antibodies or immune modulators (such as INTERFERON) to treat brain tumors. The goal of immunotherapy is to stimulate the body's immune system to fight the brain tumor more effectively. Agents that open the blood-brain barrier are being combined with chemotherapy drugs that do not normally cross the blood-brain barrier. Some chemotherapeutic agents are implanted directly in the tumor in "wafers" saturated with the drug for slow release.

Unconventional chemotherapy drugs　In addition to developing and testing new chemotherapy drugs, many researchers are testing unconventional drugs not normally used for chemotherapy. For example, growth factor inhibitors prevent the effects of growth factors that tumors make to promote their own growth. Angiogenesis inhibitors prevent the formation of new blood vessels necessary to feed the tumor, and hypoxic cell sensitizers make tumor cells more sensitive to radiation.

See also BRAIN TUMOR SOCIETY; CHILDHOOD CANCERS.

brain-stem glioma   See BRAIN CANCER.

brain tumors   See BRAIN CANCER.

Brain Tumor Society   A nonprofit organization that provides information about brain tumors and related conditions for patients and their families. They offer a patient/family telephone network, educational publications, funding for research projects, and access to support groups for patients.

The society's goal is to find a cure for brain tumors and to improve the quality of life of brain tumor patients and their families. The group provides educational information and access to social support. It raises funds for carefully selected scientific research projects; works to improve clinical care; educates the medical community, patients, and families about brain tumors; raises public awareness; and facilitates early diagnosis and treatment. For contact information, see Appendix I.

BRCA1/BRCA2   The abbreviation for two genes (Breast Cancer 1 and Breast Cancer 2) that normally help to suppress cell growth. A person who inherits either gene in an altered form has a higher risk of getting BREAST CANCER, OVARIAN CANCER, FALLOPIAN TUBE CANCER, and possibly PROSTATE CANCER, LIVER CANCER, or COLORECTAL CANCER. Experts believe that the inherited alterations in the *BRCA1* and *BRCA2* genes are responsible for nearly all cases of familial ovarian cancer and about half of all cases of familial breast cancer.

The likelihood that breast and/or ovarian cancer is associated with *BRCA1* or *BRCA2* is highest in families with

- a history of multiple cases of breast cancer
- cases of both breast and ovarian cancer
- one or more family members with two primary cancers (original tumors at different sites)
- an Ashkenazi (Eastern European) Jewish background

However, not every woman in such families carries an alteration in *BRCA1* or *BRCA2*, and not every cancer in such families is linked to alterations in these genes.

Two new studies suggest that people who inherit *BRCA1* mutations are at an increased risk of not only breast and ovarian cancer but may be implicated in a number of other cancers as well, including prostate and colon cancer. However, the absolute magnitude of the increase in risk of these other cancers is small. Several studies have examined the association of *BRCA1* with other cancers, particularly prostate cancer and colon cancer, but the results have been mixed.

In a 2002 study, experts estimated cancer risk rates among 11,847 people from families that had a history of breast and/or ovarian cancer and had at least one member who was a *BRCA1* mutation carrier. The researchers found small but statistically significant increases in the risk of colon, liver, pancreatic, uterine, and cervical cancers among female *BRCA1* mutation carriers, compared with the general population. In male *BRCA1* mutation carriers, there was a slightly elevated risk of prostate cancer. However, this increase was seen only in men younger than age 65.

In the second study, researchers used a different method to estimate *BRCA1*-related cancer risks among 483 mutation carriers identified through a cancer risk counseling program. Some of the subjects had participated in the first study. Over their lifetimes, *BRCA1* mutation carriers had an estimated 73 percent risk of breast cancer and 41 percent risk of ovarian cancer, compared with risks of 13 percent and 2 percent, respectively, in the general population. In addition, mutation carriers had a small increase in risk of colon, pancreatic, and gastric cancers. Although the risk of fallopian tube cancer increased 120-fold, the authors point out that this cancer is extremely rare in the general population.

Cause

Genes are small pieces of DNA, the material that acts as a master blueprint for all the cells in the body. A person's genes determine such things as hair or eye color, height, skin color, and how chemical substances in the body are created. Any mistakes in a gene that interferes with its job can lead to disease.

The *BRCA1* and *BRCA2* genes produce a chemical substance that helps the body prevent cancer. Most women have two normal copies of both the *BRCA1* and *BRCA2* genes, both of which produce this cancer-preventing substance. However, some women have a genetic defect in one copy of their two *BRCA1* and *BRCA2* genes, which means they do not produce a normal amount of this cancer-fighting substance. These women are at very high risk of getting breast or ovarian cancer.

According to estimates of lifetime risk, about 13.2 percent (132 out of 1,000 individuals) of women in the general population will develop breast cancer, compared with estimates of 36 to 85 percent (360 to 850 out of 1,000) of women with altered *BRCA1* or *BRCA2* genes. This means that women with an altered *BRCA1* or *BRCA2* gene are three to seven times more likely to develop breast cancer than women without alterations in those genes. Lifetime risk estimates of ovarian cancer for women in the general population indicate that 1.7 percent (17 out of 1,000) will get ovarian cancer, compared with 16 to 60 percent (160 to 600 out of 1,000) of women with altered *BRCA1* or *BRCA2* genes.

People inherit one copy of each of their genes from their mothers and a second copy of each gene from their fathers. If one parent has a defective *BRCA1* or *BRCA2* gene, there is a 50 percent chance the child may inherit the defective copy, and a 50 percent chance the child may inherit the normal copy. If a person inherits a defective *BRCA1* or *BRCA2* gene, then each of that person's children likewise has a 50 percent chance of inheriting it.

Women with an inherited alteration in one of these genes have an increased risk of developing ovarian or breast cancers at a young age (before menopause) and often have multiple close family members with the disease. These women also may have a higher chance of developing colon cancer.

Men and BRCA Genes

Men with an altered *BRCA1* or *BRCA2* gene also have an increased risk of breast cancer (primarily if the alteration is in *BRCA2*), and possibly prostate cancer. Alterations in the *BRCA2* gene have also been associated with an increased risk of LYM-PHOMA, MELANOMA, and cancers of the pancreas, gallbladder, bile duct, and stomach in some men and women.

BRCA1 *vs.* BRCA2

Some evidence suggests that there are slight differences in patterns of cancer between people with *BRCA1* alterations and people with *BRCA2* alterations, and even between people with different alterations in the same gene. Studies suggest that the risk of breast and ovarian cancer is higher in those who inherit the *BRCA1* gene than in the *BRCA2* gene.

Another study found that alterations in a certain part of the *BRCA2* gene were associated with a higher risk for ovarian cancer in women and a lower risk for prostate cancer in men than alterations in other areas of *BRCA2*.

Most research related to *BRCA1* and *BRCA2* has been done on large families with many affected individuals. Estimates of breast and ovarian cancer risk associated with *BRCA1* and *BRCA2* alterations have been calculated from studies of these families. Because family members share a proportion of their genes and, often, their environment, it is possible that the large number of cancer cases seen in these families may be partly due to other genetic or environmental factors. Therefore, risk estimates that are based on families with many affected members may not accurately reflect the levels of risk in the general population.

Racial Risk

Specific gene alterations have been identified in different ethnic groups. In Ashkenazi Jewish families, about 2.3 percent (23 out of 1,000 persons) have an altered *BRCA1* or *BRCA2* gene. This rate is about five times higher than that of the general population. Three particular alterations in *BRCA1* or *BRCA2* have been found to be most common in the Ashkenazi Jewish population. It is not known whether the increased frequency of these alterations is responsible for the increased risk of breast cancer in Jewish populations compared with non-Jewish populations.

Other ethnic and geographic populations, such as Norwegian, Dutch, and Icelandic people, also have a higher rate of certain genetic alterations in *BRCA1* and *BRCA2*. This information about genetic differences between ethnic groups may help health-care providers determine the most appropriate genetic test to select.

Genetic Testing

A simple blood test will reveal alterations in a person's *BRCA1* or *BRCA2* gene, but the testing is expensive (ranging from several hundred to several thousand dollars; not all insurance policies cover the test). To protect their privacy, some people may choose to pay for the test even when their insurer would be willing to cover the cost.

In a family with a history of breast and/or ovarian cancer, it is usually most informative to first test a family member who has the disease. If that person is found to have an altered *BRCA1* or *BRCA2* gene, the specific change is referred to as a "known mutation." Other family members can then be tested to see if they also carry that specific alteration. In this scenario, a positive test result indicates that a person has inherited a known mutation in *BRCA1* or *BRCA2* and has an increased risk of developing certain cancers. However, a positive result provides information only about a person's risk of developing cancer—it cannot tell whether cancer will actually develop.

Other genetic changes While it is possible to test for *BRCA 1* and *2* mutations, there are also other changes in these genes that are not well understood. One study found that 10 percent of women who underwent *BRCA1* and *BRCA2* testing had an ambiguous genetic change.

Because everyone has genetic alterations that do not increase the risk of disease, it is sometimes not known whether a specific change affects a person's risk of developing cancer. As more research is conducted and more people are tested for *BRCA1* or *BRCA2* alterations, scientists will learn more about these genetic alterations and cancer risk.

If the Test Is Positive

If a patient tests positive for altered *BRCA1* or *BRCA2* genes, there are several possible approaches to take. Careful monitoring for symptoms of cancer may lead to an earlier diagnosis, when treatment is more effective. Surveillance methods for breast cancer may include mammography and a clinical breast exam. For ovarian cancer, surveillance methods may include trans-

vaginal ultrasound, CA-125 blood testing, and clinical exams.

Preventive surgery Patients may also choose prophylactic surgery in which the doctor removes as much of the at-risk tissue as possible in order to reduce the chance of developing cancer. Preventive MASTECTOMY (removal of healthy breasts) and preventive SALPINGO-OOPHORECTOMY (removal of healthy fallopian tubes and ovaries) are no guarantee against developing these cancers. Because not all at-risk tissue can be removed by these procedures, some women have developed breast cancer, ovarian cancer, or a type of cancer similar to ovarian cancer even after prophylactic surgery.

Exercise Patients with a mutant gene also may choose to lower breast cancer risk by exercising regularly and limiting alcohol consumption. Research results on the benefits of these behaviors are based on studies in the general population; the effects of these actions in people with *BRCA1* or *BRCA2* alterations are not yet known.

Tamoxifen Some patients may consider preventive drugs such as tamoxifen, which was shown to lower the risk of invasive breast cancer by 49 percent in women at increased risk for developing the disease. However, few studies have been done to see whether tamoxifen is effective in women with a *BRCA1* or *BRCA2* mutation. One study found that tamoxifen reduced the incidence of breast cancer by 62 percent in women with alterations in *BRCA2,* but the results showed no reduction in breast cancer incidence with tamoxifen use among women with *BRCA1* alterations.

Genetic Discrimination

Genetic discrimination occurs when people are treated differently by their insurance company or employer because they have a gene alteration that increases their risk of a disease. People who undergo genetic testing to find out whether they have an alteration in their *BRCA1* or *BRCA2* gene may be at risk for genetic discrimination. A positive genetic test result may affect a person's health insurance coverage. For example, people with a positive result may be denied coverage for medical expenses related to their genetic condition, dropped from a current health plan, or unable to qualify for new insurance. Some insurers view the affected individual as a potential cancer patient whose medical treatment would be costly to the insurance company.

The Health Insurance Portability and Accountability Act (HIPAA) of 1996 provides some protection for people who have employer-based health insurance, because it prohibits group health plans from using genetic information as a basis for denying coverage if a person does not currently have a disease. However, the act does not prohibit employers from refusing to offer health coverage as part of their benefits, or prevent insurance companies from requesting genetic information.

In 2000 the Department of Health and Human Services released the HIPAA National Standards to Protect Patients' Personal Medical Records. This regulation covers medical records maintained by health-care providers, health plans, and health-care clearinghouses. Although the standards are not specific to genetic information, they provide the first comprehensive federal protection for the privacy of health information.

A person who tests positive for a *BRCA1* or *BRCA2* alteration may also experience genetic discrimination in the workplace if an employer learns about the test result. Although there are currently no federal laws specific to genetic nondiscrimination, some protection from discrimination by employers is offered through the Americans with Disabilities Act of 1990 (ADA). In 1995 the Equal Employment Opportunity Commission expanded the definition of "disabled" to include individuals who carry genes that put them at higher risk for genetic disorders. The extent of this protection, however, has not yet been tested in the courts. Several states also have laws that address genetic discrimination by employers and health insurance companies. The degree of discrimination protection varies from state to state. Therefore, the decisions that people make about genetic testing while living in one state may have repercussions in the future if they move to another area.

breakthrough pain   Intense increases in pain that occur with rapid onset even when painkillers are being used. Breakthrough pain can occur spontaneously or in relation to a specific activity.

breast cancer   One of the most common types of cancer among women in the United States, second only to SKIN CANCER. More than 180,000 women and more than 1,000 men are diagnosed with breast cancer in the United States each year. Scientists are making progress in their fight against breast cancer, developing better treatments, noting reduced death rates, and improving quality of life for patients.

Risk Factors

Although the exact causes of breast cancer are not known, studies show that the risk of breast cancer increases as a woman gets older. This disease is uncommon in women under age 35; most breast cancers occur in women over age 50, and the risk is especially high for women over age 60. Breast cancer also occurs more often in Caucasian women than African-American or Asian women. Research has shown that the following conditions increase a woman's chances of getting breast cancer:

- *Age.* The most important factor in the risk for breast cancer is a woman's age. The older a woman is, the greater her chance of getting breast cancer. A woman's chance of having breast cancer by age 30 is 1 out of 2,525; by age 40 it is 1 out of 217; by age 50, 1 out of 50; by age 60, 1 out of 24; by age 70, 1 out of 14; by age 80, it is 1 out of 10.

- *Personal history.* Women who have had breast cancer face an increased risk of getting breast cancer in their other breast.

- *Family history.* A woman's risk for developing breast cancer increases if her mother, sister, or daughter had breast cancer, especially at a young age.

- *Breast changes.* Atypical hyperplasia or lobular carcinoma in situ (LCIS) may increase a woman's risk for developing cancer.

- *Genetic alterations.* Changes in certain genes (*BRCA1*, *BRCA2*, and others) increase the risk of breast cancer.

- *Estrogen.* Evidence suggests that the longer a woman is exposed to estrogen (whether made by her body, taken as a drug, or delivered by a patch), the more likely she is to develop breast cancer. For example, risk is somewhat increased among women who began menstruation at an

early age (before age 12), experienced menopause late (after age 55), never had children or
had the first child after about age 30, or took hormone replacement therapy for long periods of
time. Each of these factors increases the amount
of time a woman's body is exposed to estrogen.

- *DES (diethylstilbestrol).* This synthetic form of
estrogen was used between the early 1940s and
1971. Women who took DES during pregnancy
to prevent certain complications are at a slightly
higher risk for breast cancer. This does not
appear to be the case for their daughters who
were exposed to DES before birth.

- *Breast density.* Breasts with a high proportion of
lobular and ductal tissue appear dense on mammograms. Breast cancers nearly always develop
in lobular or ductal tissue (not fatty tissue),
which is why cancer is more likely to occur in
breasts that with a lot of dense tissue than in
breasts with a lot of fatty tissue. In addition,
when breast tissue is dense, it is more difficult for
doctors to see abnormal areas on a mammogram.

- *Radiation therapy.* Women whose breasts were
exposed to radiation during RADIATION THERAPY
before age 30, especially those who were treated
with radiation for HODGKIN'S DISEASE, are at an
increased risk for developing breast cancer.
Studies show that the younger a woman was
when she received her treatment, the higher her
risk for developing breast cancer later in life.

- *Alcohol.* Studies suggest that women who have
three or more drinks per day have twice the
usual risk of developing breast cancer. One to
two (eight ounces) drinks a day is not associated
with an increased risk for breast cancer. Taking a
folate supplement can help lower the risk for
breast cancer if a woman drinks alcohol.

Most women who develop breast cancer have
none of the risk factors listed above, other than the
risk that comes with growing older. Scientists are
conducting research into the causes of breast cancer to learn more about risk factors and ways of
preventing this disease.

Prevention

Women should talk with their doctors about factors that can affect their chances of getting breast
cancer. Some risk factors, such as family history,
genetic patterns, and age of menstruation and
childbirths, cannot be altered. But some choices,
such as breast-feeding a child, eating a healthy
diet, getting plenty of exercise, taking preventive
drugs, and avoiding alcohol, may lower risk. In
addition, women at risk for inheriting a breast cancer gene can consider preventive surgery or more-
frequent mammograms and exams.

Exercise Recent studies suggest that regular
exercise may decrease the risk in younger women
and decrease the chance of cancer recurring in
women who have breast cancer. Other studies suggest that women with cancer who exercise live
longer than those who do not.

Diet Some evidence suggests a link between
diet and breast cancer. Ongoing studies are looking
at ways to prevent breast cancer through changes
in diet or with dietary supplements, but it is not yet
known whether specific dietary changes will actually prevent breast cancer.

BRCA genes Research also has led to the
identification of mutations in certain genes that
increase the risk of developing breast cancer.
Women with a strong family history of breast cancer may choose to have a blood test to see if they
have inherited a change in the *BRCA1* or *BRCA2*
gene. If they have inherited the gene, some
women choose preventive surgery or medications
to lower their risk, or more frequent mammograms
and exams.

Preventive drugs Scientists are looking for
drugs that may prevent the development of breast
cancer. In one large study, the drug tamoxifen
reduced the number of new cases of breast cancer
among women at an increased risk for the disease.
Doctors are now studying how another drug called
raloxifene compares to tamoxifen. This study is
called STAR (Study of Tamoxifen and Raloxifene).

Prophylactic mastectomy Some women at
very high risk for breast cancer choose to have one
or both breasts removed *before* disease occurs.
While this does not completely eliminate the risk
(some tiny bits of breast tissue always remain), it
does lower the risk considerably—to less than 5
percent. While some people consider this a controversial and radical step to avoid breast cancer,
some women who are at high risk believe it is a

worthwhile step. Insurance companies may or may not cover the surgery.

Symptoms

Early breast cancer usually does not cause pain or any other symptoms, but as it grows it can cause the following changes:

- a lump or thickening in or near the breast or in the underarm area
- a change in the size or shape of the breast
- nipple discharge or tenderness
- the nipple inverted into the breast
- ridges or pitting of the breast (the skin looks like the skin of an orange)
- a change in the way the skin of the breast, areola, or nipple looks or feels

Mammograms

Women should have regularly scheduled screening mammograms and clinical breast exams. A screening mammogram, which looks for breast changes in women who have no signs of breast cancer, is the best tool available for finding breast cancer early. Mammograms can often detect a breast lump before it can be felt, and a mammogram can show small deposits of calcium (called MICROCALCIFICATIONS) that may be an early sign of cancer.

The NATIONAL CANCER INSTITUTE recommends that women in their 40s or older get screening mammograms every one to two years. Women who are at increased risk for breast cancer should seek medical advice about when to begin having mammograms and how often to be screened. (For example, a doctor may recommend that a woman at increased risk begin screening before age 40 or change her screening intervals.) The following strong risk factors may be used to justify yearly screening in women between 40 and 50 and perhaps even regular mammography at an earlier age (30 to 35):

- previous breast cancer
- *BRCA1* or *BRCA2* mutations
- mother, sister, or daughter with a history of breast cancer

- atypical hyperplasia found on any previous breast biopsy
- at least 75 percent of breast classified as dense tissue on mammogram at age 45 to 49
- two or more previous breast biopsies, even if the results are benign

If an area of the breast looks suspicious on the screening mammogram, additional mammograms may be needed. Depending on the results, the doctor may advise the woman to have a biopsy. Although a mammogram is the best method for finding breast abnormalities early, it is not perfect. Physicians reading mammograms may miss some cancers that are present (false negative) or may raise an alarm about findings that then turn out not to be cancer (false positive). In addition, detecting a tumor early does not guarantee that a woman's life will be saved, because some fast-growing breast cancers may already have spread to other parts of the body before being detected. Nevertheless, studies show that mammograms reduce the risk of dying from breast cancer. Most doctors recommend that women in their 40s and older have mammograms regularly, every 1 to 2 years.

Some women perform monthly breast self-exams to check for any changes in their breasts. When doing a breast self-exam, it is important to remember that each woman's breasts are different, and that changes can occur because of aging, the menstrual cycle, pregnancy, menopause, or taking birth control pills or other hormones. It is normal for the breasts to feel a little lumpy and uneven, especially right before or during a menstrual period. Women over 40 should be aware that even if they examine their own breasts each month, they still need to have regularly scheduled screening mammograms and clinical breast exams performed by a health professional.

Diagnosis

Diagnosis of breast cancer includes a careful physical exam, personal and family medical history, together with one or more of the following breast exams:

- *Clinical breast exam.* The doctor should carefully feel the breast and the tissue around it and examine the size and texture of any lumps. Benign lumps often feel different from cancerous ones. A lump that moves easily is probably benign.

- *Mammography*
- *Ultrasonography.* Using high-frequency sound waves, ultrasounds can show whether a lump is a fluid-filled cyst (not cancer) or a solid mass (which may or may not be cancer). This exam may be used along with mammography.

Based on these exams, the doctor may decide that no further tests are needed and no treatment is necessary. In such cases, the doctor may need to check the woman regularly to watch for any changes. However, in some cases the doctor needs more information and will schedule a BIOPSY of fluid or tissue removed from the breast. A woman's doctor may refer her for further evaluation to a surgeon or other health-care professional who has experience with breast diseases.

These doctors may perform a FINE-NEEDLE ASPIRATION, a needle biopsy, or a surgical biopsy. In a *fine-needle aspiration,* the doctor inserts a thin needle to remove fluid or cells from a breast lump. If the fluid is clear, it may not need to be checked by a lab.

In a *needle biopsy,* the doctor removes tissue with a needle from an area that looks suspicious on a mammogram but that cannot be felt. Tissue removed in a needle biopsy goes to a lab to be checked by a pathologist for cancer cells.

There are two types of surgical biopsy. In an *incisional biopsy,* the surgeon cuts out a sample of a lump or suspicious area; in an *excisional biopsy,* the surgeon removes all of a lump or suspicious area and an area of healthy tissue around the edges. A pathologist then examines the tissue under a microscope to check for cancer cells.

Types of Breast Cancer

When cancer is found, the pathologist can tell what kind of cancer it is (whether it began in a duct or a lobule) and whether it is invasive (has invaded nearby tissues in the breast). Special lab tests of the tissue help the doctor learn more about the cancer. For example, hormone (estrogen and progesterone) receptor tests can help determine whether hormones help the cancer to grow. If test results show that hormones do affect the cancer's growth (a positive test result), the cancer is likely to respond to hormonal therapy. This therapy deprives the cancer cells of estrogen.

Lobular carcinoma in situ (LCIS)   This refers to abnormal cells in the lining of a lobule that seldom become invasive cancer. However, their presence is a sign that a woman has an increased risk of developing breast cancer. This risk of cancer is increased for both breasts. Some women with LCIS may take tamoxifen, which can reduce the risk of developing breast cancer; others may choose not to have treatment but simply return to the doctor regularly for checkups. Occasionally, women with LCIS may decide to have preventive surgery to remove both breasts to try to prevent cancer from developing, a technique called prophylactic mastectomy. (In most cases, in this situation removal of underarm lymph nodes is not necessary.)

Ductal carcinoma   The most common type of breast cancer, it begins in the lining of the milk ducts.

Ductal carcinoma in situ (DCIS)   Also called "intraductal carcinoma," this refers to abnormal cells growing in the lining of a milk duct. In this type of precancer, the abnormal cells have not spread beyond the duct to invade the surrounding breast tissue, but women with DCIS are at an increased risk of getting invasive breast cancer. Some women with DCIS have breast-sparing surgery followed by radiation therapy, or they may choose to have a mastectomy with or without breast reconstruction to rebuild the breast. Underarm lymph nodes are not usually removed. Women with DCIS may want to consider taking tamoxifen to reduce the risk of developing invasive breast cancer.

Lobular carcinoma   This type of breast cancer, which seldom becomes invasive, features abnormal cells in the lobules. Lobular carcinoma in situ increases a woman's risk of developing breast cancer in either breast.

Inflammatory breast cancer   This is an uncommon type of locally advanced breast cancer in which the breast looks red, swollen, and warm because cancer cells block the lymph vessels in the skin of the breast. The skin of the breast may also show the pitted appearance called *peau d'orange*

(French for "skin of an orange"). The nipple might be retracted or leak fluid, and there may be swollen lymph nodes under the arm or above the collarbone. Inflammatory breast cancer generally grows rapidly, and the cancer cells often spread to other parts of the body.

Stages of Breast Cancer

In most cases, the most important factor determining prognosis is the stage of the disease, which is based on the size of the tumor and whether the cancer has spread.

Stage 0: Sometimes called noninvasive carcinoma or carcinoma in situ.

Stage I: An early stage of breast cancer in which the cancer has spread beyond the lobe or duct and invaded nearby tissue. Stage I means that the tumor is no more than about an inch across and cancer cells have not spread beyond the breast.

Stage II: This is still considered an early stage of breast cancer. The cancer has spread beyond the lobe or duct and invaded nearby tissue. In this stage, either the tumor in the breast is less than one inch across and the cancer has spread to the lymph nodes under the arm; or the tumor is between one and two inches (with or without spread to the lymph nodes under the arm); or the tumor is larger than two inches but has not spread to the lymph nodes under the arm.

Stage III: Also called locally advanced cancer, in this stage, the tumor in the breast is large (more than two inches across) and the cancer has spread to the underarm lymph nodes; or the cancer is extensive in the underarm lymph nodes; or the cancer has spread to lymph nodes near the breastbone or to other tissues near the breast.

Stage IV: This is metastatic cancer. The malignancy has spread beyond the breast and underarm lymph nodes to other parts of the body.

Recurrent cancer Recurrent cancer means the disease has returned in spite of the initial treatment. Usually this occurs when undetected cancer cells remained somewhere in the body after treatment. Most recurrences appear within the first two or three years after treatment, but breast cancer can recur many years later. Cancer that returns only in the area of the surgery is called a local recurrence. If the disease returns in another part of the body, the distant recurrence is called metastatic breast cancer. The patient may have one type of treatment or a combination of treatments for recurrent cancer.

Other Tests

Other tests are sometimes done on the tumor to help the doctor predict whether the cancer is likely to progress. A sample of breast tissue may be checked for a gene (the human epidermal growth factor receptor-2 or HER-2 gene) that is associated with a higher risk that the breast cancer will come back. The doctor may also order special exams of the bones, liver, or lungs, because breast cancer may spread to these areas.

Treatment

Breast cancer may be treated with local or body-wide therapy. Some patients have both kinds of treatment. Local therapy, such as surgery and radiation, is used to remove or destroy breast cancer in a specific area such as the breast or, when breast cancer has spread, the lung or bone.

Systemic treatments are used to destroy or control cancer throughout the body. Chemotherapy, hormonal therapy, and biological therapy are systemic treatments. Some patients have systemic therapy to shrink the tumor before local therapy. Others have systemic therapy to prevent the cancer from coming back, or to treat cancer that has spread.

Surgery This is the most common treatment for breast cancer. There are several types of surgery. The doctor can explain each type, discuss and compare their benefits and risks, and describe how each will affect the woman's appearance. Surgery causes short-term pain and tenderness in the area of the operation, so women may need to talk with their doctor about pain management. The skin over the surgical area may be tight, and the muscles of the arm and shoulder may feel stiff. Because nerves may be injured or cut during surgery, a woman may have numbness and tingling in the chest, underarm, shoulder, and upper arm ("postmastectomy pain syndrome"). These feelings usually go away within a few weeks or months, but some women have permanent numbness.

Breast-conserving surgery, or breast-sparing surgery, is an operation to remove the cancer but not the breast. *Lumpectomy* and *segmental mastectomy* (also called *partial mastectomy*) are types of breast-sparing surgery. After breast-sparing surgery, most women receive radiation therapy to destroy cancer cells that remain in the area.

In a *lumpectomy,* the surgeon removes the breast cancer and some normal tissue around it. (Sometimes an excisional biopsy serves as a lumpectomy.) Often, some of the lymph nodes under the arm are removed.

A *mastectomy* is an operation to remove the breast (or as much of the breast as possible). BREAST RECONSTRUCTION, performed either at the same time as the mastectomy or in a later surgery, is often an option. Women considering reconstruction should discuss this with a plastic surgeon before having a mastectomy.

After a mastectomy, some women have some permanent loss of strength in muscles in the arms, chest, or shoulder, but for most women, reduced strength and limited movement are temporary. The doctor, nurse, or physical therapist can recommend exercises to help a woman regain movement and strength in her arm and shoulder.

In *segmental mastectomy,* the surgeon removes the cancer and a larger area of normal breast tissue around it. Occasionally, some of the lining over the chest muscles below the tumor is removed as well. Some lymph nodes under the arm may also be removed.

Simple (or total) mastectomy is the removal of the whole breast and possibly lymph nodes under the arm.

In a *modified radical mastectomy,* the whole breast, most of the lymph nodes under the arm, and often the lining over the chest muscles are removed. The smaller of the two chest muscles is also taken out to help in removing the lymph nodes.

Radical mastectomy is the removal of the breast as well as the surrounding lymph nodes, muscles, fatty tissue, and skin. Formerly considered the standard for women with breast cancer, it is rarely used today. In rare cases, radical mastectomy may be suggested if the cancer has spread to the chest muscles.

In most cases of *axillary lymph node dissection,* the surgeon also removes LYMPH NODES under the arm to help determine whether cancer cells have entered the lymphatic system. This is called an axillary lymph node dissection.

Removing the lymph nodes under the arm slows the flow of lymph. In some women, after surgery and removal of lymph nodes, fluid builds up in the arm and hand and causes swelling (LYMPHEDEMA). To prevent this, women need to protect the arm and hand on the treated side from injury or pressure, even years after surgery. This is why women should not have blood pressure taken or injections given on the side where lymph nodes have been removed. Doctors will discuss how women should handle any cuts, scratches, insect bites, or other injuries to the arm or hand. Also, they should contact the doctor if an infection develops in that arm or hand.

A *sentinel lymph node biopsy* is offered at many cancer centers. Researchers are hoping that this procedure may reduce the number of lymph nodes that must be removed during breast cancer surgery. Before surgery, the doctor injects a radioactive substance near the tumor, which then flows through the lymphatic system to the first lymph nodes where cancer cells are likely to have spread (the "sentinel" nodes). This injection can be momentarily quite painful, but the burning lasts for only a few minutes. The doctor uses a scanner to locate the radioactive substance in these sentinel nodes. Sometimes the doctor also injects a blue dye near the tumor. The dye travels through the lymphatic system to collect in the sentinel nodes. The surgeon makes a small incision and removes only the nodes with radioactive substance or blue dye. A pathologist checks the sentinel lymph nodes for cancer cells; if no cancer cells are detected, it may not be necessary to remove additional nodes. If sentinel lymph node biopsy proves to be as effective as the standard axillary lymph node dissection, the new procedure could prevent the risk of lymphedema.

Radiation therapy Women who have had a lumpectomy will almost always be candidates for radiation therapy after the surgery has healed.

Such therapy is used to kill any remaining cancer cells. The radiation may be directed at the breast by a machine or may come from radioactive material in thin plastic tubes that are placed directly in the breast (implant radiation). Some women have both kinds of radiation therapy.

In external radiation therapy, the patient usually goes to the hospital five days a week for several weeks. For implant radiation, a woman stays in the hospital for several days while the implants remain in place; they are removed before the woman goes home.

Radiation therapy, alone or with chemotherapy or hormonal therapy, is sometimes used before surgery to destroy cancer cells and shrink tumors. This approach is most often used in cases in which the breast tumor is large or not easily removed by surgery.

During radiation therapy women may be extremely tired, especially after several treatments. This feeling may continue for a while after treatment is over. Resting is important, but research has suggested that trying to stay reasonably active can help fend off fatigue.

It is also common for the skin in the treated area to become red, dry, tender, and itchy, and the breast may temporarily feel heavy and hard. Toward the end of treatment, the skin may become moist; exposing this area to air as much as possible will help the skin heal. These effects of radiation therapy on the skin are temporary, and the area gradually heals once treatment is over. However, there may be a permanent change in the color of the skin.

Chemotherapy   This is the use of drugs to kill cancer cells. CHEMOTHERAPY for breast cancer is usually a combination of drugs that may be given in a pill or by injection. Most patients, depending on which drugs are given and on their general health, can have chemotherapy as an outpatient. However, some women may need to stay in the hospital during their treatment.

Women who are still menstruating may still be able to get pregnant during treatment. Because the effects of chemotherapy on an unborn child are not known, it is important for a woman to talk with her doctor about birth control before treatment begins. After treatment, some women

regain their ability to become pregnant, but in women over the age of 35, infertility is likely to be permanent.

Hormonal therapy   This keeps cancer cells from getting the hormones they need to grow by changing the way such hormones work, or by eliminating these hormones through surgical removal of the ovaries, which make them. The side effects of hormonal therapy depend on the kind of drug or treatment.

Tamoxifen, which blocks the cancer cells' use of estrogen but does not stop estrogen production, is the most common hormonal treatment. Tamoxifen may cause hot flashes, vaginal discharge or irritation, nausea, and irregular periods. Women who are still menstruating and having irregular periods may become pregnant more easily when taking tamoxifen.

Serious side effects of tamoxifen are rare and include blood clots in the veins, a slightly higher risk of stroke, and cancer of the uterine lining. Any unusual vaginal bleeding should be reported to the doctor.

Young women whose ovaries are removed to deprive the cancer cells of estrogen experience menopause immediately, and the symptoms are likely to be more severe than symptoms associated with natural menopause.

Biological therapy   This is a treatment designed to enhance the body's natural defenses against cancer. For example, Herceptin (trastuzumab) is a monoclonal antibody that targets breast cancer cells that have too much of a protein known as human epidermal growth factor receptor-2 (HER-2). By blocking HER-2, Herceptin slows or stops the growth of these cells. Herceptin may be given by itself or along with chemotherapy.

The side effects of biological therapy depend on the types of substances used. Rashes or swelling at the injection site are common, and flulike symptoms also may occur. These and other side effects generally become less severe after the first treatment. Less commonly, Herceptin can also cause damage to the heart that can lead to heart failure. It can also affect the lungs, causing breathing problems that require immediate medical attention. For these reasons, women are checked carefully for heart and lung problems before taking Herceptin.

Treatment Options

A woman's treatment options depend on a number of factors, including her age and menopausal status, her general health, the size and location of the tumor and the stage of the cancer, the results of lab tests, and the size of her breast. Certain features of the tumor cells (such as whether they depend on hormones to grow) are also considered before settling on a particular treatment.

Women with early stage breast cancer (Stage 0 through II) may have breast-sparing surgery followed by radiation therapy to the breast, or they may have a mastectomy, with or without breast reconstruction to rebuild the breast. Both approaches are equally effective. Sometimes radiation therapy is also given after mastectomy. The choice of breast-sparing surgery or mastectomy depends mostly on the size and location of the tumor, the size of the woman's breast, certain features of the cancer, and how the woman feels about preserving her breast.

With either approach, lymph nodes under the arm usually are removed. Many women with stage I and most with stage II breast cancer have chemotherapy and/or hormonal therapy after primary treatment with surgery or surgery and radiation therapy. This added treatment is called ADJUVANT THERAPY.

Chemotherapy given to shrink a tumor before surgery is called NEOADJUVANT THERAPY. Physicians give chemotherapy to try to destroy any remaining cancer cells and prevent the cancer from recurring in the breast or elsewhere.

Patients with stage III breast cancer usually have both local treatment to remove or destroy the cancer in the breast and chemotherapy or hormonal therapy to stop the disease from spreading. The local treatment may include surgery and/or radiation therapy to the breast and underarm. Chemotherapy may be given before local therapy to shrink the tumor or afterward to prevent the disease from recurring in the breast or elsewhere.

Women who have stage IV breast cancer will be given chemotherapy and/or hormonal therapy to destroy cancer cells and control the disease. They may have surgery or radiation therapy to control the cancer in the breast. Radiation may also be useful to control tumors in other parts of the body.

Rehabilitation

Rehabilitation is an important part of breast cancer treatment. Each woman recovers differently, depending on the extent of the disease, type of treatment, and other factors.

Exercising the arm and shoulder after surgery can help a woman regain motion and strength in these areas and can also reduce pain and stiffness in the neck and back. Carefully planned exercises should be started as soon as the doctor says the woman is ready, often within a day or so after surgery. Exercising begins slowly and gently and can even be done in bed. Gradually, exercising can be more active, and regular exercise becomes part of a woman's normal routine. (Women who have a mastectomy and immediate breast reconstruction need special exercises, which the doctor or nurse will explain.)

Often, lymphedema after surgery can be prevented or reduced with certain exercises and by resting with the arm propped up on a pillow. If lymphedema occurs, the doctor may suggest exercises and other ways to deal with this problem. For example, some women with lymphedema wear an elastic sleeve or use an elastic cuff to improve lymph circulation. The doctor also may suggest other approaches, such as medication, manual lymph drainage, or use of a machine that gently compresses the arm.

Regular follow-up exams are important after breast cancer treatment. A woman who has had cancer in one breast should report any changes in the treated area or in the other breast to her doctor right away. Because a woman who has had cancer in one breast is at risk of getting cancer in the other breast, mammograms are an important part of follow-up care.

breast cancer genes   See *BRCA1/BRCA2*.

breast-conserving surgery   An operation to remove the BREAST CANCER but not the breast itself. Types of breast-conserving surgery include LUMPECTOMY (removal of the lump), quadrantectomy (removal of one quarter of the breast), and segmental MASTECTOMY (removal of the cancer as well as some of the breast tissue around the tumor and the lining over the chest muscles below the tumor).

breast reconstruction   The surgical rebuilding of a breast during or after MASTECTOMY. Almost every woman who chooses mastectomy is eligible for the surgical reconstruction of a breast mound. The procedure often can be started during surgery to remove the breast; alternatively, breast reconstruction by a plastic surgeon can take place after recovery from the mastectomy.

There are two basic types of breast reconstruction: those that use a saline implant and those that use tissue moved from another part of the woman's body (flap surgery). Whichever type of reconstruction is planned, most surgeons today perform mastectomy using a skin-sparing technique that leaves almost no scar. In this technique, the surgeon removes the inner breast tissue and the nipple, but leaves the shell of surrounding skin.

A woman can begin discussing reconstruction as soon as she has been diagnosed with cancer, because ideally, the surgical oncologist and the plastic surgeon should work together to develop a strategy for reconstruction. After evaluating the woman's health, the plastic surgeon will explain which reconstructive options are most appropriate based on the patient's age, health, anatomy, tissues, and goals. The woman should ask the plastic surgeon to explain the risks and benefits of each type of reconstruction. The surgeon should also give information about the anesthesia, the facility where the surgery will be performed, and the costs. In most cases, health insurance policies will cover most or all of the cost of post-mastectomy reconstruction.

Breast Implants

A breast implant is a silicone shell filled with a saltwater solution (saline). (The shell may also be filled with silicone gel. Because of concerns about the safety of silicone-gel-filled breast implants, the U.S. Food and Drug Administration (FDA) allows a woman to have a gel-filled implant only if she is participating in an approved study. Women interested in having silicone implants should talk with their doctor about the FDA's findings and the availability of silicone implants. Saline-filled implants are available on an unrestricted basis.)

Following mastectomy, the plastic surgeon inserts a saline-filled "expander" beneath the skin and chest muscle. Through a tiny valve buried beneath the skin, saltwater solution is periodically injected every few weeks or months to gradually fill the expander, stretching the skin. After the skin over the breast area has stretched sufficiently, the expander is removed in a second operation, so that a permanent implant can be inserted. (Some expanders are designed to be left in place as the final implant so that this subsequent surgery is not required.)

The nipple and the areola can be reconstructed in a subsequent tattooing procedure, if the woman wishes.

Some patients do not require preliminary tissue expansion before receiving an implant. For these women, the surgeon will proceed with inserting an implant as the first step.

Flap Reconstruction

An alternative approach to implant reconstruction involves creation of a skin flap using tissue taken from another part of the body, such as the back, abdomen, or buttocks. In one type of flap surgery, the tissue remains attached to its original site, retaining its blood supply. The skin, fat, and muscle that comprise the flap are tunneled beneath the skin to the chest, creating a pocket for an implant or, in some cases, creating the breast mound itself without need for an implant.

In a TRAM flap procedure (short for "transverse rectus abdominis myocutaneous" flap), the surgeon creates a breast mound using tissue removed from another part of the body—usually the abdomen.

Flap vs. Saline Implants

Flap surgery is more complex than the skin expansion/saline implant procedure. Scars will be left at both the tissue donor site and at the reconstructed breast, and recovery will take longer than with an implant. On the other hand, when the breast is reconstructed entirely with a woman's own tissue, the results are generally more natural and there are no concerns about implants breaking or leaking. In some cases, the woman may have the added benefit of an improved abdominal contour (a "tummy tuck") with flap surgery.

While saline implants require a simpler initial surgery, patients may then need to undergo a second surgery to replace the expander with a permanent implant. Moreover, saline implants generally last only about 10 years, so that a new implant would eventually have to be inserted during yet another procedure. Flap surgery is more painful and may involve major abdominal surgery but does not require a second operation.

If only one breast is to be removed and reconstructed, many surgeons recommend an additional operation to enlarge, reduce, or lift the opposite one to match the reconstructed breast. Unfortunately, this procedure may leave scars on an otherwise normal breast and may not be covered by insurance.

Depending on the extent of the surgery, a woman is usually released from the hospital in two to five days. Many reconstruction options require surgical drains to remove excess fluids from surgical sites immediately after the operation, but these drains are removed within the first week or two after surgery. Most stitches are removed in a week to 10 days.

It may take up to six weeks to recover from a combined mastectomy and reconstruction or from a flap reconstruction alone. If implants are used without flaps, and reconstruction is done apart from the mastectomy, recovery time may be shorter.

Reconstruction cannot restore normal sensation to the breast, but in time some feeling may return. Most scars will fade substantially over time—it may take as long as one to two years—but they will never disappear entirely.

In general, patients should refrain from any overhead lifting, strenuous sports, and sexual activity for three to six weeks following reconstruction. The reconstructed breast may have a different appearance. It may feel firmer and look rounder or flatter than it did before. It will not exactly match the opposite breast. For most mastectomy patients, however, breast reconstruction dramatically improves their appearance and quality of life following surgery.

Risks

There are general risks associated with any surgery and specific complications associated with this procedure. General risks, which are relatively uncommon, may include bleeding, fluid collection, excessive scar tissue, or problems with anesthesia. Women who smoke may face greater difficulties since nicotine can delay healing, resulting in conspicuous scars and prolonged recovery.

Occasionally, complications are severe enough to require a second operation. If an implant is used, there is a remote possibility that an infection will develop, usually within the first two weeks following surgery. In some of these cases, the implant may need to be removed for several months until the infection clears. A new implant can later be inserted.

The most common problem, called "capsular contracture," occurs if the scar (or capsule) around the implant begins to tighten. This squeezing of the soft implant can make the breast feel hard. Capsular contracture can be treated in several ways and sometimes requires either removal or "scoring" of the scar tissue, or removal or replacement of the implant.

Reconstruction has no known effect on the recurrence of disease in the breast, nor does it generally interfere with chemotherapy or radiation treatment, should cancer recur. The surgeon may recommend continuation of periodic mammograms on both the reconstructed and the remaining normal breast. If the reconstruction involves an implant, the patient should go to a radiology center where technicians have experience with the special techniques required to get a reliable X-ray of a breast with an implant.

Breslow's staging A method used to describe MELANOMA, developed by Dr. Alexander Breslow.

Brief Pain Inventory A questionnaire used to measure pain.

Brompton cocktail A mixture of drugs (heroin, cocaine, and morphine) in syrup, alcohol, and chloroform water used to treat extreme cancer pain. Introduced in the early 20th century, doctors began using the mixture again in English hospices during the 1970s. Since that time, it has been abandoned again with the advent of powerful modern painkillers.

bronchiolalveolar lung cancer See LUNG CANCER.

bronchography An X-ray examination of the bronchial tubes used to diagnose LUNG CANCER. After a local anesthetic is given, a catheter is inserted through the nose for the administration of contrast dye; once the dye has outlined the bronchial tubes, the X-rays are taken. The procedure takes less than an hour in a doctor's office.

bronchoscopy Examination of the larger airways (trachea and bronchi) using an instrument called a bronchoscope.

Burkitt cell acute lymphocytic leukemia See LEUKEMIA.

Burkitt's leukemia See LEUKEMIA.

Burkitt's lymphoma A cancer that is rare in most parts of the world—with about only 100 new cases a year diagnosed in the United States—but that is the most common childhood cancer in Central Africa. It is one of the most aggressive of all human cancers and causes large tumors in the abdomen or the jaw. Although in the early stages the cancer responds well to CHEMOTHERAPY, if it is untreated, it is rapidly fatal.

Burkitt's lymphoma is a type of NON-HODGKIN'S LYMPHOMA, a general term for cancers that develop in the lymphatic system. It was first described in Africa by David Burkitt in 1958.

Symptoms usually include a large lesion in the jaw that expands rapidly over a period of a few weeks to invade the bony cavity containing the eyeball. It may occasionally spread to other parts of the head. An abdominal mass often develops as well, and the bone marrow and central nervous system may be involved.

Diagnosis is made by incisional biopsy, and treatment involves radiation therapy of the jaw and eye areas; abdominal involvement requires systemic chemotherapy. Central nervous system tumors require a combination of both types of treatment.

CA 15-3 A marker in the blood for malignant tumors that may be measurable in some patients with recurrent BREAST CANCER. CA 15-3 has been evaluated for its ability to determine diagnosis, prognosis, monitor therapy, and predict recurrence of breast cancer after surgery and RADIATION THERAPY. Multiple studies have shown that the incidence of high levels of CA 15-3 in the blood increases with more advanced stages of disease. However, until there is better evidence of clinical benefit, experts say that present data are insufficient to recommend routine use of the CA 15-3 test.

Nine percent of women with stage I and 19 percent of women with stage II breast cancer have high CA 15-3 levels. The incidence of abnormal values increases to 38 percent and 75 percent for patients at stage III and IV, respectively. However, low CA 15-3 levels do not mean that breast cancer has *not* spread, and a given CA 15-3 level cannot be used to determine the stage of disease.

When CA 15-3 is evaluated before surgery in patients with primary breast cancer, levels have not correlated with prognosis. Still, very high CA 15-3 levels tend to indicate advanced disease, and a value five to 10 times normal could alert a physician that the patient's cancer has spread. CA 15-3 levels are highest in patients whose breast cancer has spread to the liver or bone.

CA 19-9 A tumor marker in the blood that appears in some patients with cancers of the stomach, bile duct, pancreas, and colon or rectum. CA 19-9 has become known as the PANCREATIC CANCER antigen.

Several other noncancerous conditions can also result in higher-than-normal CA 19-9 levels, including cirrhosis, pancreatitis, gallstones, and cholecystitis. For this reason, routine evaluation of a person's CA 19-9 levels is not recommended. However, they are useful in monitoring a patient's known cancer.

CA 27-29 A tumor marker found in the blood of most patients with BREAST CANCER that is similar to CA 19-9. A search for this marker along with other procedures (such as mammograms) can be used to check for breast cancer recurrence in women with stage II and III cancer.

CA 27-29 levels also can rise in the presence of cancers of the liver, colon, stomach, kidney, lung, ovary, pancreas, and uterus. Higher levels also occur during nonmalignant conditions, such as pregnancy, ovarian cysts, benign breast disease, kidney disease, and liver disease.

CA 125 A protein produced by a variety of cells, sometimes found at an increased level in the blood, other body fluids, or tissues, suggesting the presence of some types of cancer—especially OVARIAN CANCER. High levels of CA 125 are found in 80 percent of women with epithelial ovarian cancer, and also in cancer of the uterus, cervix, pancreas, liver, colon, breast, lung, or digestive tract. These high levels also may suggest that cancer has spread or recurred.

The CA 125 blood test is approved by the U.S. Food and Drug Administration to monitor patients with ovarian cancer, but it is considered experimental as a screening test. The test is not recommended as a general screen for ovarian cancer because it is possible to have normal levels and yet still have cancer. It is also possible to have high levels of CA 125 caused not by cancer but by noncancerous conditions such as liver disease, pelvic inflammatory disease, peritonitis, pancreatitis, and endometriosis.

cachexia   The medical term for "wasting," the loss of body weight and vital muscle mass common among patients with cancer. Wasting makes therapy harder to tolerate; studies suggest that patients who lose more than five percent of their original weight have a worse prognosis than those who do not lose weight.

About half of all cancer patients suffer serious weight loss and malnutrition that makes survival harder, but experts say there are ways to head it off. Unfortunately, with the vast majority of patients, quite often nutrition is an afterthought.

Tumors themselves can cause the wasting, particularly if they occur in the gastrointestinal system, but treatment also is often a cause. Radiation and some CHEMOTHERAPY drugs can cause NAUSEA, APPETITE LOSS, mouth sores, difficulty swallowing, dry mouth, or strangely altered taste.

Nausea is the best-known side effect, although for many patients it is periodic, striking for a few days and then abating until the next treatment. While antinausea drugs developed in the last decade bring relief to many patients, some of the most potent are very expensive and not covered by all insurance plans, so clinics may not give them until a patient complains.

The altered-taste problem, however, is often a surprise because doctors seldom warn patients it may occur. Some patients develop an aversion to a particular food, complaining that meat tastes rotten or bread tastes like sawdust. Others notice a metallic taste in their mouths so unpleasant that they simply cannot bear to eat. These sensations together with a sore or dry mouth that makes chewing difficult can result in many patients going days with very little food, risking electrolyte imbalances.

Once wasting is diagnosed, doctors may try different medications to stimulate appetite, but it is far better to prevent the problem before a patient gets very sick. Sucking lemon wedges or lemon drops and keeping hydrated can cut the metallic taste, and eating crackers, sherbet, or rice when nauseated can help.

caffeine   Caffeine has been both praised and accused for preventing—or causing—cancer, but no definitive conclusions have yet been reached. While one recent study suggested that topical caffeine lotions might prevent skin damage from sun exposure, another study appears to indicate that caffeine might repress the repair of genetic mutations caused by low levels of radiation.

Older studies suggesting a link between caffeine and PANCREATIC CANCER have been disproved.

Caffeine as a Skin Cancer Preventive

Laboratory mice slathered with caffeine developed fewer skin tumors than untreated animals, according to a 2002 study at Rutgers University. A skin lotion spiked with caffeine or with another compound found in green TEA cut the number of skin tumors in half among hairless mice exposed to high levels of ultraviolet radiation. Unlike sunscreen lotions, which protect against SKIN CANCER by preventing the skin from absorbing ultraviolet rays from the Sun (a blocking effect), the caffeine's cancer protection works in the cells after exposure to the ultraviolet rays (a biological effect). Rays from the Sun can cause genetic changes in the skin that can lead to skin cancer. Scientists said caffeine apparently blocks this action by causing abnormal cells to kill themselves, a type of programmed cell suicide that prevents the development of abnormal growths. The caffeine appears to selectively cause the abnormal cells to die but does not affect the normal cells. The next step in studying the topical effects of caffeine will be to use the solution on people who are highly susceptible to skin cancer.

Radiation and Caffeine

A second Denver study added caffeine to hamster cells that had been exposed to alpha radiation (implicated in some cases of lung cancer) and gamma radiation. The caffeine-soaked, irradiated cells sustained similar amounts of genetic damage to cells without added caffeine. In the absence of caffeine, however, cells exposed to alpha radiation exhibited fewer mutations. The findings suggest that cell mutations induced by alpha radiation can be repaired during cellular division, but that caffeine can interfere with the body's repair mechanisms.

calcification   Deposits of calcium in the tissues. *Macrocalcifications* are large deposits of calcium that are usually not related to cancer. MICROCALCIFICATIONS are specks of calcium that may be found in an area of rapidly dividing cells, which may be a sign of cancer when many are grouped together. Calcification in the breast can be seen by MAMMOGRAPHY but cannot be detected by physical examination.

calcium   A diet rich in calcium may help reduce the risk of some types of colon cancer, according to a 2002 study by the NATIONAL CANCER INSTITUTE. At the same time, another study suggested that too much calcium could be linked to PROSTATE CANCER.

In the colon cancer study, researchers found that people with a higher calcium intake had a lower risk of "left-sided" colon cancer. (Doctors often characterize colon cancer on the side where it originates, such as "left-side," "right-side," or "middle." Calcium did not affect cancers involving the latter two.) Men and women who got between 700 and 800 mg of calcium in their diets each day had a 40 to 50 percent lower risk of left-sided colon cancer than those who had less than 500 mg of calcium a day.

Researchers found that even a modest increase in calcium intake among people with low-calcium diets seemed to provide some protection against colon cancer. People who already had a high-calcium diet (more than 700 mg a day) did not receive any benefits from adding calcium supplements. The study traced the diets and colon cancer history of about 88,000 women in the Nurses' Health Study and 47,000 men in the Health Professionals Follow-Up Study.

The authors suggest that calcium reduces colon cancer risk by slowing cell growth that, when uncontrolled, can lead to cancer. Other scientists think that calcium might help bind fatty acid and bile acid within the colon, preventing them from irritating the colon lining.

Calcium-rich foods include

- 1 cup of milk—300 mg
- 1/2 cup of broccoli—35 mg
- 1/2 cup of spinach—120 mg
- 1.5 oz. of cheddar cheese—300 mg
- 8 oz. of low-fat yogurt—300–415 mg
- 1 cup of calcium-fortified orange juice—300 mg

Prostate Cancer

While calcium appears to lower the risk of colon cancer, other studies suggest too much dietary calcium can boost the risk for prostate cancer. In a 2000 Harvard University study, scientists observed a moderate increase in the risk of prostate cancer associated with higher intake of dairy foods and dairy calcium. This could be because calcium can reduce the body's level of vitamin D, which has been shown to protect the prostate. Vitamin D slows down the growth of many types of cells and can prevent the progression of cancer to a more advanced stage.

Researchers emphasized that their study only suggests a possible link between calcium and prostate cancer, and they are not recommending any dietary changes. Not all studies see a link between calcium and prostate cancer, and most men never get too much calcium—which would be above 1,000 mg a day for men 50 or younger, and 1,200 mg a day for those over 50. Calcium may be a concern only for men who get more than 2,000 milligrams a day.

Cancell/Entelev   A liquid (also known as Sheridan's Formula, Jim's Juice, Crocinic Acid, and Cantron) that has been distributed as an alternative treatment for cancer, but that has not been approved by the U.S. Food and Drug Administration (FDA) for use in the United States.

In 1989 the principal manufacturers of Cancell/Entelev were permanently prohibited from distributing the mixture, which was judged to be an unapproved new drug by the FDA.

It has been produced in various forms primarily by two manufacturers since the late 1930s. The FDA has listed the components of Cancell/Entelev as the chemicals inositol, nitric acid, sodium sulfite, potassium hydroxide, sulfuric acid, and catechol. However, the exact composition of Cancell/Entelev is unknown. Independent tests on one form of Cancell/Entelev found 12 different compounds, none of which are known to be effective in treating any form of cancer.

In 1978 and 1980, the National Cancer Institute (NCI) conducted animal studies on Cancell/ Entelev and determined that the mixture lacked substantial anticancer activity. Samples of Cancell/Entelev were also tested under NCI's In Vitro Anticancer Drug Discovery Program in 1990 and 1991. On the basis of negative results from these studies, NCI researchers concluded that no further study of Cancell/Entelev was necessary.

cancer A general term for more than 200 diseases caused by the overgrowth of abnormal cells, each with its own type of treatment. Basal cell and SQUAMOUS CELL CARCINOMA OF THE SKIN are the most common cancers, but these are almost never fatal. LUNG CANCER is the leading cause of cancer-related death in both men and women. Although prostate and BREAST CANCER occur more often, early detection and treatment have been much more successful, resulting in falling death rates.

Cancer is second only to heart disease as the leading cause of death in the United States—and soon it is expected to surpass heart disease as the number one killer. About 1.2 million new cancer cases are diagnosed each year in this country, and about 500,000 Americans will die. About 33 percent of Americans will develop cancer at some time in their lives. Over the past generation, the death rate from heart disease, stroke, and other conditions has decreased, but death from cancer still rises, largely because of the steep increase in cases of lung cancer.

Cancer is largely a disease of older adults; about two out of every three cancer deaths occurs in those over 65. Race is also strongly linked to cancer risk; African-American men have had a much higher increase in cancer death rates than Caucasian men. Cancer death rates for African-American women have risen modestly, but less than the rates for all men. Caucasian women have not experienced any significant change in cancer death rates.

Regardless of race, poor people are more likely to die of cancer than wealthy people. Experts estimate that the five-year cancer survival rate among poor Americans is 10 percent to 15 percent lower than that for people in higher socioeconomic groups. The lower rate for the wealthy could be related to better diet, more exercise, less stress, and better access to top-quality health care and early diagnosis.

Cause

All cancers begin in cells, which make up tissues, which make up the organs of the body. In a healthy adult, millions of cells grow and divide each day to replace dying cells or to repair injury. If the genetic material of cells becomes damaged as a result of heredity, smoking, pollutants, or simply bad luck, the cells can start dividing at a much faster rate. When this process goes awry, new cells form when the body does not need them, and old cells do not die when they should. These extra cells can form a mass of tissue called a tumor, which can be benign or malignant.

Cancer cells can invade and damage nearby tissues and organs; at the same time, tiny cancer cells can break away from the main malignant tumor and enter the bloodstream or the lymphatic system, spreading to distant sites. That is how cancer cells spread from the original (primary) tumor to form new tumors in other organs. The spread of cancer is called metastasis.

Some tumors secrete hormones or enzymes that disrupt the body's normal functions. As tumors grow, they develop networks of blood vessels and begin robbing the body of essential nutrients.

Doctors can tell whether a tumor is benign or malignant by examining a small sample of cells under a microscope in a procedure called a BIOPSY.

Heredity

Almost all types of cancer are caused by alterations in DNA, the genetic material that is a blueprint that controls how cells behave. In some cases, the DNA may be changed by the activation of ONCOGENES (mutated genes that cause cells to grow out of control) or by the disabling of suppressor genes (genes that keep cells from dividing too rapidly).

Most damage to genes is believed to be caused by environmental factors, such as exposure to chemicals, radiation, smoke and pollution, diet, or viruses. In addition, cell mutations may simply occur by mistake, as cells normally divide. Mutations also can be inherited, which is why many cancers run in families.

Prevention

As researchers begin to unravel the various risk factors associated with different cancers, they have begun to develop suggestions for how to avoid cancer. People can reduce the risk of cancer by limiting their exposure to substances that are known to promote cancer, such as cigarette smoke and alcohol. Improving the diet, taking antioxidant vitamins, and getting lots of exercise can also help.

Treatment

Scientists have made great strides in understanding and treating cancer. Even when cancer cannot be prevented, advances in screening and early detection have made it possible to diagnose it at the earliest possible stage. As a general rule, the smaller and more confined a tumor is at the time of diagnosis, the better the chance of achieving a permanent cure.

Statistics

Many people with cancer are living longer than ever before. Since the 1950s, the overall survival rate has more than doubled, but the usefulness of cancer statistics depends on how they are interpreted and used. It has been widely reported that the lifetime risk of developing breast cancer is one in eight—a frightening thought for women who misinterpret that statistic to mean that at any time, they have a one in eight chance of having breast cancer. The actual chance of developing breast cancer changes throughout a woman's life, so that for a 20-year-old woman the risk of developing the disease within the next 10 years is only one in 2,500; the risk for a 50-year-old woman is about one in 39.

Because heredity, ethnicity, reproductive history, lifestyle factors, and other risk factors all contribute to an individual's risk, cancer statistics are useful when used for broad perspective but not for an individual situation.

"Incidence" describes the number of new cases of cancer developed by a specific population group within a set period of time—usually a year. For example, the total 2001 U.S. incidence of TESTICULAR CANCER was about 7,200 men. Incidence rate is the number of new cases in a population. The incidence rate usually is expressed in terms of the number of cases per 100,000 people. For example, the incidence rate for testicular cancer in the United States is about four new cases per 100,000 men, often stated simply as four per 100,000.

"Prevalence" refers to the *total* number of people with cancer, or who have a particular risk factor for cancer at a particular moment in time among the entire population. For large groups of people, prevalence is estimated by collecting information from a smaller subset of people and then extrapolating that information. For example, scientists have estimated that the prevalence of the *BRCA-1* gene in the total population is between 0.04 percent and 0.2 percent, meaning that much less than 1 percent of the total population has this breast-cancer-susceptibility gene.

"Morbidity" is a state of illness; "mortality" pertains to death. "Mortality rate" is the number of people in a group who die of cancer within a set period of time (usually a year). A cancer mortality rate usually is expressed in terms of deaths per 100,000 people. For example, the mortality rate for STOMACH CANCER in the United States in 1930 was 28 (28 deaths per 100,000 people); this dropped to 4 by 1992, meaning that only 4 Americans out of every 100,000 died of stomach cancer in 1992.

Prognosis

Patients with cancer usually want to know what the course of their disease will be, or what their chances of recovery are. While physicians may base a prognosis on statistics, each patient is different and is affected by many factors such as age, general health, type and stage of cancer, and effectiveness of treatment.

While a prognosis may help explain the seriousness of a disorder or guide treatment decisions, it cannot be used to predict accurately how one person in particular will fare.

Many cancer patients are familiar with the "five-year survival rate" that used to be considered a "cure" (that is, experts used to think if a cancer patient survived for five years, he or she was cured). Today, scientists commonly use five-year survival as the standard statistical basis for defining when a cancer has been successfully treated.

The five-year survival rate includes anyone who is living five years after a cancer diagnosis. This includes those who are cured, those in remission, and those who still have cancer and are undergoing treatment. For example, when COLORECTAL CANCER is detected early, the five-year survival rate is 92 percent, meaning that 92 percent of all colorectal cancer patients whose cancer is detected early live at least five years after diagnosis.

When calculating the overall five-year survival rate for a particular cancer, the experience of everyone with that diagnosis is weighted equally. For example, a 90-year-old man and a 30-year-old man who have the same cancer will be grouped together. The 90-year-old may die of other causes within the five-year period due to normal life expectancy, and this can affect the data. A more statistically accurate view of survival is the relative five-year survival rate, which compares cancer patients' survival rate with the survival rate of the general population, taking into account differences in age, gender, race, and other factors. In this case, the 30-year-old and the 90-year-old would be treated as statistically different.

Cancer Care, Inc. A national nonprofit agency that since 1944 has offered free support, information, financial assistance, and practical help to people with cancer and their loved ones. Services are provided by oncology social workers and are available in person, over the telephone, and through the agency's Web site.

As the oldest and largest national nonprofit agency devoted to offering professional services, Cancer Care has helped more than two million people nationwide through its toll-free counseling line and teleconference programs, its office-based services, and Internet support. All services are provided free and are available to people of all ages, with all types of cancer, at any stage of the disease. Cancer Care's reach, including its cancer awareness initiatives, also extends to family members, caregivers, and professionals, providing vital information and assistance.

A section of the Cancer Care Web site and some publications are available in Spanish, and staff can respond to calls and e-mails in Spanish. For contact information, see Appendix I.

cancer centers A type of institution dedicated to treating and researching cancer, as designated by the NATIONAL CANCER INSTITUTE (NCI). The designation *cancer center* refers to an institution with a scientific agenda distinct from that of a "comprehensive" or "clinical" cancer center. "Cancer centers" may have a narrow research focus such as in basic science, population research, epidemiology, diagnosis, immunology, or other areas.

A CLINICAL CANCER CENTER conducts research in clinical oncology, and may or may not do basic or prevention research. A COMPREHENSIVE CANCER CENTER conducts a wide range of basic research, clinical research, and prevention, control, behavioral, and population-based research.

The Cancer Centers Program of the NCI supports cancer research programs in about 60 institutions across the United States through Cancer Center Support Grants.

cancer clusters The occurrence of a higher-than-expected number of cases of cancer within a group of people, a geographic area, or a period of time. Cancer clusters may be suspected when people report that several family members, friends, neighbors, or coworkers have been diagnosed with the same or related cancers.

In the 1960s one of the best-known cancer clusters was identified, involving many cases of MESOTHELIOMA (a rare cancer of the lining of the chest and abdomen). Researchers traced this outbreak to exposure to ASBESTOS, which was used heavily in shipbuilding during World War II and in manufacturing industrial and consumer products.

Suspected cancer clusters are investigated by epidemiologists who study environmental science, lifestyle factors, and biostatistics to try to determine whether a suspected cluster represents a true excess of cancer cases. A suspected cancer cluster is more likely to be a true cluster, rather than a coincidence, if it involves many cases of a specific type of cancer (rather than several different types), a rare type of cancer, or more cases than usual of a certain type of cancer in an age group that is not usually affected.

Because most cancers are likely to be caused by a combination of factors related to heredity and environment (including behavior and lifestyle), studies of suspected cancer clusters usually focus on these two issues. Researchers are just starting to understand how heredity and the environment affect cancer. The Cancer Mortality Maps & Graphs Web site (http://cancer.gov/atlasplus/) of the NATIONAL CANCER INSTITUTE (NCI) offers interactive maps, graphs, text, tables, and figures showing geographic patterns and time trends of cancer death rates between 1950 and 1994 for more than 40 cancers. It also provides interactive mortality charts and graphs, mortality maps, and links to related domestic and international Web sites, including a link to the online publication of NCI's *Atlas of Cancer Mortality in the United States: 1950–94.*

Through its Health Hazard Evaluation Program, the National Institute for Occupational Safety and Health (NIOSH) investigates potentially hazardous working conditions, including suspected cancer clusters, when requested by employers, employees, or their representatives. The NIOSH Web site is located at www.cdc.gov/niosh/homepage.html.

CancerFax A service sponsored by the NATIONAL CANCER INSTITUTE (NCI) that provides NCI fact sheets on various cancer topics (in English or Spanish) via fax machine. CancerFax does not provide listings of clinical trials.

CancerFax can be accessed 24 hours a day, seven days a week by anyone in the United States, by dialing (800) 624-2511, toll-free, from a touch-tone phone or from the telephone on a fax machine (the machine must be set to touch-tone dialing) and following the recorded instructions. Anyone calling from outside the United States may use the local number: (301) 402-5874. For a fact sheet that explains how to use CancerFax, consumers may call the CANCER INFORMATION SERVICE at (800) 4-CANCER.

Cancer Genetics Network A national network of eight centers specializing in the study of inherited predisposition to cancer, together with the Informatics Technology Group, which provides supporting information. The network supports collaborative investigations into the genetic basis of cancer susceptibility, and into how to integrate this new knowledge into medical practice and address psychosocial, ethical, legal, and public health issues.

The network includes

- Carolina-Georgia Cancer Genetics Network Center (Duke University Medical Center, Emory University, and the University of North Carolina/Chapel Hill)
- Georgetown University Medical Center's Cancer Genetics Network Center (Georgetown University Lombardi Cancer Center, Washington, D.C.)
- Mid-Atlantic Cancer Genetics Network Center (Johns Hopkins University and the Greater Baltimore Medical Center)
- Northwest Cancer Genetics Network (Fred Hutchinson Cancer Research Center in Seattle and the University of Washington School of Medicine in Seattle)
- Rocky Mountain Cancer Genetics Coalition (University of Utah, University of New Mexico, and the University of Colorado)
- Texas Cancer Genetics Consortium (M.D. Anderson Cancer Center, Health Science Center at San Antonio, Southwestern Medical Center at Dallas, and Baylor College of Medicine)
- University of Pennsylvania Cancer Genetics Network
- UCI-UCSD Cancer Genetics Network Center (University of California/Irvine and the University of California/San Diego)
- Informatics Technology Group

Cancer Hope Network A nonprofit organization that provides individual support to cancer patients and their families by matching them with trained volunteers who have undergone and recovered from a similar cancer experience. Matches are based on the type and stage of cancer, treatments used, side effects experienced, and other factors. Through this matching process, the network tries to provide support and hope, to help patients and family members look beyond the diagnosis and cope with treatment.

This unique program was built in the belief that matching cancer patients with someone who had recovered from a similar experience could make a real difference in their own fight. It is available to all cancer patients and their loved ones from anywhere in the United States at no cost. After a patient contacts the office and discusses her or his situation, the office matches the patient with a volunteer who has recovered from the same cancer experience. Staff makes a match based on the type of cancer, treatment, side effects experienced, and other factors such as age or gender.

Patients may contact the group at any point, and the program can benefit patients at all stages of their cancer experience. Ideally the network recommends a match before the patient begins treatment, which gives the patient a chance to discuss any fears and questions about treatment.

Volunteers are former patients who have survived a cancer experience and who want to help others as they deal with the disease; they have been off treatment for at least one year and have gone through extensive training before their first patient visit. For contact information, see Appendix I.

Cancer Information and Counseling Line　A toll-free telephone service that is part of the psychosocial program of the AMC Cancer Research Center. Professional counselors provide up-to-date medical information, emotional support through short-term counseling, and resource referrals to callers nationwide between the hours of 8:30 A.M. and 5 P.M. MST. Individuals may also submit questions about cancer and request resources via e-mail. For contact information, see Appendix I.

Cancer Information Service (CIS)　A service sponsored by the NATIONAL CANCER INSTITUTE that interprets research findings for the public and provides personalized responses to specific questions about cancer. Consumers can reach the CIS by calling 1-800-4-CANCER or 1-800-422-6237 or by visiting the Web site (http://cis.nci.nih.gov).

Cancer Legal Resource Center　An organization that provides information and educational outreach on cancer-related legal issues to people with cancer and others impacted by the disease. The center, a joint program of Loyola Law School and the Western Law Center for Disability Rights, provides outreach to cancer support groups, cancer survivors, and caregivers. It also provides speakers for outreach programs at hospitals, community centers, cancer organizations, and places of employment.

When necessary, the center refers patients to volunteer attorneys and other professionals. The center is presently working with major cancer centers in Los Angeles but accepts calls from the greater Los Angeles area, Orange County, and outside California.

The center also trains law students to appreciate and understand the legal needs of people battling cancer and of cancer survivors. For contact information, see Appendix I.

CancerMail　CancerMail is a service of the NATIONAL CANCER INSTITUTE that provides cancer information via e-mail. To obtain a contents list, consumers can send an e-mail to cancermail@cips.nci.nih.gov with the word *help* in the body of the message. CancerMail will respond by sending a contents list via e-mail. Instructions for ordering documents through e-mail are also provided.

CancerNet　A NATIONAL CANCER INSTITUTE Web site that offers educational materials and information on a wide range of cancer topics, including treatment options, clinical trials, reducing cancer risk, coping with cancer, support groups, and financial assistance. CancerNet can be accessed at http://cancernet.nci.nih.gov.

cancer of unknown primary origin　A type of cancer that has been diagnosed but in which the place where the cells first started growing is unknown.

Cancer Research Foundation of America (CRFA)　A nonprofit group that seeks to prevent cancer by funding research and providing educational materials on early detection and nutrition. The group focuses on cancers that can be prevented through lifestyle changes or early detection followed by prompt treatment, including cancers of the breast, cervix, colon/rectum, lung, prostate, skin, and testicles.

When CRFA began its work 16 years ago, prevention was not regarded as a major strategy in the war against cancer. Scientists primarily focused on discovering new cancer treatments rather than thinking about ways to prevent the disease from ever developing.

Today, prevention research is recognized as essential to the fight against cancer. Now that scientists better understand how tumors develop, they are learning ways that people can reduce their cancer risks. Since its inception, the foundation has provided funding to more than 200 scientists at more than 100 leading academic institutions across the country. For contact information, see Appendix I.

Cancer Survivors Network A telephone- and Internet-based service for cancer survivors, their families, caregivers, and friends. The telephone component may be reached at (877) 333-HOPE and provides survivors and families access to prerecorded discussions. The Web-based component offers live online chat sessions, virtual support groups, prerecorded talk shows, and personal stories. Cancer Survivors Network is supported by the AMERICAN CANCER SOCIETY. For contact information, see Appendix I.

cancerTrials A Web site sponsored by the NATIONAL CANCER INSTITUTE that provides information and news about cancer research studies. The primary mission of cancerTrials is to help people consider clinical trials as an option when making cancer care decisions. Consumers can access cancerTrials at http://www.cancer.gov/clinicaltrials.

candidiasis A condition in which yeast (*Candida albicans*) grows out of control in moist skin areas of the body as a side effect of CHEMOTHERAPY. Also called thrush or moniliasis, the condition usually affects the mouth, but rarely it can spread throughout the entire body.

The yeast that causes candidiasis naturally grows in both the vagina and the mouth, where it is usually kept under control by bacteria present in the body. However, the yeast may grow if the bacteria are destroyed, which may occur when a person takes drugs that affect the immune system.

Candida can also grow around the genitals or other moist areas of the body, such as the skin folds in the groin or under the breasts. It also may crop up with diaper rash in infants. Candidal infection of the penis (which occurs more often among uncircumcised men) may be transmitted from an infected partner.

Symptoms
Infection of the interior of the mouth causes sore, white-colored raised patches that usually do not cause pain, but can alter taste. In skin folds or with diaper rash, candidal infection forms an itchy red rash with flaky white patches; there may be burning or stinging.

Treatment
Antifungal drugs will usually clear up the infection, but it may recur. Those with a tendency toward this type of infection should keep the skin dry. Compresses with Burow's solution (an antiseptic water-based product), plenty of air, and infrared heat lamps to dry the affected parts may help.

Yogurt (18 oz. daily serving) that contains lactobacillus acidophilus reduces the colonization of the vagina and mouth and is effective in preventing recurrent yeast infections.

Candlelighters Childhood Cancer Foundation A nonprofit organization that provides information, peer support, and advocacy for families affected by pediatric cancers. Publications, an information clearinghouse, and a network of local support groups are available. The foundation also provides a list of organizations to which eligible families may apply for financial assistance.

The foundation was established in 1970 by concerned parents of children with cancer. Today more than 43,000 members include children with cancer, survivors of childhood cancer, family members, bereaved families, health-care professionals, and educators. For contact information, see Appendix I.

CaP CURE (Association for the Cure of Cancer of the Prostate) A nonprofit organization that provides funding for research projects to improve methods of diagnosing and treating PROSTATE CANCER. It also offers printed resources for prostate cancer survivors and their families. The mission of CaP CURE is to find a cure for prostate cancer.

CaP CURE is the largest private source of funding for prostate cancer research in the world, raising more than $165 million for research and funding more than 1,000 medical research projects worldwide since it was founded in 1993. CaP CURE's advocacy has had a significant impact on cancer research: The group helped to increase government funding for prostate cancer research from $60 million to $430 million, organized the first National Cancer Summit and March on Washington, and sponsored more than 80 clinical trials. For contact information, see Appendix I.

capsaicin   A component of cayenne and red pepper used on the skin to treat peripheral nerve pain, such as post-mastectomy pain syndrome. The use of capsaicin is also being studied as a way of controlling pain following CHEMOTHERAPY or RADIATION THERAPY.

carcinoembryonic antigen (CEA)   A substance that occurs in everyone's blood, but that is sometimes found at higher levels in the blood of people with certain cancers.

A blood test of CEA is typically used to monitor COLORECTAL CANCER when the disease has spread, and to check for recurrence after treatment. However, a wide variety of other cancers can produce high levels of this tumor marker, including cancers of the breast, lung, pancreas, stomach, cervix, bladder, kidney, thyroid, liver, and ovary. High CEA levels can also occur in patients with noncancerous conditions such as inflammatory bowel disease, pancreatitis, and liver disease. Tobacco use can also contribute to higher-than-normal levels of CEA.

carcinoembryonic antigen assay (CEA assay)   A lab test that measures CARCINOEMBRYONIC ANTIGEN (CEA), a substance that is sometimes found at higher levels in the blood of people who have certain cancers.

carcinoembryonic antigen peptide-1 (CAP-1)   A protein that can stimulate an immune response to certain tumors.

carcinogens   Substances known to cause cancer in humans. More than 80,000 chemicals are registered for use in commerce in the United States, and an estimated 2,000 new ones are introduced annually for use in everyday items such as foods, personal care products, prescription drugs, household cleaners, and lawn care products. The effects of many of these chemicals on human health are unknown, yet people and the environment may be exposed to them during their manufacture, distribution, use, and disposal or as pollutants in our air, water, or soil.

The National Toxicology Program was established in 1978 by the U.S. Department of Health and Human Services to coordinate toxicological testing programs and identify potential carcinogens. Every two years, the toxicology program releases its "Report on Carcinogens." The report identifies substances such as metals, pesticides, drugs, and natural and synthetic chemicals that are "known" or are "reasonably anticipated" to cause cancer, and to which a significant number of Americans are exposed. The report was first ordered by Congress in 1978 to determine if cancers were caused by exposure to substances in the environment, or from use of agents such as food additives, pesticides, or pharmaceuticals.

In the most recent report, released in 2002, a total of 228 known or potential carcinogens are listed. Among the substances and agents under review as potential carcinogens for the 2004 version are workplace lead and napthalene, an ingredient in mothballs. Three viruses also may be added: hepatitis B and C, which are linked to liver cancer, and HUMAN PAPILLOMAVIRUSES, which cause CERVICAL CANCER.

In addition to discussing substances and exposure circumstances that may lead to cancer, the biannual reports also contain information received from other federal agencies relating to estimated exposures and exposure standards or guidelines.

Known Human Carcinogens

There are a number of new carcinogens that were added to the 2002 report, including the following:

- *Estrogen.* This reproductive hormone, a component of hormone replacement therapy, causes breast and uterine tumors. A number of steroidal estrogens had made previous lists as "reasonably anticipated carcinogens," but all estrogens are now listed as a group.

- *Nickel and nickel compounds.* The metal causes lung and nasal cancer, chiefly from occupational exposure in refiners and welders.

- *Beryllium and beryllium compounds.* Another workplace toxin, the element leads to lung cancer.

- *Wood dust.* Produced in furniture making and other industrial settings, it causes cancer of the nasal cavities.

- *Ultraviolet radiation.* Ultraviolet light in general is known to cause skin cancer. Tanning lamps, which rely on UV radiation, are known carcinogens.

The full list of carcinogens includes

- aflatoxins
- alcoholic beverage consumption
- 4-aminobiphenyl
- analgesic mixtures containing phenacetin
- arsenic compounds, inorganic
- asbestos
- azathioprine
- benzene
- benzidine
- beryllium and beryllium compounds
- 1,3-butadiene
- 1,4-butanediol dimethylsulfonate (Myleran)
- cadmium and cadmium compounds
- chlorambucil
- 1-(2-Chloroethyl)-3-(4-methylcyclohexyl)-1-nitrosourea (MeCCNU)
- bis(Chloromethyl) ether and technical-grade chloromethyl methyl ether
- chromium hexavalent compounds
- coal tar pitches
- coal tars
- coke oven emissions
- cyclophosphamide
- cyclosporin A (Ciclosporin)
- diethylstilbestrol
- dyes metabolized to benzidine
- environmental tobacco smoke
- erionite
- estrogens
- ethylene oxide

- melphalan
- methoxsalen with ultraviolet A therapy (PUVA)
- mineral oils (untreated and mildly treated)
- mustard gas
- 2-naphthylamine
- nickel compounds
- radon
- silica, crystalline (respirable size)
- smokeless tobacco
- solar radiation
- soots
- strong inorganic acid mists containing sulfuric acid
- sunlamps or sunbeds
- tamoxifen
- 2,3,7,8-tetrachlorodibenzo-p-dioxin (TCDD); "dioxin"
- thiotepa
- thorium dioxide
- tobacco smoking
- ultraviolet radiation, broad spectrum UV radiation
- vinyl chloride
- wood dust

Probable Carcinogens

The National Toxicology Program also provides a list of substances that it "reasonably anticipates" are carcinogenic. Newest additions to the list include several forms of vinyl, PCBs, urethane, and acrylamide, a molecule generated in frying, baking, and other high-temperature cooking. Acrylamide has been on the list of likely carcinogens since the sixth report, released in 1991. The U.S. Food and Drug Administration has released acrylamide levels in scores of foods, including french fries and potato chips, and plans to test hundreds more foods.

The full list includes

acetaldehyde
2-acetylaminofluorene
acrylamide
acrylonitrile
Adriamycin® (doxorubicin hydrochloride)

2-aminoanthraquinone

o-aminoazotoluene

1-amino-2-methylanthraquinone

2-amino-3-methylimidazo[4,5-f]quinoline (IQ)

amitrole

o-anisidine hydrochloride

Azacitidine (5-azacytidine, 5-AzaC)

benz[a]anthracene;
   benzo[b]fluoranthene; benzo[j]fluoranthene;
   benzo[k]fluoranthene; benzo[a]pyrene

benzotrichloride

bromodichloromethane

2,2-bis-(bromoethyl)-1,3-propanediol

butylated hydroxyanisole (BHA)

carbon tetrachloride

ceramic fibers

chloramphenicol

chlorendic acid

chlorinated paraffins

1-(2-chloroethyl)-3-cyclohexyl-1-nitrosourea
   bis(chloroethyl) nitrosourea

chloroform

3-chloro-2-methylpropene

4-chloro-o-phenylenediamine

chloroprene

p-chloro-o-toluidine and p-chloro-o-toluidine
   hydrochloride

chlorozotocin

basic red

cisplatin

p-cresidine

cupferron

dacarbazine

danthron (1,8 dihydroxyanthraquinone)

2,4-diaminoanisole sulfate

2,4-diaminotoluene

dibenz[a,h]acridine; dibenz[a,j]acridine; dibenz85
   [a,h]anthracene;

7H-dibenzo[c,g]carbazole; dibenzo[a,e]pyrene;
   dibenzo[a,h]pyrene dibenzo[a,i]pyrene; dibenzo-
   [a,l]pyrene

1,2-dibromo-3-chloropropane

1,2-dibromoethane (ethylene dibromide)

2,3-dibromo-1-propanol

tris(2,3-dibromopropyl) phosphate

1,4-dichlorobenzene

3,3'-dichlorobenzidine and 3,3'-dichlorobenzidine
   dihydrochloride

3,3'-dichlorobenzidine and 3,3'-dichlorobenzidine
   dihydrochloride)

dichlorodiphenyltrichloroethane (DDT)

1,2-dichloroethane (ethylene dichloride)

dichloromethane (methylene chloride)

1,3-dichloropropene

diepoxybutane

diesel exhaust particulates

diethyl sulfate

diglycidyl resorcinol ether

3,3'-dimethoxybenzidine

4-dimethylaminoazobenzene

3,3'-dimethylbenzidine

dimethylcarbamoyl chloride

1,1-dimethylhydrazine

dimethyl sulfate

dimethylvinyl chloride

1,6-dinitropyrene; 1,8-dinitropyrene

1,4-dioxane

disperse blue

dyes metabolized to 3,3'-dimethoxybenzidine;
   dyes metabolized to 3,3'-dimethylbenzidine

epichlorohydrin

ethylene thiourea

di(2-ethylhexyl) phthalate

ethyl methanesulfonate

formaldehyde (gas)

furan

glasswool (respirable size)

glycidol

hexachlorobenzene

hexachlorocyclohexane isomers

hexachloroethane

hexamethylphosphoramide

hydrazine and hydrazine sulfate

hydrazobenzene

indeno[1,2,3-cd]pyrene

iron dextran complex

isoprene

Kepone (chlordecone)

lead acetate; lead phosphate

lindane and other hexachlorocyclohexane isomers

2-methylaziridine (propylenimine)

5-methylchrysene

4,4'-methylenebis(2-chloroaniline)

4-4'-methylenebis(N,N-dimethyl)benzenamine

4,4'-methylenedianiline and 4,4'-methylenediani-
   line dihydrochloride

methyleugenol
methyl methanesulfonate
N-methyl-N′-nitro-N-nitrosoguanidine
metronidazole
Michler's ketone [4,4′-(dimethylamino)benzophe-
    none]
mirex
nickel (metallic)
nitrilotriacetic acid
o-nitroanisole
6-nitrochrysene
nitrofen (2,4-Dichlorophenyl-p-nitrophenyl ether)
nitrogen mustard hydrochloride
2-nitropropane
1-nitropyrene
4-nitropyrene
N-nitrosodi-n-butylamine
N-nitrosodiethanolamine
N-nitrosodiethylamine
N-nitrosodimethylamine
N-nitrosodi-n-propylamine
N-nitroso-n-ethylurea
4-(N-nitrosomethylamino)-1-(3-pyridyl)-1-
    butanone
N-nitroso-n-methylurea
N-nitrosomethylvinylamine
N-nitrosomorpholine
N-nitrosonornicotine
N-nitrosopiperidine
N-nitrosopyrrolidine
N-nitrososarcosine
norethisterone
ochratoxin A
4,4′-oxydianiline
oxymetholone
phenacetin
phenazopyridine hydrochloride
phenolphthalein
phenoxybenzamine hydrochloride
phenytoin
polybrominated biphenyls (PBBs)
polychlorinated biphenyls (PCBs)
polycyclic aromatic hydrocarbons (PAHs)
procarbazine hydrochloride
progesterone
1,3-propane sultone
â-propiolactone
propylene oxide

propylthiouracil
reserpine
safrole
selenium sulfide
streptozotocin
styrene-7,8-oxide
sulfallate
tetrachloroethylene (perchloroethylene)
tetrafluoroethylene
tetranitromethane
thioacetamide
thiourea
toluene diisocyanate
o-toluidine and o-toluidine hydrochloride
toxaphene
trichloroethylene
2,4,6-trichlorophenol
1,2,3-trichloropropane
ultraviolet A, B and C radiation
urethane
vinyl bromide
4-vinyl-1-cyclohexene diepoxide
vinyl fluoride

carcinoid   A type of usually benign tumor most often found in the gastrointestinal system (usually the appendix) and sometimes in the lungs. When malignant, it can spread to other organs (especially the liver), where it can cause carcinoid syndrome. This syndrome may include attacks of flushing, severe diarrhea, low blood pressure, bronchospasm, and light-headedness. These symptoms are caused by the production of serotonin and histamine.

Injections with octreotide (Sandostatin) can inhibit the release of serotonin and histamine and relieve many of the symptoms. Some patients develop heart failure from associated heart valve disease.

Treatment of advanced carcinoid disease may require surgery, CHEMOTHERAPY, radiation, and hepatic artery occlusion.

Carcinoid Cancer Foundation, Inc.   A nonprofit organization chartered in 1968 to encourage and support research and education on CARCINOID tumors and related neuroendocrine tumors. For contact information, see Appendix I.

carcinoma A general term that refers to cancer that starts in the cells lining or covering practically every tissue in the body. (For example, the term *carcinoma of the breast* could be substituted for BREAST CANCER.)

carcinoma in situ Cancer that involves only the cells in which it began and that has not spread to neighboring tissues.

carcinosarcoma A malignant tumor with features of CARCINOMA and SARCOMA (cancer of connective tissue, such as bone, cartilage, or fat).

carotenoid A substance found in yellow and orange fruits and vegetables and in dark green, leafy vegetables that may reduce the risk of developing cancer. The most widespread pigments in the natural world, carotenoids play an important role in the colorful appearance of many plants and animals, including red peppers, tomatoes, paprika, flamingos, canaries, ladybugs, and salmon. They are also widely used to tint manufactured products such as soft drinks (although in such low concentrations that they do not produce much nutritional benefit).

The most common natural carotenoid is BETA-CAROTENE, a yellow-orange pigment that produces the color in yellow fruits and vegetables such as carrots or sweet potatoes. It is easily converted by the human body into vitamin A.

In the past few years scientists have found that many different carotenoids appear to prevent several different kinds of cancer. For example, a 2000 study suggested that LUTEIN (a carotenoid found in spinach, broccoli, lettuce, tomatoes, oranges and orange juice, carrots, celery, and greens) may reduce the risk of COLORECTAL CANCER. An earlier study found a link between LYCOPENE (a carotenoid found in tomato-based foods) and a reduced risk of PROSTATE CANCER. An October 2000 Harvard University study found that a diet featuring many different carotenoids was associated with a 32 percent drop in cases of LUNG CANCER. The study tracked the diets of more than 124,000 men and women from 1984 to 1996 and focused on alpha-carotene, as opposed to beta-carotene, which had been the focus of earlier studies.

It is now possible to buy individual carotenoid supplements, such as lutein pills, but experts warn that scientists still do not really understand how carotenoids can prevent cancer or whether they interact with other substances. Although studies reinforce the idea that fruits and vegetables may help prevent a wide variety of cancers, results for supplements (especially beta-carotene) have been more ambiguous. For example, one study on beta-carotene and alpha-tocopherol (a form of vitamin E) published in the *New England Journal of Medicine* in 1994 found that smokers who received beta-carotene supplements had an 8 percent higher mortality and an 18 percent *higher* incidence of lung cancer than did smokers who received placebo. Similar findings came from another study that examined the effects of beta-carotene and retinol, a form of vitamin A. (See also DIET.)

cartilage (shark and bovine) Bovine (cow) cartilage and shark cartilage have been studied as treatments for cancer and other medical conditions for more than 30 years, and many cartilage products are sold in the United States as dietary supplements.

Although more than a dozen clinical studies of cartilage as a treatment for cancer have been conducted since the early 1970s, relatively few results have been reported in peer-reviewed scientific journals. Only three human studies on the effectiveness of cartilage as a treatment for cancer have been published, and the results are inconclusive. Additional clinical trials of cartilage as a treatment for cancer are now being conducted. At present, therefore, federal cancer researchers do not recommend the use of bovine or shark cartilage as a treatment for cancer.

At least some of the interest in cartilage as cancer treatment arose from the mistaken belief that sharks, whose skeletons are made primarily of cartilage, cannot get cancer. Although reports of malignant tumors in sharks are rare, a variety of cancers have been detected in these animals.

Mechanism of Action
Although proponents have suggested that cartilage may kill cancer cells directly or stimulate the immune system to kill cancer, only limited evidence has been reported to support these ideas.

However, there is more substantial evidence to suggest that cartilage may block the formation of new blood vessels (ANGIOGENESIS), which tumors need for unrestricted growth. The absence of blood vessels in cartilage led to the hypothesis that cartilage cells produce substances that inhibit blood vessel formation. Several substances that have antitumor activity have been identified in cartilage.

To conduct clinical drug research in the United States, researchers must file an Investigational New Drug (IND) application with the Food and Drug Administration. To date, IND status has been granted to at least four groups of investigators to study cartilage as a treatment for cancer.

Side Effects

The side effects associated with cartilage therapy are generally described as mild to moderate. Inflammation at injection sites, FATIGUE, NAUSEA, labored breathing, fever, dizziness, and scrotal swelling have been reported after treatment with bovine cartilage.

Nausea, vomiting, abdominal cramping and/or bloating, constipation, low blood pressure, high blood sugar, generalized weakness, and high blood levels of calcium have been associated with the use of powdered shark cartilage. (The high level of calcium in shark cartilage may contribute to the development of high blood levels of calcium). In addition, one case of hepatitis has been associated with the use of powdered shark cartilage.

Castleman's disease An unusual disorder in which noncancerous growths develop in LYMPH NODE tissue. Rarely, patients develop systemic Castleman's disease, which behaves as a malignant disorder with fever, enlarged lymph nodes, enlarged liver and spleen, and lung and brain involvement. Some patients also develop KAPOSI'S SARCOMA or LYMPHOMA. Treatment may require corticosteroids and CHEMOTHERAPY.

causes of cancer Scientists have identified many factors that contribute to the development of cancer, including ALCOHOL, BACTERIA AND VIRUSES, poor DIET, toxins in the environment, excessive ESTROGEN exposure, heredity, sedentary lifestyle, SMOKING, and sun exposure. Avoiding these risk factors whenever possible could have a significant effect on an individual's chance of getting cancer. (See also CARCINOGENS.)

cell phones Although there have been reports linking brain tumors with wireless cell phones, available scientific evidence does not show that any health problems are associated with using wireless phones. On the other hand, there is also no proof that wireless phones are absolutely safe.

Wireless phones emit low levels of radiofrequency energy (RF) in the microwave range while being used and when in the standby mode. Whereas high levels of RF can affect health by heating tissue, exposure to low-level RF that does not produce heating effects causes no known adverse health effects. Many studies of low-level RF exposures have not found any biological effects.

Two American studies published in December 2000 by major medical journals and a study from Denmark published in February 2001 add new weight to the evidence that regular use of handheld cell phones appears to be safe, at least in the short term. The two American studies were based on interviews with U.S. hospital patients from 1994 to 1998 about cell-phone use. One of the studies was conducted by the American Health Foundation (AHF) and published in 2000 in the *Journal of the American Medical Association*. It compared the cell-phone use of 469 BRAIN CANCER patients at five academic medical centers with that of 422 patients who did not have cancer. The other study, sponsored by the National Cancer Institute (NCI), and published in *The New England Journal of Medicine* 2000, involved 782 patients, at three medical centers, who had brain cancer and 799 patients who had other ailments. All three studies found that no matter how they analyzed the data, the people who used cellular phones were no more likely to have cancer than nonusers. However, the average exposure (more than 100 total hours for the cell phone users in the NCI study and about three years for the AHF and Danish studies) was still low compared with what may be common use patterns in the future.

Although some studies have suggested that some biological effects may occur, such findings have not been confirmed by additional research. In some cases, other researchers have had trouble reproducing the studies or determining the reasons for inconsistent results.

Most human studies show no indication of an increased brain tumor risk among persons who had used handheld cellular phones compared to those who had not used them. More important, there was no evidence of increasing risk with increasing years of use or average minutes of use per day, nor did brain tumors among cellular phone users tend to occur more often than expected on the side of the head on which the person reported holding his or her phone. Specifically, there was no indication of increased risk associated with use of a cell phone for one hour or more per day, for five or more years, or for cumulative use of more than 100 hours. These findings pertain to all three tumor types considered (glioma, meningioma, and acoustic neuroma).

However, because no one knows how many years it takes for brain cancer to develop, researchers say longer-term studies are essential. As people use the phones for 10 years or 20 years, it is possible that there may be some damage with long-term exposure. In the United States alone, the number of users nearly doubled in three years, from 55 million in 1997 to 107 million in 2000. In addition, Americans spent 50 percent more time on the phone in 1999 than they did in 1996, according to industry statistics. Many people now use their cellular phone as their primary phone line. These changes in use patterns have occurred since the study information was collected, making it difficult to say with certainty that using cellular phones is safe. Typical use now may well exceed the average among study participants. Since this research looked primarily at analog phones, digital phone use also needs to be examined.

What Consumers Can Do

There are also some things consumers can do to ensure cell-phone safety, according to the FDA. First, consumers can find out how much energy is emitted by their phones. Under Federal Communications Commission safety standards, cell phones sold in the United States are allowed to emit no more than 1.6 watts of energy per kilogram of tissue (the "specific absorption rate," or SAR, which is the amount of radiation absorbed by the body). That standard was set far below the absorption level demonstrated to cause any biological change in lab animals The SAR gives only the maximum emission from a phone, which occurs when the user reaches the outer limits of a transmission tower's range (emissions are lower near a tower). The SAR for a cell phone can be obtained if the consumer has the FCC ID number of the phone or device and if it was produced and marketed after 2000. For information on finding the SAR, consumers can visit the FCC cell-phone Web page at: http://www.fcc.gov/oet/rfsafety/sar.html, or the FDA cell-phone Web page at http://www.fda.gov/cellphones/qa.html#6

In addition, consumers can use a headset, place the phone away from the body, and minimize time spent on the phone. Consumers also can switch to a model with a remote antenna outside the car. The FDA does not evaluate or recommend "cell-phone shields" that purport to block cell-phone radiation.

The U.S. Federal Communications Commission (FCC) and the FDA each regulate wireless telephones. The FCC ensures that all wireless phones sold in the United States follow safety guidelines that limit radiofrequency energy. The FDA monitors the health effects of wireless telephones. Each agency has the authority to take action if a wireless phone produces hazardous levels of energy.

Center to Reduce Cancer Health Disparities (CRCHD)   An office of the NATIONAL CANCER INSTITUTE (NCI) dedicated to directing the implementation of the institute's Strategic Plan to Reduce Health Disparities. The center also houses NCI's Office of Special Populations Research, which coordinates research that addresses cancer-related concerns for medically underserved and other vulnerable populations. For contact information, see Appendix I.

central nervous system cancers   Tumors of the central nervous system, which include brain-stem glioma, craniopharyngioma, medulloblastoma, and meningioma.

See also BRAIN CANCER.

ceramide A type of fat produced in the body that may cause some types of cells to die. Ceramide is being studied in cancer treatment.

c-erbB-2 Another name for the ONCOGENE HER-2/NEU.

cervical cancer Each year about 15,000 women in the United States learn that they have cancer of the cervix, the lower, narrow part of the uterus that opens into the vagina. Scientists believe that some abnormal changes in cells on the cervix are the first step in a series of slow changes that can lead to cancer years later; this is why cells on the surface of the cervix sometimes appear abnormal but are not yet cancerous.

Over the years, doctors have used different terms to refer to abnormal changes in the cells on the surface of the cervix. The most common term now used is squamous intraepithelial lesion (SIL); changes in these cells can be divided into two categories—low grade or high grade.

Low-grade SIL This refers to early changes in the size, shape, and number of cells on the surface of the cervix. Although some low-grade lesions go away on their own, others may become more abnormal. Precancerous low-grade lesions are also called mild dysplasia or cervical intraepithelial neoplasia 1 (CIN 1). Such early changes in the cervix most often occur in women between the ages of 25 and 35, but they can appear in other age groups as well.

High-grade SIL In this type of cervical cell abnormality there are many precancerous cells that look very different from normal cells. As in low-grade SIL, these precancerous changes involve only cells on the surface of the cervix. The cells will not become cancerous and invade deeper layers of the cervix for many months or years. High-grade lesions also may be called moderate or severe dysplasia, CIN 2 or 3, or carcinoma in situ. They appear most often in women between the ages of 30 and 40, but they can occur at other ages as well.

If abnormal cells spread deeper into the cervix or into other tissues or organs, it is called cervical cancer, or invasive cervical cancer. Cervical cancer occurs most often in women over the age of 40.

Risk Factors

There are certain risk factors that increase the chance that cells in the cervix will become abnormal or cancerous. In many cases, cervical cancer develops when a person has two or more risk factors that act together. Risk factors include:

Sexual patterns Women who have sex before age 18 or who have had many sexual partners have a higher risk of developing cervical cancer. Women also are at increased risk if their partners began having sexual intercourse at a young age, have had many sexual partners, or were previously married to women who had cervical cancer. This may be related to the fact that some sexually transmitted viruses can trigger changes in cervical cells that can lead to cancer.

Human papillomaviruses (HPVs) Some sexually transmitted HPVs cause genital warts (condylomata acuminata); other HPV viruses that do not cause visible genital warts *do* cause to grow in the cervix abnormal cells that play a role in cancer development. Some experts believe that up to 90 percent of all cervical cancers are caused by these viruses. Women with HPV or whose partners have HPV have a higher-than-average risk of developing cervical cancer.

However, most women who are infected with HPV do not develop cervical cancer, and the virus is not present in all infected women. For these reasons, scientists believe that other factors—such as the genital herpes virus—may act together with HPVs to cause cervical cancer. Further research is needed to learn the exact role of these viruses and how they act together with other factors in the development of cervical cancer.

Smoking Although scientists are not sure why, it appears that SMOKING increases the risk of cancer of the cervix. The risk appears to increase with the number of cigarettes a woman smokes each day and with the number of years she has smoked.

DES Women whose mothers were given the drug DIETHYLSTILBESTROL (DES) during pregnancy to prevent miscarriage are at increased risk. This drug was used from about 1940 to 1970 but was then discontinued because of its link to cancer. A rare type of vaginal and cervical cancer has been found in a small number of women whose mothers used DES.

Immune problems Several reports suggest that women whose immune systems are weakened are more likely than others to develop cervical cancer. For example, women who have the human immunodeficiency virus (HIV) that causes AIDS are at increased risk. Organ transplant patients, who receive drugs that suppress the immune system to prevent rejection of the new organ, are also more likely than other women to develop precancerous lesions.

Birth control pills Some researchers believe that there is an increased risk of cervical cancer in women who use oral contraceptives, but no solid proof has ever been found that indicates the Pill directly causes cancer of the cervix. This relationship is hard to prove because the two main risk factors for cervical cancer—sex at an early age and multiple sex partners—may be more common among women who use the Pill than among those who do not.

Nevertheless, oral contraceptive labels warn of this possible risk and advise women who use them to have yearly PAP TESTS.

Geography It appears that where a woman lives may have something to do with her risk of developing cervical cancer. Despite a threefold reduction in cervical cancer mortality nationwide in the past 50 years, certain areas of the country have experienced persistently higher mortality rates. These high-risk areas include counties stretching from Maine southwest through Appalachia to the Texas/Mexico border, many southeastern states, and the Central Valley of California.

Symptoms

Precancerous changes of the cervix usually do not cause any symptoms, which is why they are not detected unless a woman has a pelvic exam and a Pap tests (a lab analysis of cells scraped from the cervix). Symptoms usually do not appear until abnormal cervical cells become malignant and invade nearby tissue.

When this happens, the most common symptom is abnormal bleeding, which may begin and end between regular menstrual periods, or may occur after sexual intercourse, douching, or a pelvic exam. Menstrual bleeding may last longer and be heavier than usual. Bleeding after menopause also may be a symptom of cervical cancer. Increased vaginal discharge is another symptom of cervical cancer.

Diagnosis

The pelvic exam and Pap test allow the doctor to detect abnormal changes in the cervix. COLPOSCOPY is a common test used to check the cervix for abnormal areas. The doctor applies a vinegarlike solution to the cervix and then uses an instrument to look closely at the cervix. The doctor may then coat the cervix with an iodine solution (a procedure called the Schiller test). Healthy cells turn brown; abnormal cells turn white or yellow. These procedures may be done in the doctor's office. The doctor may do a biopsy, removing a small amount of cervical tissue for examination by a pathologist.

In order to check inside the opening of the cervix (an area that cannot be seen during colposcopy), the doctor may perform endocervical curettage, using a curette to scrape tissue from inside the cervical opening.

If these tests do not definitively reveal whether the abnormal cells are present only on the surface of the cervix, the doctor will remove a larger, cone-shaped sample of tissue. This procedure, called CONIZATION or cone biopsy, allows the pathologist to see whether the abnormal cells have invaded tissue beneath the surface of the cervix. Conization also may be used as treatment for a precancerous lesion if the entire abnormal area can be removed.

In a few cases, it may not be clear whether an abnormal Pap test or a woman's symptoms are caused by problems in the cervix or in the lining of the uterus. In this situation, the doctor may do dilation and curettage (D & C). The doctor stretches the cervical opening and uses a curette to scrape tissue from the lining of the uterus as well as from the cervical canal. Like conization, this procedure requires local or general anesthesia and may be done in the doctor's office or in the hospital.

Once cervical cancer has been diagnosed, the doctor will want to learn how far it has spread. Blood and urine tests are usually done, and the doctor also may do a pelvic exam in the operating room with the patient under anesthesia. During this exam, the doctor may perform a cystoscopy (viewing the bladder with a thin, lighted instrument) or proctosigmoidoscopy (checking the rectum and lower part of the intestine with a lighted instrument).

Because cervical cancer may spread to the bladder, rectum, lymph nodes, or lungs, the doctor may order X-rays or tests to check these areas. The doctor also may check the intestines and rectum using a barium enema. To look for lymph nodes that may be enlarged because they contain cancer cells, the doctor may order a CT or CAT scan, a series of X-rays analyzed together by a computer to produce detailed pictures of areas inside the body. Other procedures that may be used to check organs inside the body are ultrasonography and MRI.

The stages of cervical cancer include

Stage I: The cancer cells are present only within the cervix.

Stage II: The tumor has spread into surrounding structures such as the upper part of the vagina or nearby lymph nodes.

Stage III: The tumor has spread to surrounding structures such as the lower part of the vagina, nearby lymph nodes, the outer layer of the womb, or to nearby structures within the pelvic area. Sometimes a tumor that has spread to the pelvis may press on one of the ureters, which may cause urine to build up in the kidney.

Stage IV: The tumor has spread beyond the pelvic area, or to the bladder or bowel. This stage includes tumors that have spread into the lungs, liver, or bone, although these are not common.

Treating Precancerous Conditions

Treatment for a precancerous lesion of the cervix depends on the grade, whether the woman wants to have children, and the woman's age and general health. A woman with a low-grade lesion may not need further treatment, especially if the abnormal area was completely removed during biopsy, but she should have a Pap test and pelvic exam regularly. When a precancerous lesion requires treatment, the doctor may remove it with cryosurgery (freezing), cauterization, conization, or laser surgery to destroy the abnormal area without harming nearby healthy tissue. In some cases, a woman may have a hysterectomy, particularly if abnormal cells are found inside the opening of the cervix. This surgery is more likely to be done when the woman does not want to have children in the future.

Treating Cancerous Lesions

The choice of treatment for cervical cancer depends on the location and size of the tumor, the extent of the disease, and the woman's age and general health. Cervical cancer is treated with some combination of surgery, radiation therapy, chemotherapy, or biological therapy.

Surgery The aim of surgery is to remove abnormal tissue in or near the cervix. If the cancer is only on the surface of the cervix, the doctor may destroy the cancerous cells using methods similar to those chosen to treat precancerous lesions. If the disease has invaded deeper layers of the cervix but has not spread beyond the cervix, the doctor may remove the tumor but leave the uterus and the ovaries. In other cases, however, a woman may need to—or may choose to—have a hysterectomy, especially if she is not planning to have children in the future. In a hysterectomy, the doctor removes the entire uterus (including the cervix). Sometimes the ovaries and fallopian tubes also are removed. In addition, the doctor may remove lymph nodes near the uterus to learn whether the cancer has spread to these organs.

Radiation therapy Internal or external radiation therapy, stops cancer cells from growing. Radiation therapy is given at a hospital or clinic five days a week for five or six weeks. Internal radiation is administered by inserting a capsule containing radioactive material directly in the cervix and left in place for one to three days; the treatment may be repeated several times over the course of one or two weeks. The patient stays in the hospital while the implants are in place.

Chemotherapy At least five different studies have shown that adding the chemotherapy drug cisplatin to surgery and radiation reduces the risk of cancer returning.

Biological therapy Biological therapy (using substances to help the body's immune system) may be used to treat cancer that has spread from the cervix to other parts of the body. Interferon is the most common form of biological therapy for cervical cancer; it may be used in combination with chemotherapy. Most patients who receive interferon are treated as outpatients.

Follow-up treatment Regular pelvic exams, Pap tests, and other lab tests are very important for any woman who has been treated for either precancerous changes or for cancer of the cervix.

Prognosis

Nearly all women with precancerous changes of the cervix or very early cancer of the cervix can be cured. Researchers continue to look for new and better ways to treat invasive cervical cancer.

Prevention

A yearly pelvic exam and Pap test is the best way to diagnose most precancerous conditions so that they can be treated before cancer develops, or to find invasive cancer at an early, curable stage. In a pelvic exam, the doctor checks the uterus, vagina, ovaries, fallopian tubes, bladder, and rectum for abnormal shape or size. The Pap test is a simple, painless way to detect abnormal cells in and around the cervix.

Women should have regular checkups, including a pelvic exam and a Pap test, if they are or have been sexually active or if they are age 18 or older. Those who are at increased risk of developing cancer of the cervix should be especially careful to follow their doctor's advice about checkups. Women who have had a HYSTERECTOMY should ask their doctor's advice about having pelvic exams and Pap tests.

Some research has shown that vitamin A may play a role in stopping or preventing cancerous changes in cells like those on the surface of the cervix. Further research with forms of vitamin A may help scientists learn more about preventing cancer of the cervix.

cervical intraepithelial neoplasia (CIN) A general term for the growth of abnormal cells on the surface of the cervix. Numbers from 1 to 3 may be used to describe how much of the cervix contains abnormal cells.

See also CERVICAL CANCER.

cheek cancer See MOUTH CANCER.

chemoembolization A palliative procedure used to treat LIVER CANCER in which the blood supply to the tumor is blocked surgically or mechanically and anticancer drugs are administered directly into the tumor. This permits a higher concentration of drug to be in contact with the tumor for a longer period of time.

During chemoembolization, CHEMOTHERAPY drugs are injected directly into the artery that supplies blood to the tumor. The artery is then blocked off ("embolized") with a mixture of oil and tiny particles, or a substance called Gelfoam depriving the tumor of oxygen and nutrients. Because the drugs are injected directly at the tumor site, the dosage can be 20 to 200 times greater than that achieved with standard chemotherapy injected into a vein in the arm. Because no blood washes through the tumor, the drugs stay in the tumor for a much longer time—up to a month. In addition, the procedure causes fewer side effects because the drugs are trapped in the liver instead of circulating throughout the body.

After the procedure, the patient may experience pain, fever, and nausea lasting a few hours to a few days. There also may be slight hair loss. Serious complications from chemoembolization are rare. In less than 3 percent of the procedures, the tumor killed by the procedure may become infected.

chemotherapy The use of toxic drugs to control cancer by interfering with the growth or production of malignant cells. There are more than 50 different chemotherapy drugs given either alone or—more typically—in combinations. The type of treatment a patient is given depends on the type of cancer, its location, what the cancer cells look like under the microscope, and how far they have spread.

How It Works

Chemotherapy drugs interfere with the ability of cancer cells throughout the body to divide and reproduce themselves. While normal cells typically divide in very controlled ways, malignant cells grow and reproduce in a rapid, haphazard way. Chemotherapy drugs are taken up by rapidly dividing cells—which include cancerous cells and also some healthy cells that normally divide quickly, in the lining of the mouth, the BONE MARROW, the hair follicles, and the digestive system. However, while healthy cells can repair the damage caused by chemotherapy, cancer cells cannot—and so they eventually die.

Chemotherapy drugs damage cancer cells in different ways. If a combination of drugs is used, each drug is chosen because of its different effects. Chemotherapy must be carefully planned so that it destroys more and more of the cancer cells during the course of treatment but does not destroy the normal cells and tissues. With some types of cancer, chemotherapy can destroy all the cancer cells and cure the disease.

Chemotherapy may be given after surgery or RADIATION THERAPY (adjuvant therapy) to reduce the chance of cancer returning. If any cancer cells remain after surgery or radiation that are too small to see, they can be destroyed by the chemotherapy. If a cure is not possible, chemotherapy may be given to shrink and control a cancer, or reduce the number of cancer cells and try to prolong a good quality of life.

Chemotherapy can be given before surgery (neo-adjuvant therapy) to shrink a tumor and make it easier to remove and prevent its spread. This is usually done when a cancer cannot be removed easily during an operation. Chemotherapy can also be used in this way before or during radiation therapy.

High-dose chemotherapy For some types of cancer with a high risk of recurrence, a course of very high-dose chemotherapy is given after an initial dose of standard chemotherapy. As very high doses of chemotherapy normally destroy the bone marrow, the bone marrow is replaced after the chemotherapy has been given. This is done using stem cells collected from bone marrow or blood. These stem cells may be collected from the patient (autologous) before the high-dose treatment, or from a donor (allogenic) whose cells are a good match. This type of treatment is useful only in a few types of cancer.

How It Is Given

Chemotherapy may be given in different ways, depending on the type of cancer and the particular chemotherapy drugs used.

Intravenous Chemotherapy is often given by injection into a vein, which generally takes from half an hour to a few hours, or sometimes a few days. If it takes only a few hours, the drugs may be given on an outpatient basis; otherwise they are given on an inpatient basis.

Ports/pumps Chemotherapy can be given by IV through catheters, ports, and pumps. A catheter is a soft, thin, flexible tube that is inserted into the body and remains there throughout treatment. Patients who need many IV treatments often have a catheter to avoid frequent needles. Drugs can be given and blood samples can be drawn through the same catheter. A catheter placed in a large vein, usually in the chest, is called a central venous catheter. A catheter placed in a vein in the arm is called a peripherally inserted central catheter. Catheters can also be placed in an artery or in other locations, such as an intrathecal catheter, which delivers drugs into the spinal fluid, or intracavitary catheter, which is placed in the abdomen, pelvis, or chest. Drugs given in this way tend to stay in the area in which they are given and do not affect cells in other parts of the body.

Sometimes the catheter is attached to a port—a small, round plastic or metal disk placed under the skin, which is also used throughout treatment.

A pump (either external or internal) is used to control how fast the drug goes into a catheter or port. Catheters, ports, and pumps cause no pain if they are properly placed, although a patient is aware of them.

Pills Some drugs are given as tablets or capsules and are absorbed into the blood and thus carried around the body so that they can reach all the cancer cells.

Creams Chemotherapy creams may be used for some cancers of the skin. They are put on the affected area of skin in a thin layer and may need to be used regularly for up to a few weeks. They may cause some soreness or irritation of the skin in the affected area but act only on local cells and so do not cause side effects in other parts of the body.

Frequency

How often and how long a patient gets chemotherapy depends on the type of cancer, the treatment goals, the particular drugs, and how the patient's body responds to treatment. Patients may get treatment every day, every week, or every month. In any case, chemotherapy is often given in cycles of treatment periods with rest periods in between, to give the body a chance to produce healthy new cells and regain strength.

Chemotherapy on the Job

Most people can continue working while receiving chemotherapy, although they may need to change their work schedule if the drugs make them feel tired or sick. Federal and state laws require employers to let patients work a flexible schedule to meet treatment needs. Social workers and congressional or state representatives can provide information on state and federal laws protecting employees.

Side Effects

Great progress has been made in preventing and treating some of chemotherapy's common as well as rare serious side effects. Many new drugs and treatment methods destroy cancer more effectively while doing less harm to the body's healthy cells. Different chemotherapy drugs cause different side effects. These side effects may vary among patients and from treatment to treatment. Side effects are not a sign of whether the treatment is working or not.

Almost all side effects are short term and will gradually disappear once the treatment has stopped. The main areas of the body that may be affected by chemotherapy are those where normal cells rapidly divide and grow, such as the lining of the mouth, the digestive system, skin, hair, and bone marrow.

However, sometimes chemotherapy can cause permanent changes or damage to the heart, lungs, nerves, kidneys, reproductive organs, or other organs. Certain types of chemotherapy may have delayed effects (such as a second type of cancer) that does not appear until many years later. Patients need to balance their concerns about permanent effects with the immediate threat of cancer.

Fatigue, infection, and unusual bleeding are all common side effects due to the fact that chemotherapy lowers the number of blood cells produced by the bone marrow—white blood cells essential for fighting infections, red blood cells that carry oxygen, and platelets to help clot the blood and prevent bleeding.

Fatigue   This is the most common side effect of chemotherapy, related to low blood cell counts, stress, depression, poor appetite, lack of exercise, direct side effect of chemotherapy and many other factors. If the level of red blood cells gets too low, patients may become tired and lethargic. Because the amount of oxygen being carried around the body is lower, patients also may become breathless. These are all symptoms of anemia (a lack of hemoglobin in the blood). People with anemia may also feel dizzy and light-headed and have aching muscles and joints. The tiredness will fade away gradually once the chemotherapy has ended, but some people find that they still feel tired for a year or more afterward.

Fatigue caused by chemotherapy can appear suddenly and is not like normal tiredness. It has been described as a total lack of energy, making patients feel worn out and so drained that rest does not always relieve it.

Oncologists order regular blood tests to measure hemoglobin during chemotherapy, and injections of erythropoetin to boost red cell production or a blood transfusion can be given if the hemoglobin falls too low. The extra red cells will very quickly pick up the oxygen from the lungs and take it around the body so that patients feel more energetic and less breathless. Some studies have also suggested that moderate physical exercise (such as walking) can help prevent fatigue.

Nausea/vomiting   Although many patients fear the nausea and vomiting that have historically been side effects of chemotherapy, modern drugs have made these far less common.

Because of very effective antinausea medications, many people do not get sick this way at all, and if they do, it is quite mild. If patients are going to feel sick, it will usually begin from a few minutes to several hours after chemotherapy, depending on the drugs given. The sickness may last for a few hours or for several days. Doctors can prescribe antisickness drugs (antiemetics) to stop or reduce nausea and vomiting. Low doses of steroids also can be helpful in reducing these side effects. Antiemetics may be given by injection with the chemotherapy and as tablets to take at home afterward. Common anti-nausea medications include serotonin antagonists (ondansetron, granisetron, dolasetron), prochlorperazine, and lorazepan.

Infections If the number of white cells in the blood is low, a patient will be more likely to get an infection because these cells fight off bacteria. For this reason, oncologists order regular blood tests to show the number of white cells in the blood. If patients get an infection when their white blood cell level is very low, they may need antibiotics given directly into the bloodstream. Sometimes, drugs called growth factors can help the bone marrow make more white blood cells.

Growth factors (such as neupogen) are sometimes given after chemotherapy treatment to stimulate the bone marrow to produce new white cells quickly, thereby reducing the risk of infection. The blood cells are usually at their lowest level from seven to 14 days after the chemotherapy treatment, although this will vary depending on the type of chemotherapy.

Bleeding If the number of platelets in the blood gets too low, it can lead to bruising and nosebleeds, or heavier bleeding from minor cuts or grazes. Patients who develop unexplained bleeding or bruising need to contact a doctor as a platelet transfusion may be required. Regular blood tests are used to count the number of platelets in the blood.

Digestive problems Some chemotherapy drugs can reduce the appetite for a while. Steroids and progestational agents (Megace) can help to boost the appetite. Some chemotherapy drugs can affect the lining of the digestive system, and this may cause diarrhea for a few days. More rarely, some chemotherapy drugs can cause constipation.

Sore mouth Some drugs can cause sores in the throat and mouth. If this happens, it usually occurs about five to 10 days after treatment and will clear up within three to four weeks. Anticancer drugs also can make these tissues dry and irritated or cause them to bleed. Patients who have not been eating well since beginning chemotherapy are more likely to get mouth sores.

In addition to being painful, mouth sores can become infected by the many germs that live in the mouth. Every step should be taken to prevent infections, because they can be hard to fight during chemotherapy and can lead to serious problems.

Cleaning the teeth regularly and gently with a soft toothbrush will help to keep the mouth clean. If the mouth is very sore, gels, creams, or pastes can be painted over the ulcers to reduce the soreness.

Chemotherapy also can alter taste; food may seem more salty, bitter, or metallic. Normal taste will come back after the chemotherapy treatment ends.

Hair loss Hair loss is one of the most well-known side effects of chemotherapy. Although a few drugs do not cause hair loss (or cause little loss of hair) most do cause partial or complete hair loss for a time. Some chemotherapy can damage hair and make it brittle. If this happens, the hair may break off near the scalp a week or two after the chemotherapy has started.

The amount of hair lost depends on the type of drug or combination of drugs used, the dose given, and the person's individual reaction to the drug. If hair loss happens, it usually starts within a few weeks of beginning treatment, although rarely it can start within a few days. Body hair may be lost as well, and some drugs even trigger loss of the eyelashes and eyebrows. Hair lost as a result of chemotherapy will grow back after treatment is finished.

Skin/nail changes Some drugs can affect the skin, making it drier or slightly discolored. These changes may be worsened by swimming, especially in chlorinated water. The drugs may also make skin more sensitive to sunlight during and after treatment.

Nails may grow more slowly, and white lines may appear. Nails also may become more brittle and flaky.

Nerves Some chemotherapy drugs can affect the nerves in the hands and feet, causing tingling, numbness, or a sensation of pins and needles known as peripheral neuropathy. This feeling gradually fades away after chemotherapy ends, but if it becomes severe it can damage the nerves permanently.

Nervous system Some drugs can cause feelings of anxiety and restlessness, dizziness, sleeplessness, headaches, or concentration and memory problems. Other drugs can lead to a loss of the ability to hear high-pitched sound or cause a continuous ringing in the ears known as tinnitus.

Vaccinations Travelers should keep in mind that patients undergoing chemotherapy should not have any "live virus" vaccines, including polio, measles, rubella (German measles), MMR (measles, mumps, and rubella), BCG (tuberculosis), yellow fever, and typhoid medicine. Other vaccines, such as diphtheria, tetanus, flu, pneumonia, hepatitis B, hepatitis A, rabies, cholera, and typhoid injection, should not cause problems for chemotherapy patients.

Radiation recall Some people who have had radiation therapy develop a skin problem during chemotherapy called radiation recall during, or shortly after the time certain anticancer drugs are given. The skin over an area that had received radiation turns red and may blister and peel. This reaction may last hours or even days.

Kidney/bladder problems Some anticancer drugs can irritate the bladder or cause temporary or permanent damage to the bladder or kidneys. When a patient takes certain anticancer drugs, his or her urine may turn orange, red, green, or yellow, or take on a strong or medicine-like odor for 24 to 72 hours. Patients should always drink plenty of fluids to ensure good urine flow and help prevent problems.

Flu symptoms Symptoms of the flu may bother some patients a few hours to a few days after chemotherapy, especially if they are receiving chemotherapy together with biological therapy. Aching muscles and joints, headache, fatigue, nausea, fever, chills, and poor appetite may last from one to three days. An infection or the cancer itself can also cause these symptoms.

Fluid retention The body may retain fluid during chemotherapy. This may be due to hormonal changes from therapy, the drugs themselves, or the cancer. Patients may need to avoid table salt and foods that have a lot of salt. If the problem is severe, a doctor may prescribe a diuretic to help the body get rid of excess fluids.

Infertility Some chemotherapy treatments may cause temporary or permanent infertility. And yet, while chemotherapy may reduce fertility, it is still possible for a woman to become pregnant during treatment. Vomiting and diarrhea that often accompany chemotherapy can make birth control pills less effective. Female partners of a man having chemotherapy may also become pregnant. However, pregnancy should be avoided during chemotherapy because there is a risk that the drugs may harm the baby.

Some drugs will have no effect on a woman's fertility, but some may stop the production of eggs by the ovaries. This will also trigger the symptoms of menopause. During chemotherapy, a woman's menstrual periods may become irregular and stop, and there may be hot flashes, dry skin, and vaginal dryness. In about a third of women, the ovaries start producing eggs again and menstruation returns to normal after treatment. Usually, the younger the woman, the more likely she is to become fertile again after treatment.

Some chemotherapy drugs will have no effect at all on a man's fertility, but others may reduce the number of sperm or affect their ability to reach and fertilize a woman's egg. However, men will still be able to have an erection and orgasm and should use a reliable method of contraception during treatment.

Men who have not completed their family before chemotherapy may be able to bank some of their sperm for later use. If this is desired, several sperm samples are produced over a few weeks before treatment. These are then frozen and stored so that they can be used later to fertilize an egg. If chemotherapy does cause infertility, some men will remain infertile after their treatment has stopped, while others find their sperm returns to normal levels and their fertility returns, although it may take a few years.

Cost

The cost of chemotherapy varies with the kinds and doses of drugs used, how long and how often they are given, and whether they are given at home, in an office, or in the hospital. Most health insurance policies cover at least part of the cost of many kinds of chemotherapy. There are also organizations that will help with the cost of chemotherapy and with transportation costs. Nurses and social workers have information about these organizations. In some states, Medicaid (which makes health-care services available for people with financial need) may help pay for certain treatments.

chewing tobacco   See SMOKELESS TOBACCO.

childbirth and cancer   Because long-term exposure to ESTROGEN has been linked to the development of BREAST CANCER, women who have had many children have a lower risk of developing this type of cancer. Women who have never had children have a higher risk.

See also INFERTILITY AND CANCER.

childhood cancers   Cancer is the number one disease killer of children—more than genetic anomalies, cystic fibrosis, and AIDS combined. About 8,600 children in the United States were diagnosed with cancer in 2001, and about 1,500 of them died from the disease that year. Still, cancer is relatively rare in this age group, with only about one or two children developing the disease each year for every 10,000 children in the United States.

There has been an increase in the incidence of children diagnosed with all forms of invasive cancer since the 1980s. In 1975 there were 11.4 cases per 100,000 children; in 1998 there were 15.2 cases per 100,000 children. However, death rates have declined dramatically and survival increased for most childhood cancers in that period. For example, the five-year survival rate for all childhood cancers combined increased from 55.7 percent in the period from 1974 to 1976 to 77.1 percent in the period from 1992 to 1997. These improvements were due to significant advances in treatment, resulting in cure or long-term remission for a substantial proportion of children with cancer.

Over the last half of the 20th century, progress in childhood cancer diagnosis and treatment has transformed a once uniformly fatal disease into a group of malignancies that are now curable in most children. For example, LEUKEMIA survival rates have increased from just over 60 percent in the mid-1970s to near 80 percent in the mid-1990s.

Causes

The causes of childhood cancers are largely unknown. A few conditions, such as Down syndrome, genetic problems, and ionizing radiation exposures, explain a small percentage of cases. Many scientists have suspected many environmen-

tal causes of childhood cancer, but these factors have been difficult to identify, partly because cancer in children is rare and partly because it is so difficult to identify past exposure levels in children. In addition, each of the distinctive types of childhood cancers develops differently and has a potentially different cause.

Scientists do know that children treated with CHEMOTHERAPY and RADIATION THERAPY for certain forms of childhood and adolescent cancers, such as HODGKIN'S DISEASE, BRAIN CANCER, SARCOMAS, and others, may develop a second primary malignancy. They also know what does *not* cause childhood cancer: Low levels of radiation exposure from RADON were not significantly associated with childhood leukemias, nor was ultrasound use during pregnancy linked with childhood cancer. Residential magnetic field exposure from power lines was not significantly associated with childhood leukemias, nor were on-the-job exposures of parents.

Although scientists suspect that pesticides may be linked to the development of certain forms of childhood cancer, results have been inconsistent and have not yet been validated by physical evidence of pesticides in the child's body or environment.

Several studies have found no link between maternal cigarette SMOKING before pregnancy and childhood cancers, but increased risks were related to the father's prenatal smoking habits in studies in the United Kingdom and China.

Little evidence has been found to link specific viruses or other infectious agents to the development of most types of childhood cancers, although scientists are exploring the role of exposure of very young children to some common infectious agents that may protect children from, or put them at risk for, certain leukemias.

Recent research has shown that children with AIDS have an increased risk of developing certain cancers, predominantly NON-HODGKIN'S LYMPHOMA, KAPOSI'S SARCOMA, and LEIOMYOSARCOMA (a type of muscle cancer).

Specific genetic syndromes, such as the Li-Fraumeni syndrome, neurofibromatosis, and several others, have been linked to an increased risk of specific childhood cancers.

The role of a mother's exposure to birth control pills, FERTILITY DRUGS, and DIETHYLSTILBESTROL is being studied in several ongoing trials.

Types of Childhood Cancers

Among the 12 major types of childhood cancers, leukemia and brain cancer account for more than half of the new cases.

Leukemia About a third of childhood cancers are leukemias (cancers of the BONE MARROW and tissues that make up the blood cells). About 2,700 children younger than 15 years were diagnosed with leukemia in 2001. Leukemia triggers the production of too many abnormal white cells. These cells invade the marrow and crowd out normal healthy blood cells, making the patient susceptible to ANEMIA, infection, and bruising. The most common type in children is acute lymphoblastic leukemia, which is highly treatable. Today about 70 percent of affected children are cured.

Brain cancer Tumors of the brain and spinal cord are the most common types of solid tumors in children. Some tumors are benign, and some children can be cured by surgery, but because of the difficulty in diagnosing and treating brain tumors, there has been less dramatic progress in treating them than other childhood malignancies. Today 20 percent of all primary brain tumors occur in children younger than 15, with a peak in incidence between the ages of 5 and 10 years. Brain tumors are more common in boys than in girls.

Bone cancers Cancer usually spreads to the bones from other sites, but some types originate in the skeleton. The most common BONE CANCER in children is osteogenic sarcoma.

Bone cancer in children occurs most often during adolescent growth spurts; 85 percent of affected teenagers have tumors on their legs or arms, half of them around the knee. Ewing's sarcoma differs from osteosarcoma in that it affects the bone shaft, and tends to be found in bones other than the long bones of the arm and the leg, such as in the ribs. Between 1950 and 1980s, child deaths from bone cancer dropped by 50 percent.

Lymphomas This type of cancer begins in the lymph system, the body's circulatory network designed to filter out impurities. There are two general types of lymphoma: Hodgkin's disease and non-Hodgkin's lymphoma. Non-Hodgkin's lymphoma is more common in children; it can occur in the tonsils, thymus, bone, small intestine, spleen, or in lymph glands. The disease can spread to the central nervous system and the bone marrow. Today treatments can cure many children, and promising new treatments are being developed.

Neuroblastoma This type of tumor is found only in children and begins in the adrenal glands near the kidneys. Neuroblastoma usually appears in very young children.

Rhabdomyosarcoma The most common soft tissue sarcoma in children, this extremely malignant tumor originates in muscles, usually in the head and neck area (including the eyes), the genitourinary tract, or in the arms and legs. Although rhabdomyosarcoma tends to spread quickly, its symptoms are easy to spot compared to other forms of childhood cancer.

Wilms' tumor This rapidly developing tumor of the kidney most often appears in children between the ages of two and four. The characteristics of WILMS' TUMOR in children are different from those of KIDNEY CANCER in adults. In children the disease often spreads to the lungs; in the past, the death rate from this cancer was extremely high. However, treatments combining surgery, radiation therapy, and CHEMOTHERAPY have been very effective in controlling the disease. As a result, cure rates for Wilms' tumor have improved.

Retinoblastoma This hereditary malignant eye tumor occurs in infants and young children, accounting for just 2 percent of childhood cancer. This disease is the first cancer for which researchers identified a tumor suppressor gene.

Other Other rare forms of childhood cancers include GERM CELL CANCER, THYROID CANCER, malignant MELANOMA, TESTICULAR CANCER, and primary cancers in the kidney, liver, and lung.

Childhood vs. Adult Cancers

Cancer in children and young people has different characteristics from cancer in adults. For example, young patients often have a more advanced stage of cancer when first diagnosed. While only about 20 percent of adults with cancer show evidence that the disease has already spread when it is diagnosed, 80 percent of children's cancer has already invaded distant sites at diagnosis.

While most adult cancers are linked to lifestyle factors such as smoking, diet, or exposure to cancer-causing agents, the causes of most childhood cancers are unknown.

Adult cancers primarily affect the lung, colon, breast, prostate, and pancreas, while childhood cancers usually affect the white blood cells (leukemias), brain, bone, the lymphatic system, muscles, kidneys, and nervous system.

While most adult cancer patients are treated in their local communities, cancers in children are rarely treated by family physicians or pediatricians. A child with cancer must be diagnosed precisely and treated by physicians and clinical and laboratory scientists who have special expertise in managing the care of children with cancer. Such teams are found only in major children's hospitals, university medical centers, and cancer centers.

Childhood Cancer Survivor Study (CCSS) A study that was created to learn about the long-term effects of cancer and its therapy on CHILDHOOD CANCER survivors (http://www.cancer.umn.edu/ltfu#CCSS). This knowledge may be useful in designing future treatments that increase survival and minimize harmful health effects. In addition, the CCSS serves to educate survivors about the potential impacts of cancer diagnosis and treatment on their health.

The CCSS includes 14,000 childhood cancer survivors diagnosed with cancer before the age of 20 between 1970 and 1986 and approximately 3,500 siblings of survivors, who serve as control subjects for the study. The study includes 27 participating centers in the United States and Canada and is coordinated by investigators at the University of Minnesota. Initiated in 1993, the study was funded by the NATIONAL CANCER INSTITUTE for continuation through 2004.

Long-term survivors of childhood cancer are at risk of developing second cancers and of experiencing organ dysfunction, reduced growth and development, decreased fertility, and early death. The degree of risk of late effects may be influenced by various treatment-related factors such as the intensity, duration, and timing of therapy, as well as by individual characteristics such as the type of cancer diagnosis, the person's sex, age at time of treatment, and genetic factors such as the child's family history of cancer.

children's cancer centers Hospitals or units in hospitals that specialize in the diagnosis and treatment of cancer in children and adolescents. A childhood CANCER CENTER should be staffed by trained pediatric ONCOLOGISTS and other specialists who work as a team, including pediatric surgeons, specialist surgeons, radiation oncologists, pathologists, nurses, consulting pediatric specialists, psychiatrists and psychologists, oncology social workers, nutritionists, and home health-care professionals. Together, these professionals offer comprehensive care.

Because childhood cancer is relatively rare, it is important to seek centers that specialize in the treatment of children with cancer. Specialized cancer programs at comprehensive, multidisciplinary cancer centers follow established step-by-step guidelines for treatment carried out using a team approach. The team of health professionals is involved in designing the appropriate treatment and support program for the child and the child's family. In addition, these centers participate in specially designed and monitored research studies that help develop more effective treatments and address issues of long-term childhood cancer survival.

The Pediatric Oncology Branch (POB) of the NATIONAL CANCER INSTITUTE (NCI) conducts clinical trials for a wide variety of childhood cancers at the Warren Grant Magnuson Clinical Center at the National Institutes of Health in Bethesda, Maryland. There is no charge to patients for services provided at the center. Children, teenagers, and young adults with newly diagnosed or recurrent cancer may be referred to the POB. To refer a patient with cancer, the patient's doctor should call the POB's toll-free number at 1-877-624-4878 between 8:30 A.M. and 5 P.M. and ask for the attending physician. The attending physician will discuss the case with the patient's doctor, determine whether the patient is eligible for treatment at the NCI, and help arrange the referral. The POB can also be reached on the Internet at www-dcs.nci.nih.gov/branches/pedonc/index.html.

POB attending physicians also are available to provide a second opinion about a patient. The patient, family, or physician can contact the POB to arrange for a second opinion. POB staff can offer assistance in cases where a diagnosis is difficult and can aid in developing an appropriate treatment plan.

Alternatively, a family's pediatrician or family doctor often can provide a referral to a comprehensive children's cancer center. Families and health professionals also can call the NCI's Cancer Information Service at 1-800-4-CANCER to learn about children's cancer centers that belong to the Children's Cancer Study Group and the Pediatric Oncology Group. All of the cancer centers that participate in these groups have met strict standards of excellence for childhood cancer care.

Some health plans cover part or all of the cost of care at children's cancer centers, but benefits vary from plan to plan. Questions or concerns about health-care costs should be discussed with a medical social worker or the hospital or clinic billing office. Financial assistance and resources to cover health-care costs may be available.

Children's Hospice International A nonprofit organization founded in 1983 to promote HOSPICE support through pediatric care facilities, to encourage the inclusion of children in existing and developing hospice and home-care programs, and to include hospice perspectives in all areas of pediatric care, education, and the public arena. The organization provides resources and referrals to children with life-threatening conditions and their families, helps to establish children's hospice programs worldwide, provides education and training for health-care providers, and advocates on behalf of children and families. For contact information, see Appendix I.

Children's Oncology Group (COG) A research group, supported by the NATIONAL CANCER INSTITUTE, that conducts clinical trials devoted exclusively to children and adolescents with cancer at more than 200 member institutions, including cancer centers at all major universities, teaching hospitals throughout the United States and Canada, and sites in Europe and Australia.

COG was formed in 2000 by the merger of four children's cancer cooperative groups in order to accelerate the search for a cure for the cancers of children and to make it possible for children with cancer, regardless of where they live, to have access to state-of-the art therapies and the collective expertise of world-renowned pediatric specialists.

cholangiosarcoma See BILE DUCT CANCER.

cholecystectomy The surgical removal of the gallbladder.

cholesteatoma See BRAIN CANCER.

chondrosarcoma See BONE CANCER.

chordoma See BONE CANCER.

choriocarcinoma A rare cancer that generally occurs in women of childbearing age in which cancer cells grow in the tissues that are formed in the uterus after conception. It is also called gestational trophoblastic disease, gestational trophoblastic neoplasia, gestational trophoblastic tumor, or molar pregnancy.

This type of cancer is more common in older women and responds well to CHEMOTHERAPY. Typically, the tumor begins within the uterus. It may invade the wall of the uterus and spread through the lymphatic system or the bloodstream. Once it has spread, it may appear in the vagina, vulva, lungs, liver, brain, and LYMPH NODES.

Choriocarcinoma may occasionally appear in men, developing in a tumor of the testicles or the pineal gland.

choroid plexus papilloma See BRAIN CANCER.

choroid plexus tumor See BRAIN CANCER.

chronic phase The early stages of chronic myelogenous LEUKEMIA. The number of mature and immature abnormal white blood cells in the bone marrow and blood is higher than normal, but lower than in the accelerated or blast phase.

cigarettes See SMOKING.

cigars See CIGAR SMOKING AND CANCER; SMOKING.

cigar smoking and cancer Studies have shown that cancers of the oral cavity (lip, tongue, mouth, and throat), larynx, lung, and esophagus—and possibly pancreatic cancer—are all associated with cigar smoking. In addition, daily cigar smokers (particularly those who inhale) have a higher risk of developing heart and lung disease. As with cigarette smoking, the more a person smokes cigars, the higher the cancer risks.

Smoking only one to two cigars per day doubles the risk for oral and esophageal cancers. Smoking three to four cigars daily can increase the risk of oral cancers to more than eight times that of a nonsmoker, while the chance of esophageal cancer is increased to four times the risk for someone who has never smoked. Both cigar and cigarette smokers have similar levels of risk for oral, throat, and esophageal cancers.

The health risks associated with occasional cigar smoking (less than daily) are not known; about three-quarters of cigar smokers are occasional smokers.

Cigars vs. Cigarettes

One of the major differences between cigar and cigarette smoking is the degree of inhalation. Almost all cigarette smokers say they inhale, while most cigar smokers do not, because cigar smoke is generally more irritating. However, cigar smokers who have a history of cigarette smoking are more likely to inhale cigar smoke.

Cigar smokers experience higher rates of lung cancer, coronary heart disease, and chronic obstructive lung disease than do nonsmokers, but not as high as the rates for cigarette smokers. These lower rates for cigar smokers are probably related to reduced inhalation.

There are other differences between cigars and cigarettes. They are different sizes and use different types of tobacco. Cigarettes usually contain less than a gram of tobacco each, whereas cigars can vary in size and shape—and can measure more than seven inches long. Large cigars typically contain between five and 17 grams of tobacco; it is not unusual for some premium cigars to contain the tobacco equivalent of an entire pack of cigarettes.

And while U.S. cigarettes are made from different blends of tobaccos, most cigars include one type of tobacco (air-cured or dried burley tobacco). In addition, large cigars can take between one and two hours to smoke, whereas most cigarettes on the U.S. market take less than 10 minutes to smoke.

Although cigar smoking occurs primarily among men between the ages of 35 and 64 who have higher educational backgrounds and incomes, most new cigar users today are teenagers and young adult men (ages 18 to 24) who smoke less than daily. Cigar use has increased nearly five times among women and appears to be increasing among adolescent women as well. Furthermore, a number of studies have reported high rates of use not only among teens but among preteens. Cigar use among older men (age 65 and older), however, has continued to decline since 1992.

c-kit receptor A protein on the surface of some cells that binds to STEM CELL factor (a substance that causes certain types of cells to grow). Altered forms of this receptor may be associated with some types of cancer.

clear cell adenocarcinoma A type of curable cancer that occurs in glandular tissue and that has been linked to the antimiscarriage drug DIETHYLSTILBESTROL (DES). This synthetic hormone was prescribed to pregnant women between 1940 and 1971—about 4 million women in the United States alone.

Before 1971 clear cell adenocarcinoma of the vagina or cervix was a rare disease, diagnosed primarily in women over age 70. In 1971, however, doctors documented several cases of this cancer in young women whose mothers had taken DES during pregnancy. This discovery led the U.S. Food and Drug Administration in 1971 to ban the use of DES during pregnancy.

Researchers estimate that approximately one in 1,000 daughters of mothers who took DES are at risk of developing the cancer, although this number may turn out to be higher as the daughters age. Fortunately, more than 80 percent of the women who have had clear cell adenocarcinoma have recovered.

So far, clear cell adenocarcinoma has been found in DES daughters between the ages of seven and 48. It is important for DES daughters and their physicians to be aware that there is no specific age after which the risk for this type of clear cell cancer is over. Today, the upper age limit for the development of the cancer is unknown.

Symptoms

Symptoms of adenocarcinoma in the vagina or cervix include bleeding or discharge not related to menstrual periods, difficult or painful urination, painful intercourse, pelvic pain, constipation, or a mass that can be felt. Even if a woman has had a HYSTERECTOMY, she still has a chance of developing adenocarcinoma in the vagina.

Diagnosis

DES daughters should have a gynecological exam once a year, including a thorough pelvic examination with careful visual examination, a cervical PAP TEST, a vaginal Pap test taken from all four sides of the vagina, and a manual inspection of the vagina. The recommended pelvic exam for a DES daughter is different from a routine exam, in which the Pap smear is taken only from the cervix.

Treatment

The most common treatment is surgery—a radical hysterectomy (removal of uterus, fallopian tubes, and one or both ovaries), vaginectomy (removal of all or part of the vagina), and LYMPHADENECTOMY (removal of surrounding lymph gland). A vaginectomy is necessary only if diagnosis includes VAGINAL CANCER. Internal and external radiation may also be used to treat the cancer, alone or in conjunction with surgery.

clear cell sarcoma of the kidney   See KIDNEY CANCER.

clinical cancer centers   A type of CANCER CENTER sponsored by the NATIONAL CANCER INSTITUTE that conducts programs in clinical research, and also may support programs in other areas such as basic research or prevention, control, and population-based research. The focus on both laboratory research and clinical research within the same institutional framework is a distinguishing characteristic of many clinical cancer centers. For contact information for individual clinical cancer centers, see Appendix II.

clinical trial   A kind of research study that compares a specific treatment currently recognized as the best available (called the "standard of care") with a new treatment that the study's researchers believe is even safer or more effective. If clinical trials prove a new treatment to be more effective than current therapies, then it may become the new standard of care.

Some patients agree to participate in clinical trials because this is a way to obtain high-quality cancer care with constant monitoring. If patients are in a study and do not receive the new treatment being tested, they will still receive the best standard treatment, which may be as good as or better than the new approach. If a new treatment approach is proven to work, patients taking this treatment in the clinical trial may be among the first to benefit. Some patients also like the idea that they are helping to further research that may benefit future patients.

On the other hand, there is no way to be sure whether the new treatment will work. New treatments being studied are not always better than (or even as good as) standard care, and they may have side effects that doctors do not expect or that are worse than those of standard treatment. Moreover, not everyone benefits from a new treatment. Even standard treatments, proven effective for many people, do not help everyone. In addition, patients in the "control" group receive only standard therapy. If patients receive standard treatment instead of the new treatment being tested, it may not be as effective as the new approach.

Clinical trials move through three phases before the final outcome leads to a potential new treatment.

Phase I

These trials are the first step in testing new treatments in patients, and are designed to determine how the treatment should be given and at what dose. Because less is known about the possible risks and benefits in phase I trials, these studies usually include only a small number of patients who would not be helped by other known treatments.

Phase II

In this phase, researchers examine possible side effects and how well the treatment works (for example, how much a tumor shrinks). Although these trials are larger than phase I trials, they still include only a small number of patients because the usefulness and the side effects of the new treatments are still unknown.

Phase III

Phase III trials compare the results for people taking the new treatment with results for people taking standard treatment to see which group has better survival rates and fewer side effects. Patients are randomly divided into each treatment group, one receiving the new treatment and the other receiving the current standard-of-care treatment. Sometimes patients do not know which group they are in.

Usually studies move into phase III testing only after a treatment has shown promise in phases I and II. Phase III trials may include many hundreds of people around the country.

Safety

Cancer clinical trials are tightly regulated and closely monitored by the federal government to make sure each phase of the study is as safe as possible. All clinical trials must follow a detailed plan (the "protocol") written by the researchers and approved by the institutional review board at each institution. This board, which includes consumers, clergy, and health professionals, reviews the protocol to try to be sure that the research will not expose patients to extreme or unethical risks.

In addition, each patient must receive all the facts about a study before deciding whether to take part, including details about treatments, tests, possible benefits, and risks. Each patient must sign an informed consent form that highlights key facts. The informed consent process continues throughout the study. (For instance, if new risks of the treatment are discovered during a trial, the patients will be told of any new findings and must sign a new consent form to stay in the study.) Signing a consent form does not mean patients are required to stay in the study; patients can withdraw at any time.

A complete list of clinical trials relating to cancer and detailed information about clinical trials are available at the Web site of the NATIONAL CANCER INSTITUTE: http://www.cancer.gov/clinical_trials/finding.

CLL   See LEUKEMIA.

cloacogenic cancer   See ANAL CANCER.

CML   See LEUKEMIA.

coactivated T cells   T cells that have been stimulated by antibodies to enhance their ability to kill tumor cells.

cobalt 60   A radioactive form of the metal cobalt, which is used as a source of radiation to treat cancer.
    See also COBALT TREATMENT.

cobalt treatment   A type of RADIATION THERAPY using the metal cobalt first employed in 1951 to treat cancer.

coenzyme Q10 (ubiquinone, or ubidecarenone) A compound produced naturally in the body that helps cells produce energy needed for cell growth and maintenance. Coenzyme Q10 is found in most body tissues, especially in the heart, liver, kidneys, and pancreas; the lowest amounts are found in the lungs. It is also an ANTIOXIDANT (a substance that protects cells from harmful chemicals called FREE RADICALS).

Studies with cancer patients have shown that coenzyme Q10 decreases the harmful effects of the CHEMOTHERAPY drug doxorubicin on the heart. However, no report of a randomized clinical trial of coenzyme Q10 as a treatment for cancer itself has been published in a peer-reviewed, scientific journal.

Coenzyme Q10 was first identified in 1957, but scientists did not consider its use as a potential cancer drug until 1961, when a deficiency of the enzyme was noted in the blood of cancer patients. Low blood levels of coenzyme Q10 have been found in patients with MYELOMA, LYMPHOMA, and cancers of the breast, lung, prostate, pancreas, colon, kidney, and head and neck.

Some studies have suggested that coenzyme Q10 stimulates the immune system and increases resistance to disease. In part because of this, researchers have theorized that coenzyme Q10 may be useful as an ADJUVANT THERAPY for cancer. Animal studies have found that coenzyme Q10 stimulated the immune system and increased resistance to disease; it also helped protect the hearts of animals given the anticancer drug doxorubicin, which can cause damage to the heart muscle.

There have been three small studies of coenzyme Q10 that seem to show a positive effect on breast cancer, but all three studies had problems with their design that may have influenced results.

No serious side effects have been reported from the use of coenzyme Q10. Some patients using coenzyme Q10 have experienced mild insomnia, higher levels of liver enzymes, rashes, NAUSEA, and upper abdominal pain. Other reported side effects have included dizziness, visual sensitivity to light, irritability, headache, heartburn, and FATIGUE.

Patients should discuss with their health-care provider possible interactions between coenzyme Q10 and prescription drugs they may be taking. Certain drugs, such as those that are used to lower cholesterol or blood sugar levels, may also reduce the effects of coenzyme Q10. Coenzyme Q10 may also alter the body's response to warfarin (a drug that prevents the blood from clotting) and insulin.

Coenzyme Q10 is used by the body as an antioxidant, which protects cells from free radicals, the highly reactive chemicals that can damage cells. Some conventional cancer therapies, such as CHEMOTHERAPY and RADIATION THERAPY, are designed to kill cancer cells in part by triggering free radicals to form. Researchers are studying whether combining coenzyme Q10 with conventional therapies is effective or harmful in fighting cancer.

Several companies distribute coenzyme Q10 as a dietary supplement, which is regulated as a food, not a drug. This means that evaluation and approval by the U.S. Food and Drug Administration are not required before marketing, unless specific health claims are made about the supplement. Because dietary supplements are not formally reviewed for manufacturing consistency, there may be variations in the composition of the supplement from one batch to another.

cold nodule Nodules that collect less radioactive material than surrounding thyroid tissue during examination of the thyroid with a scanner using radioactive material. A nodule that is "cold" does not make thyroid hormone and may be either benign or cancerous. Cold nodules are sometimes called low-functioning nodules and are often biopsied to rule out malignancy.

colectomy An operation to remove a section of the colon, performed as a treatment for COLORECTAL CANCER. An open colectomy is the removal of a section of the colon through a surgical incision made in the wall of the abdomen. Laparoscopic-assisted colectomy uses a thin, lighted tube attached to a video camera that allows the surgeon to remove the colon without a large incision.

colo-anal anastomosis A surgical procedure, used as a treatment for COLORECTAL CANCER, in which the colon is attached to the anus after the rectum has been removed. The procedure is also called a colo-anal pull-through.

colo-anal pull-through See COLO-ANAL ANASTOMOSIS.

colon cancer See COLORECTAL CANCER.

colonoscopy An examination of the inside of the colon using a thin, lighted tube (a colonoscope) inserted into the rectum. If the doctor sees any abnormal areas (tumors or polyps), tissue or an entire polyp can be removed and examined under a microscope to determine whether the tissue is malignant. Colonoscopy is a diagnostic tool used to detect COLORECTAL CANCER.

colon polyps Abnormal growths of tissue in the lining of the bowel that pose a higher risk of colon cancer.

See also COLORECTAL CANCER.

colony-stimulating factor (CSF; hematopoietic growth factors) A natural or genetically-altered protein that encourage BONE MARROW stem cells to divide and develop into white blood cells, platelets, and red blood cells. CSFs are used by doctors to help patients undergoing cancer treatment boost their blood counts. Because CHEMOTHERAPY drugs can damage the body's ability to make blood cells, patients receiving these drugs have a higher risk of developing infections, becoming anemic, and bleeding more easily.

Researchers are also studying CSFs as a way to treat some types of LEUKEMIA, metastatic COLORECTAL CANCER, MELANOMA, LUNG CANCER, and other types of cancer.

By using CSFs to stimulate blood cell production, doctors can increase the doses of anticancer drugs without increasing the risk of infection or the need for transfusion with blood products. As a result, researchers have found CSFs particularly useful when combined with high-dose chemotherapy.

Some examples of CSFs and their use in cancer therapy are the following:

- *G-CSF* (filgrastim) and *GM-CSF* (sargramostim) increase the number of white blood cells, reducing the risk of infection in patients receiving chemotherapy. They can also stimulate the production of stem cells in preparation for STEM CELL or BONE MARROW TRANSPLANTS.

- *ERYTHROPOIETIN* increases the number of red blood cells and reduces the need for red blood cell transfusions in patients receiving chemotherapy

- *Oprelvekin* reduces the need for platelet transfusions in patients receiving chemotherapy

colorectal cancer The appearance of cancerous cells either in the rectum, the colon, or the cecum (a pouch in the first part of the intestine). Because the rectum is part of the colon, colon cancer and rectal cancer are often referred to as one disease; cancers affecting either of these organs may also be called colorectal cancer.

Together, cancers of the colon and rectum are among the most common cancers in the United States; nearly 7 percent of Americans will develop colon cancer at some point in their lives. It occurs in both men and women and is most often found among people who are over the age of 50. Excluding SKIN CANCERS, colorectal cancer is the third most common cancer diagnosed in men and women in the United States. There were about 107,300 new cases of colon cancer (50,000 men and 57,300 women) and 41,000 new cases of rectal cancer (22,600 men and 18,400 women) diagnosed in 2002.

The annual death rate for colorectal cancer is 57,100. This rate has been dropping for the past 20 years, in part because there are fewer cases, they are being found earlier, and treatments have improved. Although the five-year relative survival rate is 90 percent for people whose colorectal cancer is treated at an early stage, unfortunately only 37 percent of colorectal cancers are found at that early stage. Once the cancer has spread to nearby organs or LYMPH NODES, the five-year relative survival rate drops to 65 percent. For people whose colorectal cancer has spread to distant parts of the body such as the liver or lungs, the five-year relative survival rate is a mere 8 percent.

Although the death rate has been declining since 1985, it has not declined among African Americans, for whom colon cancer takes a higher toll. A new 2002 study reveals the death rate for colorectal cancer among poor African Americans remains very high, despite a steady drop among other groups in the United States. Doctors attribute this primarily to patients not receiving initial treatment until a late stage of the disease. In the study the overall five-year survival for these patients was 19.7 percent, dramatically lower than the national average, which rose from 49.5 percent in 1974 to 61.5 percent in 1992. Previous studies show that the stage of the disease at the time of diagnosis is the most important factor in determining the outcome of colorectal carcinoma.

Risks

How general risk factors for colorectal cancer relate to a specific person's risk and to death rate is not completely clear. Some people with a number of risk factors will never develop cancer, whereas others with few or no risk factors will develop it. Nevertheless, the statistics associated with some risk factors remain consistent:

Age   Colorectal cancer is more common in people over the age of 50, although it can occur at younger ages and even in rare cases in adolescence.

Diet   Colorectal cancer seems to be associated with poor diets that are high in saturated fat and calories and low in fiber.

Alcohol   Regular drinkers significantly increase their risk of rectal cancer (but not colon cancer)—but that risk is reduced if wine makes up a third or more of weekly consumption. New research shows a clear association between rectal cancer risk and the amount of alcohol consumed.

Polyps   Polyps are benign growths on the inner wall of the colon and rectum that are fairly common in people over age 50. Some types of polyps increase a person's risk of developing colorectal cancer. A rare, inherited condition called familial polyposis causes hundreds of polyps in the colon and rectum. Unless this condition is treated, familial polyposis is almost certain to lead to colorectal cancer.

Personal medical history   Women with a history of cancer of the ovary, uterus, or breast have a somewhat higher chance of developing colorectal cancer as well. A person who has had colorectal cancer may develop this disease a second time.

Family history   First-degree relatives of a person who has had colorectal cancer are somewhat more likely to develop this type of cancer themselves, especially if the relative had the cancer at a young age. If many family members have had colorectal cancer, the chances increase even more. Genetic blood tests are now available to determine a person's risk.

Ulcerative colitis   This inflammation of the lining of the colon increases a person's chance of developing colorectal cancer.

Sedentary lifestyle   People who exercise regularly have half the risk of colon cancer (even regular brisk walking may reduce a person's risk).

Research

Research shows that colorectal cancer develops gradually from benign polyps, and that early detection and removal of polyps may help to prevent colorectal cancer. Scientists are studying possible ways to prevent colorectal cancer via smoking cessation, dietary supplements, aspirin or similar medicines, lower alcohol consumption, and increased physical activity. Some studies suggest that a diet low in fat and calories and high in fiber can help prevent colorectal cancer.

Certain tests can detect polyps, cancer, or other abnormalities, even when a person does not have symptoms:

- *Fecal occult blood test.* This checks for hidden blood in the stool. Sometimes cancers or polyps can bleed, and this test can detect small amounts of bleeding.
- *Sigmoidoscopy.* The examination of the rectum and lower colon with a lighted instrument called a sigmoidoscope.
- *Colonoscopy.* The examination of the rectum and entire colon using a lighted instrument called a colonoscope.
- *Double contrast barium enema.* This is a series of X-rays of the colon and rectum.
- *Digital rectal exam.* In this exam the doctor inserts a lubricated, gloved finger into the rectum to feel for abnormal areas.

Symptoms

Common signs and symptoms of colorectal cancer include

- abdominal discomfort (frequent gas pains, bloating, fullness, and/or cramps)
- blood (either bright red or very dark) in the stool
- bowel habit changes
- diarrhea, constipation, or a feeling that the bowel does not empty completely
- fatigue
- stools that are narrower than usual
- vomiting
- weight loss

Diagnosis

Diagnosis may include medical history, physical exam, and diagnostic tests such as X-rays of the large intestine, SIGMOIDOSCOPY, COLONOSCOPY, polypectomy (the removal of a polyp during a sigmoidoscopy or colonoscopy), or a biopsy.

A new noninvasive experimental test may one day detect colon cancer in its early stages by checking for gene mutations. The test, which screens a patient's stool for a faulty cancer-suppressor gene, could potentially be more accurate than the current fecal occult blood tests. However, investigators expect that this test will not be commercially available until 2008.

The new test is believed to be the first to reliably pinpoint colon cancer-linked gene mutations in DNA shed into feces. Although scientists had long suspected that an early colon cancer marker was present in cells shed into stool, it required several years of additional research to develop the technology to identify reliably the mutated DNA.

Staging

If the diagnosis is cancer, the doctor needs to learn the extent of disease and if and where it has spread. Knowing the stage of the disease helps the doctor plan treatment. The stages of colorectal cancer include

Stage 0: Very early cancer found only in the innermost lining of the colon or rectum.

Stage I: The cancer involves more of the inner wall of the colon or rectum.

Stage II: The cancer has spread outside the colon or rectum to nearby tissue, but not to the lymph nodes.

Stage III: The cancer has spread to nearby lymph nodes, but not to other parts of the body.

Stage IV: The cancer has spread to other parts of the body (especially the liver and/or lungs).

Recurrent: The cancer has returned after treatment. The disease may recur in the colon or rectum or in another part of the body.

Treatment

Treatment depends mainly on the size, location, and extent of the tumor, and on the patient's general health.

Surgery This is the most common treatment for colorectal cancer. Generally, the surgeon removes the tumor along with part of the healthy colon or rectum and nearby lymph nodes. In most cases, the doctor is able to reconnect the healthy portions of the colon or rectum, but if the surgeon cannot reconnect the healthy portions, a temporary or permanent COLOSTOMY is needed.

In a colostomy, the surgeon creates an opening (stoma) through the wall of the abdomen into the colon, providing a new path for waste material to leave the body. After a colostomy, the patient wears a special bag to collect body waste. Some patients need a temporary colostomy to allow the lower colon or rectum to heal after surgery, but about 15 percent of colorectal cancer patients require a permanent colostomy.

Chemotherapy This may be given to destroy any cancerous cells that may remain in the body after surgery, to control tumor growth, or to relieve symptoms. Most anticancer drugs are given by IV injection or through a catheter into a large vein. The catheter remains in place as long as it is needed. Some anticancer drugs are given by mouth.

Radiation therapy This is most often used in patients whose cancer is in the rectum. Doctors may use radiation along with chemotherapy before surgery to shrink a tumor so that it is easier to remove, or after surgery to destroy any cancer cells that remain in the treated area. Radiation therapy is also used to relieve symptoms. The radiation may be either internal or external, and some patients have both types.

Biological therapy This repairs, stimulates, or enhances the immune system's natural anticancer function. Biological therapy may be given after surgery, either alone or in combination with chemotherapy or radiation treatment. Most biological treatments are given by IV injection. Recently, two new monoclonal antibodies have been approved for treatment of metastatic COLON CANCER. The first cetuximab (Erbitux) targets the epidermal growth factor receptor expression on colon cancer cells. The second, bevacizumab (Avastin) binds to and inhibits vascular endothelial growth factor, curtailing tumor blood vessel growth.

Recurrence

Cancer will return in 10 percent to 30 percent of colon cancer patients after initial treatment, but doctors have no way of being able to say who is more susceptible. Scientists in Atlanta and Baltimore have developed a new chromosome-testing technique that may accurately predict whether cancer will return in colon cancer patients. Previous research had shown that if certain chromosome imbalances occur, cancer cells can return after treatment. The new research, led by a scientist at Emory University's Winship Cancer Institute, is the first to utilize a technique that looks at specific chromosome markers that can predict whether a patient will suffer a recurrence of colorectal cancer. The technique definitively shows where cancer cells might be able to come back and grow after chemotherapy, radiation, or surgery.

Researchers examined tumor samples taken from 180 colorectal patients from four hospitals in the United States and Europe. If two particular chromosome markers—on chromosomes 8 and 18—were present, there was a low risk of cancer recurrence, the study found. But if they lost both sets of markers, on average they had a 46 percent chance of recurrence.

The technique also could be applicable to other cancers, but researchers expressed caution because much has yet to be proven through further studies. It could be years before the test might be used in patients.

Colorectal Cancer Network   A nonprofit organization for patients, their families, and friends that offers support groups, listservs, chat rooms, and a "matching list" to connect newly diagnosed patients with long-term survivors. The group also offers an extensive library of colorectal cancer information, other relevant links, literature, awareness pins, and T-shirts. For contact information, see Appendix I.

colostomy   An opening into the colon from the outside of the body that provides a new path for waste material to leave the body after part of the colon has been removed.

colposcopy   An examination of a woman's vagina and cervix using a tubular instrument with a light source and lenses that magnify up to 25 times. Also called a vaginoscopy, this test may allow the doctor to remove tissue for a BIOPSY. The procedure lasts between 10 and 15 minutes and may be done in a doctor's office.

comedo carcinoma   A type of ductal carcinoma in situ (very early-stage BREAST CANCER).

common cold virus   A genetically engineered version of a common cold virus has been studied as a potential treatment for COLORECTAL CANCER and STOMACH CANCER. Investigators in a multicenter study reported that a therapeutic adenovirus, when injected into the artery leading to the liver, appears to kill tumors that have spread to the organ. It does this without harming healthy liver tissue.

COLORECTAL CANCER kills 50,000 people every year in the United States and typically spreads to the liver, as do stomach, pancreatic, and other forms of gastrointestinal cancer. Treatment options after spread to the liver include surgery and CHEMOTHERAPY, but these benefit only a minority of patients. This virus could become part of a new generation of chemotherapy agents that are much more selective about what they attack. Standard chemotherapy kills some healthy cells along with the cancer, but genetically engineered cold viruses are designed to kill only the cancer and not to harm healthy cells.

Although the therapy is genetically based, it is not strictly gene therapy. Normally with gene therapy, a specific gene is spliced into a deactivated virus, and the virus acts as a way to get the gene inside the body's cells. In this case, the live virus itself—without any extra gene—is used as the treatment. Rather than being injected directly into the tumor, where it might not get distributed evenly, it is injected into the liver artery, so that the flow of blood carries it throughout the organ, treating each tumor. (People with cancer that has spread to the liver typically have multiple tumors in the liver.)

Although this synthetic virus is live, it is genetically engineered to be weaker, and therefore it is not as highly infectious as a normal cold virus. It was designed to infect only cells with an abnormality in the tumor suppressor gene, p53. This abnormality may explain why those cells are susceptible to cancer to begin with. P53 is part of the body's own surveillance system, which detects and destroys most early cancers. About one-half to two-thirds of cancers have abnormal p53 function.

Most patients feel sick with a mild flu for up to a week after the injection, although not as ill as they typically feel after standard chemotherapy. Unlike most viruses used in gene therapy, this virus retains the ability to replicate. Because it copies itself, the virus is very effective at depleting the cancerous cell's resources and killing it. When the cancerous cell dies, it breaks open and releases the virus and all its copies, which can then infect other cancerous cells and start the process again.

Although the lack of p53 makes a cell aggressive and cancerous, it also means it cannot recognize when it is being infected by a virus. It makes the cell particularly susceptible to viral infection by this particular engineered virus.

The first phase of the study on this virus was conducted to determine whether the treatment is safe and what dose can be tolerated by patients. In the phase II study, investigators will treat cancer patients with the virus as well as standard chemotherapy to try to confirm the beneficial effects of the virus; the virus seems to have an additive effect with chemotherapy. It could be years before it is approved for standard treatment.

complementary and alternative medicine (CAM)

A broad group of healing philosophies, approaches and products (also referred to as integrative medicine) that are not presently considered to be part of conventional medicine.

Complementary treatment is generally considered to be therapy used in addition to conventional treatments; "alternative" treatments usually indicate it is used *instead of* conventional treatment. Conventional treatments are those that are widely accepted and practiced by the mainstream medical community.

Although there is scientific evidence for the effectiveness and safety of some CAM therapies, in general many of these therapies have not been scientifically tested. As CAM therapies are proven safe and effective through rigorous studies, they are adopted into conventional health care. Though grouped together, complementary and alternative medicines are different from each other. Complementary medicine is used together with conventional medicine. An example of complementary therapy is the use of aromatherapy to help lessen a patient's discomfort following surgery. Alternative medicine is used in place of conventional medicine. An example of alternative medicine is using a special diet to treat cancer instead of undergoing surgery, radiation, or chemotherapy that has been recommended by a conventional health care practitioner.

The National Center for Complementary and Alternative Medicine (NCCAM) has classified CAM therapies into five groups:

- alternative medical systems (for example, homeopathic medicine and traditional Chinese medicine)
- mind-body interventions, such as visualization or relaxation
- manipulative and body-based methods such as chiropractic and massage
- biologically based therapies such as vitamins and herbal products
- energy therapies such as qi gong and therapeutic touch

Research indicates that the use of CAM therapies is increasing. A large-scale study published in the November 11, 1998, issue of the *Journal of the American Medical Association* found that CAM use among the general public increased from 34 percent in 1990 to 42 percent in 1997. Several surveys of CAM use by cancer patients have been conducted with small numbers of patients. One study published in the February 2000 issue of the journal *Cancer* reported that 37 percent of 46 patients with prostate cancer used one or more CAM therapies as part of their cancer treatment. These therapies included herbal remedies, old-time remedies, vitamins, and special diets. A larger study of CAM use in patients with different types of cancer was published in the July 2000 issue of the *Journal of Clinical Oncology*. That study found that 83 percent of 453 cancer patients had used at least one CAM therapy as part of their cancer treatment. The study included CAM therapies such as special diets, psychotherapy, spiritual practices, and vitamin supplements. When psychotherapy and spiritual practices were excluded, 69 percent of patients had used at least one CAM therapy in their cancer treatment.

Cancer patients considering complementary or alternative therapy should discuss this decision with their doctor, because some complementary and alternative therapies may interfere with standard treatment or may be harmful when used with conventional treatment. It is also a good idea to become informed about the therapy, including whether the results of scientific studies support the claims that are made for it.

Unlike conventional treatments for cancer, complementary and alternative therapies are often not covered by insurance companies. Cancer patients considering complementary and alternative therapies should discuss this decision with their doctor because this may interfere with standard treatment or may be harmful when used with conventional treatment.

complete blood count (CBC) A test to check the number of red blood cells, white blood cells, and platelets in a sample of blood. Because CHEMOTHERAPY can inhibit the body's production of red blood cells, causing ANEMIA, it is important to monitor blood cell counts of cancer patients receiving this treatment. Doctors routinely order a CBC test before each chemotherapy treatment to make sure a patient's red blood cell count has not dropped too low. A CBC is one of the most important tests that people with cancer routinely take.

complete remission The disappearance of all signs of cancer in response to treatment. This does not always mean the cancer has been cured.

comprehensive cancer center A type of special cancer institution sponsored by the NATIONAL CANCER INSTITUTE (NCI) that conducts programs in all three areas of research—basic, clinical, and prevention and control—as well as programs in community outreach and education.

In 1990 there were 19 comprehensive cancer centers across the country. Today more than 40 cancer centers meet the NCI criteria for "comprehensive" status.

Each type of cancer center has special characteristics and capabilities for organizing new programs of research. To be recognized by the NCI as a comprehensive cancer center, an institution must pass rigorous peer review, perform research in the three major areas mentioned above, and must also

have a strong body of interactive research that bridges these research areas.

In addition, a comprehensive cancer center must provide outreach, education, and information directed toward and accessible to both health-care professionals and the lay community.

All NCI-designated cancer centers are reevaluated each time their grant comes up for renewal (generally every three to five years). For contact information on individual comprehensive cancer centers, see Appendix II.

computed tomography colography See VIRTUAL COLONOSCOPY.

computed tomography laser mammography An imaging test using laser technology to examine different planes of breast tissue and produce a 3-D view of the breast. The technique does not use radiation and does not require breast compression. It is available only in clinical studies and has not been approved for general use by the U.S. Food and Drug Administration.

See also DIGITAL MAMMOGRAPHY; DUCTOGRAM; MAMMOGRAPHY; THERMAL IMAGING.

cone biopsy See CONIZATION.

conization Surgery to remove a cone-shaped piece of tissue from the cervix or cervical canal. The procedure may be used to diagnose or treat CERVICAL CANCER. It is also known as a cone biopsy or cold knife cone biopsy. Conization is performed if the results of a cervical biopsy have found a precancerous condition or if there is an abnormal PAP TEST.

Because cone biopsies carry risks such as bleeding and problems with subsequent pregnancies, they have been replaced with newer technologies except in a few circumstances.

Procedure

During the biopsy under general anesthesia, the vagina is held open with a speculum as the doctor removes a cone-shaped piece of the cervix containing the area with abnormal cells. The resulting wound is stitched closed, or the wound may be left open and heat or cold used to stop bleeding.

Once the tissue has been removed, it is examined under a microscope for signs of cancer. If the abnormal cells are precancerous, a laser can be used to destroy them. If cancer is present, other tests will be needed. Surgery may be performed to remove the cervix and uterus (HYSTERECTOMY), and other treatments may be used as well.

Conization may require an overnight stay in the hospital. After the test, the patient may feel some cramps or discomfort for about a week. Women should not have sex, use tampons, or douche until after seeing their physician for a follow-up appointment a week or more after the procedure.

Risks

About one in 10 women experience temporary vaginal bleeding about two weeks after the biopsy. There is also a slight risk of infection or perforation of the uterus. In a few women, the cervical canal becomes narrowed or completely blocked, which can later interfere with the movement of sperm. This can impair a woman's fertility.

If too much muscle tissue has been removed, the procedure can lead to an incompetent cervix, which can be a problem with subsequent pregnancies. An incompetent cervix cannot seal properly to maintain a pregnancy. If untreated, the condition increases the odds of miscarriage or premature labor.

Cervical conization also may temporarily alter cervical cells, which can make a Pap smear test hard to interpret accurately for three or four months.

connective tissue cancer   See SARCOMA.

continuous hyperthermic peritoneal perfusion (CHPP)   A procedure that bathes the abdominal cavity in fluid that contains CHEMOTHERAPY drugs at a temperature warmer than the body's. This procedure appears to kill cancer cells without harming normal cells.

cordectomy   A surgical operation in which the vocal cords are removed to treat LARYNGEAL CANCER.

cordotomy   A method of relieving cancer pain by interrupting pain signals in the spinal cord. In the procedure bundles of nerves in the spinal cord are cut surgically or by radio frequency waves. Unfor-

tunately, sometimes nerves that transmit other sensations such as temperature or pressure are cut, putting a patient at greater risk of self injury.

Between 7 percent and 10 percent of patients who have had a cordotomy develop new pain. In others, the pain they already had is only temporarily relieved. While a cordotomy can relieve pain in 90 percent of patients, three months later 10 percent of patients begin to experience pain again. After one year, 40 percent of patients are again experiencing pain.

core biopsy   The removal of a tissue sample with a needle for examination under a microscope.

corticosteroids   Hormones that have antitumor activity in LYMPHOMA and lymphoid LEUKEMIA; in addition, corticosteroids may be used to manage some of the complications of cancer and its treatment, such as pain, NAUSEA, and FATIGUE. Corticosteroids also are used to relieve the cerebral swelling caused by brain tumors.

craniopharyngioma   See BRAIN CANCER.

craniotomy   A major neurological operation in which an opening is made into the skull to remove a malignant tumor.

See also BRAIN CANCER.

creosote, coal tar   A thick, oily liquid that is typically amber to black, highly flammable, and does not dissolve easily in water. It is the name used for products made of a mixture of many chemicals and created by high-temperature treatment of coal. Both the International Agency for Research on Cancer and the U.S. Environmental Protection Agency (EPA) have determined that coal tar creosote is probably a human carcinogen.

Creosote prepared from coal tar, the most common form in the U.S. workplace and at U.S. hazardous waste sites, is the most widely-used wood preservative in the United States. It is also a restricted-use pesticide. About 300 chemicals have been identified in coal tar creosote, but there may be as many as 10,000 other chemicals in the mixture as well. The major chemicals in coal tar creosote that can cause harmful health effects are polycyclic aromatic hydrocarbons (PAHs), phenol, and cresols.

Coal tar creosote is released to water and soil primarily by the wood preservation industry. Companies that preserve wood with coal tar creosote may treat their water wastes in treatment plants or release the waste water to a municipal water treatment system—the largest source of coal tar creosote in the environment. However, new restrictions from the EPA have modified treatment methods, decreasing the amount of creosote available to move into soil from waste water effluents.

Coal tar creosote components that dissolve in water may move through the soil eventually to reach and enter the groundwater; once in the groundwater, breakdown may take years. The components that are not water soluble will remain stationary in a tarlike mass, and breakdown in soil can take months. Coal tar creosote components may also be found in the soil as a result of leaking or seeping from treated timber.

Volatile chemicals in coal tar creosote may evaporate and enter the air; about 1 to 2 percent of the coal tar creosote applied to treated wood is released to the air (a smaller amount than is found in wastewater or soil).

Once coal tar creosote is in the environment, both plants and animals can absorb parts of the creosote mixture. Aquatic animals, such as crustaceans and shellfish, also accumulate coal tar creosote compounds. For instance, mussels attached to creosote-treated pilings, and snails and oysters living in water near a wood-treatment plant, had creosote in their tissues. Coal tar creosote components are also broken down by microorganisms living in the soil and natural water.

Hazardous waste sites are a major source of creosote contamination. Individuals working in the wood-preserving industry make up the largest part of the population that might be exposed to coal tar creosote. Workers who use creosote-treated wood in building fences, bridges, or railroad tracks or installing telephone poles may be exposed; those who inspect or maintain these materials, or apply asphalt or other materials containing coal tar pitch, may also be exposed. Homeowners, farmers, or landscapers who apply coal tar creosote to wood in noncommercial settings using a brush or dip procedure, or who use railroad ties or telephone poles in landscaping, or who reclaim scrap lumber from a treated structure may also be exposed. In addition, people who work or live in treated-wood houses may be exposed through the air or by direct contact with the wood. Consumers can be exposed by any contact with water, soil, air, or plant or animal tissues that contain creosotes.

SKIN CANCER and cancer of the scrotum have resulted from long exposure to low levels of these chemical mixtures, especially through direct contact with skin during wood treatment or manufacture of products treated with coal tar creosote. Cancer of the scrotum in chimney sweeps has been associated particularly with prolonged skin exposure to soot and coal tar creosote. These levels are much higher than the levels in groundwater, food, air, or soil. Exposure to coal tar products through the skin has resulted in skin cancer in animals.

Diagnosis

There is no medical test to determine exposure to coal tar creosote itself, but constituent chemicals contained in coal tar creosote (PAHs) can be found in the body and can be measured in organs, muscle, fat, blood, or urine. Urine tests are commonly done for employees in industry who work with coal tar creosote, coal tar, and coal tar pitch to monitor their exposure. The tests, available at a doctor's office, can confirm that a person has been exposed to the chemicals found in coal tar creosote, but can neither accurately predict whether the person will experience any effects nor indicate whether the chemicals came from coal tar creosote or other sources.

Since the chemicals in coal tar products remain in body tissues for long periods, urine tests may not be useful in determining when the person was exposed. Tests that measure levels of breakdown products may be more accurate in determining approximate date of exposure.

Government Regulation

The federal government has not developed regulatory standards and guidelines to protect people from the potential health effects of exposure to coal tar creosote in drinking water and food. Regulatory standards and guidelines for air and water exist for the most dangerous individual PAHs and phenols contained in coal tar creosote. The EPA has declared coal tar creosote a "restricted use" pesticide, which means it can be bought and used only by certified applicators and only for those uses covered by the applicator's certification.

In addition, coal tar creosote has been identified as a hazardous waste. The federal government has developed guidelines to protect workers from the potential health effects of coal tar products in air. The Occupational Safety and Health Administration has set a legal limit of 0.2 milligrams of coal tar pitch volatiles per cubic meter of air in a workroom.

Crohn's disease   Chronic inflammation of the gastrointestinal tract (usually the bowel), which increases the risk for colon cancer.

See also COLORECTAL CANCER.

cruciferous vegetables   A family of vegetables that contain substances that may protect against CANCER, including PHYTOCHEMICALS called INDOLES and isothiocyanates. These phytochemicals have been found to block or reduce cell damage. Cruciferous vegetables include kale, collard greens, broccoli, cauliflower, cabbage, Brussels sprouts, and turnips.

cryoablation   A cancer treatment technique in which a tumor is killed by freezing the tissue. Doctors have been attacking tumors with heat for a long time; now a few clinics around the country are turning to cold temperatures to do the same thing.

The technique is used to extend the lives of people dying from LIVER CANCER, to treat PROSTATE CANCER, and as the first nonsurgical alternative for the half-million women who have benign breast tumors removed each year. Doctors have just begun testing it as a possible scar-free way to remove early BREAST CANCER and as an alternative to open surgery for KIDNEY CANCER.

Because the delicate technique requires special training to avoid serious side effects caused by accidentally freezing healthy tissue, it is not yet a widespread treatment.

Cryoablation, first introduced in the 1960s, destroys cells by shattering their outer walls during freeze-and-thaw cycles. It used to be too risky for much use on tumors deep in the body because doctors could not see what they were freezing, causing high rates of complication. Dermatologists and gynecologists continued to freeze away easy-to-see skin or cervical growths, but other uses of cryoablation faded away.

Today it is slowly becoming more popular as a result of better medical imaging scans that allow doctors to see deep inside the body while they work. This allows a doctor to place a needle that emits freezing gas (usually argon) in a tumor or organ and literally watch until ice encases the growth.

The first approved use of this therapy was in patients whose COLORECTAL CANCER had spread to the liver and become inoperable. Cryoablation for this type of cancer is not curative, but it may give the patient some time; about 20 percent of patients survive five years.

For prostate cancer, cryoablation proved more difficult; poor aim causes serious side effects in the rectum, and inconsistent freezing can miss cancer. But after years of research a recent study suggests that careful cryoablation techniques may be as effective as radioactive seed implants in treating prostate cancer. Unfortunately, like other prostate treatments, cryoablation can cause impotence.

A cryoablation system designed to destroy benign breast tumors (fibroadenomas) also has been recently approved, and scientists are now studying whether the technique might successfully treat breast cancer, too. In one study, 25 women had small cancers frozen, and three weeks later they had a LUMPECTOMY (standard surgery) to determine if there were any cancer cells left lurking around the edges of the tumor. Scientists hope that cryoablation might someday replace lumpectomies for certain women.

Patients considering approved uses of cryoablation should pick an experienced cryosurgeon, because it requires a great deal of training and practice to avoid complications.

cryosurgery   The surgical destruction of tissue using below-freezing temperatures. The standard agent for this type of surgery is liquid nitrogen; carbon dioxide is less often used. The liquid nitrogen is applied to the skin with a cotton-tipped applicator (or using a Cryospray unit) for five to 30 seconds.

Dressings are not usually needed after treatment. Skin cancers such as BASAL CELL CARCINOMA and some in situ squamous cell carcinomas may be treated with cryosurgery. Because it involves minimal scarring, it is especially helpful for cosmetic reasons.

Complications may include hypopigmentation or, less often, scarring. Some malignant lesions treated with aggressive cryosurgery have had reported cure rates of 95 percent.

cryptorchidism   A condition in which one or both testicles fail to move from the abdomen, where they develop before birth, into the scrotum. Known commonly as "undescended testicles," cryptorchidism may increase the risk for development of TESTICULAR CANCER.

culdoscopy   A visual examination of a woman's genital organs as a way of diagnosing OVARIAN CANCER, ENDOMETRIAL CANCER, and FALLOPIAN TUBE CANCER. The doctor views the internal organs and pelvic tissue using a culdoscope (a lighted tubular instrument) that is inserted through an incision in the vaginal wall.

curcumin   A yellow pigment of the spice turmeric that is being studied in cancer prevention.

cutaneous breast cancer   Cancer that has spread from the breast to the skin.

cutaneous T-cell lymphoma   A disease in which certain cells of the lymph system (called T lymphocytes) become cancerous and affect the skin. This disease is also called mycosis fungoides. The malignant T-lymphocytes initially involve the skin, but can spread into lymph nodes and other organs. As it advances further, it can enter the bloodstream, triggering a leukemic phase called Sézary syndrome, causing generalized reddened, hot skin. At times, skin lesions may become ulcerated and infected.

Treatment

Treatment includes total skin electron-beam (superficial) radiation, topical chemotherapy, oral psoralen with ultraviolet A activation (PUVA),

bexarotene (a retinoid medication), denileukin diftitox (Ontak), photophoresis (cells treated outside the body and re-injected), and systemic CHEMOTHERAPY.

cyclamate   See ARTIFICIAL SWEETENERS.

cystectomy   Surgical removal of the bladder as a way of treating BLADDER CANCER. If the cancer has spread, other organs may also be removed during cystectomy, including prostate and seminal vesicles in men, or uterus, ovaries, fallopian tubes, and urethra in women.

cystography   A scan of the bladder, using a contrast dye X-ray, that can be used to diagnose BLADDER CANCER. During the procedure, a catheter is inserted and dye administered through the catheter into the bladder. Once the bladder is full, the catheter is removed and X-rays are taken.

cystosarcoma phyllodes (CSP)   A type of large, bulky tumor found in breast tissue that grows quickly but that is usually benign. CSP is also called phyllodes tumor.

cystoscopy   An examination of the bladder to diagnose BLADDER CANCER. During the procedure, the cystoscope, a lighted tubular instrument, is inserted through the urethra into the bladder. Cells can be removed for examination, and small tumors also can sometimes be removed through the tube. The exam is performed under anesthesia in a hospital.

cytokines   A class of substances that are produced by cells of the immune system and can affect the immune response. Cytokines can also be produced in the laboratory by recombinant DNA technology and given to people to affect immune responses, such as INTERFERONS and INTERLEUKINS.

cytomegalovirus (CMV)   A virus that may be carried in an inactive state for life by healthy individuals. In people with a suppressed immune system, such as those undergoing BONE MARROW TRANSPLANTS or those with LEUKEMIA or LYMPHOMA or HIV, it can cause a severe pneumonia or retinal damage.

In addition, recent research suggests that CMV may actually be linked to the development of some types of cancer. Proteins from CMV have been found in about 85 percent of colorectal polyps and colorectal cancer samples, but not in normal surrounding tissue, according to Alabama researchers.

cytotoxic T cells   A type of white blood cell that can directly destroy specific cells. T cells can be separated from other blood cells, grown in the laboratory, and then given to a patient to destroy tumor cells. Certain CYTOKINES can also be given to a patient to help form cytotoxic T cells.

D

D & C See DILATION AND CURETTAGE.

DCIS See BREAST CANCER.

deodorants See ANTIPERSPIRANTS AND BREAST CANCER.

dermatofibrosarcoma protuberans A slow-growing type of tumor that begins as a hard nodule in the lower layer of the skin of the limbs or trunk of the body. It can grow into surrounding tissue but does not spread to other parts of the body.

DES See DIETHYLSTILBESTROL.

desmoid tumor A tumor of the tissue that surrounds muscles, usually in the abdomen. A desmoid tumor rarely spreads to other parts of the body. Desmoid tumors are also called aggressive fibromatosis, especially when the tumor grows outside the abdomen.

desmoplastic small round cell tumor A rare, aggressive cancer that usually affects boys and usually is located in the abdomen.

DHL See LYMPHOMA.

diagnosis There are many different tests and screens that can diagnose the presence of cancer. These include

- BARIUM ENEMA
- BIOPSY
- BONE SCAN
- BRONCHOSCOPY
- CBC (COMPLETE BLOOD COUNT)
- COLONOSCOPY
- COLPOSCOPY
- computed tomography (CT scan)
- DIGITAL RECTAL EXAM
- FECAL OCCULT BLOOD TEST
- MRI (MAGNETIC RESONANCE IMAGING)
- MAMMOGRAPHY
- PAP TEST (Papanicolaou smear)
- PET scans (positron emission tomography)
- PROSTATE-SPECIFIC ANTIGEN BLOOD TEST
- radionuclide scanning
- SIGMOIDOSCOPY
- ultrasound
- X-rays

DIEP flap A type of BREAST RECONSTRUCTION in which blood vessels (called "deep inferior epigastric perforators, or DIEP), together with the skin and fat connected to them, are removed from the lower abdomen and used for reconstruction. Abdominal muscle is left in place.

diet Many experts believe that diet plays a role in the development of cancer. People may eat too many cancer-causing foods, such as broiled or preserved meats, or not eat enough cancer-preventing foods, such as certain ANTIOXIDANT-containing fruits and vegetables, and green TEAS.

The striking differences in cancer rates among countries, changes in these rates among migrating populations, and rapid changes within countries indicate that some aspect of lifestyle or environment is primarily responsible for the common cancers that occur in Western countries.

Many experts have emphasized the role of dietary fat as a key factor in the development of cancer because national consumption is correlated with international differences in cancer rates. However, detailed analyses in large prospective studies have not found that such fat plays an important role. Instead, early age of first menstrual period, physical inactivity, and weight gain as an adult have been shown to be important determinants of BREAST CANCER and COLON CANCER.

Although the percentage of calories from fat in the diet does not appear to be related to risk of colon cancer, greater risks have been seen with higher consumption of red meat, suggesting that factors other than fat may be important.

While many studies have found that eating lots of fruits and vegetables is associated with a lower risk of many cancers, recent prospective studies suggest these associations may have been overstated. Present data most strongly support a benefit of higher folic acid (a constituent of fruits and vegetables) consumption in reducing risks of colon and breast cancers. The benefits of FOLIC ACID appear strongest among people who regularly drink ALCOHOL, which itself is associated with increased risk of these cancers.

Numerous other aspects of diet are suspected to influence the risks of cancers in Western countries, but for the moment the evidence is unclear. Two decades of effort in developing, evaluating, and refining methods of dietary assessment have laid the groundwork for further insights into the role of diet in cancer etiology that will emerge from the more than 30 large prospective studies that are currently under way.

Cancer Prevention

Still, experts recommend a diet rich in fruits, vegetables, and whole grains to help reduce the risk of tumor development. While no single food or nutrient will remove the risk of cancer, following healthy guidelines can reduce a person's chances of developing certain types of cancer. Experts recommend that to lower the risk of cancer, people should eat a plant-based diet with plenty of roughage and a variety of natural, whole grain

foods. They should avoid high-fat diets, barbecued (burned) food, and smoked, pickled, salted, or cured food.

Certain foods rich in complex carbohydrates and fiber contain substances that can inhibit tumor formation and have been associated with a reduced risk of several types of cancer.

For example, CRUCIFEROUS VEGETABLES contain sulforaphane, as well as other plant chemicals such as dithiolthiones, which may produce enzymes that help block damage to cell DNA. The cruciferous vegetables include broccoli, cauliflower, kale, brussel sprouts, and cabbage.

Garlic and onions have sulfur compounds (allyl sulfides) that trigger enzymes that may help remove carcinogens from the body.

Citrus fruits are rich in vitamin C and flavonoids, which may help inhibit cancer cell growth.

Soy foods are high in ISOFLAVONES, which block some hormonal activity in cells. Diets high in SOY PRODUCTS have been associated with lower rates of cancers of the breast, endometrium, and prostate.

Tomatoes and tomato sauce are high in the phytochemical LYCOPENE, a powerful antioxidant. A diet high in tomatoes has been associated with a decreased risk of cancers of the stomach, colon, and prostate.

Following the steps below will also decrease cancer risk.

Avoid saturated fats There is some evidence that people whose diets are high in saturated fat (more than 10 percent of total calories) have a higher cancer risk than those who do not consume that much saturated fat.

Eat a plant-based diet Many experts believe that adding more plant-based foods is the dietary cornerstone to preventing many types of cancer. That is because fruits, vegetables, and other plant-based foods typically are low in saturated fats (the fats found in meats, butter, and cheese that are linked to an increased risk of cancer) and high in fiber, which may be associated with a lower risk of colon cancer. A plant-based diet is the best source of phytochemicals—natural substances in fruits and vegetables that seem to protect against certain types of tumors. A plant-based diet would include six to 11 servings of breads, grains, and cereals; two to four servings of fruit, and three to five servings of vegetables. "Five a Day" (five servings of fruits and vegetables each day) is the goal of the NATIONAL CANCER INSTITUTE's dietary guidelines for cancer prevention. According to the NCI, if everyone followed the "5 a Day" guidelines, cancer incidence could decline by at least 20 percent.

Consume roughage   A high-fiber diet is a good way to reduce the risk of COLORECTAL CANCER. Fiber is found in all plant-based foods, including fruits, vegetables, grains, breads, and cereals, but is not available in meat, milk, cheese, or oils. White flour is not recommended because its refining process removes almost all of the fiber from grains.

Fiber can be either soluble or insoluble. Soluble fibers dissolve in water and are found in highest amounts in fruits, legumes, barley, and oats. They generally slow down digestion time so that nutrients are completely absorbed. Soluble fibers also bind with bile acids in the intestines and carry them out of the body. Since bile acids are made from cholesterol, soluble fiber can lower a person's cholesterol levels. Studies linking high bile-acid concentrations and colon cancer have led some scientists to suspect that binding bile acids may be one way that fiber helps prevent colon cancer.

Insoluble fibers are found in vegetables, whole-grain breads, and whole-grain cereals. They increase the bulk of stool, help to prevent constipation, and remove bound bile acids. Insoluble fiber also increases the speed at which food moves through the gastrointestinal system.

Some scientists believe that a high-fiber diet reduces the risk of colon or other cancers because fiber can bind potentially cancer-causing agents in the intestines and speed the transit time so harmful substances do not stay in the body. New research published in the spring of 2003 strengthened the notion that a high-fiber diet may protect against colon cancer. Long-standing recommendations for high-fiber diets had been criticized in the early 2000s after a handful of carefully conducted studies failed to find a benefit. But experts say two major studies published in May 2003 in *The Lancet* (one on Americans and the other on Europeans) indicate that previous research may not have examined a broad enough range of fiber consumption or a wide enough variety of fiber sources to show an effect. A link between cancer and lack of fiber is particularly complicated to discover because there are various types of fiber, all of which could act differently.

In the American study, investigators compared the daily fiber intake of 3,600 people who had precancerous growths in the colon with the intake of around 34,000 people who had no growths. People who ate the most fiber had a 27 percent lower risk of precancerous growths than those who ate the least. In the European study, the largest one ever conducted on nutrition and cancer, scientists examined the link in more than 500,000 people in 10 countries. They were followed for an average of four years, and 1,065 of them developed colorectal cancer. Those who ate the most fiber (about 35 grams a day) had about a 40 percent lower risk of colorectal cancer compared with those who ate the least (about 15 grams a day), the study found.

How Much Fiber?

While Americans eat about 16 grams of fiber a day and Europeans eat about 22 grams, the latest studies indicate fiber intake needs to be about 30 grams a day to protect against colon cancer.

There are 2 grams of fiber in a slice of whole meal bread; a banana has 3 grams, and an apple has 3.5 grams, the same as a cup of brown rice. Some super-high-fiber breakfast cereals have as much as 14 grams per half cup. A good way to achieve the recommended levels is to eat five fruits and vegetables each day. It is possible to increase fiber intake by eating the skins of potatoes and fruits such as apples and pears, and switching from refined foods (such as white bread and white rice) to whole-grain foods (whole-wheat breads and brown rice). Other good sources of fiber include legumes, lentils, and whole-grain cereals.

Pick low-fat foods   A high-fat diet has been associated with an increased risk of developing cancer of the prostate, colon, endometrium, and breast. Low-fat foods are usually lower in calories than high-fat foods.

There are three types of dietary fats:

- *Saturated fats*, found in animal products such as meat, milk, and cheese, have been linked to an increased risk of cancer.

- *Monounsaturated fats* are found in olive oil and canola oil.
- *Polyunsaturated fats* are found in vegetable oils.

While the latter two types of fat are less closely linked to disease, it is a good idea to limit all three kinds because overall fat intake is associated with cancer. Dietitians generally believe that tub margarine is a better choice than butter, since butter is rich in both saturated fat and cholesterol, and the hazards of saturated fats are better documented and appear to be more severe than those of hydrogenated fats in margarine. Most margarine is made from vegetable fat and has no cholesterol.

The usual recommendation is that people should get no more than 10 percent of daily calories from saturated fats, and that total fat intake should not exceed 30 percent of the day's calories.

Dietary fat can be reduced by limiting consumption of red meat, choosing low-fat or no-fat varieties of milk and cheese, removing the skin from chicken and turkey, choosing pretzels instead of potato chips, and decreasing or eliminating fried foods, butter, and margarine. Cooking with small amounts of olive oil instead of butter will significantly cut saturated fat intake.

Other Beneficial Substances

Every day scientists are learning the health benefits of substances in food, such as ANTIOXIDANTS, PHYTOCHEMICALS, and PHYTOESTROGENS.

Antioxidants   These substances seek out and destroy the naturally occurring toxic molecules called FREE RADICALS that can cause extensive damage to the body's cells. Such damage is thought to be involved in cancer development. Antioxidants reduce the number of free radicals, prevent tissue damage, and, quite possibly, prevent cancer. The antioxidants that have generated the most interest and research to date are vitamin C, vitamin E, BETA-CAROTENE, and selenium.

Good sources of vitamin C include citrus fruits, kiwi, cantaloupe, strawberries, peppers, tomatoes, potatoes, mangos, and cruciferous vegetables. Vitamin E can be found in green leafy vegetables, wheat germ, whole grain products, nuts, seeds, and vegetable oil. Beta-carotene often (but not always) is identified by its yellow, orange, or deep-

green color and occurs in carrots, cantaloupe, sweet potatoes, apricots, broccoli, spinach, and other green leafy vegetables. Selenium is found in seafood, meat, and grains.

Phytochemicals   These chemicals contribute to the color and flavor of vegetables and, when eaten, may suppress cancer development. Phytochemicals that may help prevent cancer include

- the antioxidant beta-carotene
- lutein in spinach, kale, and other green leafy vegetables
- limonen and phenols in citrus fruits
- allyl sulfides in garlic and onions
- sulforaphane
- indoles
- isothicyanates in broccoli, cauliflower, and other cruciferous vegetables
- limonen and phenols in citrus fruits

Phytoestrogens   These compounds bind with estrogen receptors in the body, reducing the effects of estrogen. Because estrogen has been associated with increased risk of breast, endometrial, and ovarian cancer, phytoestrogens may reduce the risk of these kinds of cancer. Phytoestrogens are found in soy products (such as tofu, soy milk, and soy burgers) and legumes.

Pesticides

Health experts recommend eating a variety of fruits and vegetables for a healthy diet. Most experts believe that consuming the small amount of synthetic pesticide residues on produce is not harmful; eating a wide variety of foods guarantees that a person will not get too much of any one additive.

Preparation

Whenever possible, consumers should choose foods that come as close to their natural state as possible—selecting whole-wheat bread instead of refined-flour breads, fresh fruits and vegetables instead of canned, unsweetened whole grain cereals rather than sugary cereals. Refined products, such as white rice and white bread, often have had the most nutritious part of the grain removed during processing. These products may then be enriched, which means that they have certain vitamins and minerals added back. Although "enriched" foods sound good, many valuable nutrients (such as fiber) removed during the refining process are never added back. In addition, many refined products include other undesirable ingredients, such as salt or fats.

Cancer-Causing Foods

Just as there are many healthy foods that protect against cancer, other foods have been linked to the development of cancer. Studies show that between 30 percent and 40 percent of all cancers are related to diet. Foods that have been shown to increase the risk of a variety of cancers include

- foods that are exposed to high temperatures, such as during grilling or broiling
- acrylamide-containing foods
- preserved meats and other cured food
- foods high in saturated fat.

High temperatures   Several recent reports suggest that eating foods cooked at high temperatures may promote cancer. When barbecuing, cancer-causing substances called polycyclic aromatic hydrocarbons are produced as fat from the meat drips onto the flames. These hydrocarbons rise up in the smoke and settle back down on the meat. For this reason, experts recommend that people limit the amount of barbecued meat in the diet; those who must barbecue should precook meat in an oven or microwave before transferring it to the barbecue.

Other foods cooked at high temperatures that have been linked to cancer include certain high-carbohydrate foods containing ACRYLAMIDE, such as french fries and potato chips and some types of bread fried or baked at high temperatures. The higher the heat at which the starches are cooked, the greater the level of acrylamide in the food. How acrylamide, previously known as an industrial chemical, forms in the cooking process remains a mystery.

Preserved food   Many types of preserved foods have been linked to the development of cancer, including hot dogs, bacon, ham, and pickled veg-

etables. Drinking a glass of orange juice when these foods are eaten may protect against some of the harmful effects.

In the 1930s, before refrigeration became common in the United States, STOMACH CANCER was the leading cause of cancer death in men, and the second leading cause in women—most likely due to the extensive eating of preserved food. Without the ability to freeze and safely store food, people relied on preserving methods such as smoking, pickling, salting, and curing. Because these types of preserved meats are less common today, the rates of U.S. stomach cancer are at an all-time low. In parts of the world where meat is still widely preserved, stomach cancer remains a major killer.

Fats   This dietary component also may promote cancer. People who typically consume a diet high in saturated fats (more than 10 percent of total calories) face higher rates of cancer than people who consume diets lower in saturated fats. There is also a relationship between high fat intake and cancers of the breast, prostate, colon, pancreas, and endometrium. OBESITY—closely related to dietary fat—also is associated with tumor production.

diethanolamine (DEA)   A substance used in cosmetics that may be linked to cancer in lab animals, according to research by the National Toxicology Program (NTP), which found an association between cancer in lab animals and the topical application of DEA and some DEA-related ingredients. The study did not establish a link between DEA and the risk of cancer in humans.

Although DEA itself is used in very few cosmetics, DEA-related ingredients are widely used in a variety of cosmetic products. These ingredients function as emulsifiers or foaming agents and generally are used at levels of 1 to 5 percent of a product's formulation.

diethylstilbestrol (DES)   A synthetic ESTROGEN-like hormone that was prescribed from the early 1940s until 1971 to prevent miscarriage. DES was one of the first inexpensive types of synthetic estrogen-like hormones available. However, in the early 1970s a link between DES and women's reproductive cancers was identified, and the U.S. Food and Drug Administration warned that DES should not be used during pregnancy.

An increased risk of the very rare clear cell carcinoma of the vagina has been observed in young daughters of women who used DES. DES daughters also may be at higher risk for developing CERVICAL CANCER because they have twice the risk of atypical cervical cells that could lead to malignancies. Some researchers believe that sons of women who took DES are prone to having undescended testicles and TESTICULAR CANCER. DES may also increase the risk of BREAST CANCER in women who used the hormone. It is listed as a known carcinogen by the National Toxicology Program.

DES also has been used as a beneficial medication to treat PROSTATE CANCER by suppressing the production of the male hormone androgen.

differentiation A term that refers to how mature the cancer cells are in a tumor. Differentiated tumor cells resemble normal cells and tend to grow and spread at a slower rate than undifferentiated or poorly differentiated tumor cells, which lack the structure and function of normal cells and grow uncontrollably.

diffuse histiocytic lymphoma See LYMPHOMA.

digestive/gastrointestinal cancer A group of cancers involving the digestive tract including ANAL CANCER, extrahepatic BILE DUCT CANCER, gastrointestinal CARCINOID tumor, COLORECTAL CANCER, ESOPHAGEAL CANCER, GALLBLADDER CANCER, LIVER CANCER, PANCREATIC CANCER, small intestine cancer, and STOMACH CANCER.

digital mammography A newer type of MAMMOGRAPHY system similar to standard mammography in that both uses X-rays to produce an image of the breast. From the patient's point of view, mammography with a full field digital mammography system is basically the same as the old screen-film system; the differences lie in the way the image is recorded, viewed by the doctor, and stored.

Digital mammography replaces large sheets of photographic film with solid-state detectors that convert X-rays into electric signals. The signals can be seen on a computer screen or printed on special films to look like regular mammograms. They are stored on a computer, and their magnification, brightness, or contrast can be changed after the exam is done to help the doctor see certain areas more clearly. Digital images can be transmitted over phone lines to another location for remote consultation with breast specialists.

A digital mammogram is commonly used in stereotactic imaging to guide breast BIOPSY because it is rapid and reliable. Early studies have shown that digital mammograms are at least as accurate as X-ray mammograms; additional work with this technique may show digital mammograms are superior.

Early in 2000, the U.S. Food and Drug Administration approved a digital mammogram system that can now be used for routine breast cancer screening. While many facilities providing mammogram services do not currently offer the digital option, it is expected to become more widely available in time. Digital mammography can legally be performed only in facilities that are certified.

digital rectal exam Physical examination of the rectum (the last few inches of the digestive tract). This is one diagnostic test for COLORECTAL CANCER and PROSTATE CANCER.

dilatation and curettage (D & C) A procedure used to dilate the cervix and scrape out the lining and contents of the uterus in order to diagnose the cause of abnormal bleeding. Cells harvested during a D & C can be examined for malignant cells under a microscope. A D & C may be used to diagnose CERVICAL CANCER or UTERINE CANCER. This fairly minor surgical procedure may be performed in the hospital or clinic using general or local anesthesia.

The Procedure

The cervical canal is widened (dilated) using a metal rod; the doctor then inserts a curette (a metal loop on the end of a long, thin handle) into the uterus and scrapes the inner layer of the uterus away. Tissue is usually collected for examination.

Uterine scraping may be done to diagnose conditions, treat irregular bleeding, or to remove fetal or placental tissue. It may be performed for bleeding between periods or after sexual intercourse, heavy menstrual bleeding, investigation of infertility, uterine fibroids, endometrial polyps, early uterine or cervical cancer, thickening of the uterus, an embedded IUD, an elective abortion, or following a miscarriage.

Risks

A D & C has relatively few risks. It can ease bleeding and can be used to diagnose problems including infection, cancer, infertility, and other disease. There is a slight risk of damage to the inner lining of the uterus, a dilated cervix that fails to return to normal size, a punctured uterus, laceration of the cervix, or scarring.

After Surgery

It is normal to experience irregular bleeding in the days following D & C, as well as pelvic cramps and back pain for a few days after the procedure. Pain can usually be managed well with medications. Tampon use is not recommended for a few weeks, and sexual intercourse is not recommended for a few days. The woman should contact her doctor if there is heavy bleeding with large clots, severe lower abdominal pain, bleeding, or high fever. The patient may resume normal activities the same day.

dioxins   A group of highly toxic substances used in a variety of industrial applications that are potent CARCINOGENS, according to the U.S. Environmental Protection Agency. The herbicide AGENT ORANGE, used during combat in Vietnam, contained small quantities of one type of dioxin. Diagnosis of dioxin poisoning is difficult, since it is hard to detect dioxin in blood or tissue, and there is no established correlation with symptoms.

Dioxin has spread well beyond its main industrial sources (paper processors, herbicide manufacturers, and garbage incinerators) and can be found today in the bodies of anyone who eats fish, meat, or dairy products. Research suggests that dioxin may affect the body's hormonal messengers system; it may affect sex hormones and insulin and could create permanent health problems for children exposed in the womb.

Symptoms

After exposure, patients experience skin, eye, and mucous membrane irritation, NAUSEA, and vomiting. After several weeks other symptoms appear, including acne, excessive hair growth, pigment abnormalities, motor weakness, and sensory impairments.

disphosphonates   See BISPHOSPHONATES.

distal pancreatectomy   Removal of the body and tail of the pancreas, which is a treatment for PANCREATIC CANCER.

diverticulosis   A condition marked by small sacs or pouches (diverticula) in the walls of the stomach or colon. When these sacs become inflamed, it causes a condition called diverticulitis.

DNR order (do not resuscitate order)   A legal directive by a physician that instructs hospital staff not to try to help a patient whose heart has stopped or who has stopped breathing. A patient can request a DNR order either by filling out an ADVANCE DIRECTIVE form or by telling the doctor that cardiopulmonary resuscitation (CPR) should not be performed. DNR orders are accepted by doctors and hospitals in all states.

drug treatments, new   Many cancer patients are living longer as a result of new treatment methods. The standard treatment approach for cancer featuring surgery, RADIATION THERAPY, and CHEMOTHERAPY is being updated with medications that target the genetic mechanics that underlie the development of cancer. Soon, researchers say, vaccines will be approved that boost the immune system to better tackle tumors, and so will gene therapy techniques that make chemotherapy drugs work better. Some say the new therapies could transform cancer from a death sentence into an easily treatable disease.

Traditional, intravenous chemotherapy drugs harm all dividing cells, which combats cancer but also affects many healthy cells, leading to hair loss, NAUSEA, and FATIGUE. New treatments such as Iressa (often given in pill form) can target cancer cells, leaving healthy cells unharmed, thereby causing fewer side effects. These new treatments have come as a result of recent biological breakthroughs, including the mapping of the 30,000 human genes.

The new approaches are a major thrust of the Georgia Cancer Coalition, a $1 billion, 10-year effort expected to use $400 million of the state's tobacco settlement funds and $600 million in private money and federal grants to fight the state's war on cancer. More than $20 million has gone so far to researchers at Emory University, Georgia Tech, and elsewhere.

Scientists are now recognizing and battling cancer not as one disease but as more than 100 variations of cell growth gone awry. The more scientists learn about the genetic problems that lead normal cells to become malignant, the more easily they can devise ways to keep healthy cells unharmed.

There have been problems along the way. Cancer researchers have previously heralded breakthroughs that turned out not to be so helpful, such as the immune stimulants INTERFERON and INTERLEUKIN 2 in the 1980s, whose side effects and weak responses blunted their usefulness.

Gene therapy, involved in some of today's novel cancer approaches, has led to deaths and safety questions in noncancer experiments. In fact, the U.S. Food and Drug Administration recently halted several gene therapy studies after children in France developed LEUKEMIA while receiving the treatment. One of the most successful drugs in the new arsenal—Gleevec, a drug for relatively rare forms of leukemia and STOMACH CANCER—attacks only cancers with one main gene defect. Most tumors have multiple genetic mistakes that will require assaults on many fronts, scientists say.

Still, many experts hope that new drugs such as Gleevec and Iressa may prove to be to cancer what penicillin was to bacterial infections. Some of the new drugs include Velcade for MULTIPLE MYELOMA, a blood plasma cancer. Tarceva is being targeted to treat LUNG CANCER. These drugs, just like Gleevec and Iressa, throw various switches to stop cancer's development.

For a regular cell to become cancerous, four basic parts of the body's anticancer arsenal must break down:

1. First, the accelerator—called the ONCOGENE—must burst out of control, causing cells to multiply quickly.

2. Then the tumor suppressor genes stop working so that there is no way for the body to stop the cells from multiplying out of control.

3. Next, a group of genes fail that normally cause abnormal cells to commit suicide (a process known as APOPTOSIS).

4. Finally, the gene controlling an energy source known as telomeres makes the cell think it has a limitless supply of fuel

Vaccines

Scientists are studying vaccines that would encourage a cancer patient's immune system to recognize and destroy cancer cells. The immune system is constantly scanning the body looking for foreign invaders, but because cancer cells originate in the body, they are usually not detected by the immune system.

In cancer vaccine technology, tumor cells are removed from the body, marked as "foreign" by adding a special gene, and then injected beneath the skin, where the immune system is on the alert. This tells the body that it has just been newly infected with cancer for the first time. The vaccine may help the body reject tumors and prevent cancer from recurring.

In contrast to vaccines against infectious diseases, cancer vaccines are designed to be injected after the disease is diagnosed, rather than before it develops. Cancer vaccines given when a tumor is small may be able to eradicate the cancer.

Early cancer vaccine studies involved primarily patients with melanoma, but today scientists are also testing the vaccines for many other types of cancer, including LYMPHOMA and cancers of the kidney, breast, ovary, prostate, colon, and rectum. Researchers are also investigating ways that cancer vaccines can be used in combination with other BIOLOGICAL RESPONSE MODIFIERS (BRMs).

In one study of PROSTATE CANCER that had spread to the bone, patients were given 13 shots of a cancer vaccine over four months. Forty-one percent who got a low dose and 70 percent who got a high dose were alive two years later, prompting researchers to plan larger trials set to start late in 2003. The vaccine, known as GVAX, is also being tested for lung, pancreas, and colon cancers.

Gene Therapy

Gene therapy alters a gene so that it stops the growth of cancer cells or makes the cancer cells more sensitive to other kinds of therapy. Inactivated viruses such as the one for the common cold usually are used as the modified gene, since they already know how to invade cells.

Some scientists are combining cancer vaccines and gene therapy to fight cancer. In this method, a cancer vaccine is developed by removing tumor cells, modifying them, and putting them back into the body. This is followed by the removal of the patient's immune cells so that a gene can be inserted to shield the cells from chemotherapy's harmful effects. That way, doctors can use chemotherapy after administering cancer vaccines in a double fight against tumors. Although human trials are years away, scientists believe the combination of approaches may be most powerful.

Other scientists at Georgia Tech are improving gene therapy by exploring creative ways of getting genes into cancer cells. Some scientists are using viral cousins of HIV (the AIDS virus) because these viruses penetrate cells so well. By altering viral proteins, these scientists can reprogram the killer viruses to safely carry a gene payload into the cancer cell.

Other scientists are using electric pulses and ultrasound to deliver the altered genes. Electrode pulses can pry cancer cells open, and electric fields can move genes through membranes. By placing electrodes on skin near tumors or inside the body during surgery, scientists are hoping they can quickly get gene "drugs" into the body. Ultrasound waves create bubbles that break cell membranes open. Researchers are hoping that they can use ultrasound to create tiny holes in cancer cells before they receive altered genes.

ductal carcinoma See BREAST CANCER.

ductal carcinoma in situ See BREAST CANCER.

ductal lavage A method used to collect cells from milk ducts in the breast so that the cells can be checked for cancer under a microscope. To obtain the cells, a hair-size catheter is inserted into the nipple; a small amount of saltwater flows into the duct and is then removed, along with breast cells. Ductal lavage may be used in addition to physical breast examination and MAMMOGRAPHY to detect BREAST CANCER.

ductogram (galactogram) A test that is sometimes helpful in determining the cause of a nipple discharge. In this X-ray procedure, a fine plastic tube is placed into the opening of the duct in the nipple. A small amount of contrast medium is injected, which outlines the shape of the duct on an X-ray image and will show whether there is a mass inside the duct.

Dukes' classification An older staging system used to describe the extent of COLORECTAL CANCER ranging from A (early stage) to D (advanced stage).

duodenal carcinoma A very rare type of intestinal cancer, located in the duodenum (upper part of the intestine), that is usually an ADENOCARCINOMA.

dysphasia Pain while swallowing, one of the first symptoms of ESOPHAGEAL CANCER (cancer of the tube connecting the throat with the stomach). It also may be a symptom of other physical problems, such as candidiasis of the esophagus or the side effects of radiation.

dysplastic nevus syndrome An often-hereditary condition characterized by groups of nevi (moles) that in some people may indicate a predisposition to malignant MELANOMA. Cancerous melanomas grow from the moles themselves, or elsewhere on the body.

Typically, only one defective gene (from one parent) is needed to cause the syndrome; each child of an affected person usually has a one in two chance of inheriting the defective gene and of being affected. A patient with dysplastic nevi and two or more primary family members with malignant melanoma has a very strong chance—almost 100 percent—of developing the cancer as well.

If a parent has dysplastic nevi without melanoma, the chance of offspring developing melanoma is less definite; however, offspring still are at higher risk than the general population.

Patients with dysplastic nevi but no family history are said to have a "sporadic" syndrome; if they have many moles, they are still at higher risk of developing malignant malanoma than the general population, but at less risk than those who inherited the problem.

Dysplastic nevi are bigger and usually more prevalent than ordinary birthmarks (there are usually more than 100 of them). While ordinary moles do not usually appear in adulthood, dysplastic nevi continue to develop throughout life. Moles also change appearance or disappear in people of all ages.

Prevention

Patients with many dysplastic nevi and a family history of melanoma should avoid the Sun and use sunscreens, examine their own skin, and see a dermatologist every six months. To spot signs of dysplastic nevi that may be becoming malignant, patients should check for the "ABCs": The blemish is *asymmetrical,* the *border* is notched or blurred (not smooth and distinct), or the *color* includes mixtures of different shades.

Treatment

Suspect birthmarks should be diagnosed by a doctor and removed.

See also SKIN CANCER.

E

edrecolomab A type of MONOCLONAL ANTIBODY used in cancer detection or therapy. Monoclonal antibodies are laboratory-produced substances that can locate and bind to cancer cells.

electrolarynx A battery-operated instrument that makes a humming sound and is used to help produce speech for a person whose voice box (larynx) has been removed, usually because of THROAT CANCER.

electromagnetic radiation Low-energy radiation that comes from the interaction of electric and magnetic fields. Sources include power lines, electric appliances, radio waves, microwaves, and others. Over the past 15 years there have been numerous studies of children and adults evaluating residential exposures to electric and magnetic fields in relation to the risk of cancer. Unfortunately, the findings have been inconsistent.

The NATIONAL CANCER INSTITUTE and the Children's Cancer Group collaborated on a large-scale investigation to determine whether exposures to magnetic fields contribute to the development of acute lymphocytic LEUKEMIA (ALL) in children under age 15. The results of the residential measurement component of this study were published in *The New England Journal of Medicine* on July 3, 1997, while the results of the interview component evaluating exposure to electrical appliances of the child's mother during pregnancy and the child after birth were published in the May 1998 issue of *Epidemiology*.

There was little evidence discovered of a relationship between risk for ALL in children and exposure to the magnetic fields of electrical appliances.

Although the data showed some association between appliance use and leukemia, there was no consistent pattern of increasing risk with increasing exposures. The scientists speculated that the magnetic fields from electrical appliances are unlikely to increase the risk of childhood ALL. This study provides one of the largest comprehensive measures of magnetic field exposure in children's residences.

Compared with electromagnetic field (EMF) exposure from power lines, the contribution of appliances to a person's total exposure to EMFs is thought to be small. Most appliances are used for short periods of time, and EMF exposures are elevated only when a person is close to the appliance. The electric appliances included in the study were electric blankets, mattress pads, heating pads, water beds, stereo or other sound systems, television and video games connected to a television, video machines located in arcades, computers, microwave ovens, sewing machines, hair dryers, curling irons, ceiling fans, humidifiers, night-lights, and electric clocks.

Brain Cancer Studies

The causes of tumors of the brain and nervous system are largely unknown, but genetic factors and a variety of environmental exposures have been implicated to varying degrees. Epidemiological studies have linked central nervous system cancers with a variety of environmental exposures (including physical, chemical, and biological agents).

Many consumers recently became concerned over the possibility that handheld cellular telephones, as well as other sources of magnetic fields, may cause BRAIN CANCER. While there is strong evidence that high doses of ionizing radiation (such as radiotherapy) can increase the risk of tumors of the central nervous system, the picture is less clear about possible risks posed by low doses of ionizing radiation or magnetic fields. Most studies of groups exposed to low doses of ionizing radiation on the job have not found an increased risk of brain cancer.

The few studies of magnetic fields and cancer of the nervous system have focused on low-frequency (50–60 Hz) fields, such as those associated with electric power lines and household appliances. There is very little information available concerning possible risks associated with microwave frequencies, such as those emitted from handheld cellular telephones (800–900 MHz).

While the possible health hazards of magnetic field exposure remain an active area of research, expert panels that have reviewed the existing evidence found it insufficient to support the conclusion that magnetic fields cause cancer.

Radar Exposure and Cancer

In 1980 the National Academy of Sciences conducted a 20-year follow-up study of 20,000 U.S. Navy personnel to determine whether sailors exposed to high-intensity microwave radiation (radar) were more likely to get cancer than 20,000 sailors with no or minimal radar exposure. The study, which was published in the July 1980 issue of the *American Journal of Epidemiology*, found no association between radar exposure and cancer.

Prevention

Government scientists recommend that anyone concerned about the possible health effects of magnetic fields may do the following to reduce exposure:

- Increase the space between a person and devices that may emit magnetic fields.
- Avoid standing too close to computers, microwave ovens, or televisions.
- Reduce the time of exposure to possible magnetic fields by turning off devices such as electric blankets when not in use.
- Avoid keeping electric alarm clocks too close to the bed.
- Discourage children from playing near high power lines or transformers.
- Avoid activities near magnetic field sources.

electroporation therapy   Treatment that generates electrical pulses through an electrode placed in a tumor to help CHEMOTHERAPY drugs enter tumor cells.

electrosurgery   A surgical technique in which cancerous tissue is scraped from the skin with a curette, and an electric needle burns a safety margin of normal skin around the tumor at the base of the scraped area. This technique is repeated twice to make sure the tumor has been completely removed.

embryonal cell cancer   A type of GERM CELL CANCER that tends to form glands or spaces and is characterized by bleeding and tissue death. It usually is found as a component of a mixed germ cell tumor. This highly malignant type of tumor is resistant to radiation therapy but responds to combination CHEMOTHERAPY.

embryonal rhabdomyosarcoma   A soft-tissue tumor that affects children and that usually begins in muscle cells in the head, neck, arms, legs, or genitourinary tract.

See also KIDNEY CANCER.

ENCORE Plus   A community-based program sponsored by the YWCA that helps women who need early detection education and breast and CERVICAL CANCER screening and support services. The program also provides women under treatment and those recovering from BREAST CANCER with a combined peer group/support and exercise program.

The ENCORE Plus program is designed to eliminate inequalities in health care experienced by many women by removing barriers to access and promoting effective community-based outreach, education, referral to clinical services, and support systems. For contact information, see Appendix I.

endocrine cancers   Tumors of the endocrine system include adrenocortical carcinoma, gastrointestinal CARCINOID tumor, islet cell carcinoma, parathyroid cancer, pheochromocytoma, pituitary tumor, and THYROID CANCER.

endometrial cancer The most common type of uterine cancer that develops in the inner layer of the lining of the uterus (the endometrium). Endometrial cancer can spread outside the uterus; cancer cells are often found in nearby LYMPH NODES, nerves, or blood vessels. If the cancer reaches the lymph nodes, cancer cells may spread to other lymph nodes and other organs, such as the lungs, liver, and bones.

There are other cancers that affect the uterine area, including uterine sarcoma, a rarer malignancy that develops in the uterine muscle (myometrium), and CERVICAL CANCER. In general, when people refer to "uterine cancer" they mean "endometrial cancer" or cancer of the lining of the uterus.

Cause

No one knows the exact causes of uterine cancer, but the disease is related to certain risk factors. Most women who have known risk factors still do not develop uterine cancer, and many who do get this disease have none of these factors. Studies have identified the following risk factors:

- *Age.* Cancer of the uterus occurs primarily in women over age 50.

- *Endometrial hyperplasia.* The risk of uterine cancer is higher if a woman has ENDOMETRIAL HYPERPLASIA, which is a benign overabundance of cells lining the uterus.

- *Hormone replacement therapy (HRT).* Women who use ESTROGEN without progesterone have an increased risk of uterine cancer; long-term use and large doses of estrogen seem to increase this risk. Because progesterone protects the uterus, women who use a combination of estrogen and progesterone have a lower risk of uterine cancer than women who use estrogen alone.

- *Obesity.* Fatty tissue produces estrogen, which may be why obese women have a higher risk of developing UTERINE CANCER. The risk of this disease is also higher in women with diabetes or high blood pressure, which are also conditions that occur in many obese women.

- *Tamoxifen.* Women taking the drug tamoxifen to prevent or treat BREAST CANCER have an increased risk of an aggressive form of uterine cancer, which appears to be related to the estrogen-like effect of this drug on the uterus. Doctors monitor women taking tamoxifen for possible signs or symptoms of uterine cancer, but the benefits of tamoxifen to treat breast cancer outweigh the risk of developing other cancers.

- *Race.* Caucasian women are more likely than African-American women to get uterine cancer.

- *Colorectal cancer.* Women who have had an inherited form of colorectal cancer have a higher risk of developing uterine cancer than other women.

- *Estrogen-related factors.* Women who have no children, begin menstruation at a very young age, or enter menopause late in life are exposed to estrogen longer and have a higher risk of uterine cancer.

Symptoms

Uterine cancer usually occurs after menopause, but it may also occur during perimenopause. Abnormal vaginal bleeding is the most common symptom of uterine cancer, which may begin with watery, blood-streaked flow that gradually contains more blood. Women should not assume that abnormal vaginal bleeding is part of menopause. Other symptoms include unusual vaginal discharge, difficult or painful urination, pain during intercourse, or pelvic pain.

Diagnosis

If a woman has symptoms that suggest uterine cancer, her doctor may order blood and urine tests, a pelvic exam, a PAP TEST, or a transvaginal ultrasound. If the endometrium looks too thick on ultrasound, the doctor can do a biopsy.

In a biopsy the doctor removes a sample of tissue from the uterine lining. This usually can be done in the doctor's office, but sometimes a woman may need to have a DILATION AND CURETTAGE (D & C). A D & C is usually done as same-day surgery with anesthesia in a hospital. A pathologist examines the tissue to check for cancer cells, hyperplasia, and other conditions.

Staging

If uterine cancer is diagnosed, the doctor needs to know the extent of the disease to plan the best treatment. Staging is a careful attempt to find out whether the cancer has spread, and if so, where. To find this out, the doctor may order blood and urine tests and chest X-rays, other X-rays, CT scans, an ultrasound test, magnetic resonance imaging (MRI), SIGMOIDOSCOPY, or COLONOSCOPY.

In most cases, the most reliable way to stage this disease is to remove the uterus (HYSTEREC- TOMY). After the uterus has been removed, the surgeon can check to see if the cancer has invaded the muscle of the uterus and can check the lymph nodes and other organs in the pelvic area for signs of cancer.

Stage I: The cancer is only in the body of the uterus and not in the cervix.

Stage II: The cancer has spread from the body of the uterus to the cervix.

Stage III: The cancer has spread outside the uterus, but not outside the pelvis (and not to the blad- der or rectum). Lymph nodes in the pelvis may contain cancer cells.

Stage IV: The cancer has spread into the bladder or rectum, or it has spread beyond the pelvis to other parts of the body.

Treatment

The choice of treatment depends on the size of the tumor, the stage of the disease, whether female hormones affect tumor growth, and the tumor grade, which is an explanation of how closely the cancer cells resemble normal cells and suggests how fast the cancer is likely to grow. Low-grade cancers are likely to grow and spread more slowly than high-grade cancers. The doctor also considers other factors, including the woman's age and gen- eral health.

Surgery Most women with uterine cancer are treated with a hysterectomy, including the removal of both fallopian tubes and both ovaries. (This procedure is called a bilateral SALPINGO- OOPHORECTOMY.) The doctor may also remove the lymph nodes near the tumor to see if they contain cancer. If cancer cells have reached the lymph nodes, it may mean that the disease has spread to other parts of the body. If cancer cells have not spread beyond the endometrium, the woman may not need to have any other treatment. The

length of the hospital stay may vary from several days to a week.

Radiation therapy Some women have RADIA- TION THERAPY, in which high-energy rays are used to kill cancer cells in the treated area. Some women with stage I, II, or III uterine cancer need both radiation therapy and surgery. They may have radiation before surgery to shrink the tumor or after surgery to destroy any cancer cells that remain in the area. Also, the doctor may suggest radiation treatments for the small number of women who cannot have surgery.

Doctors use both external and internal types of radiation therapy to treat uterine cancer. In external radiation therapy, a woman usually is treated as an outpatient receiving radiation treat- ments from a machine outside the body five days a week for several weeks. This schedule helps protect healthy cells and tissue by spreading out the total dose of radiation. In internal radiation therapy, tiny tubes containing a radioactive sub- stance are inserted through the vagina and left in place for a few days while a woman is hospital- ized. To protect others from radiation exposure, the patient may not be able to have visitors, or may have visitors only for a short period of time while the implant is in place. Once the implant is removed, the woman is not radioactive. Some patients need both external and internal radia- tion therapies.

Hormonal therapy If a hormone receptor test indicates that the tumor has hormone receptors, the woman is more likely to respond to HORMONAL THERAPY. Hormonal therapy usually involves taking a type of progesterone as a pill. The doctor may use hormonal therapy for women with uterine cancer who are unable to have surgery or radiation ther- apy, or for women whose cancer has spread to the lungs or other distant sites. It is also given to women with recurrent uterine cancer.

New Research

Scientists are currently studying the effectiveness of radiation therapy after surgery, as well as differ- ent combinations of surgery, radiation, and chemotherapy. Other trials are studying new drugs, new drug combinations, and biological ther- apies. Some of these studies are designed to find ways to reduce the side effects of treatment and to improve the quality of women's lives.

endometrial hyperplasia   An increase in the number of cells in the lining of the uterus. Although this increase in cells is not a malignant condition, it may sometimes develop into cancer. Heavy menstrual periods, bleeding between periods, and bleeding after menopause are common symptoms of hyperplasia. It is most common after age 40.

Unless the lining of the uterus sheds regularly, tissues and glands will build up and may later become a breeding ground for abnormal cells. Any woman of childbearing age who has missed more than two consecutive periods but is not pregnant needs to investigate the reason.

Unopposed estrogen activity may lead to endometrial hyperplasia. Such activity can occur during adolescence and in the years before menopause, when women may have many cycles without ovulation. Polycystic ovary syndrome is another condition in which women do not ovulate and have unopposed estrogen. Similarly, hormone replacement therapy with estrogen without progesterone may lead to endometrial hyperplasia.

To prevent endometrial hyperplasia from developing into cancer, a woman's doctor may recommend surgery to remove the uterus (HYSTERECTOMY) or treatment with progesterone and regular follow-up exams.

Types

Some cases of hyperplasia are more advanced than others. *Mild hyperplasia,* known as *cystic glandular hyperplasia* or *cystic endometrial hyperplasia,* is characterized by an excess of tissue with normal endometrial cells. This kind of hyperplasia is always caused by too much estrogen and rarely develops into cancer.

When mild hyperplasia is not treated, it may lead to *adenomatous hyperplasia without atypical cells.* This benign condition refers to a buildup of glandular cells (the glandular endometrial cells are growing but are still non-cancerous). This kind of hyperplasia rarely develops into cancer.

In *atypical adenomatous hyperplasia* (also called *severe hyperplasia* or *carcinoma in situ* either a small area on the endometrium or the entire lining consists of cells that are abnormal. The cells seem to be more aggressive but may still be harmless. It still is not malignant, but more women with severe hyperplasia may go on to develop uterine cancer.

Risk Factors

Women who are 25 to 50 pounds overweight are three times as likely to develop hyperplasia; women who are more than 50 pounds overweight are nine times as likely to develop hyperplasia. Women at higher risk also include those who have always had irregular periods or who have diabetes. Other potential causes of excess estrogen include environmental toxins, certain herbs (such as ginseng), hormone-fed meats and poultry, certain cosmetics made from estrogen, and hormonal contraceptives that contain estrogen.

A postmenopausal woman with an intact uterus on unopposed estrogen replacement therapy is also at risk for developing hyperplasia. An estrogen/progesterone combination therapy can reverse as many as 96.8 percent of all postmenopausal hyperplasia cases.

Diagnosis

This diagnosis can be made only by the pathologist who examines a sample of tissue removed from the thickened endometrium by a procedure such as endometrial biopsy, D & C, or HYSTEROSCOPY.

Treatment

In younger women particularly, severe hyperplasia can be reversed with hormonal therapy. Adding progesterone by taking a progestin or resuming ovulation (spontaneously or with medications) can eliminate hyperplasia. If this does not work, a D & C is the next logical step. A hysterectomy is not necessary unless the hyperplasia persists after the lining is removed. If severe hyperplasia persists and keeps redeveloping despite hormone replacement and a repeat D & C, then a hysterectomy may be required.

endoscopic retrograde cholangiopancreatography   A type of internal ultrasound test used to visualize the pancreatic duct, hepatic duct, common bile duct, duodenal papilla, and gallbladder, and used to diagnose PANCREATIC CANCER, BILE DUCT CANCER, or GALLBLADDER CANCER.

In this procedure, a thin lighted tube called an endoscope is passed through the patient's mouth and down into the first part of the small intestine. A catheter is then inserted through the endoscope into the bile and pancreatic ducts. After injecting dye through the catheter into the ducts, the physician can take X-rays to show whether the ducts are narrowed or blocked.

endoscopy   Examination of the inside of organs and cavities using a flexible instrument with a lighted tube and optical system (endoscope). During an endoscopy, a doctor can take photographs or remove tissue for a BIOPSY to check for malignant cells. Typically, endoscopy can be performed in a doctor's office or on an outpatient basis.

There are a number of different endoscopic procedures that can be performed to identify various types of cancer, including: BRONCHOSCOPY, COLONOSCOPY, COLPOSCOPY, CYSTOSCOPY, duodenoscopy, ENDOSCOPIC RETROGRADE CHOLANGIOPANCREATOGRAPHY, esophagoscopy, gastroscopy, HYSTEROSCOPY, LAPAROSCOPY, MEDIASTINOSCOPY, otoscopy, protoscopy, SIGMOIDOSCOPY, and thoracoscopy.

endothelioma   Any benign or malignant tumor that begins in endothelial tissue. The endothelium is the single layer of cells lining the heart, blood vessels, and lymphatic vessels.

environmental estrogens   A wide variety of natural compounds and man-made chemicals that mimic natural hormones. Both types may affect the endocrine system, and synthetic estrogens have been linked to growth, reproductive, and other health problems in wildlife and laboratory animals. They may also affect human health.

Environmental estrogens are known by a wide variety of names, including endocrine modulators, ecoestrogens, environmental hormones, xenoestrogens, hormone-related toxicants, endocrine-active compounds, and phytoestrogens. These terms all describe the function of endocrine disruptors.

While some believe these environmental compounds can affect human health, development, and reproduction, this has not yet been scientifically proven. Although the issue of the safety of environmental estrogens is controversial, many scientists around the world have reached a tentative conclusion that environmental chemicals do interfere with biological systems, causing adverse effects in wildlife but unclear effects in humans. Preventing exposure—especially in children—is the most effective away of protecting against environmental threats.

Environmental estrogens can affect the endocrine system in many ways. They can alter hormonal functions by:

- mimicking the sex steroid hormone estrogen by binding to hormone receptors or influencing cell signaling pathways
- blocking or altering hormonal actions. Chemicals that block or antagonize hormones are labeled antiestrogens or anti-androgens
- altering production and breakdown of natural hormones (chemicals that do this are called environmental disrupters or modulators)
- modifying the production and function of hormone receptors

Environmental estrogens are the most studied of all the endocrine disrupters. Natural compounds capable of producing an estrogen response, such as the PHYTOESTROGENS, occur in a variety of plants. Many synthetic chemicals that also mimic estrogen are commercially manufactured for a specific purpose or produced as a by-product. People are exposed to these substances throughout their lives, in food, air, water, soil, and household products including detergents, drugs, lubricants, cosmetics, PESTICIDES, and plastics. The human health risks that may be associated with these low-level yet constant exposures are still largely unknown and highly controversial. Indirect exposure occurs when chemicals are released into the air and water. Drinking water may be contaminated by chemicals, and chemical breakdown products may be found in industrial discharge and sewage.

Some proven environmental estrogens used as pesticides (such as DDT, toxaphene, and dicofol) have been banned in most Western industrial countries but are still used in many developing nations. Other proven estrogenic compounds are still being used worldwide in plastics manufacturing (phthlates) and to combat pest plants and insects (endosulfan).

Even though some of the more harmful substances have been banned in certain areas, humans are still vulnerable to their effects because they and their breakdown products remain in the environment. The human body itself carries some of these chemicals in fat and tissue and can pass them along to offspring during pregnancy and breast-feeding.

Soil, water, and animals remain contaminated with some of these persistent pollutants. For example, DDD and DDE (breakdown products of DDT) are found worldwide. The airborne pollutant toxaphene, a pesticide banned in the United States since 1982, is still found in soil, the fat tissue of seals and Baltic salmon, and in places like the Arctic and Scandinavia, where it was never even used.

Scientists are concerned because wildlife and laboratory studies associate reproductive and developmental problems in animals with exposure to high concentrations of synthetic environmental estrogens. Many animals living in or near contaminated areas have health problems, including fish, frogs, salamanders, alligators, turtles, birds, and marine mammals.

The most convincing evidence that synthetic chemicals can act like hormones comes from the experience of pregnant women who took DIETHYL-STILBESTROL (DES) during the 1950s. A strong synthetic estrogen banned since the 1970s, DES is far more potent than other environmental estrogens. It was given to pregnant women during critical fetal development to prevent miscarriages. Offspring of women who took the drug have more reproductive problems and cancer than those not exposed to DES in the womb. Laboratory studies confirmed that DES causes reproductive problems and cancer in male and female mice.

No one really knows whether long-term exposure to low levels of environmental estrogens and other hormones causes health problems in adult wildlife and humans. It may be that developing fetuses and embryos, whose growth and development is highly controlled by the endocrine system, may be the most vulnerable to and may have the most lasting effects from environmental estrogens.

At present, scientists strongly disagree among themselves about how dangerous environmental estrogens may be. Some strongly believe that wildlife and laboratory evidence show that synthetic chemicals that act like estrogens have the potential to cause (and may already have caused) severe health problems. Many believe there may be reason for concern but call for more research to clarify issues. They believe a better understanding of how environmental estrogens may impact the endocrine system will help identify the most harmful substances and lead to less human and wildlife exposure to these compounds.

Others remain skeptical, believing that scientific data are inconclusive. Pointing to the lack of strong cause-and-effect evidence, they advocate more research and believe policy decisions should be put off until more is known about the subject.

environmental factors There is clear evidence that many environmental factors may contribute to cancer development, playing a role in more than half of all cancers. Sun exposure and SMOKING are the major contributors, accounting for about 40 percent of all deaths. All other environmental contributors (excluding diet) combined account for less than 10 percent. Some of these other contributors include pesticides, air pollution, and asbestos, as well as:

- *chemicals* used in some cleaning agents, paint solvents, and deodorizers;
- *radon*, a naturally occurring, invisible gas that enters a building through cracks in the foundation. Once it is concentrated indoors, anyone who inhales the gas is at higher risk of developing LUNG CANCER. Radon test kits are available at hardware stores.

Environmental CARCINOGENS enter the body mainly through breathing but also by absorption through the skin or by ingestion (such as eating contaminated food).

Once in the body, the substance can either remain in one place (asbestos, for example, stays in the lungs), or be absorbed systematically. Once it enters the body, the carcinogen travels through the body in the blood and can undergo chemical changes that make it more or less toxic. Eventually, the carcinogen finds its way into individual cells and can cause mutations that lead to cancer.

The cancer risk posed by environmental factors becomes greater with increased exposure, either in one large toxic dose or in small-dose exposures over a long period of time.

Since it is not ethical to intentionally expose people to environmental carcinogens, information about their effects is gathered in four ways.

- *Epidemiological studies.* Cancer incidence within large population groups is measured by comparing subgroups with different exposure levels to the environmental carcinogen. For example, in any population group, when people who smoke are compared to people who do not smoke, the smokers have a higher rate of lung cancer.

- *Natural experiments.* If people are exposed accidentally to harmful levels of an environmental factor, they can be compared to the general population to see if the exposure caused an increased cancer risk. For example, children who lived near the site of the Chernobyl nuclear accident have a higher risk of THYROID CANCER due to exposure to radioactive iodine fallout.

- *Animal studies.* By exposing rats or mice to dosages of a suspected carcinogen over time and measuring the effects, scientists make assumptions about what effect that carcinogen might have on humans. Although extrapolations based on animal data are not certain, this method can help assess human risk for factors that cannot be tested in any other way.

- *Lab tests.* Some tests using bacteria or cells can determine if a suspected carcinogen can alter DNA and screen for possible carcinogens.

Using these methods and their knowledge of the prevalence of a carcinogen, scientists can estimate the cancer risk of a particular substance. For example, studies have shown that certain pesticides may promote tumor growth in the breast tissue of rats, but the amounts of these pesticides present in food consumed by people are so small that they are not believed to contribute very much to human breast cancer. This assumption has been supported by studies that compared the amount of pesticide residue in a woman's blood to her risk of developing breast cancer.

Studies of the risks associated with environmental factors are used to help regulate the use of proven carcinogens, make people aware of the risks, and encourage preventive measures to avoid exposure to those factors that pose the greatest risks.

Top 10 List of Environmental Links to Cancer

Exposure to the Sun and cigarette smoking pose the greatest risk of developing cancer, according to the U.S. Environmental Protection Agency. Other factors contribute much less significantly to cancer development. The list below shows the approximate lifetime risk of developing cancer due to different environmental exposures.

RISK FACTOR
1. Excessive sun exposure: 1 in 3
2. Cigarette smoking (one pack or more per day): 8 in 100
3. Natural radon in indoor air at home: 1 in 100
4. Outside radiation: 1 in 1,000
5. Secondhand tobacco smoke: 7 in 10,000
6. Human-made chemicals in home indoor air: 2 in 10,000
7. Outdoor air, industrialized areas: 1 in 100,000
8. Human-made chemicals in drinking water: 1 in 100,000
9. Human-made chemicals in foods (including pesticides): 1 in 100,000 or less
10. Chemicals at uncontrolled hazardous-waste sites: 1 in 10,000 to 100,000

These figures can be compared to the lifetime risk of death from a fall (four in 1,000) and the lifetime risk of death by drowning (three in 1,000).

eosinophilic leukemia   See LEUKEMIA.

ependymal tumors   See BRAIN CANCER.

ependymoblastoma   See BRAIN CANCER.

ependymoma   See BRAIN CANCER.

epidermal growth factor receptor   See HER1.

epidermoid cancer of mucous membranes A type of cancer that is strongly associated with SMOKING or ALCOHOL and that affects the lining of the upper air and food passages. Also known as an aerodigestive tract cancer, this type of malignancy usually remains in the area where it arose, although it may spread to nearby LYMPH NODES in the neck.

epidermoid carcinoma Another name for SQUA-MOUS CELL CARCINOMA OF THE SKIN.

epithelioma An older term for CARCINOMA.

Epstein-Barr virus A virus that causes infectious mononucleosis and that has also been linked to many human cancers, including BURKITT'S LYM-PHOMA, HEAD AND NECK CANCER, HODGKIN'S DISEASE, and an aggressive form of BREAST CANCER. The Epstein-Barr virus alters the function of a cellular protein that normally suppresses the movement of malignant cells. When this natural brake on cell migration is disabled by the virus, cancerous cells can spread.

More than 90 percent of adults show signs of previous viral infection with Epstein-Barr. Adolescents infected with the acute phase of the virus can develop infectious mononucleosis, but usually the body's natural immune response forces the virus to revert to its latent phase—where it hides inside the nucleus of immune cells without producing any symptoms. Although the virus is endemic in humans, most cells infected by it never become malignant. Other genetic factors are required to trigger development of cancer.

Should cancer develop, however, the risk of spreading may be higher in people who previously had been exposed to the virus.

erb B-2 See ONCOGENES.

erb-38 immunotoxin A toxic substance linked to an antibody that attaches to tumor cells and kills them.

erythroplakia Sores or inflamed areas in the mouth that are considered to be precancerous. In its early stages, erythroplakia does not cause pain but can be identified by a dentist during a routine exam. Any sore in the mouth that lasts longer than two weeks should be examined by a dentist or doctor.

This condition occurs equally among men and women, usually over age 60; it is most common among people who smoke or drink heavily.

erythropoietin Produced in the adult kidney, this COLONY-STIMULATING FACTOR triggers the production of red blood cells. It is a type of growth factor that can reverse ANEMIA in cancer patients.

esophageal cancer A cancer that begins in the esophagus and falls into one of two major categories, squamous cell carcinoma or ADENOCARCI-NOMA, depending on the type of malignant cells.

Squamous cell carcinomas begin in the squamous cells lining the esophagus, usually appearing in the upper and middle parts of the esophagus. Adenocarcinomas usually develop in the glandular tissue in the lower part of the esophagus.

Esophageal cancer can spread to the LYMPH NODES or almost any other part of the body, including the liver, lungs, brain, and bones.

Cause

The exact causes of esophageal cancer are not known, but there are a number of risk factors that increase a person's risk:

- *Age.* Esophageal cancer is more likely to occur as people get older. Most people who develop esophageal cancer are over age 60.

- *Gender.* This type of cancer is more common in men than in women.

- *Smoking.* Using cigarettes or smokeless tobacco is one of the major risk factors for esophageal cancer (especially squamous cell cancer)

- *Alcohol.* Chronic or heavy ALCOHOL abuse is a major risk factor for esophageal cancer. People who use both alcohol and tobacco have an especially high risk.

- *Barrett's esophagus.* Long-term irritation resulting from gastric reflux, which occurs when stomach acid backs up into the esophagus, can increase the risk of esophageal cancer. Eventually, irritated cells may change and begin to resemble the cells that line the stomach. This condition, known as Barrett's esophagus, is premalignant and may develop into adenocarcinoma of the esophagus.

- *Irritation.* Significant irritation or damage to the lining of the esophagus resulting from swallowing caustic substances such as lye, increases the risk of developing esophageal cancer.

- *Medical history.* Patients who have had other types of HEAD AND NECK CANCER have a higher chance of developing a second cancer in this area, including squamous cell esophageal cancer.

Still, most people with one or even several of these factors do not get the disease, and most people who do get esophageal cancer have none of the known risk factors.

Prevention

The best way to prevent esophageal cancer is to quit (or never start) SMOKING cigarettes, to stop using smokeless tobacco, and to drink alcohol only in moderation.

Symptoms

Early esophageal cancer usually does not cause symptoms, but as the cancer grows, symptoms may include

- cough that is chronic or brings up blood
- hoarseness
- pain in the throat or back, behind the breastbone, or between the shoulder blades
- swallowing problems
- vomiting
- weight loss (severe)

Diagnosis

A medical history and physical exam may be followed by a BARIUM SWALLOW (esophagram), a series of X-rays of the esophagus. In this test, the patient drinks a barium-containing liquid that coats the inside of the esophagus. The barium makes any changes in the shape of the esophagus show up on the X-rays.

The doctor also may order an esophagoscopy (also called endoscopy), an examination of the inside of the esophagus using a thin, lighted tube called an endoscope. If an abnormal area is found during this test, the doctor can collect cells and tissue through the endoscope for examination under a microscope.

Staging

A patient with esophageal cancer must be staged to find out whether the cancer has spread and, if so, to what parts of the body. Knowing the stage of the disease helps the doctor plan treatment.

Stage I: The cancer is found only in the top layers of cells lining the esophagus.

Stage II: The cancer involves deeper layers of the lining of the esophagus, or it has spread to nearby lymph nodes, but has not spread to other parts of the body.

Stage III: The cancer has invaded through the wall of the esophagus, and may have spread to tissues or lymph nodes near the esophagus, but has not spread to other parts of the body.

Stage IV: The cancer has spread to other parts of the body, including the liver, lungs, brain, and bones.

Treatment

Treatment for esophageal cancer depends on a number of factors, including the size, location, and extent of the tumor, and the patient's general health. Many different combinations of treatments may be used to control the cancer and improve the patient's quality of life by reducing symptoms.

Surgery is the most common treatment, usually involving the removal of the tumor along with all or a portion of the esophagus, nearby LYMPH NODES, and other tissue in the area. (An operation to remove the esophagus is called an ESOPHAGEC-TOMY.) If a healthy part of the esophagus remains, the surgeon connects it to the stomach so the patient is still able to swallow. Sometimes a plastic tube or part of the intestine is used to make the connection. The surgeon may also widen the opening between the stomach and the small intestine to allow stomach contents to pass more easily into the small intestine.

RADIATION THERAPY involves the use of high-energy rays to kill cancer cells. A plastic tube may need to be inserted into the esophagus to keep it open during radiation therapy. This procedure is called intraluminal intubation and dilation. Radiation therapy may be used alone or combined with CHEMOTHERAPY as primary treatment instead of surgery, especially if the size or location of the tumor would make an operation difficult. Doctors may also combine radiation therapy with chemotherapy to shrink the tumor before surgery. Even if the tumor cannot be removed by surgery or destroyed entirely by radiation, radiation therapy can often help relieve pain and make swallowing easier.

Laser therapy is the use of high-intensity light to destroy tumor cells and ease a block in the esophagus when the cancer cannot be removed by surgery. The relief of a blockage can help to reduce symptoms, especially swallowing problems. Photodynamic therapy (PDT) is a type of laser therapy in which drugs that are absorbed by cancer cells are exposed to a special light so that they become active and destroy the cells. The doctor may use PDT to relieve symptoms of esophageal cancer such as difficulty swallowing.

esophageal speech Speech produced by trapping air in the esophagus and forcing it out again. It is used by people whose voice boxes (larynxes) have been removed.

See also ESOPHAGEAL CANCER; LARYNGEAL CANCER.

esophagectomy The surgical removal of the esophagus, or part of it, as a way of treating ESOPHAGEAL CANCER. After surgery, the remaining part of the esophagus is attached to the stomach so that swallowing is still possible.

esophagitis Inflammation of the esophagus as a direct result of taking CHEMOTHERAPY drugs for cancer. Esophagitis can lead to bleeding, painful ulcers, and infection. Sores in the esophagus, most often temporary, usually develop between five and 14 days after a patient starts receiving chemotherapy. They generally heal completely once chemotherapy is finished.

Symptoms

Symptoms include chest pain or a burning feeling in the throat that can be heavy or sharp. Pain from esophagitis may be constant or intermittent. These may be worsening of the chest pain when swallowing or a feeling of food sticking in the chest after swallowing. Less often, there may be blood in the vomit or stools.

Prognosis

In most cases symptoms begin to improve within a week or two after the chemotherapy treatment, but it can take weeks for symptoms to go away completely. Patients about to undergo treatment with chemotherapy should inform the doctor about past herpes infections. In some cases it may be important to use the antibiotic acyclovir to prevent herpes virus from causing a deep infection.

esophagus, cancer of See ESOPHAGEAL CANCER.

estrogen A family of hormones that promote the development and maintenance of female sex characteristics. It is one of the hormones produced by the body that is primarily responsible for directing endometrial cells to multiply or proliferate. While proliferation is necessary during the "buildup" phase of the endometrium's cycle, the effects need to be constrained by other hormones, such as progesterone. If estrogen stimulation continues unchecked, this can cause ENDOMETRIAL HYPERPLASIA. This condition is a known risk factor for the later development of ENDOMETRIAL CANCER.

Historically, menopausal women took replacement estrogen to counteract the effects of menopause, but a NATIONAL CANCER INSTITUTE (NCI) study published in 2003 found that women who took estrogen were significantly more likely to develop OVARIAN CANCER than those not on the hormone. The study tracked thousands of women for nearly two decades and found that women who took estrogen were, on average, one-and-a-half times more likely to develop ovarian cancer, a particularly lethal form of cancer. That risk increased the longer a woman took the medicine: women on estrogen for 20 years or beyond were three times more likely to develop ovarian cancer than those who did not take the pills. Previous studies had presented conflicting evidence about the link between estrogen and ovarian cancer.

The report came one week after federal authorities halted another study of hormone replacement therapy after research showed that the pills were doing more harm than good and were causing conditions the medicine was once believed to prevent, such as heart disease. That study looked at women who took a combination of two hormones, estrogen and progestin.

Those drugs have been prominent in the medicine cabinets of millions of American women since the 1940s, originally designed to ease the short-term symptoms of menopause, such as hot flashes and night sweats. Over time, hormones also emerged as a treatment of choice to help women avoid heart disease and osteoporosis. This change resulted in women increasing the period that they used the drugs from a few months to, in some cases, decades. Eventually, an estimated 8 million women in the United States were regularly taking estrogen.

Now, with two studies in one week undermining long-held beliefs about hormones, doctors are reevaluating their recommendations to patients, who have flooded clinics with urgent phone calls. Many experts believe the new studies will mean the end of long-term hormone use.

Estrogen alone is the hormone of choice for women who have undergone hysterectomies, while other women on hormone-replacement therapy typically take a hormone drug called Prempro, which includes both estrogen and progestin.

Specialists theorize that because ovarian tissue is especially sensitive to hormones, altering them after menopause may increase cancer risk. An animal study cited in the NCI report found that estrogen stimulated growth of cancer cells in rabbits. Conversely, other hormonal changes (such as taking birth control pills) are known to provide protection against cancer. While the estrogen study monitored a substantial number of patients for an extended period, it probably will not provide the definitive answer about use of the hormone. That will come from the ongoing Women's Health Initiative, the same study that concluded that the combination therapy Prempro could be perilous to patients' health.

estrogen receptor   A protein found on some cancer cells to which ESTROGEN will attach, prima-

rily in BREAST CANCERS. Breast cancer cells that do not have the receptor molecule to which estrogen will attach are called "estrogen receptor negative." (ER-).

Breast cancer cells that are ER- do not need the hormone estrogen to grow and usually do not respond to anti-estrogen therapy that blocks these receptor sites. Breast cancer cells that have a receptor molecule to which estrogen will attach are called "estrogen receptor positive." These cells do need estrogen to grow and will usually respond to anti-estrogen therapy that blocks these receptor sites. TAMOXIFEN is one type of anti-estrogen treatment given to women who have ER+ tumors.

Testing

A lab test can determine if breast cancer cells have estrogen receptors. If the cells are found to be ER+, this information may influence how the breast cancer is treated.

estrogen receptor downregulator (ERD)   A new type of hormonal treatment for breast cancer that stops the estrogen receptor from working, first approved in April 2002 by the U.S. Food and Drug Administration (FDA). The first ERD, fulvestrant (Faslodex), was approved to treat hormone-receptor-positive metastatic BREAST CANCER in post-menopausal women who no longer responded to hormonal therapy such as tamoxifen (Nolvadex).

When the FDA approved Faslodex, it referred to the drug as an estrogen receptor antagonist (that is, a drug that blocks estrogen's effects) without known estrogen-promoting effects. However, Faslodex is commonly known as an ERD.

ERDs work by attaching to the hormone receptors on breast cancer cells, blocking them, and causing them to break down and stop working. Breast cancer cells with hormone receptors grow and multiply when estrogen attaches to the receptors. Breast cancer cells may have hormone receptors for estrogen, progesterone, or both. If the cancer cells have receptors, the tumor is called "hormone receptor positive." If there are no hormone receptors, it is "hormone receptor negative." Hormonal therapies work only if the cancer cells have estrogen or progesterone receptors. A woman's pathology report usually includes the results of a test that shows whether the tumor has hormone receptors.

ERDs work differently from other hormone therapies. In addition to binding to and blocking estrogen receptors, ERDs also stop or slow down the growth of breast cancer cells by breaking down the receptors. With fewer hormone receptors available, fewer cells receive the signal telling them to grow, and the overgrowth of cancer cells can be slowed or stopped.

ERDs vs. SERMs

ERDs are different from SERMs (SELECTIVE ESTROGEN-RECEPTOR MODULATORS) such as tamoxifen, and different also from AROMATASE INHIBITORS, such as Arimidex, Femara, and Aromasin, in the way they work, their side effects, and the way they are given.

Faslodex, the only ERD currently approved by the FDA, is given in an injection into the buttocks once a month in the doctor's office. All other hormone therapies for postmenopausal women are taken orally.

In general each hormonal therapy is given to women with metastatic breast cancer as long as the cancer is responding and the side effects are acceptable.

Side Effects

Treatments that decrease estrogen's effect on breast cells may also cut back estrogen's effect on the rest of the body, which can trigger menopause-related symptoms such as hot flashes. Faslodex is associated with relatively mild menopause-like side effects, similar to the side effects of the aromatase inhibitor Arimidex. Most of the side effects are experienced by fewer than 20 percent of women. They include NAUSEA, vomiting, constipation, diarrhea, stomach pain, headaches, back pain, hot flushes, and throat pain.

European Organisation for Research and Treatment of Cancer (EORTC)   An international non-profit group that conducts, coordinates, and stimulates laboratory and clinical research in Europe to improve the management of cancer. Because comprehensive research in this field is often beyond the means of individual European laboratories and hospitals, the organization brings together multidisciplinary, multinational efforts of basic research scientists and clinicians from the European continent.

The ultimate goal of the EORTC is to improve the standard of cancer treatment in Europe through the development of new drugs and innovative approaches, and to test more effective treatments with drugs, surgery, and radiation therapy.

The organization was founded as an international organization under Belgian law in 1962 by eminent oncologists working in the main cancer research institutes of the countries now in the European Union and Switzerland. It was named "Groupe Européen de Chimiothérapie Anticancéreuse" (GECA); it became the European Organisation for Research and Treatment of Cancer in 1968. For contact information, see Appendix I.

Ewing's sarcoma   See BONE CANCER.

Exceptional Cancer Patient, Inc. (EcaP)   A non-profit organization that emphasizes the importance of the mind-body connection in health care for cancer patients and others with chronic illnesses.

Exceptional Cancer Patients was founded in 1978 by Bernie Siegel, M.D., and successfully operated for many years; it was acquired in 1999 by the Mind-Body Wellness Center in order to advance the organization and its principles. Today it is owned and operated by Meadville Medical Center and MMC Health Systems, Inc. It offers comprehensive, integrative, "whole person" programs in a traditional medical setting. Through a combination of outcome-based clinical studies and basic science research, the center promotes healing in mind, body, and spirit.

The center provides resources, comprehensive professional training programs, and interdisciplinary retreats to help people facing the challenges of cancer discover their inner healing resources. For contact information, see Appendix I.

excisional biopsy   A surgical procedure in which an entire lump or suspicious area is removed and then examined under a microscope for diagnosis.

See also BIOPSY.

exenteration   The surgical removal of the vagina, uterus, and cervix as a treatment for advanced VAGINAL CANCER or CERVICAL CANCER. If the cancer has spread, the surgeon also may need to remove the lower colon, rectum, or bladder.

exercise   A growing body of research suggests that even moderate exercise can both help prevent the development of a wide variety of cancers and prevent them from recurring. This research is so important that the AMERICAN CANCER SOCIETY (ACS) is putting a new emphasis on exercise as a way to reduce cancer risk. The five-year update of the organization's nutrition and activity guidelines says the evidence now is convincing that exercise reduces risk of COLORECTAL CANCER and BREAST CANCER, probably fights against ENDOMETRIAL CANCER, and may help against other forms of cancer as well.

The latest research says activity apparently works directly to lower the risk and provides an added indirect benefit if the exercise also keeps a person's weight down. Experts believe that weight control, through proper nutrition or physical activity, independently reduces risk. If everyone exercised and controlled weight, the number of Americans who died of cancer would drop by about one-third, and about an equal number of new cases could be prevented. The society's minimum recommendation for cancer prevention in adults is at least 30 minutes of moderate activity, such as a brisk walk, five days a week. That is in line with the surgeon general's recommendations for overall good health and the American Heart Association's recommendations for cardiovascular health.

Being active can control weight, improving energy metabolism and reducing blood levels of insulin. Physical activity helps to prevent adult-onset diabetes, which has been associated with increased risk of cancers of the colon, pancreas and possibly other sites, according to the ACS report. Risks of some forms of cancer can be double among the overweight and obese, but the data are cloudy because studies have not uniformly defined these conditions.

Forty-five minutes or more of moderate to vigorous activity five or more days a week may further decrease breast and colon cancer risk. Vigorous activity can range from jogging to martial arts, basketball, or masonry work. This much exercise can reduce the risk of colon cancer by almost half and breast cancer by a third.

Exercise helps the body function properly so that food gets used optimally, builds lean muscle, and burns calories. Exercise reduces blood levels of ESTROGEN, a hormone that has been linked to higher breast cancer risk in postmenopausal women. Exercise also reduces other hormones that can raise the risk of colon cancer and speeds the passage of material through the bowel before any cancer-causing agents can linger against the bowel wall.

A sedentary lifestyle contributes to obesity, and obesity is a risk factor for cancers of the prostate, breast, ovary, endometrium, gallbladder, and colon. Exercise alone reduced the risk of breast cancer and prostate cancer in some studies.

The ACS guidelines also call for children and adolescents to do at least 60 minutes a day of moderate-to-vigorous physical activity, five days a week. The goal is to create lifetime habits that will keep youngsters from joining the 55 percent of American adults who now are overweight or obese.

Another study found that physically fit people are less likely to die of cancer, including cancers related to SMOKING, even if they smoke. How *much* exercise is enough is controversial, however. While some studies say that 30 minutes of exercise a day—not even at one time—is enough, others indicate the benefit may come only with more prolonged and vigorous exercise.

In one study that found that fitness may provide protection against cancer death, researchers followed 25,892 men aged 30 to 87, who took treadmill tests to determine the most exercise they could do. The men were followed for an average of 10 years. In this time, there were 133 deaths from cancers related to smoking and 202 deaths from other cancers. The fittest men had a 55 percent lower risk of all types of cancer death than did low-fit men, and moderately fit men had a 38 percent lower risk. To be moderately fit, a person would have to run 20 to 40 minutes, three to five times a week. To be most fit, a person would have to be at the recreationally competitive level. The most-fit men had a 46 percent lower risk, and moderately fit men had a 34 percent lower risk, of cancers unrelated to smoking. These diseases include cancers of the colon and prostate, and LEUKEMIA, which affects white blood cells.

The most-fit men had a 66 percent lower risk and the moderately fit men a 43 percent lower risk of cancers related to smoking, such as cancers of the lung and mouth.

If the least-fit smokers had become fit, they would have reduced their death risk by 13 percent, a statistical analysis in the study concluded.

Although the most-fit men were least likely to smoke, almost 10 percent of them did, as did 20 percent of moderately fit men and 33 percent of sedentary men. The most-fit and moderately fit smokers were still less likely to die than were the sedentary smokers, which means that high-fit smokers have a lower risk. Still, exercise is no substitute for giving up smoking—nonsmokers who were the most physically fit had the lowest risk of dying of cancer.

Researchers theorized that the heavy breathing that comes with vigorous activity clears the lungs of some cancer-causing chemicals associated with smoking, and that fitness may help the body in other ways, such as by improving defensive systems that may keep tumors from forming. It is also possible that fit men were more careful about their own health and saw doctors more often, so their cancers were diagnosed earlier, when the chance of successful treatment was greater.

A separate study has found no reduction in cancer risk from less-intense activity. Researchers at Britain's Royal Free and University College Medical School followed 7,588 men aged 40 to 59 for an average of almost 19 years. The British scientists found a reduced risk of all cancer only with moderately vigorous or vigorous activity; there was no benefit with less work, and the more strenuous the activity, the greater was the benefit, the study found.

exocrine cancer   See PANCREATIC CANCER.

extragonadal germ cell tumor   A primary GERM CELL CANCER located outside of the testicles (or ovaries). These tumors may not respond as well to therapy as primary testicular tumors.

extravasation   Leaking of a chemotherapy drug out of the vein and into the skin.

eye cancer   Cancers of the eye are rare types of malignancy, accounting for just about 2,208 cases in the United States in 1999. The two most common types of eye cancer are intraocular MELANOMA, and retinoblastoma in children under the age of two. Cancer may occur in the eyelid, in the conjunctiva, the iris, the retina, the eyeball, or the eye socket.

Secondary intraocular cancers have spread to the eye from another part of the body. The most common cancers that spread to the eye are breast and lung cancers; usually, these cancers spread to the part of the eyeball called the uvea.

General Symptoms

Symptoms of eye cancer may include a protruding eyeball, pain, double vision, or drooping eyelids. Although these symptoms can be caused by many other conditions, rarely they are caused by a malignant growth.

Diagnosis

To diagnose eye cancer, a doctor may measure how far the eye protrudes or use a special lamp that reveals the rear portions of the eye, the cornea, and the iris. Other diagnostic tools include ophthalmoscopy, angiography with contrast dyes to highlight the eye's appearance, various scans, or a needle biopsy.

Eyelid Tumors

A tumor that appears on the eyelid may be a harmless benign cyst or an inflamed stye—or it could be some type of malignancy (either a BASAL CELL CARCINOMA, squamous cell, sebaceous cell, or malignant melanoma). Malignant eyelid tumors can be completely removed, and the eyelid can be repaired with plastic surgery techniques. Additional cryotherapy (freezing therapy) and radiation are sometimes required after surgery.

The most common type of eyelid cancer is basal cell carcinoma, which usually affects the lower eyelids. Most basal cell carcinomas can be cured with surgery. But when a patient ignores or denies the existence of this tumor, it can invade behind the eye and become difficult or impossible to remove. In these cases doctors may offer radiation and chemotherapy to try to control or destroy the tumor. If left untreated, basal cell carcinomas can grow around the eye and into the orbit, sinuses, and brain. They almost never spread to other parts of the body.

Melanoma of the eyelid is a relatively rare tumor making up less than one percent of eyelid cancers. If the disease has not spread, the tumor can be surgically removed; some doctors also will remove LYMPH NODES near the tumor to determine if the cancer has spread.

Squamous carcinomas of the eyelid can locally invade the eye socket and sinuses but rarely spread elsewhere in the body. If the tumor remains small, it usually can be cured by surgical removal. These tumors are usually flat, with inflamed edges.

Sebaceous cell carcinoma can occur for months as a persistent nonresponsive blepharitis or conjunctivitis, which is why diagnosis of this type of eyelid cancer can be difficult.

Unlike a benign inflammatory tumor, such as a stye, which quickly becomes large, painful, and full of pus, sebaceous carcinomas are relatively pain free and continue to grow over time, causing eyelash loss. Once the diagnosis is made, the tumor must be completely removed.

Conjunctival Tumors

These tumors grow on the actual surface of the eye, and they include pigmented conjunctival tumors, melanoma and primary acquired melanosis (PAM) with atypia, squamous conjunctival neoplasia, conjunctival LYMPHOMA, and KAPOSI'S SARCOMA. The most common conjunctival cancers are squamous carcinoma, malignant melanoma, and lymphoma.

Squamous carcinomas that appear on the surface of the eye rarely spread to other parts of the body, but they can invade around the eye into the eye socket and sinuses. Malignant melanomas can start as moles or begin as newly formed pigmentation. A simple biopsy can determine whether a pigmented conjunctival tumor is a mole, a primary acquired melanosis, or conjunctival melanoma. Both squamous carcinomas and malignant conjunctival melanomas should be removed or destroyed.

Lymphomas also can occur on the eye's surface. These tumors resemble salmon-colored patches on the eye and can be a sign of lymphoma throughout the body. Doctors need to perform special immunology and genetic tests on lymphoid tumors of the eye to determine if the tumor is benign or malignant. Patients with lymphoid conjunctival tumors should have a complete medical checkup and be followed by a hematologist-oncologist.

Small tumors on the surface of the eye can be completely removed with surgery, but if they are either squamous carcinomas or melanomas, additional cryotherapy may be needed. When melanomas are found in many different spots on the eye, they can be hard to treat, and they may not be controlled by surgical removal and freezing therapy. Studies are currently assessing the effectiveness of CHEMOTHERAPY eyedrops, which treat the entire surface of the eye, for these patients. Systemic lymphomas can usually be treated with standard chemotherapy, which is also likely to cure the lymphoma in the eye. If the eye is the only place the lymphoma has appeared, external beam RADIATION THERAPY may be used.

Iris Tumors

Tumors may grow either within or behind the iris (the colored part of the eye). Though many iris tumors turn out to be simply benign cysts or moles, malignant melanoma also can occur in this area. High-frequency ultrasound is the only way to tell how deeply a tumor extends within and through the iris. Blood vessels within the tumor, a deformed pupil, or the development of a cataract beneath the lesion are signs that the tumor is malignant.

Most pigmented iris tumors do not keep growing, but they are photographed and monitored. If an iris melanoma does grow, it can damage the eye (usually causing glaucoma). Most small iris melanomas can be surgically removed; medium-sized melanomas can also be removed, but plaque radiotherapy may be considered instead for these tumors. Although a cataract will probably develop, vision will probably be unharmed since the radiation plaque is far from the central retina. Large melanomas can be hard to treat successfully while saving the eye. Many of these tumors cause untreatable glaucoma that may require removal of the eye.

Choroidal Tumors

Malignant melanomas can grow within the eye, beginning in the blood vessel layer (choroids) beneath the retina. In North America this type of eye cancer occurs in only six out of a million people. Most patients have no symptoms; the cancer is discovered on routine eye examination. If patients do have symptoms, they usually include seeing flashes of light, distorted vision or loss of vision, and the presence of "floaters." Eye cancer specialists can correctly diagnose an intraocular melanoma 96 percent of the time. These tumors include the choroidal melanoma, nevus, and nevus of ota.

Small melanomas are usually watched to see if they grow before treatment is begun. Medium-sized melanomas are usually treated with either radiation therapy or removal of the eye. No one knows if either of these treatments is better at preventing the spread of cancer cells, and both methods will harm the patient's vision. Initial studies suggest the two are equally good at preventing cancer spread for the first five years after treatment. Large melanomas are typically treated by removal of the eye, because the amount of radiation needed to kill a large tumor is too strong for the eye to tolerate. Although some patients with large melanomas can be treated with eye-sparing radiation, within months to several years many patients experience discomfort and poor vision and must have the eye removed.

Patients with a nevus of ota have increased amounts of pigment and pigment-producing cells in various parts of the eye. These patients are at greater risk for developing intraocular and central nervous system melanomas. Although intraocular melanomas are more common in these patients, it is still believed to occur in less than 4 percent of cases. Patients with a nevus of ota should be periodically examined by an eye-care specialist and a neurologist.

Retinal Tumors

Retinoblastoma is a type of cancer that can affect the retina and is the most common intraocular cancer of childhood, affecting about 300 children in the United States each year. More than 90 percent of these children can be cured with early detection and treatment.

Retinoblastoma was the first cancer to be directly associated with a genetic abnormality. Retinoblastoma can occur spontaneously, or it can be inherited. If a child inherits the genetic mutation, there is a 45 to 50 percent chance that a sibling will also have retinoblastoma. If there is no family history and no mutation is found, the risk of having a second child with retinoblastoma is between 2 and 5 percent. The average age of children with retinoblastoma is 18 months. More than 75 percent of children with these tumors have a white pupil, poorly aligned eyes, or a red and painful eye usually due to glaucoma. The tumor is treated with either eye-sparing radiation or (more recently) chemotherapy. Although retinoblastomas are usually cured by radiation, the treatment has been linked to the development of second cancers later in the child's life. Several studies are evaluating the use of chemotherapy to shrink the tumors before treating them with lasers or freezing them.

Optic Nerve Tumors

Cancers that affect the optic nerve include melanoma, melanocytoma, meningioma, and circumpapillary metastasis.

Orbital Tumors

Tumors and inflammation can occur behind the eye, causing the eye to bulge outward. Various scans and ultrasounds can help determine a diagnosis; most orbital tumors are diagnosed with biopsy. Orbital tumors may include lymphangioma, cavernous hemangioma, meningioma, mucocele, rhabdomyosarcoma, orbital pseudotumor, adenoid cystic carcinoma, and periocular hemangioma of childhood.

When possible, orbital tumors should be completely removed. If they cannot be removed without causing too much damage to other important structures around the eye, a piece of tumor may be removed and sent for evaluation. If tumors cannot be removed during surgery, most can be treated with radiation therapy. In some cases, orbital seed radiotherapy may be used to treat any remaining tumor. A few rare orbital tumors require removal of the eye.

fallopian tube cancer The rarest of all types of female reproductive cancers, making up just 0.3 percent to 0.5 percent of all GYNECOLOGIC CANCERS. Only 1,500 to 2,000 cases have been reported throughout the world. Fallopian tube cancer develops from cells inside the fallopian tubes (the twin tubes connecting the ovaries and the uterus).

There are several forms of cancer that may originate in the fallopian tube; the most common is ADENOCARCINOMA; more rare types include LEIO-MYOSARCOMA and TRANSITIONAL CELL CARCINOMA.

Most of the time, cancer found in the fallopian tubes did not originate there, but spread from other sites in the body (usually an ovary or the endometrium). In fact, between about 80 percent and 90 percent of cancers involving the tube have spread from the ovary, uterus, endometrium, appendix, or colon. It is often difficult for a surgeon to reliably determine if an adenocarcinoma has originated in the fallopian tube or the ovary, because the cells from these neighboring organs appear so similar. Fallopian tube cancer is so rare that even a major cancer center may see no more than a few cases over many years.

Cause

Very little is known about the origins of cancer of the fallopian tube. These cancers typically appear in middle-aged women who have had children, and often after menopause. Some experts suspect there may be a genetic factor involved.

Risk Factors

Because fallopian tube cancer is so rare, scientists have not been able to determine any specific environmental or lifestyle factors that increase the risk of this malignancy. Currently, researchers are trying to find out whether there is some inherited tendency to develop the illness. In particular, there is some evidence that women who have inherited a mutation in the BRCA1 gene (a gene linked to breast and ovarian cancer) also have an increased risk of developing fallopian-tube cancer.

Symptoms

There may not be any symptoms early in the disease. When fallopian tube cells become malignant, the resulting tumor slowly grows, eventually distending the inner passageway of the fallopian tube and causing pelvic pain. Over time, the tumor also can invade the wall of the fallopian tube, penetrate the tube's outer surface and spread throughout the pelvis and abdomen. When symptoms do appear, they may include the following:

- vague abdominal discomfort
- watery, clear or blood-tinged discharge from the vagina
- abdominal pressure or cramping
- lump or mass in the abdomen
- increased abdominal swelling without weight gain elsewhere
- abdominal swelling that does not improve with diet or exercise
- feelings of pressure on the bowel or bladder
- sensation that the bowel or bladder cannot be completely emptied

Diagnosis

Cancer of the fallopian tubes is not easy to diagnose because of the lack of symptoms early in the disease. The diagnosis of fallopian tube cancer is rarely suspected until the condition is discovered during surgery for another reason.

If this type of cancer is suspected, the doctor conducts an internal pelvic examination to determine the shape, size and position of the pelvic organs. Blood tests and an ultrasound of the pelvis may be ordered.

Staging

As in all cancers, once the tumor is removed the doctor determines the stage to plan treatment. Fallopian tube cancer staging is as follows:

Stage 0: This represents an in situ cancer that is only minimally aggressive and has not spread beyond the fallopian tubes.

Stage I: Growth of the tumor is limited to the fallopian tubes.

Stage II: The tumor involves one or both fallopian tubes and has spread to the pelvis.

Stage III: The tumor involves one or both fallopian tubes and also has spread outside the pelvis.

Stage IV: The tumor involves one or both fallopian tubes with distant metastases.

Treatment

Almost always, aggressive surgery entails a HYSTERECTOMY and removal of both tubes and both ovaries, together with a selection of abdominal and pelvic lymph glands. Patients in the advanced stages of the disease are normally also given CHEMOTHERAPY (typically paclitaxel [Taxol] and CISPLATIN) or RADIATION THERAPY.

However, if the disease is diagnosed early, is limited to one fallopian tube, and occurs in a young woman who wants to remain fertile, the surgeon may simply remove the fallopian tube and ovary on the affected side (a SALPINGO-OOPHORECTOMY), as well as the omentum (fatty tissue beneath the bottom of the stomach and including part of the bowel) and LYMPH NODES in the pelvis.

Prognosis

The prognosis for recovery depends on the stage of the disease at the time of diagnosis. The earlier stages of this illness carry a very good prognosis, but statistics are limited because the condition is so rare. If the cancer is only growing along the inside passageway of the tube, 91 percent of patients survive for at least five years after diagnosis. However, if the cancer has penetrated below the lining and involves the wall of the fallopian tube, the five-year survival rate drops to 53 percent. For tumors

that have spread entirely through the wall to involve the tube's outer surface, the five-year survival rate is less than 25 percent.

Prevention

Because experts know very little about the risk factors for fallopian tube cancer, there is no way to prevent it. Eventually, scientists hope to develop screening blood tests that can identify women who are at higher-than-average risk of developing fallopian tube cancer or ovarian cancer, either by identifying *BRCA1* mutations or measuring levels of a tumor marker called CA 125 in the blood.

familial adenomatous polyposis (FAP) An inherited condition that predisposes a patient to developing COLON CANCER. The syndrome is characterized by numerous polyps that form on the inside walls of the colon and rectum, significantly increasing the risk of colon cancer.

Typically, the polyps usually begin to appear at about 16 years, but may first appear as young as age seven, or may not appear until age 36. By age 35, however, 95 percent of individuals with familial adenomatous polyposis (FAP) have polyps.

Cause

FAP is caused by mutations in the APC gene, and between 75 and 80 percent of patients with FAP have an affected parent, and the children of an affected person have a 50 percent risk of inheriting the altered APC gene.

Prenatal testing is possible if a disease-causing mutation is identified in an affected family member; however, prenatal testing for typically adult-onset disorders is uncommon and requires careful genetic counseling.

Diagnosis

Genetic testing for APC can detect disease-causing mutations in up to 95 percent of patients. Molecular genetic testing is most often used in the early diagnosis of at-risk family members and to confirm the diagnosis of FAP in patients with equivocal findings (that is, who have fewer than 100 adenomatous polyps).

FAP is diagnosed if an individual has more than 100 colorectal adenomatous polyps, or fewer than 100 polyps AND a relative with FAP.

Attenuated FAP (AFAP) is considered as a possible diagnosis in an individual with many colonic adenomatous polyps or a family history of colon cancer in people under age 60 years with multiple adenomatous polyps.

Other symptoms that may help establish the clinical diagnosis of FAP or AFAP include: gastric polyps, duodenal adenomatous polyps, osteomas, dental abnormalities, congenital hypertrophy of the retinal pigment epithelium (CHRPE), soft tissue tumors (specifically epidermoid cysts and fibromas), desmoid tumors, and associated cancers. While none of these findings is included in the diagnostic criteria, their presence may suggest FAP.

Treatment

Surgery is usually required to prevent the development of colon cancer. Without the removal of the colon (COLECTOMY), colon cancer is inevitable in these patients. The average age of colon cancer in untreated individuals is 39 years.

familial atypical multiple mole melanoma   See MELANOMA.

Familial Ovarian Cancer Registry   See GILDA RADNER FAMILIAL OVARIAN CANCER REGISTRY.

familial polyposis   See FAMILIAL ADENOMATOUS POLYPOSIS.

family history   Many types of cancers tend to run in families; close relatives of someone who has cancer have a higher risk of getting that particular cancer.

In some cases, the increased risk among family members is caused by sharing genes that are known to contribute to cancer. The *BRCA1* and *BRCA2* genes, for instance, contribute to BREAST CANCER. In some cases, DNA-based testing can be used to confirm a specific mutation as the cause of the inherited risk, and to determine whether family members have inherited the mutation.

In addition, family members may share exposure to CARCINOGENS in the environment, such as cigarette smoke, or environmental pollutants in a particular geographic area. Anyone who has a family history of cancer needs to be particularly vigilant about getting appropriate screening tests.

Identifying a person with an increased risk of cancer can be helpful because he or she can then take steps to try to prevent the development of the disease. For example, a woman at risk for breast cancer could take tamoxifen or choose a prophylactic MASTECTOMY. A person at higher risk for colon cancer could schedule more frequent colonoscopies.

See also FAMILY RISK ASSESSMENT PROGRAMS.

family risk assessment programs   Special programs often offered at many cancer centers in which patients at high risk for developing certain types of cancer receive intensive counseling, preventive programs, and risk assessments. Common family risk assessment programs exist for BREAST CANCER, PROSTATE CANCER, LIVER CANCER, and MELANOMA.

Fanconi's anemia   A rare and often fatal inherited disease in which the BONE MARROW fails to produce red blood cells, white blood cells, platelets, or a combination of these cells. The disease may transform into MYELODYSPLASTIC SYNDROME or LEUKEMIA.

Fanconi's syndrome   See FANCONI'S ANEMIA.

fatigue   The most common side effect experienced by cancer patients. An overwhelming tiredness may accompany surgery, radiation, CHEMOTHERAPY, or BIOLOGICAL THERAPY. Although it occurs most frequently in those undergoing treatment, fatigue may continue after treatment is over.

While scientists are not sure of its exact cause, some researchers believe fatigue may be caused by the waste products produced as a tumor shrinks, or it may be related to the energy the body needs to fight cancer. Others believe fatigue may be related to interruptions in the signals sent through the nervous system. A low blood count, sleep disturbances, stress, depression, poor diet, infection, or medication side effects can all contribute to this exhaustion.

Symptoms

The symptoms of cancer-related fatigue are different from normal feelings of being tired. Fatigue can begin suddenly and can be all-consuming; naps may not help. Fatigue can be physically and emotionally draining on the patient as well as the family. General weakness may be accompanied by limb heaviness, decreased ability to concentrate, sleeplessness, and/or irritability.

Diagnosis

Patients who experience this type of extreme tiredness should consult a health-care provider, who will conduct a few simple tests, including a blood count to check for ANEMIA or infection, and a physical examination.

Treatment

There are several things patients can do to help manage symptoms of fatigue. It is important to eat healthy, appetite-stimulating foods. The complex carbohydrates found in pasta, fresh fruits, and whole grain breads provide long-lasting energy. Studies have shown that a moderate amount of exercise may actually help improve energy level.

Sleep is also important. Patients should go to bed at a regular time each night and follow a regular routine.

If the patient is anemic, many studies have shown the effectiveness of ERYTHROPOETIN (Procrit, Aranesp) injections.

fecal occult blood test   A test that checks stool samples for traces of blood that cannot be seen with the naked eye. Also called a stool guaiac or hemoccult test.

See also COLORECTAL CANCER.

fertility drugs   Drugs taken by women to improve the chances of getting pregnant have in the past been linked to a higher risk of cancer. However, recent major studies have found that fertility drugs do not increase the risk of cancer of the ovaries. Scientists suspect that some women who receive fertility treatments develop ovarian cancer because of underlying conditions that cause infertility, not because of the treatments themselves.

Doctors write more than 1.4 million prescriptions for any of eight different fertility medications a year. In order to harvest as many eggs as possible for a cycle of in vitro fertilization (IVF), women are given drugs to stimulate egg maturation in the ovary. Scientists had worried for years that this ovarian stimulation could lead to cancer of the breast, uterus, or ovaries, especially if a woman experienced several cycles of IVF in her lifetime.

However, a recent study published in the *American Journal of Epidemiology* looked at more than 12,000 women and found no link. In the study, investigators collected interview data on infertility and fertility drug use from eight case-control studies conducted between 1989 and 1999 in the United States, Denmark, Canada, and Australia. The studies included 5,207 women with ovarian cancer and 7,705 women without OVARIAN CANCER.

Results showed that women who spent more than five years trying to conceive were at a 2.7-fold higher risk for ovarian cancer than those who tried for less than one year—but women who had used fertility drugs were no more likely to develop ovarian cancer than those who had never used the drugs. Instead, the infertile women who were most likely to develop ovarian cancer were those whose infertility resulted from endometriosis or from "unknown" causes.

A separate July 2002 study in Britain of more than 5,000 women likewise found that the incidence of breast, uterine, and ovarian cancers in women who used fertility drugs was no greater than expected for the general population.

fiber   Material that is found in all plant-based foods, including fruits, vegetables, grains, breads, and cereals but is not available in meat, milk, cheese, or oils. Fiber can be either soluble or insoluble.

Soluble fiber   This type of fiber dissolves in water and is found in highest amounts in fruits, legumes, barley, and oats. It generally slows down digestion time so that nutrients are completely absorbed. Soluble fibers also bind with bile acids in the intestines and carry them out of the body. Since bile acids are made from cholesterol, soluble fiber can lower a person's cholesterol levels. Studies linking high bile-acid concentrations and COLORECTAL CANCER have led some scientists to suspect that binding bile acids may be one way that fiber helps prevent colon cancer.

Insoluble fiber This type of fiber, found in vegetables, whole-grain breads, and whole-grain cereals, increases the bulk of stool, helps to prevent constipation, and removes bound bile acids. Insoluble fiber also increases the speed at which food moves through the gastrointestinal system, so harmful substances do not stay in the body. Some scientists believe that this too reduces the risk of colon or other cancers.

Both types of fiber are important for cancer prevention. Everyone should eat at least 25 grams of fiber each day (about twice the amount most Americans currently consume). A good way to do this is to eat five fruits and vegetables each day. It is possible to increase fiber intake by eating the skins of potatoes and fruits such as apples and pears, and switching from refined foods (such as white bread and white rice) to whole-grain foods (whole-wheat breads and brown rice). Other good sources of fiber include legumes, lentils, and whole-grain cereals.

See also DIET.

fibroadenoma The most common solid tumor of the breast. Fibroadenomas are benign rubbery growths that do not contain fluid and are not related to the development of BREAST CANCER. They range in size from those that cannot be felt but which may show up on a mammogram to large growths that can be easily felt. On a mammogram, a fibroadenoma will appear as a smooth area with distinct edges.

Most fibroadenomas get smaller over time, but some may grow larger and cause discomfort. They are usually found in women under age 25 and are more common in African-American women than in Caucasians. Because most masses in young women are benign, most doctors recommend simply watching the growth. In older women, however, doctors usually recommend a biopsy.

A fibroadenoma may be removed surgically if required but can usually be left alone.

fibroid A benign smooth-muscle tumor (also called a leiomyoma) usually appearing in the uterus or gastrointestinal tract. Uterine fibroids are common benign tumors that grow in the muscle of the uterus, primarily in women in their forties.

Women may have many fibroids at the same time. As a woman reaches menopause, fibroids are likely to become smaller, and sometimes they disappear, but in any case, they do not develop into cancer.

Usually, fibroids cause no symptoms and need no treatment, but in certain locations, some sizable fibroids can cause bleeding, vaginal discharge, and frequent urination. Women with these symptoms should see a doctor. If fibroids cause heavy bleeding, or if they press against nearby organs and cause pain, the doctor may suggest surgery or other treatment.

fibrosarcoma of bone See BONE CANCER.

fibrosarcoma of soft tissue A type of soft tissue SARCOMA that begins in fibrous tissue, which holds bones, muscles, and other organs in place.

financial issues Treating cancer can be very expensive, but health insurance plans will usually cover much of the cost. Patients who belong to an HMO or PPO should become familiar with their provider choices and their financial responsibility if they receive care "out of network" from a doctor not covered by the health plan.

Cancer patients who do not have insurance should contact their local Social Security office to determine if they qualify for supplemental security income (SSI) or SOCIAL SECURITY DISABILITY INSURANCE (SSDI). The medical requirements and disability determination process are the same under both programs. However, while eligibility for SSDI is based on employment history, SSI is based on financial need.

Free Hospital Care

Cancer patients without insurance also can get care from hospitals that receive federal grants from Hill-Burton Funds, which allow hospitals and nursing homes to provide low-cost or no-cost medical care. To receive a listing of hospitals or nursing homes participating in the Hill-Burton program, patients can call (800) 638-0742.

Prescription Drugs

Most major pharmaceutical companies have patient assistance programs offering a free three-month supply of medication to those who cannot afford their prescriptions. To obtain guidelines and a listing of participating companies, patients can call the Pharmaceutical Manufacturers' Association at (800) 762-4636. The medication request must be completed by a physician.

Free Air Transportation

Many nonprofit agencies offer free air transportation for patients traveling to treatment centers, relying on private pilots who donate their time and use of their own planes. Patients can obtain a list of these services at http://www.aircareall.org. In addition, major airlines sometimes offer reduced or no-cost travel through an assistance program.

Local Transportation

To assist a patient with local travel to and from treatments, the hospital social worker may be able to provide van service or cab/bus vouchers. Some local AMERICAN CANCER SOCIETY offices run volunteer transportation programs or provide funds to reimburse travel expenses. Some communities offer special vans for those who qualify due to illness or disability. Local nursing homes, park districts, or YMCAs also may offer van transportation to local hospitals. In addition, many communities offer seniors reduced-fare taxi service within the community.

Temporary Housing

Temporary housing is sometimes required by cancer patients who must travel for consultation or treatment, or for family members who visit hospitalized patients. The American Cancer Society may be able to arrange a low-cost hotel room for those receiving treatment. In addition, many hospitals negotiate discount rates at local hotels or provide dormitory-style housing.

The National Association of Hospitality Houses (call 800-542-9730) provides referral information to anyone in need of lodging while undergoing treatment away from home. RONALD MCDONALD HOUSES located near many larger hospitals throughout the country offer low-cost accommodations to families with children in treatment.

Utilities

Assistance programs are offered by many gas, electric, water, and phone companies for cancer patients who may have difficulty paying monthly bills. Many states have regulations that prohibit companies from turning off utilities; a doctor or social worker may need to write letters describing why the services are medically necessary. The regulations do not lessen a patient's responsibility for paying bills, but may allow families more time or lower monthly payments. In an emergency situation, local help lines and social service agencies may be able to provide one-time emergency help with utility bills.

Home Care/Respite

Some insurance plans offer coverage for home care ranging from skilled nursing to companions. If companion care is not a covered benefit, patients can contact various agencies for assistance.

Respite care allows the caregiver a few hours each week to take a break while someone watches over the patient. Many caregivers use this time to run errands, take care of personal health needs, or just unwind. Local respite caregivers can be located by calling the National Respite Locator at (800) 773-5433. The locator service can also provide a listing of qualifying conditions.

In addition, the National Federation of Interfaith Volunteer Caregivers, a not-for-profit group that oversees 400 regional offices, sends volunteers into the homes of people who need care, company, and supervision. They can be reached at (800) 350-7438.

Medical Supplies

The Cancer Fund of America at (800) 578-5284 can provide nonprescription medical needs such as nutritional supplements or incontinence supplies. Items available vary as the group receives donated products from companies. Patients or family members can call and be placed in their database for specific needs.

Food Programs

Meals on Wheels coordinates thousands of programs throughout the United States dedicated to delivering meals to those who are homebound. Some programs require a small donation; eligibility is determined by each program. For a local referral to Meals on Wheels, patients can contact the national office at (616) 530-0929.

Viatical Settlement Companies

Viatical companies purchase a patient's life insurance policy at a discounted rate, providing money for patients to use however they want. In general, any life insurance policy (group or individual) can be sold, but the rate of return and eligibility criteria vary with each company. However, patients should consider tax implications and the effect of a viatical settlement on assistance programs.

A free brochure, "Viatical Settlements: A Guide for People with Terminal Illnesses," is available at the Federal Trade Commission at (202) 326-2222. The National Viatical Association at (202) 347-7361 offers a listing of viatical companies.

Life Insurance Loans

LifeWise Family Financial Security, Inc., allows patients to take out a loan against their existing life insurance policy if their life expectancy is five years or less. There is no obligation to repay the loan but the option is available. If a patient chooses not to repay the loan, the life insurance policy proceeds are the sole source of repayment. All surplus funds are remitted to the patient's family. LifeWise has counselors available to answer any questions, and publishes *The Financial Resource Guide: A Comprehensive, Step-by-Step Reference for Individuals Facing Life-Threatening or Terminal Illnesses.* Counselors or a copy of the guide are available at (800) 219-7385.

fine-needle aspiration The removal of tissue or fluid with a needle for examination under a microscope, also called a needle BIOPSY.

five-year survival rate The percentage of people with a given cancer who are expected to survive five years or longer with the disease. Although the rates are based on the most recent information available, they may include data from patients treated several years earlier.

While statistically valid, five-year survival rates may not reflect advances in cancer treatment, which often occur quickly. They should not be seen as a predictor in an individual case.

flap surgery See BREAST RECONSTRUCTION.

folate See FOLIC ACID.

folate antagonist A substance that blocks the activity of folate (FOLIC ACID). Folate antagonists are used to treat cancer and are also called antifolate. The chemotherapy drug methotrexate is a folate antagonist.

folic acid (folate) A B-complex vitamin being studied as a cancer prevention agent.

follicular cell thyroid cancer See THYROID CANCER.

follicular large cell lymphoma See NON-HODGKIN'S LYMPHOMA.

follicular thyroid cancer See THYROID CANCER.

formaldehyde A colorless, strong-smelling gas that is widely used to manufacture building materials and household products and that is classified as a human CARCINOGEN linked to nasal and LUNG CANCER, BRAIN CANCER, and LEUKEMIA.

It is especially common as an adhesive resin in pressed wood products. There are two types of formaldehyde resins: urea formaldehyde (UF) and phenol formaldehyde (PF). Both types can release formaldehyde gas; products made of phenol formaldehyde generally emit lower levels.

In the home, formaldehyde may be found in glues, wood products, preservatives, permanent-press fabrics, paper product coatings, and certain insulation materials. Formaldehyde gas can be emitted by building products made with formaldehyde resins, such as particle board used as sub-flooring or shelves, fiberboard in cabinets and furniture, plywood wall panels, and foamed-in-place urea-formaldehyde insulation.

Some products that once contained formaldehyde are either no longer used or have been reformulated to contain less formaldehyde.

Workers can be exposed to formaldehyde during production or treatment of materials. Healthcare professionals, pathology and histology technicians, and teachers and students who handle preserved specimens are potentially at high risk. Consumers can be exposed to formaldehyde in building materials, cosmetics, home furnishings, and textiles.

Formaldehyde has caused cancer in laboratory animals and may cause cancer in humans; there is no known threshold level below which there is no threat of cancer. The risk depends upon amount and duration of exposure.

Prevention

The risk of exposure to formaldehyde may be lowered in a variety of ways, including:

- buying "low-emitting" wood products, or products made from phenol formaldehyde (such as oriented strand board or softwood plywood)
- increasing ventilation after bringing new sources of formaldehyde into the home
- using other products such as lumber, metal, or solid wood furniture
- avoiding foamed-in-place insulation containing formaldehyde, especially urea-formaldehyde foam insulation
- enclosing unfinished pressed-wood surfaces of furniture, cabinets, or shelving with laminate or water-based sealant
- washing durable-press fabrics before use.
- maintaining moderate temperatures and low (30 to 50 percent) relative humidity levels

Formaldehyde Measurement

In cases where accuracy is important, only trained professionals should measure formaldehyde because of the difficulty of obtaining good data. Do-it-yourself formaldehyde measuring devices are available, but the results may not be accurate due to weather conditions, ventilation rates, and other factors.

free radicals   Highly charged destructive forms of oxygen, generated by each cell in the body, that destroy cellular membranes through the oxidation process. Free radicals can also damage important cellular molecules, such as DNA or lipids, in other parts of the cell.

Because free radicals are essential to many reactions in the body (they are generated by the immune system to fend off microbes and help the digestive system break down food), they should

not be entirely destroyed. It is only when their levels become too high that damage can occur.

Free radical damage can be offset by molecules called ANTIOXIDANTS, which neutralize free radicals before they can damage cells. Antioxidants include BETA-CAROTENE, selenium, and vitamins E and C. While there are no guarantees regarding the effectiveness of dietary supplements containing such antioxidants, many doctors believe in and recommend them to their patients.

fruits   A diet rich in fruits, vegetables, and whole grains is believed to help reduce the risk of tumor development. Fruits, vegetables, whole grains, and other plant-based foods contain fiber, complex carbohydrates, and other substances that can inhibit tumor formation. Citrus fruits are rich in vitamin C and flavonoids, which may help inhibit cancer cell growth.

Many experts believe that adding more plant-based foods is the best dietary insurance against many types of cancer. That is because fruits, vegetables, and other plant-based foods typically are low in saturated fats (mostly animal fats—found in meats, butter, and cheese—which have been linked to an increased risk of cancer) and high in fiber, which may be associated with a lower risk of COLORECTAL CANCER.

Fiber is found in all plant-based foods, including fruits, and can be either soluble or insoluble. Soluble fiber is found in highest amounts in fruits. It dissolves in water and also binds with bile acids in the intestines and carries them out of the body. Since bile acids are made from cholesterol, soluble fiber can lower a person's cholesterol levels. Studies linking high bile-acid concentrations and colon cancer have led some scientists to suspect that binding bile acids may be one way that fiber helps prevent colon cancer.

Antioxidants

These substances seek out and destroy the naturally occurring toxic molecules called FREE RADICALS that can cause extensive damage to the body's cells. This damage is thought to be involved in cancer development. Antioxidants reduce the number of free radicals, prevent tissue damage and, quite possibly, prevent cancer. The antioxidants that have generated the most interest and research to date are

- *Vitamin C.* Good sources of vitamin C include citrus fruits, kiwi, cantaloupe, strawberries, peppers, tomatoes, potatoes, mangos.

- *Beta-carotene.* It often (but not always) is identified by its yellow, orange, or deep-green color. It is found in carrots, cantaloupe, sweet potatoes, and apricots.

- *Phytochemicals.* These plant chemicals contribute to the color and flavor of fruits and vegetables and may suppress cancer development. Among the PHYTOCHEMICALS that may help prevent cancer are limonen and phenols, both found in citrus fruits.

Bioflavonoids   Chemical compounds related to vitamin C that have demonstrated an ability to slow down cancer growth and may be able to protect normal, healthy cells. These naturally occurring plant compounds act primarily as plant pigments and ANTIOXIDANTS.

Lemons, grapes, plums, grapefruit, cherries, blackberries, and rosehips are some of the richest dietary sources of bioflavonoids. Additional sources include other citrus fruits, green peppers, broccoli, tomatoes, and herb TEA (especially stinging nettle tea). Bioflavonoids belong to a large group of more than 2,000 phytochemicals called phenols that are known to be very powerful antioxidants. Many studies have identified their unique role in protecting vitamin C from oxidation in the body, thereby allowing the body to reap more benefits from vitamin C.

Different bioflavonoids tend to have different health effects on the body, but in general, a diet high in bioflavonoids is associated with a lower incidence of many diseases, including cancer. For example, green tea extract protects against the development of some types of cancer, and a recent Hawaiian study suggests that consumption of certain flavonoids cuts the risk of LUNG CANCER in half. According to the January 19, 2000, issue of the *Journal of the National Cancer Institute*, high consumption of onions, apples,

and white grapefruit were associated with significantly less lung cancer. Most of the effect was attributed to onions reducing a specific type of lung cancer called squamous cell carcinoma.

Consumption of broccoli, SOY PRODUCTS, red wine, and green or black tea had no beneficial effect on lung cancer in this study. These foods are rich sources of flavonoids, which suggests that the antioxidant effect of flavonoids is not necessarily connected to health outcomes. However, the foods may protect against other conditions.

Orange and other citrus juices contain bioflavonoid compounds that may help the body fight off cancer-causing substances. Scientists have identified several bioflavonoids from citrus that inhibit certain cytochrome P450 enzymes. Thwarting these enzymes is important, because some of them can turn cigarette smoke, pesticides, and other substances into carcinogens. Cigarette smoke and pesticides contain procarcinogens—substances that may not cause cancer in their original form but could become carcinogenic later inside the body. One P450 enzyme, known as P450 1B1, turns procarcinogens into carcinogens. It is also present at high levels in breast and prostate cancer cells and can even modify the female hormone estradiol into a possible carcinogen. Scientists have found that hesperetin, the most abundant bioflavonoid in orange juice, inhibits the P450 1B1 enzyme from metabolizing procarcinogens, reducing the chances that the body could turn these substances into carcinogens. Hesperetin's effect on enzyme P450 1B1 might lead to the development of alternatives to traditional cancer chemotherapy treatments that affect healthy as well as diseased cells. Only cells containing the enzyme P450 1B1, which are largely cancer cells, would be affected by hesperetin.

Side Effects
Anyone taking bioflavonoid supplements should inform a doctor before undergoing surgery; they may interfere with the results of some blood and urine tests.

G

galactogram   See DUCTOGRAM.

gallbladder cancer   Cancer of the tissues of the gallbladder, a pear-shaped organ lying under the liver in the upper abdomen. The gallbladder stores bile, a fluid made by the liver to help digest fat. As food is being digested in the stomach and the intestines, bile is released from the gallbladder through the bile duct, which connects the gallbladder and liver to the first part of the small intestine.

Gallbladder cancer is extremely rare, affecting only 7,100 people in the United States each year. Cancer of the gallbladder is more common in women than in men, and more common in people with gallstones.

Symptoms
Symptoms may mimic other gallbladder diseases, such as gallstones or infection; there may be no symptoms in the early stages. If symptoms do appear, they may include stomach pain, unexplained weight loss, fever, bloating, decreasing appetite, NAUSEA, or an enlarging abdominal mass. The chance of recovery and choice of treatment depend on the stage of cancer (whether it is just in the gallbladder or has spread to other places) and on the patient's general health. Itching may be caused by a buildup in the skin of bilirubin, a derivative of bile that turns the skin yellow. This symptom usually reflects advanced disease.

Cause
Scientists have not identified a clear-cut cause for gallbladder cancer. Although it occurs most often in people with a hardened gallbladder due to repeated inflammation from passing gallstones, it is extremely rare even in these patients. Since the gallbladder is not essential, people with a hardened gall bladder may consider having it removed as a preventive measure.

Diagnosis
Cancer of the gallbladder is hard to diagnose because of the gallbladder's location, hidden behind other organs in the abdomen. This is why it is sometimes not discovered until the gallbladder is removed for other reasons. If symptoms do occur, a doctor may order X-rays and other diagnostic tests; usually, however, the cancer cannot be found unless the patient has surgery to directly examine the gall bladder.

Staging
Once cancer of the gallbladder is found, more tests will be done to find out if cancer cells have spread to other parts of the body. The following stages are used to describe cancer of the gallbladder:

Localized   Cancer is found only in the wall of the gallbladder, which can be removed completely in an operation.

Unresectable   Not all of the cancer can be removed in an operation, and the cancer has spread to other nearby areas, such as the liver, stomach, pancreas, intestine, and/or local LYMPH NODES.

Recurrent   The cancer has returned after it has been treated, either to the gallbladder or elsewhere in the body.

Treatment
Unless the cancer is very small and found when the gallbladder is removed for other reasons, treatments now available are not particularly effective. In the advanced stages, pain relief and the restoration of normal bile flow from the liver into the intestines are the principal goals of therapy. Standard treatment usually includes some combination of surgery, RADIATION THERAPY, or CHEMOTHERAPY.

Surgery   If the malignancy has not spread to surrounding tissues, the most common treatment for cancer of the gallbladder is surgery. Because the gallbladder is a nonessential organ, it can be removed without significant consequences.

In early stage cancer, the doctor may remove the gallbladder (CHOLECYSTECTOMY) along with part of the liver and abdominal lymph nodes. If the cancer has spread and cannot be removed, the doctor may still perform surgery as a way of easing symptoms.

If cancer blocks the bile ducts so that bile builds up in the gallbladder, the doctor may perform a biliary bypass around the cancer, cutting the gallbladder or bile duct and sewing it directly to the small intestine.

The doctor also may choose to insert a catheter to drain bile that has built up in the area. The doctor may have the catheter drain through a tube to the outside of the body, or around the blocked area and into the small intestine.

Radiation therapy   This treatment method uses X-rays to kill cancer cells and shrink tumors. Radiation may be used alone or in addition to surgery.

Chemotherapy   Anticancer drugs can be used to kill cancer cells in the gallbladder. Chemotherapy or other drugs may be given at the same time as radiation therapy to make cancer cells more sensitive to radiation.

Clinical trials   Because most patients with gallbladder cancer are not cured with standard therapy and some standard treatments may have side effects, some patients may choose to participate in a clinical trial to find better ways to treat their cancer. Clinical trials are ongoing in many parts of the country for patients with cancer of the gallbladder. Information about clinical trials can be obtained by calling the CANCER INFORMATION SERVICE at (800) 422-6237.

gamma knife   A type of RADIATION THERAPY in which high-energy rays are aimed at a tumor from many angles in a single treatment session.

ganglioneuroma   See BRAIN CANCER.

Gardner's syndrome   A hereditary disorder featuring benign skin growths that appear during ado-lescence; the syndrome also causes thousands of polyps in the colon, as well as the stomach and upper intestine, together with bony tumors in the jaw and skull. The polyps associated with this syndrome usually appear around age 15 and eventually lead to COLORECTAL CANCER.

Cause

The condition was discovered in the 1950s by Dr. Eldon Gardner, who noticed multiple symptoms among members of two different families. Recently the gene responsible for Gardner's syndrome, which affects the growth cells in the body, has been identified. The syndrome is autosomal dominant, which means that only one defective gene from one parent is needed to cause it. Each child of an affected person usually has a one in two chance of inheriting the gene and of being affected.

Treatment

Since the inevitable outcome of this disease is colon cancer, typically about 10 to 15 years after the onset of the polyps, patients with documented Gardner's should have their colon and rectum removed. Although there is no recommended nonsurgical therapy for Gardner's, studies have shown that the colon polyps regress to a significant degree with use of sulindac (Clinoril), a nonsteroidal anti-inflammatory drug. Since other polyps may be present elsewhere, regular endoscopic examination of these areas is also recommended.

All blood relatives of a person diagnosed with Gardner's syndrome should be screened with colonoscopy. There are also genetic tests to screen younger patients who may have not yet developed the polyps.

garlic   Garlic has been used by humans as a health tonic for thousands of years. Recently several studies have shown that chemical compounds in garlic can help prevent the formation of cancerous tumors in mice.

Some studies have found that garlic can inhibit the growth of BREAST CANCER, and significantly reduces the growth of BLADDER CANCER, in mice. Recently researchers have shown that if a compound called diallyldisulphide (formed when raw garlic is cut or crushed) is injected into tumors, their size can be reduced by half. Another compound (S-allylcysteine) can stop cancer-causing agents from binding to human breast cells. Other promising areas of study include stomach and colon cancer.

Researchers think garlic may help boost the IMMUNE SYSTEM in laboratory mice, thereby reducing the growth of cancerous cells. In one study, white blood cells from garlic eaters were able to kill 139 percent more tumor cells than white blood cells from mice who did not eat garlic.

Because it is nontoxic and relatively cheap, experts do not hesitate to recommend its use. Cooks should remember to peel garlic and let it sit for 15 minutes before cooking with it for increased cancer-fighting benefits. According to nutrition experts, peeling garlic releases an enzyme called allinase that starts a series of chemical reactions. These reactions produce substances that help protect the body against cancer, but it takes 15 minutes for the protective substances to form. Peeling garlic and immediately starting to cook with it inactivates the allinase and destroys garlic's cancer-fighting properties.

See also DIET.

gastrectomy   An operation to remove all or part of the stomach.

See also STOMACH CANCER.

gastric adenocarcinoma   See STOMACH CANCER.

gastric cancer   See STOMACH CANCER.

gastric polyps   Usually benign tumors in the stomach that in most cases cause no symptoms. Hyperplastic polyps make up nearly 80 percent of all stomach polyps. Hyperplastic polyps typically cause no symptoms and need no treatment. Rarely they may bleed or become malignant and need to be removed. Hyperplastic polyps are often found during an X-ray or endoscopy of the stomach done for some other reason.

Adenomatous polyps (the second most common type) tend to be precancerous, especially if they are bigger than one centimeter. A doctor usually monitors these polyps for increase in size or evidence of precancerous changes (dysplasia).

See also STOMACH CANCER.

gastrinoma   A tumor that causes overproduction of gastric acid by secreting gastrin. These tumors are usually found in the islet cells of the pancreas but may also occur in the stomach, and other areas of the gastrointestinal tract. Gastrinomas also may spread to the LYMPH NODES and the liver.

The syndrome of excess gastric acid and gastric or duodenal ulcers is called the Zollinger-Ellison syndrome (ZES). About 20 percent of ZES is hereditary; this inherited syndrome is called multiple endocrine neoplasia-1 (MEN-1).

MEN-1 is characterized by tumors of the pituitary, pancreas (ISLET CELL TUMORS) and parathyroid; the gene responsible for this syndrome has been located on chromosome 11.

Treatment includes surgery and strong acid-inhibiting medications. If the disease is advanced, chemotherapy with or without radiation may be needed.

gastrointestinal stromal tumor (GIST)   A soft tissue SARCOMA—a rare tumor that grows from the cells that make up connective tissue, such as muscle, fat, nerves, blood vessels, bone, and cartilage—that grows anywhere along the gastrointestinal tract from the esophagus to the anus. GISTs originate in the connective tissue that supports the organs involved in digestion. Each year, between 5,000 and 10,000 men and women develop this type of tumor. Although they are most often diagnosed in people 50 years of age or older, they can occur in any age group.

Most GISTs develop in the stomach, while a smaller number will grow from the small intestine. Fewer than 20 percent arise in the esophagus, colon, and rectum, although sometimes they develop outside the intestinal tract in the abdominal cavity.

Risk Factors

People with neurofibromatosis are most at risk for developing GISTs. Other risk factors may include a type of skin disorder called familial urticaria pigmentosa. Rarely, familial GIST occurs among several family members.

Symptoms

People with early stage GIST often do not have any symptoms of the disease. Most GISTs are diagnosed after a person develops symptoms. These may include abdominal discomfort, vomiting, bloody stools or vomit, or fatigue as a result of anemia.

Diagnosis

Although there is no general screening test to check for GISTs, the earlier any tumor is discovered and treated, the better is the chance of survival. For this reason, people who notice signs or symptoms of GIST should discuss them with their doctor right away.

If there are symptoms, a doctor will take a detailed history of the patient and may perform tests such as an ultrasound, a computed tomography (CT scan), or magnetic resonance imaging (MRI).

In addition, a doctor might perform one of three types of biopsies: fine needle aspiration; core needle biopsy; and excisional or incisional biopsy.

Staging

GISTs grow differently in each patient, so it is important to determine the size and the rate at which it grows in order to determine the risk that the tumor presents to the patient. Very small GISTs (less than 1 cm) never spread, but larger GISTs (above 15 cm) virtually always spread. Doctors estimate that 30 to 50 percent of GISTs are likely to spread. The location of the tumor seems to affect the tumor's behavior in how it grows and spreads. For example, a small GIST from the small intestine may grow more quickly and be more likely to spread than a large tumor from the stomach. When a GIST metastasizes it usually spreads to the liver or peritoneal cavity (the lining of the abdominal wall) and rarely spreads to the lymph nodes.

Treatment

Until recently, the only treatment for GIST has been surgery to remove the tumor completely. However, surgery alone for larger GISTs, or for GISTs that have spread, has yielded disappointing results. Because there is a chance that malignant tumors can recur after surgery, chemotherapy or radiation are added after removing many types of cancer. However, using either chemotherapy or radiation after removing a GIST has not been shown to work in preventing the tumor from recurring.

For this reason researchers have sought new effective therapies for GIST. Gleevec (imatinib mesylate) was approved in 2002 as a chemotherapy treatment for GIST; it works by blocking an abnormal enzyme on GIST cells that plays a role in cancer growth. Because these abnormal enzymes are largely confined to cancer cells, Gleevec causes relatively little damage to normal cells while killing the cancer cells. In the study that was the basis for the drug's approval as a GIST treatment, 38 percent of tumors grew smaller by 50 percent or more, although no tumors completely disappeared.

Gleevec was approved under accelerated approval regulations and under the orphan drug program, which provides financial incentives for drugs developed to treat rare diseases (diseases that affect fewer than 200,000 patients). Accelerated approval requires continued patient follow-up and information from additional studies to evaluate whether Gleevec provides an actual clinical benefit such as improved survival.

Common side effects include fluid retention, NAUSEA and vomiting, diarrhea, skin rash, muscle cramps, liver toxicity, and lower blood cell counts. Side effects are generally mild to moderate and rarely require that Gleevec doses be decreased or interrupted for prolonged periods of time. Seven GIST patients had hemorrhage into the tumor or gastrointestinal tract that required red blood cell transfusions.

See also GASTROINTESTINAL CANCER; SARCOMA, SOFT TISSUE.

genes and cancer   Virtually every cancer is caused by mutations in DNA, the genetic material that controls how cells behave. In some cases, the DNA may be altered by the activation of ONCOGENES (mutated genes that cause cells to grow out of control) or by the disabling of suppressor genes (normal genes that control cell growth and keep cells from dividing too rapidly).

Experts believe that environmental factors, such as exposure to chemicals, radiation, smoke and pollution, saturated fat in the diet, or viruses, cause most genetic damage. In addition, cell mutations may occur by mistake as cells divide. Some mutations may be inherited, which is why many cancers run in families.

Within the past few years, researchers have identified two genes linked to an increased risk for the development of BREAST CANCER: BRCA1/BRCA2. A person who inherits one of these genes has an 80 percent chance of developing breast cancer in her lifetime.

See also FAMILY RISK ASSESSMENT PROGRAMS; HEREDITY AND CANCER.

gene therapy Experimental treatment that inserts a gene into affected cells so that it stops the growth of cancer cells or makes the cancer cells more sensitive to other kinds of therapy. Inactivated viruses such as the one for the common cold usually are used as the modified gene, since they already know how to invade cells.

Some scientists are doing research on combining VACCINES and gene therapy to fight cancer. In this method, a cancer vaccine is developed by removing tumor cells, modifying them, and putting them back into the body. This is followed by CHEMOTHERAPY, which is administered after the patient's immune cells are removed so that a gene can be inserted to shield the cells from chemotherapy's harmful effects. Although human trials are years away, scientists believe this combination of approaches may be most powerful.

Scientists are also exploring creative ways of getting genes into cancer cells. Some of them are experimenting with viral cousins of HIV (the AIDS virus) because these viruses penetrate cells so well. By altering viral proteins, the killer viruses can be reprogrammed to safely carry a gene payload into the cancer cell.

Other scientists are using electric pulses and ultrasound to deliver the altered genes. Electric pulses can pry cancer cells open, and electric fields can move genes through membranes. By placing electrodes on skin near tumors or inside the body during surgery, scientists are hoping they can quickly get gene "drugs" into the body. Ultrasound waves create bubbles that break cell membranes open. Researchers are hoping that they can use ultrasound to create tiny holes in cancer cells before they receive altered genes.

genetic markers Alterations in DNA that may indicate an increased risk of developing a specific disease or disorder.

genetic testing A type of testing that determines genetic alterations that may be linked to CANCER. Genetic testing may be sought by people affected by cancer, both newly diagnosed individuals and longtime survivors, or by those with a significant family history of cancer.

People may choose genetic testing to determine more clearly how they got cancer, to clarify risk to their children, to define the appropriateness of particular surveillance approaches, or to aid in decision making about risk-reducing prophylactic surgery.

While there are effective interventions for some cancer-causing genetic syndromes (such as multiple endocrine neoplasia type 2A, FAMILIAL ADENOMATOUS POLYPOSIS, or retinoblastoma), genetic testing is still being integrated into the management of patients with hereditary forms of common cancers such as BREAST CANCER.

See also FAMILY RISK ASSESSMENT PROGRAMS; GENES AND CANCER.

genitourinary cancers Cancer of the genital area and urinary tract, which includes BLADDER CANCER, KIDNEY CANCER, PENILE CANCER, PROSTATE CANCER, transitional cell renal pelvis and ureter cancer, TESTICULAR CANCER, URETHRAL CANCER, and WILMS' TUMOR.

geography and cervical cancer Research suggests that where a woman lives may have something to do with her risk of developing CERVICAL CANCER. Despite a threefold reduction in cervical cancer mortality nationwide in the past 50 years, certain areas of the country have experienced persistently higher cervical cancer mortality rates. These high-risk areas include counties stretching from Maine southwest through Appalachia to the Texas/Mexico border, many southeastern states, and the Central Valley of California.

germ cell cancers Tumors that begin in the cells that produce sperm or eggs. Germ cell cancers can occur virtually anywhere in the body and can be either benign or malignant. They include childhood extracranial germ cell tumor, extragonadal germ cell tumor, ovarian germ cell tumor, and TESTICULAR CANCER.

germinoma   A type of tumor that develops from cells that normally make egg cells or sperm (germ cells). Germinomas can form in the ovaries, testicles, chest, abdomen, and brain. They occur most commonly in young people.

Gerson therapy   A dietary approach to treating cancer by focusing on the role of minerals, enzymes, hormones, and other nutritional factors in restoring health. The daily regimen calls for drinking 13 glasses of juice prepared from fresh, organic fruits and vegetables, and eating vegetarian meals prepared from organically grown fruits, vegetables, and whole grains. Various supplements are given, including an iodine solution called Lugol, vitamin B_{12}, potassium, thyroid hormone, an injectable crude liver extract, and pancreatic enzymes. Regularly administered enemas (including coffee or chamomile) are recommended to detoxify the body. Salt, spices, and aluminum cookware or utensils are not used when preparing food.

Gerson therapy was named after Dr. Max B. Gerson, who initially developed this approach to treat his migraine headaches. Subsequently, consumers began to hear of his therapy in the 1930s as a treatment for a type of tuberculosis. His therapy was later used to treat other conditions, including cancer.

In a presentation before a congressional subcommittee in 1946, Dr. Gerson estimated that about 30 percent of cancer patients treated with his therapy had a favorable response. In 1947 the NATIONAL CANCER INSTITUTE (NCI) reviewed 10 cases submitted by Dr. Gerson. However, the patients were also receiving other anticancer treatments, so the NCI could not determine what was responsible for the patients' condition.

For most cancer patients, nutrition recommendations stress a well-balanced diet that includes a generous amount of fruits, vegetables, and whole-grain products. The NCI recommends that patients talk with their doctor about an appropriate DIET.

gestational trophoblastic disease   See CHORIO-CARCINOMA.

gestational trophoblastic neoplasia   See CHORIO-CARCINOMA.

giant cell tumor of the bone   See BONE CANCER.

Gilda Radner Familial Ovarian Cancer Registry
An international registry of families with two or more members who have OVARIAN CANCER that offers a help-line, education, information, and peer support for women at high risk for ovarian cancer.

The registry also is pursuing research into causes of familial ovarian cancer in hopes of identifying new genes associated with the condition and improving genetic and psychosocial counseling for individuals and families. Researchers also hope to learn whether certain lifestyle choices, such as the use of oral contraceptives or hormone replacement therapy, can reduce ovarian cancer risk in women who may be more susceptible to the disease. To further that aim, the registry collects family histories, medical records, and tissue samples from ovarian cancer patients. For contact information, see Appendix I.

Gilda's Clubs   Places where all patients with any type of cancer and their families and friends can get social and emotional support as a supplement to medical care. Free of charge and nonprofit, Gilda's Clubs offer support and networking groups, lectures, workshops, and social events in a nonresidential, homelike setting. Funding is solicited from private individuals, corporations, and foundations.

The Gilda's Club program is composed of the following elements:

- *Support and networking groups.* These include weekly wellness groups for those living with cancer, family groups for family members and friends, and monthly networking groups focusing on a particular kind of cancer or topic of common interest (PROSTATE CANCER, young adults with cancer, living solo with cancer, etc.)

- *Lectures and workshops.* Typical lecture topics, which are selected based on members' interests, include stress reduction, nutrition, talking to your children about cancer, and managing pain. Major workshop areas include art and other forms of self-expression, meditation, exercise and yoga, and cooking.

- *Social activities.* A range of gatherings such as potluck suppers with music, karaoke nights, joke fests, comedy nights, and major celebrations around special holidays.

- *Team convene.* Two-hour sessions requested at the time of diagnosis by a person with cancer or family member to create an active support network. Sessions include all significant friends and family in a member's life, who join together to help with transportation, food preparation, child care, and other necessities.

- *Family focus.* A family meeting, facilitated by a staff member, designed to enlist the entire family as a resource and help them learn together how to live with cancer. It seeks to identify and discuss family beliefs about cancer, critical family issues, and immediate practical problems as well as solutions.

- *Noogieland.* In a special area of every clubhouse, activities are conducted for children affected by cancer. Most Gilda's Clubs also have several kinds of activity for teens, who frequently volunteer in many parts of the clubhouse.

Gilda's Club is named in memory of comedian Gilda Radner, who died from OVARIAN CANCER in 1989. Gilda is best known for her work on NBC's *Saturday Night Live;* her book, *It's Always Something,* describes her life with cancer. Gilda's Club was founded by Joanna Bull, Gilda's cancer psychotherapist, with the help of Gilda's husband, Gene Wilder, Joel Siegel, and other friends.

ginseng (*Panax ginseng*) An herb with a root that some people believe may have anticancer effects. Most cancer experts in the United States have said there is insufficient evidence demonstrating that ginseng is an effective treatment for cancer, and most experts believe there is no scientific evidence that Siberian ginseng is effective in reducing the side effects of chemotherapy or radiation therapy. There have been no human studies of its safety or long-term effects. Although some practitioners claim that the herb enables chemotherapy drugs to penetrate cancer cells more easily, there has been no scientific evidence to support this.

Siberian ginseng is an herb that grows in Siberia, China, Korea, and Japan. The dried root and other underground parts of the plant are used in herbal remedies. *Siberian ginseng* should not be confused with *Asian ginseng* or *American ginseng,* which belong to a different family of herbs.

Herbalists have long prescribed Siberian ginseng for menopausal complaints and to treat cancer and reduce the toxic effects of chemotherapy and radiation therapy. After the Chernobyl nuclear reactor disaster, Russian and Ukrainian citizens reportedly received the herb to counter the effects of radiation poisoning, but few animal studies of Siberian ginseng have been published in peer-reviewed medical journals. In addition, lack of standardization of extracts, study methods, and doses makes it difficult to draw conclusions regarding effectiveness.

The AMERICAN CANCER SOCIETY has offered no official position on ginseng as a cancer treatment or preventive agent, but cautions that it has not yet been adequately tested in a scientific way. The organization noted that the studies that were conducted produced contradictory results and that ginseng products are not standardized.

Safety/Dosage
However, Siberian ginseng is on the approval list of Commission E (Germany's herbal regulatory agency). Ginseng supplements are available in tablets and liquid extracts. There is no standardization for the purity and strength of ginseng, as several different plants go by the same name. No federal agency enforces quality control over these ingredients, and studies of 54 ginseng products found that 25 percent contained no ginseng at all, and 60 percent contained only trace amounts.

The powdered or cut root can be brewed as a tea; an average dose is 2 to 3 g/day. Typically, Siberian ginseng is taken regularly for 6 to 8 weeks, followed by a 1- or 2-week break before resuming.

Health risks associated with Siberian ginseng have not been established, although side effects seem to be rare. A few cases of diarrhea and insomnia have been reported, and people with high blood pressure should avoid the supplements. There have been no studies of Siberian ginseng's long-term effects.

Gleason grading system A widely used method for classifying the aggressiveness of malignant

PROSTATE CANCER tumors by rating them from 1 to 10. A doctor will use this system to "grade" a tumor by describing how closely the tumor resembles normal tissue. The less the cancerous cells appear like normal cells, the more malignant the cancer is. Based on the microscopic appearance of a growth, pathologists may describe it as low-, medium-, or high-grade cancer. The higher the score, the higher the grade of tumor.

Two numbers (each from 1 to 5) are assigned successively to the two predominant patterns of differentiation present in the examined tissue sample; added together, these produce the Gleason score. The pathologist checks prostate tissue under a microscope to determine where the tumor is most prominent (the primary grade) and second-most prominent (secondary grade). The pathologist then gives a score from 1 to 5 for each of these two areas and adds the two together to come up with the Gleason score (the primary grade is usually the first number). The range can thus be anywhere from a low of 2 (grade 1 and grade 1) to a high of 10 (grade 5 and grade 5). However, not all Gleason scores are equal. If two men both have a combined Gleason score of 7, the breakdown of those scores may be different. If the first man's score breaks down to a primary grade 3 and a secondary grade 4 and the second man has a primary grade 4 and a secondary grade 3, the first man may have a better outlook because his cancer is more likely to be cured.

In general, however, the lower the combined Gleason score, the better. Numbers of 2, 3, and 4 indicate a well-differentiated cancer; 5 and 6 indicate a mildly aggressive cancer; grade 7 is considered moderately aggressive. High numbers (8, 9, and 10), indicate a highly aggressive tumor.

The system was devised by pathologist Dr. Donald Gleason in 1966, who invented the scale by studying the biopsies of more than 3,000 patients with prostate cancer. The Gleason score is used by pathologists throughout the world to grade prostate cancer tumors, and is considered to be quite reliable.

Prostate cancer can be graded both before and after surgery, but the grading done after a prostate gland is removed may be more accurate because the pathologist has the entire gland to assess. Grad-ing done before surgery is performed on just a sliver of tissue from a biopsy. This means that after surgery, a man's grade may change (either for the better or worse).

glial tumors   A general term for many types of tumors of the central nervous system, including astrocytomas, ependymal tumors, glioblastoma multiforme, and primitive neuroectodermal tumors.

See also BRAIN CANCER; CENTRAL NERVOUS SYSTEM CANCERS.

glioblastoma multiforme   See BRAIN CANCER.

glioma   See BRAIN CANCER.

gliosarcoma   See BRAIN CANCER.

glomus tumor   A rare, benign tumor that typically appears in the head or neck, or under the fingernails of middle-aged patients. The tumor is usually a small lesion that grows very slowly, rarely causes symptoms, and is usually surgically removed. Glomus tumors may be tender and may cause severe intermittent burning pain that can be excruciating. The exact cause of the pain is not completely understood, but nerve fibers containing the pain neurotransmitter substance P have been identified in the tumor. The tumors are usually small, red-blue nodules.

glossectomy   Surgical removal of all or part of the tongue.

See also HEAD AND NECK CANCER.

glucagonoma   See PANCREATIC CANCER.

gonioscopy   An examination of the front of the eye, using a special instrument called a gonioscope, to detect ocular MELANOMA.

grade   The grade of a tumor indicates how abnormal the cancer cells look under a microscope and how quickly the tumor is likely to grow and spread. Grading systems are different for each type of cancer, but in general, the lower the grade, the more like a normal cell and the better the prognosis. The grade of a tumor helps determine the type of treatment.

grade IV astrocytoma   See BRAIN CANCER.

graft-vs.-host disease (GVHD)   A side effect of BONE MARROW TRANSPLANTS or blood transfusions in which transplanted immune cells attack the tissues of the recipient, which are perceived as "foreign." The only transplanted tissues that contain enough immune cells to cause a problem are blood and bone marrow.

Bone marrow transplants are used to replace blood-producing cells and immune cells in patients whose cancer treatment has destroyed their own bone marrow. Because bone marrow cells are among the most sensitive to radiation and CHEMOTHERAPY, they often must be destroyed along with the cancer. Bone marrow transplants are used most often in the treatment of LEUKEMIA, although some other cancers have also been treated this way.

The most common sites of graft-vs.-host disease are the skin, liver, and gastrointestinal tract. About half of all patients receiving bone marrow that is not genetically identical to their own develop the condition.

Causes and Symptoms

Even 25 percent of those who receive genetically identical marrow can still develop GVHD. There are many different elements involved in immune reactions; testing can often identify donors who match all the major genetic elements, but there are many minor ones that will always be different. How good a match is found also depends upon the urgency of the need.

The acute form of bone marrow graft-vs.-host disease appears within two months of the transplant; the chronic form usually appears within three months. The acute disease produces a skin rash, liver problems, and bloody diarrhea. Chronic disease can produce a similar patchy skin rash, a tightening or an inflammation of the skin, lesions in the mouth, dry eyes and mouth, hair loss, liver damage, lung damage, and indigestion. Patients can die of liver failure, infection, or other severe disturbances of their system.

Treatment

Both the acute and the chronic disease are treated with cortisone drugs, immunosuppressive drugs such as cyclosporine, or with antibiotics and immune chemicals from donated blood (gamma globulin).

Prognosis

Bone marrow transplant patients who do not have a graft-vs.-host reaction gradually return to normal immune function in a year. A graft-vs.-host reaction may prolong the diminished immune capacity indefinitely, requiring supplemental treatment with immunoglobulins (gamma globulin). Somehow the grafted cells develop a tolerance to their new home after six to 12 months, and the medications can be gradually withdrawn. Graft-vs.-host disease is not the only complication of blood transfusion or bone marrow transplantation. Host-vs.-graft or rejection is also common and may require a repeat transplant with another donor organ. Infections are a constant threat in bone marrow transplant because of the disease being treated, the prior radiation or chemotherapy, and the medications used to treat the transplant.

Prevention

For transfusion patients especially likely to have graft-vs.-host reactions, the red blood cells can safely be irradiated using X-rays to kill all the white immune cells. The red blood cells are less sensitive to radiation and are not harmed by this treatment.

granulocyte colony-stimulating factor   A COLONY-STIMULATING FACTOR that triggers the production of a type of white blood cell called neutrophil. Granulocyte colony-stimulating factor is a CYTOKINE that belongs to the family of drugs called hematopoietic (blood-forming) agents.

granulocytopenia   See NEUTROPENIA.

granulosa cell tumor   A type of slow-growing, solid malignant tumor that usually affects the ovary. Granulosa cell tumors are most common in postmenopausal women. They may cause vaginal bleeding and an elevated level of the tumor marker inhibin in the blood. Between 1 and 2 percent of all ovarian tumors are granulosa cell tumors; they are associated with endometrial hyperplasia.

See also OVARIAN CANCER.

Grawitz' tumor A type of KIDNEY CANCER.

green tea See TEA.

growth factor See COLONY-STIMULATING FACTOR.

guaiac test See FECAL OCCULT BLOOD TEST.

gynecologic cancers A group of cancers that can occur in the female reproductive tract, including CERVICAL CANCER, CHORIOCARCINOMA, ENDOMETRIAL CANCER, gestational trophoblastic tumor, OVARIAN CANCER, UTERINE CANCER, VAGINAL CANCER, and VULVAR CANCER. BREAST CANCER may be included in this group.

gynecologic oncologist Cancer specialist in gynecologic ONCOLOGY, a field of medical specialization that deals with the study and treatment of malignancies arising in the female reproductive tract.

A gynecologic oncologist must first train as an obstetrician/gynecologist, then receive two to four years of structured training at a medical center in all of the types of treatment for gynecologic cancers (surgery, RADIATION THERAPY, CHEMOTHERAPY, and experimental treatments) as well as the biology and pathology of gynecologic cancer. Gynecologic oncologists practice in a variety of settings, including teaching hospitals, cancer centers, and regional and local hospitals.

The ovary, endometrium, cervix, vulva, and vagina are the sites of origin of the most common and serious gynecologic malignancies. Although they are often discussed as a group, they have significant differences in etiology, prevention, detection, treatment, and likelihood of cure.

See also SOCIETY OF GYNECOLOGIC ONCOLOGY.

H

hair dye Products used to alter the color of the hair that at one time were linked to the development of cancer. Most studies have found no link between hair dye and cancer.

Permanent hair dyes contain ammonia and peroxide. Semipermanent dyes penetrate into the hair shaft, but not as deeply as permanent dyes. Semipermanent dyes do not rinse off with water, but they do fade and wash out of hair after about five to 10 shampoos. Vegetable dyes (such as henna) deposit a coating of dye on the cuticle of the hair shaft and keep their color only with repeated applications.

Synthetic (aniline) dyes are the most popular, since they are easy to apply and their color is stable, but they can react with skin protein and trigger an allergic reaction. About 10 percent of people who use these dyes will develop an allergy to them. This is why hair dye should never be used on eyelashes or eyebrows, and why eyelash and eyebrow dyes are forbidden by the U.S. Food and Drug Administration.

Several studies appear to put to rest the fears of a possible cancer risk for people who dye their hair. (Most of the previous studies that raised concerns about hair dye were relatively small and looked at the former habits of people who had already gotten cancer.) In general, the studies showed that women who dyed their hair (even those who had used hair color for more than 20 years) were at no greater risk than those who never colored their hair. There was one exception to the findings: women who for at least 20 years used permanent black dye, the most concentrated form of hair dye, did have a higher risk for two rare types of cancer.

Those who do use black hair dyes are advised to wear rubber gloves, avoid mixing different products, leave dye on as briefly as possible, rinse scalp completely, and never dye eyebrows or eyelashes.

hair loss Known medically as alopecia, this is one of the most well known side effects of CHEMOTHERAPY. Although a few drugs do not cause hair loss (or cause little loss), most do cause partial or complete hair loss for a time. Some chemotherapy can damage hair and make it brittle. If this happens, the hair may break off near the scalp a week or two after the chemotherapy has started.

Chemotherapy works by targeting rapidly dividing cells typical of malignancies. However, some normal cells in the body also divide quickly—such as the cells responsible for growing hair.

The amount of hair lost depends on the type of drug or combination of drugs used, the dose given, and the person's individual reaction to the drug. If hair loss is going to happen, it usually begins within a few weeks of the start of treatment, although rarely it can start within a few days. Body hair may be lost as well, and some drugs even trigger loss of the eyelashes and eyebrows.

If patients do lose their hair as a result of chemotherapy, it will grow back once treatment is over.

Some people having certain types of chemotherapy may be able to prevent hair loss by using a "cold cap" that temporarily slows blood flow to the scalp and consequently decreases the amount of the drug that reaches the area. Unfortunately, the cold cap blocks the action only of certain drugs.

hairy cell leukemia See LEUKEMIA.

Halsted mastectomy See MASTECTOMY.

hand and foot syndrome A condition marked by pain, swelling, numbness, tingling, or redness of the hands or feet that sometimes occurs as a side effect of certain anticancer drugs. The syndrome is also known as palmar-plantar erythodysthesia.

head and neck cancer   A group of cancers that include hypopharyngeal cancer, LARYNGEAL CANCER, throat cancer, ORAL CANCER, metastatic squamous neck cancer, nasopharyngeal cancer, pharyngeal cancer, nasal cavity cancer, and salivary gland cancer. Cancers of the brain, eye, and thyroid usually are not included in the category of head and neck cancers, nor are cancers of the scalp, skin, muscles, and bones of the head and neck.

These cancers account for three percent of all cancer in the United States and occur more often in men and in people over 50. It is estimated that almost 38,000 American men and women will develop head and neck cancers each year.

Most head and neck cancers begin in the squamous cells that line the structures in the head and neck. Because of this, head and neck cancers are often referred to as squamous cell carcinomas, although it is possible for these malignancies to begin in other types of cells.

Cancers of the head and neck are usually identified by the area in which they begin, as listed below:

Oral Cavity (Lips and Mouth)

This cancer may begin in the lips, the front two-thirds of the tongue, the gums, the lining inside the cheeks and lips, the floor of the mouth under the tongue, the bony top of the mouth (hard palate), and the small area behind the wisdom teeth. Almost all cancers in this area are squamous cell carcinomas (cancerous cells in the outermost layer of skin). These cancers are more common in people older than 45, and men are affected two to four times more often than women. More than 90 percent of cases are related to tobacco use, although sun exposure is an additional risk factor for cancer of the lips.

Salivary Glands

Cancer in this part of the head and neck may begin in the glands under the tongue, in front of the ears, and under the jawbone, as well as in other parts of the upper digestive tract. Salivary gland cancer is rare, and may begin in any of several cell types within the salivary glands. The aggressiveness of the tumor growth and spread often is related to the cell type. The only known risk factor is exposure to radiation, although smoking may play some role in certain types of salivary gland cancer.

Throat

This cancer may start in the back third of the tongue, the tonsils, and the part of the throat that lies directly behind the mouth. Squamous cell carcinoma is the most common type of cancer found in this area, and the most important risk factors are tobacco use and heavy alcohol consumption.

Nasopharynx

Cancers of the nasopharynx may begin where the throat meets the back of the nasal cavity, and most are squamous cell cancers. Unlike other head and neck cancers, they do not seem to be linked to tobacco or alcohol use. In fact, in the United States nasopharyngeal cancer has not been associated with any particular risk factors, but in parts of northern Africa, Asia, and the Arctic region, where this cancer is more common, it has been related to infection with the Epstein-Barr virus, consumption of Cantonese salted fish, excess exposure to dusts and smoke, and excess consumption of fermented foods.

Sinuses and Nasal Cavity

Cancer found in this area may begin in the sinuses (the small hollow spaces in the bones of the head surrounding the nose) or the nasal cavity (the hollow space inside the nose). Most cancers found in the sinuses and inside the nose are squamous cell carcinomas (74 percent to 79 percent of cases). Rarely, ADENOCARCINOMAS, MELANOMAS, and LYMPHOMAS also occur in this area. These cancers often grow fairly large before they are diagnosed because the sinuses and nasal cavity have enough room for tumors to grow before they trigger symptoms.

Larynx

Also called the voice box, this short passageway is formed by cartilage just below the pharynx in the neck. The larynx contains the vocal cords and the epiglottis, which moves to cover the larynx to prevent food from entering the air passages. Most cancers in this area are squamous cell carcinomas that are related to SMOKING, heavy ALCOHOL use, or exposure to ASBESTOS. Most cases occur in people aged 55 or older, more often in men and among African Americans.

Hypopharynx

The hypopharynx is the area of the neck below the back of the throat and above the esophagus (not including the larynx). Most cancers in this region are squamous cell carcinomas related to tobacco or alcohol use. In 10 percent to 15 percent of cases, more than one cancer is found, with the second tumor usually found in the esophagus. Of all the head and neck cancers, cancers of the larynx and hypopharynx have the greatest tendency to spread, especially to other parts of the hypopharynx and to the tongue.

Lymph Nodes

Sometimes squamous cancer cells are found in the lymph nodes of the upper neck when there is no evidence of cancer in other parts of the head and neck. When this happens, the cancer is called "metastatic squamous neck cancer with unseen primary."

Causes

Tobacco (including smokeless tobacco) and alcohol use are the most important risk factors for head and neck cancers, particularly those of the oral cavity, oropharynx, hypopharynx, and larynx. Eighty-five percent of head and neck cancers are linked to tobacco use. People who use both tobacco and alcohol are at greater risk for developing these cancers than people who use either tobacco or alcohol alone. Other risk factors for cancers of the head and neck include

- *Oral cavity:* sun exposure (lip), human papillomavirus infection
- *Salivary glands:* radiation to the head and neck from diagnostic X-rays or radiation therapy
- *Paranasal sinuses and nasal cavity:* certain industrial exposures such as wood or nickel dust inhalation; tobacco and alcohol use may play less of a role in this type of cancer
- *Nasopharynx:* Asian (particularly Chinese) ancestry, Epstein-Barr virus infection, occupational exposure to wood dust, and consumption of certain preservatives or salted foods

- *Pharynx:* poor oral hygiene, mechanical irritation such as from poorly fitting dentures, and use of mouthwash that has a high alcohol content
- *Hypopharynx:* Plummer-Vinson (also called Paterson-Kelly) syndrome, a rare disorder that results from nutritional deficiencies and is characterized by severe anemia. The syndrome leads to difficulty swallowing due to webs of tissue that grow across the upper part of the esophagus
- *Larynx:* exposure to airborne particles of asbestos, especially in the workplace

Symptoms

Symptoms that are common to several head and neck cancer sites include a lump or sore that does not heal, a sore throat that does not go away, difficulty swallowing, and a change or hoarseness in the voice. Other symptoms may include the following:

- *Lips and mouth:* white or red patch; sore or bleeding on the gums, tongue, or lining of the mouth; a swelling of the jaw that causes dentures to fit poorly or become uncomfortable; earache; unusual bleeding or pain in the mouth
- *Nasal cavity and sinuses:* blocked sinuses that do not clear, chronic sinus infections that do not respond to antibiotics, nosebleeds, frequent headaches, swollen eyes, pain in the upper teeth, or problems with dentures
- *Salivary glands:* swelling under the chin or around the jawbone, numbness or paralysis of the muscles in the face, or pain in the face, chin, or neck that does not go away
- *Pharynx and hypopharynx:* ear pain, hoarseness, discomfort or difficulty in swallowing, pain in the neck, jaw, or ear, a lump or swelling in the neck, or a feeling that something is stuck in the throat
- *Nasopharynx:* trouble breathing or speaking, frequent headaches, pain or ringing in the ears, or trouble hearing
- *Larynx:* pain when swallowing, ear pain, hoarseness, pain in the neck, jaw, or ear, a lump or swelling in the neck, or a feeling that something is stuck in the throat

Diagnosis

To find the cause of symptoms, a doctor evaluates a person's medical history, performs a physical examination, and orders diagnostic tests. The exams and tests conducted may vary depending on the symptoms but may include

- *Endoscopy:* a laryngoscope is inserted through the mouth to view the larynx; an esophagoscope is inserted through the mouth to examine the esophagus; and a nasopharyngoscope is inserted through the nose so the doctor can see the nasal cavity and nasopharynx.
- *Lab tests:* blood, urine, or other substances
- *X-rays*
- *CAT and MRI scans*
- *Biopsy*

Treatment

For most head and neck cancers, the stage is determined by the tumor's size (in diameter), whether it has invaded tissues next to it, whether the cancer has spread to nearby lymph nodes, and whether the cancer has metastasized to other areas of the body. The treatment plan for an individual patient depends on a number of factors, including the exact location of the tumor, the stage of the cancer, and the person's age and general health. Treatment might include surgery, radiation, chemotherapy, or a combination of these treatments.

Oral and throat   In the early stages in which the cancer has not spread, surgery or radiation may be the only treatment needed. More advanced stages may be treated with various combinations of surgery, radiation, and chemotherapy. If caught early, this cancer has a cure rate of 90 percent to 100 percent. More advanced stages have a cure rate of 65 percent to 90 percent if the cancer has not spread to lymph nodes in the neck. Cancers with lymph-node involvement or distant metastases tend to have a poorer prognosis.

Salivary glands   In this cancer, staging is based on tumor size, spread to local lymph nodes or distant sites, and whether tumor has invaded the facial nerve or the base of the skull. Smaller, early-stage, tumors can be treated with surgery alone, but larger tumors that have spread usually require radiation after surgery. Inoperable tumors are treated with radiation or chemotherapy.

Early-stage cancer of the salivary gland often can be cured by surgery alone, but the outlook is poorest for cancers under the tongue or minor salivary glands, cancers that have invaded the facial nerve, and bulky cancers that have spread to other parts of the body.

Nasopharynx   High-dose radiation is the primary treatment, although chemotherapy and surgery can be used in patients who have a poor response to radiation. Radiation cures 80 percent to 90 percent of patients with small nasopharyngeal cancers that have not spread, but survival drops to 10 percent to 40 percent in the later stages.

Sinuses and nasal cavity   In most patients, the cancer is far advanced when it is discovered, and the danger is that the tumor will invade areas of the skull near the eye and brain. For this reason, surgery is performed to remove as much of the tumor as possible, followed by radiation. Sometimes, radiation treatment is given before surgery to shrink the tumor. Because most tumors in this area are diagnosed so late, the prognosis is often poor. In general, the cure rate is 50 percent or less.

Larynx   Small superficial cancers that have not spread to lymph nodes can be treated with radiation, laser surgery, and possibly chemotherapy. Larger tumors are treated with radiation, surgery (either a partial or a total laryngectomy), and/or chemotherapy. If the cancer is small and has not spread to the lymph nodes, the cure rate is 75 percent to 95 percent.

Hypopharynx   Most hypopharyngeal cancers have no symptoms until they reach an advanced stage. For this reason, treatment usually requires extensive surgery to remove portions of the larynx and pharynx, followed by radiation therapy. In some patients, chemotherapy has been used to shrink the size of the tumor before surgery, which may allow the surgeon to save enough of the larynx to preserve the patient's voice. Because many patients have advanced cancer at the time of diagnosis, the prognosis is often poor. Patients who continue to smoke during treatment do not respond as well, or survive as long, as patients who stop smoking.

Rehabilitation

Depending on the location of the cancer and the type of treatment, rehabilitation may include physical therapy, nutrition counseling, speech therapy, or learning how to care for the opening in the windpipe (stoma) after a laryngectomy. A patient with mouth cancer may need reconstructive surgery to rebuild the bones or tissues, or to create an artificial dental or facial part to restore swallowing ability and speech.

Patients who have trouble speaking after treatment, or who have lost their ability to speak, may need speech therapy. A speech-language pathologist may visit the patient in the hospital to plan therapy and teach speech exercises or alternative methods of speaking. Speech therapy usually continues after the patient returns home.

Eating may be difficult after treatment for head and neck cancer. Some patients receive nutrients directly into a vein after surgery, or need a feeding tube until they can eat on their own. A nurse or speech-language pathologist can help patients learn how to swallow again after surgery.

Regular follow-up care is very important after treatment to make sure the cancer has not returned, or that a second new cancer has not developed. Depending on the type of cancer, medical checkups could include exams of the stoma, mouth, neck, and throat. Regular dental exams may also be necessary. From time to time, the doctor may perform a complete physical exam, blood tests, X-rays, and CT or MRI scans.

Doctors may continue to monitor thyroid and pituitary gland function, especially if the head or neck was treated with radiation.

Prevention

People can reduce the risk of head and neck cancer by not smoking; avoiding chewing tobacco, snuff, and excessive alcohol; practicing good oral hygiene; and visiting the dentist regularly.

People who have been treated for head and neck cancer have an increased chance of developing a new cancer, usually in the head and neck, esophagus, or lungs. The chance of a second primary cancer varies depending on the original diagnosis but is higher for people who smoke. Studies have shown that continuing to smoke increases the chance of a second primary cancer for up to 20 years after the original diagnosis.

Some research has shown that isotretinoin (13-cis-retinoic acid), a substance related to vitamin A, may reduce the risk of a second primary cancer in patients who have been successfully treated for cancers of the oral cavity, oropharynx, and larynx. However, treatment with isotretinoin has not been shown to improve survival.

Helicobacter pylori   Bacteria that cause inflammation and ulcers in the stomach and that have been implicated in the development of STOMACH CANCER. Although it is difficult to give exact figures, experts believe that *H. pylori* infection may play some role in up to 40 to 60 percent of all stomach cancers. Gastric cancer is the second most common cancer worldwide, and it is most common in countries such as Colombia and China, where *H. pylori* infects more than 90 percent of the population. In the United States, where *H. pylori* is less common in young people, gastric cancer rates have been dropping since the 1930s.

How It Spreads

There seems to be a link between infection and living conditions such as poor sanitation, close contact, and overcrowding. In the United States, about 50 out of every 100 adults are infected, and these infections were probably acquired during childhood. How *H. pylori* is passed from one person to another is unclear, although the germs have been found in saliva, dental plaque, and in stools.

Once it infects someone, the *H. pylori* germ lives in the lining of the stomach, but scientists are not sure how it causes gastritis, ulcers, or cancer. Some experts believe one possibility is that the germ damages the stomach lining, allowing stomach acid to irritate the lining.

Symptoms

Some people with *H. pylori* have no symptoms. For those who have gastritis or ulcers, the most common symptoms are stomach pain, heartburn, or bleeding, which can lead to anemia. If left untreated, ulcers can become life threatening.

Diagnosis

A blood test for *H. pylori* can reveal an infection, but not whether it is current or happened in the past; the blood can remain positive for months after the germs are gone.

H. pylori infection also can be detected by special changes in the exhaled breath; the urea breath test is positive only if the person has a current infection.

The most accurate test is an endoscopy, in which small samples of the stomach lining are taken through a tube passed through the mouth into the stomach and tested for *H. pylori.*

Treatment

At the present time, doctors treat *H. pylori* infection only if the patient has an ulcer. Therapy for *H. pylori* infection involves 10 days to two weeks of one or two effective antibiotics such as amoxicillin, tetracycline, metronidazole, or clarithromycin, plus either ranitidine bismuth citrate, bismuth subsalicylate, or a proton pump inhibitor. Currently, eight *H. pylori* treatment regimens are approved by the Food and Drug Administration, although several other combinations have been used successfully. Overall, treatment with three different drugs has been more effective than with two, and longer treatment (14 days versus 10 days) results in better eradication rates.

hemangioblastoma See BRAIN CANCER; CHILDHOOD CANCERS.

hemangiopericytoma A type of cancer involving blood vessels and soft tissue.

hemangiosarcoma A rare type of soft tissue SARCOMA that can affect the blood vessels in the arms, legs, or trunk. Hemangiosarcomas make up about 2 percent of all soft tissue sarcomas.

hematemesis Vomiting blood. This symptom may be associated with several conditions, including ESOPHAGEAL CANCER, STOMACH CANCER, or benign ulcers. Sometimes individuals vomit blood swallowed after a nosebleed, or after prolonged retching due to a tear in the throat. Hematemesis can sometimes be difficult to distinguish from coughing up blood from the lungs. The vomited material may contain only a small amount of dark blood, resembling coffee grounds, or it may be full of blood, which can be a medical emergency.

In any case, vomiting blood requires immediate medical evaluation, so the patient should call a doctor or go to an emergency room. In the case of massive hematemesis, emergency intervention may include intravenous fluids, medications, blood transfusions, or other treatments. Bleeding that does not stop may require surgery.

hematologist-oncologist A doctor who specializes in treating cancers of the blood and blood-forming tissues. To become certified as a hematologist-ONCOLOGIST, after medical school a candidate must train as a specialist (internist or pediatrician) and subspecialist (medical oncologist-hematologist or pediatric oncologist-hematologist).

The American Board of Internal Medicine examines and certifies internists who choose to acquire additional education and training in the dual subspecialty of medical oncology and hematology. The American Board of Pediatrics examines and certifies pediatricians who choose to acquire additional education and training to subspecialize in pediatric oncology/hematology.

hematopoietic growth factors See COLONY-STIMULATING FACTOR.

hematuria The presence of blood in the urine, which can be caused by many kidney diseases and disorders of the genital or urinary systems.

hemochromatosis gene (HFE) A gene that, when inherited with a particular mutation, is associated with an increased risk of COLON CANCER.

Hereditary hemochromatosis is an autosomal recessive disease that is characterized by iron overload, which leads to dysfunction of the pancreas, liver, heart, and other organs. Although the disease itself is rare, the HFE gene mutations that cause the disease occur in up to 15 percent of the U.S. population. HFE gene mutations are associated with increased total body iron stores in some people.

Investigators found that two types of HFE mutations (C282Y and H63D) occurred more often among patients with colon cancer than among cancer-free control subjects. Also, subjects with any HFE gene mutation were more likely to have colon cancer than subjects with no HFE gene mutations, when the analysis was adjusted for other potential risk factors. The risk of colon cancer associated with an HFE gene mutation was independent of a family history of colon cancer.

If subsequent studies confirm that mutations in the HFE gene are a risk factor for colon cancer, testing for such mutations may allow the identification of a subgroup of individuals that might benefit from intensified COLORECTAL CANCER screening.

hemoglobin Substance contained in red blood cells that is responsible for the red blood color. Hemoglobin takes up oxygen as blood passes through the lungs, and releases it as blood passes through tissues in the rest of the body. Hemoglobin is measured in grams (g) per deciliter (dL). The normal hemoglobin ranges are 14 g/dL to 18 g/dL for men and 12 g/dL to 16 g/dL for women. However, the definition of "normal" varies from person to person.

Patients who are anemic (have low hemoglobin levels) have less oxygen to send to muscles and organs. As a result, the person with anemia feels tired and unable to do everyday activities.

Patients with LEUKEMIA, or cancer patients taking certain CHEMOTHERAPY drugs, may have low hemoglobin counts and be diagnosed with ANEMIA. This is sometimes treated with epoetin alfa (Procrit).

hemolysis A condition in which red blood cells break down and release hemoglobin. In some cancer patients undergoing CHEMOTHERAPY, this may lead to ANEMIA because the body is unable to produce more red blood cells in the BONE MARROW to replace those that were destroyed. Many types of cancer and treatments may be linked to significant hemolysis.

hemoptysis Coughing up blood, which can be a warning sign of LUNG CANCER. When this occurs, it means that small blood vessels have burst in the lung, sending blood into the sputum. (Many other kinds of lung infections, such as pneumonia or tuberculosis, also cause hemoptysis.)

hepatic arterial infusion A procedure to deliver CHEMOTHERAPY directly to the liver in cases of LIVER CANCER. Catheters are put into an artery in the groin that leads directly to the liver, and drugs are given through the catheters.

hepatoblastoma See LIVER CANCER.

hepatocellular carcinoma The most common type of liver tumor, which accounts for 80 percent to 90 percent of all LIVER CANCER. It occurs more often in men than women and occurs mostly in people 50 to 60 years old.

hepatomegaly Enlargement of the liver associated with both primary LIVER CANCER and tumors that have spread to the liver from elsewhere in the body. Liver enlargement may be diagnosed by a physical exam or scans (both ultrasound and CT).

HER1 Epidermal growth factor receptor found on the surface of some cells and to which epidermal growth factor binds, causing the cells to divide. HER1 is found at abnormally high levels on the surface of many types of cancer cells, so these cells may divide excessively in the presence of epidermal growth factor. HER1 is also known as EGFR or ErbB1.

herbicides See ENVIRONMENTAL FACTORS.

herbs as antioxidants In addition to making food tastier, herbs are an abundant source of ANTIOXIDANTS and could provide potential anticancer benefits when supplementing a balanced diet, according to government researchers. Antioxidants are a class of compounds thought to prevent certain types of chemical damage caused by an excess of FREE RADICALS (charged molecules that are generated by a variety of sources including pesticides, smoking, and exhaust fumes). Researchers believe that destroying free radicals may help fight cancer.

Herbs have higher antioxidant activity than fruits, vegetables, and some spices, including GARLIC, and some should be eaten regularly, according to scientists at the United States Department of Agriculture's Beltsville Agricultural Research Center in Beltsville, Maryland. Using various chemical tests, the scientists compared the antioxidant activity of 39 commonly used herbs grown in the same location and conditions, including 27 culinary and 12 medicinal herbs.

The herbs with the highest antioxidant activity belonged to the oregano family. In general, oregano had three to 20 times more antioxidant activity than the other herbs studied. On a per-gram fresh-weight basis, oregano and other herbs ranked even higher in antioxidant activity than fruits and vegetables, which are known to be high in antioxidants. Oregano has 42 times more antioxidant activity than apples, 30 times more than potatoes, 12 times more than oranges, and four times more than blueberries. For example, one tablespoon of fresh oregano contains the same antioxidant activity as one medium-sized apple. Other herbs also appear to contain significant amounts of antioxidants. Among the more familiar, ranked in order, are dill, garden thyme, rosemary, and peppermint. The most active phenol component in some of the herbs with the highest antioxidant activity, particularly oregano, was rosmarinic acid, a strong antioxidant.

Fruits and vegetables have long been viewed as a rich source of antioxidant compounds. Health officials have been urging consumers for years to eat more fruits and vegetables in order to gain the health benefits of antioxidants, but Westerners still tend to favor diets that are rich in fats and carbohydrates.

More recently, researchers have begun to study the health benefits of herbs and spices (herbs typically come from the leaves of plants, whereas spices come from the bark, stem, and seeds of plants). Both have been used for thousands of years to flavor foods and treat illness. In the new research, herbs carried more of an antioxidant punch than did spices such as paprika, garlic, curry, chili, and black pepper.

Herbs can be consumed in a variety of ways. Some people prefer to drink herb extracts, which can be made by adding herbs to hot water to make potent antioxidant teas, or to use concentrated herbal oils available in some health food stories. Others prefer flavoring meats and vegetables with fresh or dried herbs.

In general, fresh herbs and spices are healthier and contain higher antioxidant levels compared to their processed counterparts. For example, the antioxidant activity of fresh garlic is 1.5 times higher than that of dry garlic powder.

However, herbs should be used with moderation and are not a substitute for a balanced diet. Pregnant women in particular should consult a doctor before taking herbal supplements.

hereditary nonpolyposis colon cancer An inherited disorder in which affected individuals have a higher-than-normal chance of developing COLORECTAL CANCER and certain other types of cancer, usually before the age of 60. This disorder is also called Lynch syndrome.

heredity and cancer While many people assume that most types of cancer are inherited, in fact only 5 percent to 10 percent of the estimated one million new cases of cancer diagnosed every year are considered hereditary. In addition, inheriting a predisposition to cancer does not mean a person will definitely get the disease. Often, it is possible to minimize the genetic risk by making healthy lifestyle choices about DIET, EXERCISE, and tobacco use.

A detailed family medical history can help a doctor determine if a particular person is at risk for inherited cancers. Indicators can include

- cancer that develops 10 to 20 years earlier than a random cancer
- cancer that strikes on both sides, such as in both breasts or at two different locations in one organ
- two or more members of one generation who have the same type of cancer
- particular tumor site combinations seen within one family, especially breast-ovary or colon-uterus

See also BRCA1/BRCA2; FAMILY HISTORY; FAMILY RISK ASSESSMENT PROGRAMS; GENES AND CANCER; HEREDITARY NONPOLYPOSIS COLON CANCER.

HER-2/neu A gene that when it mutated, works like a switch that turns normal cells into cancerous ones.

Scientific evidence has mounted that the HER-2/neu gene may be altered in at least 25 percent of all BREAST CANCER tumors; patients with the altered form of the gene tend to have the most aggressive disease. Scientists also have noted the importance of HER-2/neu as a marker of tumor aggressiveness in cancers of the ovary, endometrium, and salivary glands.

HER-2/neu is an example of an ONCOGENE (cancer gene) that speeds up the growth of malignant cells. As with many oncogenes, the normal version of the HER-2/neu gene is harmless and plays a key role in early development and cell growth. Many tumors contain too many copies of the HER-2/neu gene, which may also carry genetic changes that cause the gene to be turned on constantly. Combined with other potent alterations in a cell's genes, this leads to the uncontrolled growth of cancer.

Most women today are not tested to see whether their breast cancer involves HER-2/neu or not, which will probably change as research reveals the importance of knowing HER-2/neu status, especially when considering which treatment to use on a patient. Already some studies have suggested that women with breast tumors containing HER-2/neu alterations are more likely to respond to the CHEMOTHERAPY drug Taxol.

high-dose-rate remote brachytherapy See BRACHYTHERAPY.

Hispanics/Latinos and cancer Hispanic Americans and Latinos are less likely than non-Hispanic Caucasians to develop and die from the most common cancers, but they have higher rates of certain other cancers and are more likely to have cancer detected at a later stage. This largest and fastest-growing minority in the United States has a unique cancer risk profile that requires a targeted approach to prevention, according to the AMERICAN CANCER SOCIETY. People from Cuba, Mexico, Puerto Rico, South or Central America, and other Spanish cultures—regardless of race—are considered Hispanic.

Compared to non-Hispanic Caucasians, Hispanic Americans and Latinos have lower incidence and death from all cancers combined, as well as from each of the four most common cancers (lung, breast, prostate, and colon). However, they have higher rates of certain other cancers, including cancers of the stomach, cervix, and liver, and they

are less likely to use screening tests for colon cancer, PROSTATE CANCER, and CERVICAL CANCER. In addition, this group as a whole is more likely to be overweight and less likely to EXERCISE—factors increasingly associated with cancer. Traditionally, Hispanics and Latinos have been much less likely to smoke.

All of the approaches that are most important in the general population are also important for Hispanics: preventing and treating tobacco dependence, increasing access to high quality cancer screening and appropriate follow-up care, increasing physical activity, maintaining a healthy body weight. In addition, several other approaches are particularly important for this group:

- getting PAP TESTS
- hepatitis B vaccination
- removing barriers that interfere with access to high quality screening and medical care
- delivering health messages more effectively.

Cancer Screening
Historically, Hispanic women have been the least likely of racial and ethnic groups to use screening tests, such as Pap tests, MAMMOGRAPHY, and clinical breast exams. Even though they are 40 percent less likely to be diagnosed with BREAST CANCER, Hispanic women are more likely to be diagnosed at a later stage.

The death rate from cervical cancer is 40 percent higher among Hispanic women compared to other groups, and Hispanics are much less likely than non-Hispanics to have had a FECAL OCCULT BLOOD TEST in the past year (15.4 percent versus 24.1 percent) or a SIGMOIDOSCOPY or COLONOSCOPY in the past five years (31.2 percent versus 39.2 percent). Hispanic men are less likely to have had a PSA test for the early detection of prostate cancer than Caucasian non-Hispanic men (46 percent versus 58.2 percent).

Tobacco Use
Hispanics as a group smoke far less than the national average (16 percent versus 22.8 percent), which is primarily why they have lower rates of lung and many other cancers. Between 1992 and 1999, LUNG CANCER diagnosis rates dropped an aver-

age of 3.1 percent per year among Hispanic men and women. Still, the disease remains the top cancer killer of Hispanics. U.S.-born Hispanics are more likely to smoke than those who are foreign born.

Obesity and Physical Activity

OBESITY, which raises the risk for many chronic diseases, including cancer, is on the rise among Hispanics, particularly Hispanic women. In 2001, 35.8 percent of Hispanic adults had no form of leisure time physical activity, compared to 22.9 percent of non-Hispanic Caucasians.

histiocyte non-Hodgkin's lymphoma   See NON-HODGKIN'S LYMPHOMA.

1H-nuclear magnetic resonance spectroscopic imaging   A noninvasive imaging method that measures activity at the cellular level and that provides chemical information. It is used in conjunction with MAGNETIC RESONANCE IMAGING (MRI). This imaging method is also called proton magnetic resonance spectroscopic imaging.

Hodgkin's disease   A malignant disease of the lymphatic system that is characterized by painless enlargement of LYMPH NODES, the spleen, or other lymphatic tissue. It is one of the LYMPHOMAS, which are cancers that develop in the lymphatic system (a part of the body's immune system that helps fight disease and infection). Hodgkin's disease is an uncommon lymphoma and accounts for less than 1 percent of all cases of cancer in this country. Other cancers of the lymphatic system are called NON-HODGKIN'S LYMPHOMAS.

Cause

In Hodgkin's disease, cells in the lymphatic system become abnormal, dividing too fast and growing without any control. Because lymphatic tissue is present in many parts of the body, Hodgkin's disease can start almost anywhere. It may begin in a single lymph node, a group of lymph nodes, or in other parts of the lymphatic system such as the BONE MARROW and spleen.

This type of cancer tends to spread in a fairly orderly way from one group of lymph nodes to the next group. For example, Hodgkin's disease that begins in the lymph nodes in the neck will spread first to the nodes above the collarbones, and then to the lymph nodes under the arms and within the chest. Eventually, it can spread to almost any other part of the body.

At this time, no one knows what causes Hodgkin's disease, and doctors can seldom explain why one person gets it and another does not. It is clear, however, that Hodgkin's disease is not caused by an injury and is not contagious.

Risk Factors

There are risk factors for Hodgkin's disease, but most people with these risk factors do not get the disease (and many who do have none of the known risk factors). Risk factors include

- *Age.* Hodgkin's disease occurs most often in people between 15 and 34 and in people over age 55.
- *Gender.* The disease is more common in men than in women.
- *Family history.* Siblings of those with Hodgkin's disease have a higher-than-average chance of developing the disease as well.
- *Viruses.* EPSTEIN-BARR VIRUS is an infectious agent that may be associated with an increased chance of getting Hodgkin's disease.

Symptoms

Symptoms of Hodgkin's disease may include a painless swelling in the lymph nodes in the neck, underarm, or groin; unexplained recurrent fevers; night sweats; unexplained WEIGHT LOSS; FATIGUE; and itchy skin. Early Hodgkin's disease may not cause pain.

Diagnosis

If Hodgkin's disease is suspected, the doctor will do a physical exam to see if the lymph nodes in the neck, underarm, or groin are enlarged, and will check the patient's medical history, blood tests, and body scans. The diagnosis usually depends on a BIOPSY; a surgeon will remove part or all of a lymph node so that a pathologist can examine it under a microscope to check for cancer cells. The pathologist studies the tissue and checks for Reed-Sternberg cells—large, abnormal cells that are usually found with Hodgkin's disease.

Staging

If biopsy reveals Hodgkin's disease, the doctor will need to diagnose the extent of the disease. The stage of Hodgkin's disease depends on the number and location of affected lymph nodes, whether the affected lymph nodes are on one or both sides of the diaphragm, and whether the disease has spread to the bone marrow, spleen, or places outside the lymphatic system, such as the liver.

To help stage the disease, the doctor may use additional biopsies of lymph nodes, the liver, bone marrow, or other tissue. Rarely, a surgeon may perform an operation called a laparotomy, in which an incision is made through the wall of the abdomen to remove tissue samples to check for cancer cells.

Treatment

Treatment for Hodgkin's disease depends on the stage of the disease, the size of the enlarged lymph nodes, symptoms, and the age and general health of the patient. Patients with Hodgkin's disease may be vaccinated against the flu, pneumonia, and meningitis.

RADIATION THERAPY and CHEMOTHERAPY are the most common treatments for Hodgkin's disease. Depending on the stage of the disease, treatment with radiation may be given alone or with chemotherapy. Bone marrow transplantation, peripheral STEM CELL transplantation, and BIOLOGICAL THERAPIES are being studied in clinical trials. Researchers are also exploring new ways of giving radiation therapy and chemotherapy, new drugs, and new drug combinations.

Chemotherapy for Hodgkin's disease usually consists of a combination of several drugs given alone or followed by radiation therapy. If Hodgkin's disease does not respond well to standard chemotherapy, or comes back after standard treatment, high-dose chemotherapy with stem cell support may be used.

Prognosis

Today, cancer research has led to real progress against Hodgkin's disease, with better survival rates and improved quality of life. Most people diagnosed with Hodgkin's disease can now be cured, or their disease can be controlled for many years.

Still, patients treated for Hodgkin's disease have an increased chance of developing LEUKEMIA; non-Hodgkin's lymphoma; and cancers of the colon, lung, bone, thyroid, and breast. Because of this, regular follow-up care is important.

hormonal therapy Treatment that adds, blocks, or removes hormones. To slow or stop the growth of certain cancers such as prostate and BREAST CANCER, hormones may be given to block the body's natural hormones. Sometimes surgery is needed to remove the source of hormones. Hormonal therapy is also called hormone therapy, hormone treatment, or endocrine therapy.

hormone receptor test A test to measure the amount of certain proteins, called hormone receptors, in cancer tissue. A high level of hormone receptors may mean that hormones help the cancer grow.

The degree to which a tumor is dependent or not dependent on hormones for growth is known as its "hormone receptor status." In BREAST CANCER, estrogen and progesterone receptor tests are performed during a biopsy. An estrogen receptor positive result means that the tumor appears to be stimulated by the hormone estrogen and depends on estrogen to grow. An estrogen receptor negative result indicates the tumor does not depend on estrogen to grow. Results of the receptor test helps a physician decide what treatment to recommend.

hormone replacement therapy (HRT) Hormones (ESTROGEN, progesterone, or both) given to postmenopausal women or women who have had their ovaries surgically removed, to replace the estrogen previously produced by the ovaries. Recently, in a large study, long-term use of a combination estrogen/progesterone in postmenopausal women was linked to an increased risk of BREAST CANCER, among other problems.

During menopause, a woman's body produces much lower amounts of estrogen than when she was menstruating. The resulting problems include hot flashes, bone loss, vaginal dryness, and mood swings. To ease menopausal symptoms, doctors in the past have prescribed HRT. Since HRT adds estrogen (and progesterone for women whose uterus is intact) back to the body, the risk of estrogen-fueled cancers is not insignificant.

Studies have found that a woman's risk of developing breast cancer is increased by about 40 percent if she uses postmenopausal hormones. This increased risk declines over time once a woman stops taking hormones. Overall, there is little, if any, increase in a woman's risk of breast cancer if she is a short-term user (less than five years). Links between estrogen and cancer are the reason why women who have had breast cancer, or who were at high risk, were always discouraged from taking HRT.

The largest randomized study ever to look at combined HRT in healthy postmenopausal women was stopped three years early, in July 2002, when researchers identified an increased risk of breast cancer among participants. At the time of the study, 38 percent of postmenopausal American women were on HRT.

The Women's Health Initiative (WHI) study report, along with an editorial opposing the long-term use of HRT in healthy postmenopausal women, was published in the July 17, 2002, issue of the *Journal of the American Medical Association.*

When hormone replacement was first developed, doctors simply administered estrogen alone (estrogen replacement therapy, or ERT). ERT helped relieve the symptoms of menopause and appeared to protect against heart disease and bone fractures, problems often found in older women, but doctors discovered that it also increased the risk of cancer of the uterine lining. Adding progesterone to estrogen—and calling it "hormone replacement therapy" (HRT)—seemed to protect against endometrial cancer in women with an intact uterus. Whether or not this conferred the other benefits seen with ERT, however, had not been known. The 2002 study results were important, although they do not apply to all groups, the authors reported.

For example, they do not apply to women receiving just estrogen replacement (ERT), which is still commonly given to women who have had a hysterectomy. The effects of ERT on women who no longer have a uterus are being studied in a separate WHI clinical trial, with results expected in 2005.

The 2002 study also did not look at short-term use of HRT to prevent menopausal symptoms, such as hot flashes, so it is difficult to draw conclusions about this, according to the authors.

The researchers looked at more than 16,000 healthy postmenopausal women who were part of the WHI, a trial funded by the National Institutes of Health. All of the women were between the ages of 50 and 79, and each still had a uterus. The women began taking either a combination estrogen/progesterone pill or a placebo each day, starting in the mid-1990s. The women were supposed to be followed for an average of eight and a half years, with the researchers looking at the results twice each year. The last scheduled review (May 2002) showed the results were significant enough that the trial was stopped after just over five years.

The rate of breast cancers was 26 percent higher among those receiving HRT than among those getting placebo. In those getting HRT, the rate for heart disease was 29 percent higher, stroke rates were 41 percent higher, and blood clot rates were more than twice as high.

HRT did have some benefits: the rate of colorectal cancer was 37 percent lower in the HRT group, and the rate of bone fractures was 24 percent lower. Endometrial cancer rates were about the same in both groups.

By weighing each of these factors, researchers came up with an overall "global index," which showed that the risks outweighed the possible benefits for these serious conditions.

Given these results, researchers recommended that clinicians stop prescribing HRT for long-term use. While the increased risk of breast cancer and other conditions may make HRT unsuitable for prevention in healthy people, the overall risk for each woman is still rather small. For example, the 36 percent increased risk of breast cancer is based on the fact that during one year, among 10,000 women receiving combination HRT, there will be 38 cases of breast cancer. Among 10,000 women taking a placebo, there will be 30 cases. The same holds true for heart disease (37 cases per 10,000 women per year with HRT, versus 30 cases per 10,000 women per year with placebo) and blood clots (34 cases per 10,000 women per year with HRT, versus 16 cases per 10,000 women per year with placebo). Nevertheless, there is a risk, and it would probably increase as the length of time taking combination HRT increased.

The AMERICAN CANCER SOCIETY acknowledged that decisions to take hormone replacement therapy, particularly estrogen plus PROGESTIN, will be more difficult now and recommended that women who are taking hormone replacement therapy should discuss this latest finding with their doctors.

Other studies have found an increased risk of OVARIAN CANCER with postmenopausal hormone use. A recent study that followed 44,241 postmenopausal women for approximately 20 years concluded that estrogen use is associated with an increased risk of ovarian cancer. In this study, women who used estrogen alone for 10 to 19 years were twice as likely to develop ovarian cancer as women who did not use postmenopausal hormones. For women who used estrogen for 20 or more years, the risk of ovarian cancer increased to three times that of women who did not use postmenopausal hormones. Another recent large study found an association between estrogen use and death due to ovarian cancer. In this study, the increased risk appeared to be limited to women who used estrogen for 10 or more years.

Because most studies have followed women using estrogen alone, there are currently not enough data to assess the potential effects of the estrogen-progestin combination on ovarian cancer. The above study of 44,241 postmenopausal women found that those who used estrogen in combination with progestin were not at increased risk of ovarian cancer, but the number of women in the study who had used estrogen plus progestin was small. More data are needed to determine whether estrogen-progestin has any effect on ovarian cancer risk.

hospice   A concept, rather than a place of care, that focuses on a holistic model of services designed to make a patient's final days as positive and symptom free as possible (but neither to hasten nor postpone death). It is based on a philosophy of caring that respects and values the dignity and worth of each person. Although hospices care for people approaching death, they cherish and emphasize life by helping patients and their families live each day to the fullest. There are almost 3,000 hospice and palliative care organizations in the United States.

Typically, a family member serves as the primary caregiver and, when appropriate, helps make decisions for the terminally ill individual. Hospice is a medical benefit covered by most insurance plans, enabling patients to stay home at the end of their lives and receive care from an integrated hospice team of nurses, medical social workers, physical and occupational therapists, nutritionists, home aid workers, pastoral counselors, and trained volunteers. Patients can continue to be treated by their own physician or by the hospice physician. Members of the hospice staff make regular visits to assess the patient and provide additional care or other services, and they are on call 24 hours a day, seven days a week.

The hospice team develops a care plan that meets each patient's individual needs for pain management and symptom control. The plan specifies the medical and support services required, such as nursing care, personal care (dressing, bathing), social services, physician visits, counseling, and homemaker services. It also identifies the medical equipment, tests, procedures, medication, and treatments necessary to provide high-quality comfort care.

While patients are at home, all necessary symptom-relieving medications are provided by hospice workers, along with any necessary special medical equipment. In emergencies, hospice workers take patients to a hospital or hospice inpatient unit designed to be as homelike as possible. Inpatient respite care is also available to provide a break for families.

Besides medical aid, hospice workers help patients with practical support (such as shopping) and emotional support, including life-closure, grief, and spiritual counseling. Depending on the hospice's resources, it may also provide other services such as art, touch, and music therapy.

Hospice care is available as a benefit under MEDICARE Part A, which is designed to provide patients with a terminal illness and their families with special support and services not otherwise covered by Medicare. Under the Medicare hospice benefit, beneficiaries choose to receive non-curative treatment and services for their terminal illness by waiving the standard Medicare benefits for treatment of a terminal illness. However, the beneficiary may continue to access standard Medicare benefits for treatment of conditions unrelated to the terminal illness. Medicare law states that to qualify for hospice care, a patient must have "a medical prognosis that life expectancy is six months or less if the illness runs its normal course." However, it is difficult to predict how much time is left to a patient with cancer, and beneficiaries are not restricted to six months of coverage by hospice rules.

See also HOSPICE EDUCATION INSTITUTE; HOSPICE FOUNDATION OF AMERICA; NATIONAL HOSPICE AND PALLIATIVE CARE ORGANIZATION.

Hospice Education Institute An independent nonprofit organization founded in 1985 that serves a wide range of individuals and organizations interested in improving and expanding HOSPICE and palliative care throughout the United States and around the world. The institute works to inform, educate, and support people seeking or providing care for the dying and the bereaved, or those coping with loss or advanced illness.

The institute offers a range of services including HOSPICELINK, which maintains a directory of hospice programs; a program offering small gifts to patients and their families; seminars; books; and pamphlets. For contact information, see Appendix I.

Hospice Foundation of America A nonprofit organization that promotes HOSPICE care and educates professionals and those they serve about caregiving, terminal illness, loss, and bereavement. The foundation provides leadership in the development and application of hospice and its philosophy of care. Hospice Foundation, Inc., was chartered in 1982 as a way to help raise money for hospices operating in South Florida, prior to passage of the Medicare hospice benefit. In 1990 the foundation expanded its scope in order to provide leadership on a national level in the entire spectrum of end-of-life issues.

To more accurately reflect its national scope, in 1992 the foundation opened a Washington, D.C., office and in 1994 changed its name to Hospice Foundation of America. For contact information, see Appendix I.

Hospicelink A service offered by the HOSPICE EDUCATION INSTITUTE that maintains a computerized directory of all hospice and palliative care programs in the United States. The toll-free telephone number (800-331-1620) provides referrals to hospice and palliative care programs and provides general information about the principles and practices of good hospice and palliative care. For contact information, see Appendix I.

human chorionic gonadotropin (HCG) In adults, significant elevation of levels of this hormone occurs only during pregnancy and in patients with trophoblastic tumors or nonseminomatous germ cell tumors. This allows doctors to use it as a tumor marker. One hundred percent of patients with trophoblastic tumors and 40 to 60 percent of patients with nonseminomatous germ cell tumors (including all patients with CHORIOCARCINOMA, 80 percent of patients with EMBRYONAL CARCINOMA, and 10 to 25 percent of patients with pure seminoma) have high levels of HCG. Elevated concentrations should return to normal within five to seven days after surgery if all tumor is removed. The HCG level can also rise due to abnormally low levels of testosterone or because of marijuana use.

See also TESTICULAR CANCER.

human epidermal growth factor receptor 2 See HER-2/NEU.

human papillomavirus (HPV) A virus that causes the common wart on hands and feet, as well as warts in the genital area. Infection by human papillomavirus (HPV) is believed by many researchers to be one of the most important avoidable risk factors for CERVICAL CANCER. Women infected by the HPV have a significantly higher risk for developing low and high-grade cervical lesions than women who are not infected.

Types of HPV

HPVs are a group of more than 100 types of viruses called "papillomaviruses" because they can cause warts (papillomas). Different HPV types cause different types of warts in different parts of the body, and HPV infections cause symptoms in some but not all patients. Some types cause common warts on the hands and feet, on lips or tongue; certain other types of HPV types can infect the genitals and the anal area. More than 30 types of HPV are transmitted through sexual contact, and approximately half of these have been linked to cancer. For years recognized as the major cause of cancer of the cervix (the opening to the uterus), HPV has also been associated with cancers of the vulva, vagina, anus, penis, and middle throat (including the base of the tongue and the tonsils).

Low-risk infections   Most genital warts are caused by two sexually transmitted HPV types, HPV 6 and HPV 11; these rarely develop into cancer and are called low risk viruses. The warts may appear within weeks of sexual contact with an HPV-infected person or may appear years later, or not at all.

High-risk infections   Other sexually transmitted HPVs have been linked with genital or anal cancers in women. These high risk HPV types (HPV 16, HPV 18, HPV 31, 33, HPV 35, and HPV 45) can cause growths that are usually flat and difficult to see and can lead to the development of cancer. A test for the viral DNA in the affected tissue can reveal the type of HPV that is present.

HPV and Cancer

In women, HPV infection can cause abnormal changes in the outermost layer of cells (the epithelium) covering the cervix. These abnormal cells are called squamous intraepithelial lesions (SILs) (or DYSPLASIA or CERVICAL INTRAEPITHELIAL NEOPLASIA), are not cancerous—they are precursors to cancer. SILs can be detected by a PAP TEST performed during a gynecologic examination.

Many low-grade dysplasias fade away and become normal over a period of months or years. In these patients, the Pap test result may become normal, and the HPV is considered to be latent or possibly eliminated by the patient's immune system. It is believed that a latent infection can be reactivated years after initial exposure to HPV.

In patients who develop cervical cancer, the HPV persists or is reactivated, and the SILs progress over many years, becoming increasingly abnormal and invading deeper and deeper levels of the epithelium. High-grade SILs include abnormal cells that extend through the full thickness of the epithelium, also known as carcinoma in situ—an early form of cervical cancer.

The mechanism by which HPV transforms a cell into a malignancy is probably mediated through two viral genes (E6 and E7) that are actively transcribed in HPV-infected cells. The E6 and E7 proteins bind to and inactivate the host cell's tumor suppressor gene products, leading to uncontrolled growth.

Risk Factors

Risk factors for HPV infection (and thus for cervical cancer) include having sex at an early age (before age 16), multiple sexual partners, sex with a partner who has had multiple partners, and unprotected sex at any age. Infection with a high-risk type of HPV such as HPV-16, increases the risk of developing abnormal cells (SILs) caused by HPV that will develop into cancer. SMOKING, using oral contraceptives, infection with other sexually transmitted diseases or with the HIV virus, or giving birth to many children, may act together with HPV in some way to increase the probability that abnormal cells will lead to cancer.

Symptoms

When HPV infects the skin of the external genital organs and the anal area, the virus often causes raised bumpy warts ranging from barely visible to several inches across.

Diagnosis

A patient whose Pap test result is abnormal is referred for COLPOSCOPY (examination of the cervix and vagina with a magnifying instrument). The doctor takes biopsy specimens from abnormal areas, and the tissue is examined to determine the grade of the abnormality and detect the presence of cancer.

New tests can directly identify the DNA from HPVs, and identify the exact HPV type that is causing an infection. However, it is not clear how treatment would be affected by knowing the exact type of HPV. HPV testing and typing are not presently routinely recommended, and most health care providers do not do this testing.

Treatment

There is currently no cure for human papillomavirus infection, but the warts and abnormal cell growth caused by these viruses can be effectively destroyed, to prevents them from developing into cancer.

A high-grade SIL may be treated with a laser, LOOP ELECTROSURGICAL EXCISION PROCEDURE, CRYOSURGERY, surgical excision (including CONE BIOPSY), or CHEMOTHERAPY. Genital warts may be treated with some of these same procedures.

human T-cell leukemia virus-I (HTLV-I)   This virus causes a rare type of chronic lymphocytic LEUKEMIA known as human T-cell leukemia. However, leukemia does not appear to be contagious.

Hürthle cell neoplasm   See THYROID CANCER.

hybridoma   A human-made cell produced by joining a healthy white blood cell and a malignant white blood cell. A hybridoma can be used to produce limitless amounts of a specific antibody (MONOCLONAL ANTIBODY) designed to find specific proteins on cancer cells. When used with CHEMOTHERAPY drugs, the antibodies can be used to attack cancer cells.

hydatidiform mole   This relatively rare condition is characterized by tissue that forms around a fertilized egg that normally would have developed into the placenta, but instead develops as an abnormal cluster of cells (also called a molar pregnancy). Instead of a normal embryo, this grapelike mass forms inside the uterus after fertilization. A hydatidiform mole triggers a positive pregnancy test and in some cases can become cancerous.

A hydatidiform mole (*hydatid* means "drop of water" and *mole* means "spot") occurs in about one out of every 1,500 pregnancies in the United States, although in some parts of Asia the incidence may be as high as one in 200. Molar pregnancies are most likely to occur in very young pregnant women and pregnant women over age 45. Some women who have had one molar pregnancy will have a second one.

If not removed, about 15 percent of moles can become cancerous, burrowing into the uterine wall and causing serious bleeding. Another 5 percent will develop into fast-growing cancers called

CHORIOCARCINOMAS. Some of these tumors spread very quickly outside the uterus to other parts of the body. Fortunately, cancer developing from these moles is rare and highly curable.

Cause

A molar pregnancy occurs when cells of the chorionic villi (tiny projections that attach the placenta to the lining of the uterus) do not develop correctly. Instead, they turn into watery clusters that cannot support a growing baby.

A partial molar pregnancy includes an abnormal embryo that does not survive. In a complete molar pregnancy there is a small cluster of clear blisters or pouches that do not contain an embryo.

Scientists are not sure what triggers the formation of a hydatidiform mole; some believe it is caused by problems with the chromosomes in either the egg or sperm, or both. It may be associated with poor nutrition, or a problem with the ovaries or the uterus. A mole sometimes can develop from placental tissue that is left behind in the uterus after a miscarriage or childbirth.

Symptoms

Women with a hydatidiform mole will have a positive pregnancy test and often believe they have a normal pregnancy for the first three or four months. However, in these cases the uterus grows abnormally fast, triggering vaginal bleeding by the end of the first trimester. The woman may also have hyperthyroidism (overproduction of thyroid hormones causing symptoms such as weight loss, increased appetite, and intolerance to heat). Sometimes the grapelike cluster of cells itself will be shed with the blood during this time. Other symptoms may include severe nausea and vomiting and high blood pressure. As the pregnancy progresses, the fetus will not move and there will be no fetal heartbeat.

Diagnosis

The physician may not suspect a molar pregnancy until after the third month or later. First, a doctor will rule out a tubal pregnancy, and then check the levels of human chorionic gonadotropin (HCG), a hormone that is normally produced by a placenta or a mole. Abnormally high levels of HCG together with the symptoms of vaginal bleeding, lack of fetal heartbeat, and an unusually large uterus all indicate a molar pregnancy. An ultrasound of the uterus to make sure there is no living fetus will confirm the diagnosis.

Treatment

It is extremely important to make sure that all of the mole is removed from the uterus, since the tissue is potentially cancerous. Often, the tissue is naturally expelled by the fourth month of pregnancy, but in other cases the doctor will give the woman a drug called oxytocin to trigger the release of the mole. If this is ineffective, a vacuum aspiration can be performed to remove the mole.

If the woman is older and does not want any more children, the uterus can be surgically removed because of the higher risk of cancerous moles in this age group. Because of the cancer risk, the physician will continue to monitor the patient for at least two months after the end of a molar pregnancy.

Since invasive disease is usually signaled by high levels of HCG that do not go down after the pregnancy has ended, the woman's HCG levels will be checked every two weeks for two months. If the levels do not return to normal by that time, the mole may have become cancerous. If the HCG level is normal, the woman's HCG will be tested each month for six months, and then every two months for a year.

If the mole was cancerous, treatment includes removal of the cancerous tissue and CHEMOTHERAPY. If the cancer has spread to other parts of the body, radiation will be added. Specific treatment depends on how advanced the cancer is.

Women should make sure not to become pregnant within a year after HCG levels have returned to normal. If a woman were to become pregnant sooner than that, it would be difficult to tell whether the resulting high levels of HCG were caused by the pregnancy or a cancer from the mole.

Prognosis

A woman with a molar pregnancy often goes through the same emotions and sense of loss as does a woman who has a miscarriage. Most of the time, she truly believed she was pregnant and now has suffered a loss of the baby she thought she was carrying. In addition, there is the added worry that the tissue left behind could become cancerous.

In the unlikely case that the mole is cancerous, the cure rate is almost 100 percent. As long as the uterus is not removed, it still is possible to have a child at a later time.

hydrazine sulfate   A chemical that has been studied as an antitumor agent and as a treatment for the CACHEXIA (loss of muscle mass and body weight) associated with advanced cancer.

It has been claimed that hydrazine sulfate limits the ability of tumors to obtain glucose, which is a type of sugar used by cells to create energy. But there is only limited evidence from animal studies that hydrazine sulfate has anticancer activity, and it has shown no antitumor activity in randomized clinical trials.

Hydrazine sulfate also has been shown to increase the incidence of lung, liver, and breast tumors in laboratory animals, suggesting it may cause cancer. Data concerning its effectiveness in treating cancer-related cachexia are inconclusive. Hydrazine sulfate is commercially available in the United States, but its use outside of clinical trials has not been approved by the Food and Drug Administration.

5-hydroxyindoleacetic acid (5HIAA)   A breakdown product of serotonin that is excreted in the urine. Serotonin is a hormone and neurotransmitter found in many body tissues; both serotonin and 5HIAA are produced in excess amounts by CARCINOID tumors. As a result, measuring the levels of these substances in urine is a way to test for carcinoid tumors.

hyperalimentation   The intravenous administration of a highly nutritious solution for patients who have problems eating. Nutritional support is an important part of the care of many cancer patients, who may, for many reasons, have trouble eating. Others may have problems absorbing nutrients. Hyperalimentation can be performed either through tubes (enteral feeding) or intravenously (total parenteral nutrition).

hypercalcemia   An abnormally high level of calcium in the blood. Between 10 and 20 percent of all cancer patients have hypercalcemia, which is the most common life-threatening metabolic disorder associated with the disease.

According to the NATIONAL CANCER INSTITUTE, it is seen most often in patients with tumors of the lung (25 percent to 35 percent of them have it) and breast (20 percent to 40 percent), but it also occurs in cancers of the head and neck, kidney, and certain cancers of the blood, particularly malignant MYELOMA.

Cancer causes hypercalcemia in two circumstances: when a tumor destroys bony tissue as it invades the bone or when cancer cells secrete substances that increase calcium levels (humoral hypercalcemia of malignancy). Because immobility causes an increase in the loss of calcium from bone, cancer patients who are weak and spend most of their time in bed are more prone to hypercalcemia. In addition, cancer patients may be dehydrated because they often do not eat and drink enough, and because they often suffer from nausea and vomiting. Dehydration reduces the ability of the kidneys to remove excess calcium from the body, contributing to hypercalcemia. Hormones and diuretics that increase the amount of fluid released by the body can also trigger hypercalcemia.

Symptoms

Many patients with mild hypercalcemia have no symptoms; instead, their condition is discovered during routine lab tests. If symptoms do appear, they may include appetite loss, nausea, vomiting, constipation, abdominal pain, and a bowel blockage. If the kidneys are involved, the individual will have to urinate frequently during both the day and night and will be very thirsty.

As calcium levels rise, the symptoms become more serious. Stones may form in the kidneys and waste products can build up. Blood pressure rises, the heart rhythm changes, and muscles get weaker. The patient may experience mood swings, confusion, psychosis, and, eventually, coma and death.

Treatment

The treatment of hypercalcemia depends on how high the calcium level is, but rapid reduction is important because the condition can be life threatening. If the patient has normal kidney function, fluids can be given intravenously to clear the excess

calcium. If the kidneys are not working well, acute hemodialysis is the safest and most effective method to reduce dangerous calcium levels.

Loop diuretics such as furosemide can be given after the patient begins drinking. These drugs inhibit calcium reabsorption in the kidneys and boost urine production.

For cancer patients, drugs that inhibit long-term bone loss, such as calcitonin, biphosphates, and plicamycin, can help control excess calcium levels. Anti-inflammatory agents such as steroids are helpful with some cancers.

hyperkeratosis Thickening of the outer layer of the skin caused by too much keratin (a protein component of the outer skin layer). The most common types of hyperkeratosis are corns and calluses caused by pressure or friction. Hyperkeratosis is often seen in scaly conditions such as warts or eczema; at some point, the skin thickenings may become malignant.

hyperplasia An increase in the production and growth of normal cells in skin tissue. It can result in a thickened outer layer of the skin. While not in itself a cancerous condition, it may become cancerous in some cases.

hyperthermic perfusion A procedure in which a warmed solution containing anticancer drugs is used to bathe, or is passed through the blood vessels of, the tissue or organ containing the tumor.

hypopharyngeal cancer A disease in which cancer cells are found in the tissues of the hypopharynx, the bottom part of the throat (also called the pharynx). The pharynx is a hollow tube about five inches long that starts behind the nose and becomes part of the esophagus, the tube that goes to the stomach. Air and food pass through the pharynx on the way to the windpipe or the esophagus. Hypopharyngeal cancer usually starts in the squamous cells that line the throat.

Symptoms

Symptoms include persistent sore throat, trouble swallowing, a lump in the neck, a change in voice, or ear pain.

Diagnosis

To diagnose symptoms of hypopharyngeal cancer, a doctor will feel the throat and examine the tissues by inserting a thin lighted tube, called an endoscope, down the throat. If abnormal tissue is discovered, the doctor will do a biopsy of the tissue to see if there are any cancer cells.

Staging

Stage I: The cancer is in only one part of the hypopharynx and has not spread to lymph nodes in the area.

Stage II: The tumor is either between 2 and 4 centimeters and has not spread to the larynx *or* is found in more than one area of the hypopharynx or in nearby tissues.

Stage III: One of the following is found.

- The tumor is in only one area of the hypopharynx and is 2 centimeters or smaller; cancer also has spread to a single lymph node on the same side of the neck and the lymph node is 3 centimeters or smaller; or

- Cancer is in more than one area of the hypopharynx, is in nearby tissues, or is larger than 2 centimeters but not larger than 4 centimeters and is not in the larynx; cancer has also spread to a single lymph node on the same side of the neck and the lymph node is 3 centimeters or smaller; or

- The tumor is larger than 4 centimeters or has spread to the larynx; cancer may have spread to a single lymph node on the same side of the neck and the lymph node is 3 centimeters or smaller.

Stage IV: Stage IV is divided into stages IVA, IVB, and IVC.

- In stage IVA, the tumor can be any size and has spread to nearby soft tissue, connective tissue, the thyroid, or the esophagus; cancer may be found either in one lymph node on the same side of the neck (the lymph node is 3 centimeters or smaller) or in one or more lymph nodes anywhere in the neck (all of these lymph nodes are 6 centimeters or smaller); or it is in only one area of the hypopharynx, is 2 centimeters or smaller, and has also spread to one or more lymph nodes anywhere in the neck (all of these lymph nodes are 6 centimeters or smaller); or it is in more than one area of the hypopharynx, is in nearby tissue, or is larger than 2 centimeters but not larger than 4 centimeters and has not spread to the larynx; cancer has spread to one or more lymph nodes anywhere in the neck (all of these lymph nodes are 6 centimeters or smaller); or it is larger than 4 centimeters or has spread to the larynx; or cancer has also spread to one or more lymph nodes anywhere in the neck (all of these lymph nodes are 6 centimeters or smaller).

- In stage IVB, the tumor either has spread to nearby soft tissue, connective tissue, blood vessels, the thyroid, or the esophagus and may have spread to lymph nodes of any size; or it is of any size and has spread to lymph nodes that are larger than 6 centimeters.

- In stage IVC, cancer has spread beyond the hypopharynx to other parts of the body.

Recurrent: This means that the cancer has returned after it has been treated, either in the hypopharynx or in another part of the body.

Treatment

Treatment of cancer of the hypopharynx depends on its location, stage, the patient's age and overall health and may involve surgery and/or radiation. CHEMOTHERAPY is being tested in clinical trials.

Surgery In this common treatment method, a doctor may remove the larynx and part of the throat in an operation called a laryngopharyngectomy. If the cancer has spread to the lymph nodes, they also may be removed.

Radiation therapy Radiation may be used to kill cancer cells and shrink tumors. Giving drugs with the RADIATION THERAPY to make the cancer cells more sensitive to radiation (radiosensitization) is being tested in clinical trials. If smoking is stopped before radiation therapy is started, a patient has a better chance of surviving longer.

Because radiation to the thyroid or the pituitary gland may change the way the thyroid gland works, the doctor may test the thyroid gland before and after therapy to make sure it is working properly.

Prognosis

The chance of recovery depends on where the cancer is in the throat, the stage, and the patient's general state of health.

See also THROAT CANCER.

hysterectomy A surgical procedure involving the removal of the uterus, usually including the cervix but not necessarily the ovaries and fallopian tubes. One in four women in the United States has a hysterectomy by the age of 60. It is a lifesaving operation when performed to stop the growth of cancers of the uterus, ovaries, or cervix. Each year U.S. doctors perform about 500,000 hysterectomies.

This procedure, first performed in 1872, became popular in the 1890s and was by 1975 the second most commonly performed operation in America. There are several basic types of hysterectomy:

- *Total (simple) hysterectomy*—the uterus and cervix are removed, but the ovaries and fallopian tubes are left intact.

- *Total hysterectomy with bilateral salpingo-oophorectomy*—removal of uterus and cervix, plus both ovaries and fallopian tubes. (There are also variations on these two operations, such as removing only one ovary or part of one ovary; in some cases, the fallopian tubes may be left intact.)

- *Radical hysterectomy*—usually performed for cancerous conditions, this procedure involves the removal of the uterus, ovaries, fallopian tubes, the upper portion of the vagina, and the pelvic lymph nodes. However, even in this extensive procedure, the ovaries may be preserved if they are definitely not involved in the illness.

- *Subtotal hysterectomy*—only the body of the uterus is removed, leaving the cervix in place. In most cases, the fallopian tubes and the ovaries are preserved as well. Subtotal hysterectomy was performed commonly through the 1950s, but physicians became worried about cervical cancer and began to recommend total hysterectomy. However, total hysterectomy usually involves shortening the vagina, which can make sex painful, and some women rely on cervical stimulation for orgasm. If a woman chooses subtotal hysterectomy, she will still need yearly Pap smears to check for cervical abnormalities.

Vaginal Hysterectomy

In laparoscopically assisted vaginal hysterectomy, a few small abdominal incisions allow the surgeon to insert a laparoscope and specially designed instruments to detach and remove the uterus through the vagina. These operations are very popular with patients because of their reduced recovery time and minimal scarring, but they have been shown to have a higher complication rate than traditional vaginal or abdominal techniques.

Controversy

In the past, medical experts often thought of the uterus as something a woman did not need once she was past childbearing years, and it was sometimes removed during fibroid surgery to eliminate the chance of UTERINE CANCER. Today, however, many doctors suspect the uterus may play a role in regulating hormones and do not advise removing it unless it is completely necessary.

For many women, the biggest problem with a hysterectomy is the loss of fertility. Some experience a loss of sexual desire, although this problem appears treatable with hormone therapy. Some studies suggest that up to 40 percent of women experience a decrease in sexual response after the operation, which may be related to a testosterone deficiency that can develop if the ovaries are removed. (Most hysterectomies spare the ovaries, however, thus sparing ovarian hormonal function.) This problem can be treated with hormones, including the use of natural testosterone creams applied vaginally. Since contractions of the uterus can contribute to orgasm, some women report that they have more difficulty reaching a satisfying orgasm.

hysterography An examination of the uterus using an X-ray and contrast dye, which is inserted into the vagina and uterus. A hysterography may help in the diagnosis of ENDOMETRIAL CANCER.

hystero-oophorectomy Surgical removal of the uterus and the ovaries in the treatment of OVARIAN CANCER, ENDOMETRIAL CANCER, and FALLOPIAN-TUBE CANCER.

See also HYSTERECTOMY.

hysteroscopy   An examination in which a doctor checks the uterus and fallopian tubes for cancer and other abnormalities by placing a thin pen-sized device through the cervical canal to inspect the inside of the uterus. The procedure can be used both to diagnose and treat problems. Modern hysteroscopes are so thin that they can fit through the cervix with minimal or no dilation.

This procedure usually takes place in an operating room under general anesthesia. It can also be done in a doctor's office with or without sedation. Local anesthesia minimizes discomfort, and afterward most women are able to get up and return to their normal activities immediately.

Because the inside of the uterus is not naturally inflated, it must be artificially distended to allow better visualization. By inserting gas or liquid through the hysteroscope, a doctor can separate the uterine walls and check for malignancies, fibroids, polyps, scarring, or abnormal shape. Hysteroscopy is usually performed during the first half of the menstrual cycle in order to avoid interrupting a possible pregnancy.

For diagnostic purposes the scope is used to view the inside of the uterus, but it is also possible to remove polyps, cut adhesions, and remove tissue to check for cancer cells. In many situations, operative hysteroscopy may offer an alternative to hysterectomy.

I Can Cope program   A patient education program supported by the AMERICAN CANCER SOCIETY that is designed to help patients, families, and friends cope with the day-to-day issues of living with cancer. For contact information, see Appendix I.

Id1   A recently discovered cancer-causing gene that controls the switch for tumor blood vessel growth, known as ANGIOGENESIS. Id1 helps fuel tumor growth by providing a needed blood source to tumor cells. The Id1 gene is associated with MELANOMA and cancers of the breast, head and neck, brain, cervix, prostate, pancreas, and testicles.

ileostomy   An opening into the ileum (part of the small intestine) from the outside of the body. An ileostomy provides a new path for waste material to leave the body after part of the intestine has been removed.

See also COLORECTAL CANCER.

immune system   A complex network of cells and organs that work together to defend the body against attacks by germs. The immune system functions by distinguishing between healthy cells and cancer cells and trying to kill the latter. If the immune system is not working properly, cancer may develop. Biological therapies are designed to repair, stimulate, or enhance the immune system's responses so that they will better be able to fight cancer.

Cells in the immune system secrete two types of proteins: antibodies and CYTOKINES. *Antibodies* respond to antigens (invaders) by recognizing and latching on to them. Specific antibodies match specific antigens. *Cytokines* are substances produced by some immune system cells to communicate with other cells. Types of cytokines include lymphokines, INTERFERONS, INTERLEUKINS, and COLONY-STIMULATING FACTORS. Cytotoxic cytokines attack cancer cells directly.

Immune system cells include

- B cell lymphocytes, which mature into plasma cells that secrete antibodies (immunoglobulins). Each type of B cell makes one specific antibody, which recognizes one specific antigen.
- T cell lymphocytes, which directly attack infected, foreign, or cancerous cells. They also regulate the immune response by signaling other immune system defenders through production of lymphokines.
- Natural killer cells, which produce powerful chemical substances that bind to and kill any foreign invader. They attack without first having to recognize a specific antigen.

immunosuppression   Suppression of the body's IMMUNE SYSTEM and its ability to fight infections or disease. Immunosuppression may be deliberately induced with drugs, as in preparation for bone marrow transplants to prevent rejection of the donor tissue. It may be caused by certain diseases such as LYMPHOMA, or as a result of treatment with CHEMOTHERAPY drugs.

immunotherapy   A technique in treating cancer that uses the body's own IMMUNE SYSTEM to help fight disease. Although cancer cells are foreign and abnormal, they can elude the body's immune system defenses by hiding within a normal cell. Immunotherapy tries to get the body to reject the cancer cell in the same way it would try to reject a transplanted organ. (Some experts believe that the immune system actually does often kill cancer cells throughout a person's lifetime, before they form into a tumor, but that during times of lowered immunity the malignant cells win out.)

Immunotherapy drugs are designed to activate a patient's white blood cells so that they attack the malignant cells. Approved immunotherapy drugs include alpha interferons 2-A (Roferon-A) and 2-B (Intron-A), bacillus Calmette-Guérin (Theracys), denileukin diftitox (Ontak), interleukin-2 (Proleukin), levamisole (Ergamisol), rituximab (Rituxan), trastuzumab (Herceptin), and yttrium-90 radiolabeled carcinoembryonic-antigen antibody.

implant radiation   See BRACHYTHERAPY.

indolent non-Hodgkin's lymphoma   See NON-HODGKIN'S LYMPHOMA.

indoles   A group of plant chemicals that bind to cancer-causing chemicals, activating enzymes that destroy the chemicals and prevent damage to cells. Indoles fall within a much larger group called organosulfur compounds, which are found in CRUCIFEROUS VEGETABLES such as broccoli, bok choy, cabbage, kale, Brussels sprouts, and turnips.

induction therapy   Treatment designed to be used as a first step toward shrinking a tumor and to evaluate response to other drugs. Induction therapy is followed by additional treatment to eliminate any remaining cancer.

infants and cancer   Cancer during the first year of life represents 10 percent of all cancer diagnosed in children under age 15. Every year there are an average of 233 cases of infant cancer per million infants, which is 12 percent higher than the rate for infants the age with the next-highest incidence (age 2). Babies of both sexes are diagnosed with cancer at about the same rate, making this the only age group of children under 15 in which boys are not diagnosed at a higher rate than girls.

A type of BRAIN CANCER called neuroblastoma is the most common type of cancer in infants (28 percent of all cases); the next most common type is LEUKEMIA (17 percent of all cases). About 13 per-

cent of all infant cancers are central nervous system malignancies; about 6 percent of cases are malignant germ cell, and another 6 percent are malignant soft tissue tumors.

The prognosis for infants diagnosed with cancer is often worse than it is for older children. For example, the five-year relative survival rate for children under age 15 with acute lymphoid leukemia is well over 70 percent, but for infants with the same disease, the survival rate is just 33 percent. On the other hand, infants with neuroblastoma appear to survive longer than do older children; more than 80 percent of infants with neuroblastoma survive for at least five years, whereas only about 45 percent of older children with this cancer survive for at least five years.

See also CHILDHOOD CANCERS.

infection   Cancer patients undergoing CHEMOTHERAPY are at greater risk for developing life-threatening infections because the drugs affect the BONE MARROW, inhibiting production of infection-fighting white blood cells. The blood cells are usually at their lowest level from seven to 14 days after the chemotherapy treatment, although this will vary depending on the type of chemotherapy.

As the number of white cells in the blood falls, patients will be more likely to get an infection. For this reason, oncologists order regular blood tests to show the number of white cells in the blood. Patients whose immune system has not recovered quickly enough may need to wait until the white cell count has improved to have their next chemotherapy treatment.

Treatment

If patients get an infection when their white blood cell level is very low, they may need antibiotics given directly into the bloodstream. Sometimes drugs called growth factors can help the bone marrow make more white blood cells. Growth factors are sometimes given after chemotherapy treatment to stimulate the bone marrow to produce new white cells quickly, thereby reducing the risk of infection.

Prevention

Chemotherapy patients can prevent a great many infections by being very careful not to injure themselves and not to eat potentially tainted food. Patients should wash their hands often during the day, especially before meals, and after using the toilet or touching animals. The rectal area should be cleaned gently but thoroughly after each bowel movement.

Patients should avoid crowds during those periods when their white counts are lowest, and they should stay away from people with contagious diseases such as colds, the flu, measles, or chicken pox. Patients should also avoid contact with children who have recently received live-virus vaccines such as chicken pox or oral polio, since they may be contagious to people with a low blood cell count.

Patients should be careful to avoid breaking the skin when using scissors, knives, or razors and should not squeeze or scratch pimples or insect bites. Cuts and scrapes that do occur should be cleaned daily until healed with warm water, soap, and an antiseptic. Good oral hygiene and daily baths can help prevent infections, and lotion or oil can soften and heal skin that has become dry and cracked. Protective gloves should be worn when gardening or cleaning up after others.

Patients should avoid contact with animal litter boxes and waste, birdcages, and fish tanks, and avoid standing water in birdbaths, flower vases, or humidifiers. They should not get any immunizations, such as flu or pneumonia shots, before checking with a doctor, and they should avoid raw fish, seafood, meat, or eggs.

Symptoms of Infection

Patients on chemotherapy should call a doctor right away if they have any of the following symptoms:

- fever over 100°F
- chills (especially shaking chills)
- sweating
- loose bowel movements
- frequent urgency to urinate or a burning feeling during urination
- severe cough or sore throat
- unusual vaginal discharge or itching
- redness, swelling, or tenderness, especially around a wound, sore, ostomy, pimple, catheter site, or the rectal area

- sinus pain or pressure
- earaches, headaches, or stiff neck
- blisters on the lips or skin
- mouth sores

infertility and cancer   Cancer survivors typically have more problems with fertility than do people who have never had cancer; birthrates among cancer survivors are only 40 percent to 85 percent of the expected rates. Moreover, certain cancers (especially TESTICULAR CANCER) can severely impair sperm production. However, while some cancer treatments (drugs and radiation) can cause sterility or reduced fertility in men and women, preliminary evidence suggests that cancer therapy in general does not affect the ability to reproduce and to produce healthy children as severely as had been previously thought. At the same time, new methods are being devised to reduce the effects of cancer treatments on fertility and on pregnancies already in progress when a cancer is discovered.

In one recent study, researchers found that while higher rates of miscarriage and lower birth weights were observed among the offspring of former patients, there are still a large number of live births, births of healthy children, a lack of congenital abnormalities, and very low cancer rates in offspring.

The closer radiation treatments are to a person's reproductive organs, the higher the risk for infertility. While it may take as long as five years after RADIATION THERAPY, sperm production in men may eventually recover. Alkylating agents or other drugs that can harm reproductive function tend to affect fertility more severely in men than in women. However, new combinations of cancer drugs are helping to improve fertility rates.

Today, as millions of men and women of childbearing age and younger survive cancer, the question of reproduction is arising as a paramount consideration in planning treatment. Among the issues are the ability to preserve fertility while curing the disease and the safety of pregnancy for both mothers with cancer and their future children. In a continuing study of more than 20,000 survivors of childhood cancers, the two greatest concerns mentioned by former patients two and three decades later were whether they could still have children and, if so, whether those offspring would be healthy.

Less than a generation ago, reproductive-aged women with cancer did not have much chance of a hopeful outcome, but today many cancers are no longer a death sentence. More and more women with cancer are now concerned about maintaining fertility.

Experts say that even women whose BREAST CANCERS are discovered during pregnancy no longer should be advised to terminate the pregnancy, because there are no data indicating that an abortion would benefit her outcome. The estrogen produced in pregnant women is weaker than that produced in nonpregnant women and is less likely to stimulate breast cancer growth, even if the woman's tumor is estrogen sensitive.

Today even cancers directly involving the ovaries, uterus, or cervix can sometimes be treated in ways that allow future pregnancies and healthy births. Many modern chemotherapy drugs are less damaging to ovarian function than older medications and do not induce permanent early menopause, so that a woman's fertility may return months or even years after treatment ends. Fears that potent cancer-fighting drugs will damage the DNA of a woman's eggs or a man's sperm, causing birth defects, have not been borne out by experience.

In fact, current medical literature on children born of parents previously treated for cancer, including HODGKIN'S DISEASE, LEUKEMIA, MELANOMA, and BREAST CANCER, shows no unusual numbers of birth defects or medical diseases among them compared to the general population. There is also no report of damage to the children's chromosomes.

Although there are cancers that run in families, and susceptibility to these cancers could be transmitted to patients' children, cancer treatment itself is not now considered a factor influencing genetic risk.

infiltrating ductal carcinoma   See BREAST CANCER.

infiltrating lobular carcinoma   See BREAST CANCER.

inflammatory breast cancer   See BREAST CANCER.

inflammatory carcinoma of the breast   See BREAST CANCER.

informed consent   A process in which a patient learns key facts about a clinical trial, including potential risks and benefits, before deciding whether or not to participate. Informed consent continues throughout the trial.

infusion therapy   The delivery of highly concentrated CHEMOTHERAPY drugs directly to a cancer site by an internal or external pump. Because this method administers the drug over a number of days instead of minutes, side effects can be reduced.

An external pump is carried about by the patient; an internal pump is implanted during surgery and can be refilled as needed by injection with additional doses.

Infusion therapy is used for cancers of the colon, brain, and head and neck.

in situ cancer   Early cancer that has not spread to neighboring tissue.

Institutional Review Board (IRB)   A group of scientists, doctors, clergy, and consumers at each health-care facility that oversees clinical trials to protect study participants. The board reviews and approves the action plan for every clinical trial, checking to see that the trial is well designed, does not involve undue risks, and includes safeguards for patients.

insurance coverage   The cost of treating cancer can be high, but health insurance plans will usually cover much of the cost. Cancer patients who do not have insurance should contact their local Social Security office to determine if they qualify for Supplemental Security Income (SSI) or SOCIAL SECURITY DISABILITY INSURANCE (SSDI). The medical requirements and disability determination process are the same under both programs. However, while eligibility for SSDI is based on employment history, SSI is based on financial need.

Cancer patients without insurance can also receive care from hospitals that get federal grants from Hill-Burton Funds. These grants allow hospitals and nursing homes to provide low-cost or no-cost medical care. To receive a listing of hospitals or nursing homes participating in the Hill-Burton program, patients can call (800) 638-0742.

See also FINANCIAL ISSUES.

interferon A substance that occurs naturally in the body and that boosts the body's natural response to infection and disease (BIOLOGICAL RESPONSE MODIFIER, or BRM). As their name implies, interferons *interfere* with the division of cancer cells; as a result, they can slow tumor growth.

Interferons boost the immune system's anticancer function by stimulating natural killer cells, T cells, and macrophages. In addition, interferons may act directly on cancer cells by slowing their growth or promoting their development into cells with more normal behavior.

Although interferons are normally produced by the body, they can also be produced in the laboratory for use in treating cancer and other diseases. There are several types of interferons, including interferon-alpha, -beta, and -gamma. Interferon-alpha is the type most widely used in cancer treatment.

The U.S. Food and Drug Administration has approved the use of interferon-alpha for the treatment of certain types of cancer, including hairy cell LEUKEMIA, MELANOMA, chronic myeloid leukemia, and AIDS-related KAPOSI'S SARCOMA. Studies have shown that interferon-alpha may also be effective in treating other cancers such as metastatic KIDNEY CANCER and NON-HODGKIN'S LYMPHOMA. In clinical trials researchers are exploring the use of combinations of interferon-alpha and other BRMs or chemotherapy to treat a number of cancers.

interleukins A group of natural hormonelike substances produced by white blood cells in the body and also made in the laboratory. Interleukins are a type of CYTOKINE that act as messengers, carrying signals between blood-producing cells of the immune system that help stimulate the immune system to fight cancer. They are considered to be a type of BIOLOGICAL RESPONSE MODIFIER, a substance that can improve the body's response to infection and disease. Although many interleukins have been identified, interleukin-2 (IL-2) has been the most widely studied in cancer treatment.

Researchers continue to study the benefits of interleukins to treat a number of cancers, including colorectal, ovarian, lung, brain, breast, prostate, some LEUKEMIAS, and some LYMPHOMAS.

Interleukin-1-Alpha

IL-1a is a protein that stimulates the growth and action of disease-fighting immune system cells. IL-1a triggers a number of processes related to inflammation, activates T cells, and stimulates bone marrow growth.

Interleukin-2

IL-2 enhances the ability of the immune system to kill tumor cells and may interfere with blood flow to the tumor. IL-2 is normally produced by activated T cells in the body and plays a central role in regulating the immune system. It stimulates the growth and activity of many types of cells, including several that kill cancer cells. Aldesleukin is IL-2 that is made in the laboratory for use in treating cancer and other diseases.

Treatment with IL-2 is most effective with KIDNEY CANCER and advanced MELANOMA. Although there are a number of side effects associated with IL-2, they usually fade away when treatment is completed.

Interleukin-3

IL-3 enhances the immune system's ability to fight tumor cells and stimulates the growth of many precursor bone marrow cells.

Interleukin-4

IL-4 enhances cell growth and antibody production and stimulates the production of other immune system cells.

Interleukin-5

Also known as eosinophil colony-stimulating factor, IL-5 stimulates the growth of bacteria-killing blood cells known as eosinophils.

Interleukin-6

IL-6 stimulates B cell growth.

Interleukin-11

IL-11 stimulates immune response and may reduce toxicity to the gastrointestinal system resulting from cancer treatment. It also stimulates the production of platelets.

Interleukin-12

IL-12 enhances the ability of the immune system to kill tumor cells and may interfere with blood flow to the tumor.

International Association of Laryngectomees (IAL)   A nonprofit program that assists people who have lost their voice as a result of cancer. It provides information on the skills needed by laryngectomees, works toward total rehabilitation of patients, helps form new clubs, fosters improvement in laryngectomee programs, and works to improve the minimum standards for teachers of post-LARYNGECTOMY speech.

The association is composed of about 250 member clubs and recognized regional organizations, generally known as "lost chord" or "new voice" clubs. The IAL was formed in 1952 by representatives of 13 individual clubs to help coordinate club activities. For contact information, see Appendix I.

International Myeloma Foundation   A nonprofit organization designed to provide patients and their families with information and support. The foundation conducts patient seminars, scientific workshops, and clinical conferences. It also funds a broad range of research projects around the world. For contact information, see Appendix I.

International Union Against Cancer (Union Internationale Contre le Cancer, or UICC)   The only global cancer association with member groups and activities covering all aspects of cancer control. Founded in 1933, UICC is an independent, international, nongovernmental association of 291 cancer-fighting organizations from 87 countries.

The association promotes volunteerism and collaboration against cancer and promotes a comprehensive approach to tobacco control around the world. It also promotes prevention and early diagnosis and advocates sharing research skills and information. For contact information, see Appendix I.

intraductal carcinoma   See BREAST CANCER.

intraocular melanoma   See EYE CANCER.

intraperitoneal chemotherapy   See CHEMOTHERAPY.

iridium seeds   Small bits of the element iridium that are implanted at the cancer site to irradiate malignant tumors from within.

See also BRACHYTHERAPY.

islet cell tumor   An uncommon group of tumors that begin in the distinct type of cell found in the pancreas (the islet cells). With the exception of gastrinomas (found in the pancreas), the majority of these tumors develop within the upper small intestine. Although the islet cells normally produce hormones and insulin, some of these tumors also secrete hormones in excessive amounts, causing specific symptoms.

Normal islet cells are small, isolated masses of cells that make up the Islet of Langerhans in the pancreas. When functioning normally, they secrete the protein hormones insulin and glucagon.

Tumors composed of irregular islet cells may occur alone or in a group of many tumors, ranging from 0.5 to 2 cm in diameter; most (about 90 percent) are benign. Normally, islet cells produce a wide variety of hormones that regulate a variety of bodily functions, such as blood sugar level and the production of stomach acid.

Types of Tumors

Pancreatic islet cell tumors can be benign or malignant, and they may appear in one of two forms: nonfunctioning or functioning tumors. Nonfunctioning tumors do not produce hormones; they may obstruct the shortest part of the small intestine (duodenum) or the biliary tract, which connects the liver to the duodenum and includes the gall bladder. These nonfunctioning tumors may erode and bleed into the stomach or the intestines, or they may form an abdominal mass.

Functioning tumors secrete excessive amounts of hormones, which may lead to various syndromes including low blood sugar (hypoglycemia), multiple bleeding ulcers (Zollinger-Ellison Syndrome), pancreatic cholera (Verner-Morrison Syndrome), CARCINOID syndrome or diabetes.

Insulinomas: These tumors produce insulin and cause low blood sugar.
Gastrinomas: These tumors produce gastrin, which induces gastric acid secretion.
Vipomas: These tumors produce vasoactive intestinal peptide (VIP), which causes severe diarrhea.
Glucagonomas: These tumors produce glucagons, but the symptoms of rash, tongue inflammation, constipation, blood clots, and high blood sugar are not all caused by glucagons. The causes of these symptoms are not known.
Somatostatinomas: These tumors are associated with high levels of blood sugar, gallstones, and diarrhea.

Diagnosis

The type of diagnostic test that is ordered may depend on the patient's symptoms. Some of these tests include a variety of blood tests (including glucose tolerance tests), abdominal CT scan, catheterization of the pancreas to show high hormone level in the veins (this involves putting a wire into a blood vessel and taking blood out for measurements), abdominal MAGNETIC RESONANCE IMAGING (MRI), secretin stimulation test and calcium infusion test.

Treatment

Malignant islet cell tumors tend to spread to other organs, grow aggressively, and may not be treatable. Treatment for islet cell tumors includes surgery and CHEMOTHERAPY.

Patients may be cured if tumors are surgically removed before they have spread to other organs; if malignant cells have spread to the liver, a portion of the liver also may be removed.

If the cancer is widespread, chemotherapy may be used to shrink the tumors, but these medications cannot usually cure the patient. If abnormal hormone production is causing problems, medications may be given to counteract their effects. (For example, GASTRINOMA-induced overproduction of gastrin triggers oversecretion of stomach acid; medications that block acid secretion can ease symptoms).

isoflavones Plant compounds found in SOY PRODUCTS that may help prevent cancer. Isoflavones are very similar to the human ESTROGEN hormone in chemical shape and properties but are much weaker than the human form.

Scientists do not agree how isoflavones in soy can reduce the risk of BREAST CANCER, because the biological action of isoflavones is still not fully understood. Studies show that at certain levels in the body, isoflavones may mimic human estrogen—but they also may block estrogen in the body. Moreover, isoflavones work differently in different parts of the human body. The effect of isoflavones also depends on other factors, such as how many estrogen receptors there are, and the level of human estrogen in the body.

Isoflavones are believed to work differently in premenopausal women than they do in postmenopausal women. Research suggests that eating soy products may decrease the risk of breast cancer in premenopausal women. Dietary isoflavones can affect menstrual cycle length, which is one of the risk factors for breast cancer. Some experts believe that Asian women have a lower risk for breast cancer because they have longer menstrual cycles and lower estrogen concentrations in their bodies.

One recent study did confirm that a DIET rich in plant estrogens might protect against breast cancer; the study showed that the lower the risk of breast cancer, the higher the level of PHYTOESTROGENS in the urine.

Animal studies also suggest that isoflavones are natural anticancer agents that are involved in regulating cell growth as well as cell death.

On the other hand, there is little proof that soy intake decreases the risk of breast cancer in postmenopausal women.

Soy Products

Not all soy foods contain isoflavones. Soy foods that are made from soy protein concentrate may have little or no isoflavones. Currently, experts recommend that people should consume 30 to 50 mg of isoflavones each day to reduce risk of cancer. Below is a list of soy products and their isoflavone content:

- Soy milk: 30 mg isoflavones in 8 ounces
- Soy Nuts: 60 mg isoflavones in $1/4$ cup

- Tempeh: 35 mg isoflavones in $1/4$ cup
- Tofu: 35 mg isoflavones in $1/2$ cup

These amounts are estimates; consumers should read labels to learn the exact amount of isoflavones in a product.

Contraindications

Consumers should also understand that soy foods and isoflavone extracts (pills or tablets) are not the same. While there is little danger of overdosing on soy foods, experts do not know the safe maximum dosage for isoflavone supplements, or whether an overdose is dangerous.

Women who have been diagnosed with estrogen-receptor-positive breast cancer should be cautious about eating too much soy, because plant estrogens in soybeans may act like estrogen in the body and encourage growth of this cancer.

Women taking tamoxifen should talk to their physician regarding soy intake, because tamoxifen works by attaching to estrogen receptor sites. To get the most benefit from tamoxifen, experts recommend women restrict their intake of weak plant estrogens. Women who are not taking tamoxifen or who do not have a history of estrogen-positive breast cancer may find that weak plant estrogens protect against breast cancer.

Japanese populations and cancer   See ASIAN/PACIFIC ISLANDERS AND CANCER.

juvenile myelomonocytic leukemia   See LEUKEMIA.

Kaposi's sarcoma (KS) A malignant condition characterized by skin tumors that is the most common cancerous manifestation of AIDS (acquired immunodeficiency syndrome). Kaposi's sarcoma was named for Dr. Moritz Kaposi who first described the condition in 1872. For decades Kaposi's sarcoma was considered to be a rare disease that primarily affected men of Mediterranean or Jewish descent, organ transplant patients, or young-adult African men. In the last 20 years, however, most Kaposi's cases have developed as a result of infection with the human immunodeficiency virus (HIV), the virus that causes AIDS, especially among homosexual men. In fact, about 95 percent of Kaposi's sarcoma cases in the United States are found in homosexual and bisexual men. In patients with AIDS, Kaposi's sarcoma is highly aggressive and causes widespread tumors.

Cause

The cause of this disorder is unknown, although there is some evidence that it may be the result of a sexually transmitted infectious agent other than HIV.

Symptoms

Kaposi's sarcoma typically causes tumors below the skin, or in the mucous membranes of the mouth, nose, or anus. The tumors appear as raised blotches that may be purple, brown, or red. Sometimes the disease causes painful swelling, especially in the legs, groin, or skin around the eyes.

Although the skin lesions may be disfiguring, they usually are not life threatening or disabling. Usually the lesions cause no symptoms, although some patients experience painful lesions. If the disease also involves the lungs, liver, gastrointestinal tract, or LYMPH NODES, other symptoms may develop. Tumors in the gastrointestinal tract, for example, can cause bleeding, whereas tumors in the lungs may cause breathing problems.

There are several types of Kaposi's sarcoma. These differ in which symptoms they cause, which organs they affect, how aggressively the cancer grows and spreads, the risk factors and other personal characteristics of patients, the treatment most effective against them, and the likelihood of survival.

Classic Kaposi's Sarcoma

The classic form of Kaposi's sarcoma usually develops in Italian men or Jewish men of Eastern European origin between ages 50 and 70. Classic KS is quite rare, even in these ethnic and age groups. Patients typically have one or more lesions on the legs, ankles, or the soles of the feet. The lesions slowly enlarge, and new lesions may develop over the course of 10 to 15 years. Pressure from the lesions can block lymph vessels, causing swelling that may be painful. Lesions can also develop in the gastrointestinal tract, lymph nodes, and elsewhere in the body, although they rarely cause symptoms.

African (Endemic) Kaposi's Sarcoma

African (or endemic) Kaposi's sarcoma is a common form of the disease that develops in people living in equatorial Africa and accounts for 9 percent of all the cancers seen among Ugandan men. In many cases this disease is identical to classic KS, although it usually appears in much younger men. Typically, African KS causes skin lesions that do not produce symptoms and do not spread to other parts of the body. However, more aggressive cases do occur, and some tumors may spread from the skin to the underlying bone.

Another form of the disease strikes children before puberty. It affects three times as many boys as girls and usually involves the lymph nodes and other organs. In most cases it is fatal within three years.

Transplant-Related (Acquired) Kaposi's Sarcoma

Transplant-related (or acquired) Kaposi's sarcoma refers to the form of the disease developed by patients whose IMMUNE SYSTEMS have been suppressed after an organ transplant. Typically, transplant patients take medication to prevent their immune system from recognizing a newly transplanted organ as foreign to the body. Because these drugs weaken the body's defenses, other diseases or infections can overwhelm the patient. Kaposi's sarcoma is 150 to 200 times more likely to develop in transplant patients than among the general population. While transplant-related KS often affects only the skin, in some cases the disease can spread to the mucous membranes or other organs.

AIDS-Related (Epidemic) Kaposi's Sarcoma

AIDS-related (or epidemic) Kaposi's sarcoma appears in people who are infected with HIV, which destroys the immune system, making the body unable to fight infections. Certain diseases occur so often in people with AIDS that they are considered "AIDS-defining conditions"—that is, their presence in a person infected with HIV is a clear sign that full-blown AIDS has developed.

The Centers for Disease Control and Prevention has identified certain cancers as AIDS-defining diseases, including Kaposi's sarcoma, LYMPHOMA (especially NON-HODGKIN'S LYMPHOMA and primary central nervous system lymphoma), ANAL CANCER, and invasive CERVICAL CANCER. Many other kinds of cancer may be more likely to develop in people with HIV infection. About four out of 10 patients with AIDS will develop cancer at some time during their illness.

In most cases, epidemic KS causes widespread lesions that erupt at many places on the body soon after AIDS develops. The purple lesions of epidemic KS may appear on the skin and the mouth. In time they may thicken into plaques or nodules and may affect the lymph nodes and other organs, usually the gastrointestinal tract and lung (where they may cause severe internal bleeding), liver, and spleen.

When they are diagnosed, some people with epidemic KS have no symptoms besides lesions, especially if their only lesions develop on the skin. Eventually, in almost all cases, epidemic KS spreads throughout the body. Extensive lung involvement by KS can be fatal. More often, however, patients die of other AIDS-related complications such as infections. KS causes or contributes to death in perhaps 30 percent of AIDS cases.

Risk Factors

The two major causes of KS are

- *Human herpesvirus 8.* This virus (also called Kaposi's sarcoma–associated herpes virus) is transmitted in the United States by sexual contact. The major risk factor is sexual activity with multiple partners among male homosexuals. It is also transmitted by transplantation of an organ that carries the virus. The virus is probably not transmitted by blood transfusion. In Africa, where this virus is very common, it is probably also passed from mothers to their babies.
- *Immune deficiency.* Usually caused by HIV infection, it can also be seen in patients who are receiving immune-suppressive therapy because of an organ transplant

Treatment

Treatment should include an antiretroviral agent such as zidovudine, which will not affect the tumors but will diminish the degree to which the immune system is suppressed. Antiretroviral agents may also boost the effectiveness of other drugs that do affect Kaposi's. Localized lesions respond well to RADIATION THERAPY, CRYOTHERAPY, surgical removal, or injection with vinblastine, bleomycin, or interferon-alfa. Oral administration of interferon-alpha is effective in about half of patients with mild Kaposi's. In more severe cases, intravenous chemotherapy is often required.

New research is also investigating the use of the drug THALIDOMIDE as a treatment for the lesions of Kaposi's. Thalidomide, used in the 1950s and 1960s as a sedative in pregnant women, led to birth defects in newborns of mothers who took the drug. The most common birth defects were shortened arms and legs, which could have been caused by thalidomide's effect on blood vessels. Scientists subsequently showed that thalidomide was an inhibitor of ANGIOGENESIS, the process by which new blood vessels help supply a tumor with nutrients to grow and spread.

Of the 20 patients enrolled in a study on thalidomide treatment for Kaposi's, eight showed a 50 percent decrease in the number of nodular lesions seen on their skin, according to scientists at the National Cancer Institute. Two patients had no change in their lesions, and seven patients got worse.

Thalidomide has also been shown, in early clinical trials, to be active against MULTIPLE MYELOMA, a bone marrow disease.

Prognosis

The outcome in adult patients with AIDS and Kaposi's sarcoma depends on the activity of the HIV disease and the degree to which the person's immune system is compromised.

Karnofsky Performance Status (KPS) A standard way of measuring the ability of cancer patients to perform ordinary tasks. The scores range from 0 to 100, with a higher score indicating a better ability to carry out daily activities. KPS may be used to determine a patient's prognosis, to measure changes in functioning, or to decide if a patient could be included in a clinical trial.

keratosis See ACTINIC KERATOSIS.

kidney cancer Cancer of the kidneys affects more than 28,000 Americans each year. The kidneys are two reddish brown bean-shaped organs located just above the waist whose main function is to filter blood and produce urine to rid the body of waste. Most kidney cancers occur in only one kidney, although 2 percent to 4 percent of patients have tumors in both kidneys.

Types of Kidney Cancer

Several types of cancer can develop in the kidney, but the most common type among adults is *renal cell cancer*. About 85 percent of all kidney cancers are renal cell carcinomas. *Transitional cell cancer (carcinoma)* is a less common type of kidney cancer

that affects the renal pelvis and is similar to cancer that occurs in the bladder.

WILMS' TUMOR is the most common type of kidney cancer in children, but it is different from adult kidney cancer. As kidney cancer grows, it may invade organs near the kidney, such as the liver, colon, or pancreas. Other types of childhood kidney cancers include clear cell SARCOMA, rhabdoid tumor, and neuroepithelial tumor.

Clear cell sarcoma of the kidney is a primary kidney tumor. It can spread to the lung, bone, brain, and soft tissue. A child with clear cell sarcoma of the kidney may be treated with surgery to remove the kidney. This may be followed by RADIATION THERAPY to the abdomen and lung (if cancer has spread to the lung), which may be followed by CHEMOTHERAPY. Rhabdoid tumor of the kidney is a type of cancer that grows and spreads quickly. At diagnosis, children are usually younger than 12 months of age and may have fever, blood in the urine, and advanced cancer. This tumor type tends to spread to the lungs and the brain. Rhabdoid tumor is usually treated with surgery to remove the kidney followed by chemotherapy. Neuroepithelial tumors of the kidney spread quickly, so that by the time they are diagnosed they often have spread to the outer layer of the kidney, the veins of the kidney, and to other parts of the body.

Cause

About 85 percent of kidney cancers are sporadic (nonfamilial) clear cell carcinoma. About 23,500 new cases are diagnosed each year. With identification of the gene that causes this cancer, scientists are hoping to develop new methods to improve the diagnosis and treatment of the disease and to make it possible to develop a blood or urine test that can detect kidney cancer early, when it is most treatable.

The damaged gene responsible for sporadic clear cell carcinoma of the kidney is a tumor suppressor gene located on the short arm of chromosome 3. Normally, the protein produced by the gene restrains cell growth, but when the gene is damaged it becomes inactivated. The gene appears to cause kidney cancer when a patient inherits two damaged copies of the gene.

The gene responsible for sporadic clear cell carcinoma is the same gene that causes the inherited cancer syndrome VON HIPPEL-LINDAU'S DISEASE, which leads to multiple tumors, including cancers of the kidney, eye, brain, spinal cord, and adrenal gland.

Risk Factors

The risk of kidney cancer increases with age and occurs most often between the ages of 50 and 70, affecting almost twice as many men as women. It is more common among urban populations and in certain areas around the world, such as the United States and Scandinavia, and it is also somewhat more common among African-American men than Caucasian men. Other risk factors include

- SMOKING. Smokers are twice as likely to develop kidney cancer as nonsmokers, and the longer a person smokes, the higher the risk. However, the risk of kidney cancer decreases for those who quit smoking.
- OBESITY. Being overweight may increase the risk of developing kidney cancer, especially in women, although scientists do not know why.
- occupation. Coke oven workers in steel plants have above-average rates of kidney cancer, and there is some evidence that asbestos in the workplace increases the risk of some kidney cancers.
- radiation. Women who have been treated with radiation therapy for uterine problems may have a slightly higher risk of kidney cancer, as do patients exposed to thorotrast (thorium dioxide), a radioactive substance used in the 1920s with certain diagnostic X-rays.
- phenacetin. Heavy, long-term use of this painkiller has been linked to kidney cancer, but it is no longer sold in the United States.
- dialysis. Patients on long-term kidney dialysis have a higher risk of developing kidney cancer.
- von Hippel-Lindau's disease. People who have this inherited disorder are at higher risk of developing kidney cancer. Isolating the gene for this disease may lead to better ways to diagnose, treat, and even prevent some kidney cancers.

Symptoms

Kidney cancer usually causes no obvious symptoms until the tumor grows, which then triggers intermittent bloody urine, or a lump in the kidney area. Other, less common, symptoms may include fatigue, loss of appetite and weight, recurrent fevers, pain in the side that does not go away, and a general feeling of poor health. Less often, there may be high blood pressure or anemia. Only the doctor can tell the difference between a kidney infection and kidney cancer. Usually, early cancer does not cause pain.

Diagnosis

Many kidney tumors are found accidentally on X-rays or ultrasounds performed for other reasons; a third of all patients show evidence that the tumor has spread by the time the cancer is diagnosed.

In addition to a general checkup, the doctor may perform blood and urine tests, assess the abdomen for lumps, and order scans of the kidneys and nearby organs, such as:

- intravenous pyelogram. This is a series of X-rays of the kidneys, ureters, and bladder illuminated with dye.
- arteriography. A series of X-rays of the blood vessels made more visible with dye injected into a large blood vessel through a catheter. X-rays show the dye as it moves through the network of smaller blood vessels in and around the kidney.
- CT, MRI, and PET scans
- ultrasounds. Tests that can show the difference between diseased and healthy tissues.

If test results suggest kidney cancer, a BIOPSY may be the only definite way to diagnose cancer. In a biopsy, the doctor inserts a thin needle into the tumor to withdraw a sample of tissue, which is examined under a microscope to check for cancer cells and properly stage the extent of the disease.

Staging

Staging is a way to find out the extent of cancer and whether it has spread. In kidney cancer, staging is based on the size of the tumor within the kidney, whether it has spread to the nearby blood vessels or lymph nodes, or beyond. To stage kidney cancer, the doctor may use more scans and studies of the tissues and blood vessels. Tumor cells are studied under the microscope to determine the cell type, because certain cell types are more aggressive than others. Knowing the cell type helps determine treatment. Cell types include: clear cell, granular cell, papillary, and sarcomatoid. Clear cell is the most common type of renal cell carcinoma. Sarcomatoid is the most aggressive, growing and spreading quickly; it has a poor prognosis.

Stage I: The tumor is confined within the kidney and is 7 cm (2 $^3/_4$ inches) or smaller. It has not extended to the nearby blood vessels and has not spread to lymph nodes or distant sites.

Stage II: The tumor is confined within the kidney but is bigger than 7 cm (2 $^3/_4$ inches). It has not extended to the nearby blood vessels and has not spread to lymph nodes or distant sites.

Stage III: Any tumor that has spread into the nearby blood vessels or adrenal gland, or spread to a single lymph node in the region of the original tumor. It has not spread to distant sites.

Stage IV: Any tumor that has spread out of the capsule that surrounds the kidney, upper ureter, and adrenal gland, or has spread to more than one regional lymph node, or to distant sites.

Treatment

Treatment for kidney cancer depends on the stage of the disease and the patient's general health, but it usually includes surgery, radiation therapy, BIO-LOGICAL THERAPY, chemotherapy, HORMONAL THERAPY, or ARTERIAL EMBOLIZATION. The outlook for people with early stage kidney cancer is good because kidney cancer is often cured if it is found and treated before it has spread.

Unlike other cancers, renal cell carcinomas occasionally shrink partially or completely without treatment; this occurs in less than 1 percent of cases. This trait is thought to be due to the activity of the immune system of the patient as it tries to fight the tumor. This observation led to speculation that the immune system is capable of causing complete elimination of renal cell carcinoma, although this has not been shown to be effective treatment. Also, the regression is generally short and the tumor grows back.

Surgery The removal of the kidney, nephrectomy, is the most common treatment for cancer there. Kidney cancer tends to grow out of the kidney and into the nearby blood vessels, making sur-

gical removal extremely difficult. It often spreads early and does not have to grow extremely large before it can spread to distant sites. Most often, the surgeon removes the whole kidney along with the adrenal gland and the tissue around it, together with some lymph nodes (radical nephrectomy). Removal of only the kidney itself is called a simple nephrectomy; removal of just the part of the kidney containing the tumor is called a partial nephrectomy. (It is difficult to remove the entire tumor without removing the entire affected kidney, although this may be attempted in specific situations.) After the operation, a pathologist examines the border of normal tissue (the "surgical margin") around the tumor to see if there are any tumor cells at the margin, which would increase the risk of recurrent disease at a later date.

If the tumor has spread, the goal of surgery is usually to relieve symptoms and not cure the disease, although recent studies have shown that surgical removal of the affected kidney in patients with metastatic renal cell carcinoma, followed by biological therapy, may prolong survival.

Arterial embolization is sometimes used before an operation to make surgery easier, or to ease pain or bleeding if the tumor is inoperable. In this procedure, small pieces of a special material are injected through a catheter to clog the main renal blood vessel, shrinking the tumor by depriving it of blood and other substances it needs to grow.

Radiation therapy Radiation has not been very effective as the primary treatment for renal cell carcinoma, though it has been used to ease symptoms for patients with end-stage kidney cancer. It is sometimes used after surgery if there are cancer cells in the margin in order to destroy any remaining malignant cells that may be left behind. However, radiation therapy is controversial because there has been no proven benefit for the use of local radiation in this case. Radiation therapy for kidney cancer is given on an outpatient basis five days a week for several weeks.

Biological therapy Interleukin-2 (IL-2) and interferon are used to treat advanced kidney cancer by strengthening the patient's immune system. The response rates have varied, but some patients have achieved complete remissions following treatment with IL-2. Vaccine therapy is experimental and is available only at a limited number of research institutions.

Immunotherapy has been used in clinical trials as adjuvant therapy for patients whose cancer has not spread after surgery, but it has not proven beneficial in these patients.

Chemotherapy Although useful in the treatment of many other cancers, chemotherapy drugs have not been very effective against kidney cancer. Many types of chemotherapy medications have been used for renal cell carcinoma in various combinations in the past, but kidney cancer is highly resistant to chemotherapy. Two specific chemotherapy drugs that exhibit minimal activity against kidney tumors are vinblastine and floxuridine. They are most often used to ease symptoms in patients with stage IV renal cell carcinoma. Chemotherapy has also been combined with immunotherapy drugs such as interferon. Researchers continue to study new drugs and new drug combinations that may be more useful.

Hormonal therapy A small number of patients with advanced kidney cancer may be treated with hormones to try to control the growth of cancer cells. More often, hormones are used only to ease pain.

Recurrence

After surgery, 20 percent to 30 percent of patients will relapse within the first three years. The most common site of distant spread is to the lungs, although sometimes the cancer spreads to the opposite kidney.

Kidney Cancer Association (KCA) A nonprofit membership organization made up of patients, family members, physicians, researchers, and other health professionals interested in KIDNEY CANCER. The KCA, which was founded in 1990 by a small group of patients and doctors in Chicago, acts as an advocate on behalf of patients with the federal government, insurance companies, and employers. The KCA has provided information to Congress and other institutions about patient needs and health-care policies. For contact information, see Appendix I.

Klinefelter's syndrome A sex chromosome disorder that leads to low levels of male hormones, sterility, breast enlargement, and small testes. Men who have Klinefelter's syndrome have an extra X chromosome (XXY), which causes the symptoms, and are at greater risk of developing TESTICULAR CANCER.

Krukenberg tumor A tumor in the ovary caused by the spread of STOMACH CANCER.

lacrimal gland tumor   A usually benign growth in the tear gland located in the upper outer part of the eye socket. Less than 10 percent of tumors in the lacrimal gland are cancerous. (See also EYE CANCER.)

lacrimation   A side effect of some types of CHEMOTHERAPY (such as 5-fluorouracil) in which excess tears are produced by the tear ducts.

lactate dehydrogenase (LDH)   An enzyme normally found in the blood that is produced by many tissues. At higher-than-normal levels, it is considered to be a nonspecific tumor marker, indicating possible malignancies such as TESTICULAR CANCER, NON-HODGKIN'S LYMPHOMA, Ewing's sarcoma, some types of LEUKEMIA, and other cancers. High LDH levels also may indicate the recurrence of cancer after treatment. However, it is also possible for cancer to recur without an increase in LDH. Nonmalignant causes of an elevated LDH are common and include trauma and several nonmalignant blood disorders (such as hemolytic ANEMIA).

laetrile   A purified form of the chemical amygdalin, a substance found in the pits of many fruits and in numerous plants, which some people have used as a cancer treatment. However, laetrile has exhibited little anticancer activity in animal studies and no anticancer activity in human clinical trials, and it is not approved for use in the United States.

Used as a poison in ancient Egypt, laetrile was first used as a cancer treatment in Russia in 1845. In the United States its use began in the 1920s, when some people thought that the cyanide contained in laetrile might fight cancer. In the 1970s laetrile gained popularity as an anticancer agent, and by 1978 more than 70,000 individuals in the United States were reported to have been treated with it.

The term "laetrile" is an acronym (from "laevorotary" and "mandelonitrile") used to describe amygdalin, a plant compound that contains sugar and produces cyanide. Laetrile has been used for cancer treatment both as a single agent and in combination with a metabolic therapy program that consists of a specialized diet, high-dose vitamin supplements, and pancreatic enzymes.

In the United States researchers must file an Investigational New Drug (IND) application with the U.S. Food and Drug Administration (FDA) to conduct clinical drug research using human subjects. In 1970 an application for an IND to study laetrile was filed by the McNaughton Foundation in San Ysidro, California. Although the request was approved at first, it was later rejected because animal research suggested that laetrile was probably not effective, and because there were questions about how the proposed study was to be conducted. Laetrile supporters viewed this reversal as an attempt by the U.S. government to block access to new and promising cancer therapies, and so they increased pressure to legalize the drug. Court cases in Oklahoma, Massachusetts, New Jersey, and California challenged the FDA's role in determining which drugs should be available to cancer patients. Consequently, laetrile was legalized in more than 20 states during the 1970s. In 1980 the U.S. Supreme Court overturned decisions by the lower courts, reaffirming the FDA's position that drugs must be proven to be both safe and effective before they could be sold. As a result, the use of laetrile as a cancer therapy is not approved in the United States, although in Mexico it continues to be manufactured and administered as an anticancer treatment.

Although the names laetrile, Laetrile, and amygdalin are often used interchangeably, they are not the same product. The chemical composition of U.S.-patented Laetrile (mandelonitrile-beta-glucuronide), a semisynthetic derivative of amygdalin, is different from the laetrile/amygdalin produced in Mexico (mandelonitrile beta-D-gentiobioside), which is made from crushed apricot pits. Mandelonitrile, which contains cyanide, is a structural component of both products.

Laetrile can be taken as a pill or by injection. It is commonly given intravenously at first, followed by dosages in pill form. The incidence of cyanide poisoning is much higher when laetrile is taken by mouth because intestinal bacteria and some commonly eaten plants contain enzymes that activate the release of cyanide after laetrile has been ingested.

Side Effects

The side effects associated with laetrile treatment are much the same as the symptoms of cyanide poisoning, including nausea and vomiting, headache, dizziness, bluish skin discoloration, liver damage, low blood pressure, droopy upper eyelid, difficulty walking due to damaged nerves, fever, mental confusion, coma, and death. These side effects are increased if the patient takes laetrile and then immediately eats raw almonds or crushed fruit pits, high doses of vitamin C, or fruits and vegetables that contain beta-glucosidase (such as celery, peaches, bean sprouts, and carrots).

laparoscopy A type of surgical procedure in which a viewing tube with camera is inserted through a small incision to allow a doctor to examine internal organs on a video monitor. Other small incisions can be made nearby so that instruments can be inserted to perform procedures. Laparoscopy plays a role in the diagnosis, staging, and treatment of a variety of cancers. It is less invasive than regular open abdominal surgery (LAPAROTOMY) and usually involves less pain, less risk, less scarring, and faster recovery. Because laparoscopy is so much less invasive than traditional abdominal surgery, patients can leave the hospital sooner.

Since the late 1980s, laparoscopy has been a popular diagnostic and treatment tool. It was first used with cancer patients in 1973, to observe and biopsy the liver.

However, the future use of laparoscopy to remove completely cancerous growths and surrounding tissues is uncertain, since scientists are not sure if it is as effective as open surgery in complex situations.

Diagnosis

As a diagnostic procedure, laparoscopy is useful in taking biopsies of abdominal or pelvic growths, as well as lymph nodes. It allows the doctor to examine the abdominal area, including reproductive organs, appendix, gallbladder, stomach, and the liver.

Cancer Staging

Laparoscopy can be used to determine the extent of the spread of certain cancers, including:

Liver cancer Laparoscopy is an important tool for isolating LIVER CANCER or for determining if cancer elsewhere in the body has spread to this organ. Laparoscopy can identify up to 90 percent of malignant lesions that have spread to the liver from a cancer located elsewhere in the body. While computerized tomography (CT) can find cancerous lesions that are 0.4 cm in size, laparoscopy is capable of locating lesions that are as small as 0.04 cm.

Pancreatic cancer Laparoscopy has been used to evaluate pancreatic cancer for years.

Esophageal and stomach cancers Laparoscopy has been found to be more effective than MAGNETIC RESONANCE IMAGING (MRI) or CT scans in diagnosing the spread of cancer from these organs.

Hodgkin's disease Some patients with HODGKIN'S DISEASE have surgical procedures to evaluate lymph nodes for cancer; laparoscopy is sometimes chosen instead of laparotomy for these procedures. In addition, when the spleen is removed in patients with Hodgkin's disease, laparoscopy is the standard surgical technique used.

Prostate cancer Patients with PROSTATE CANCER may have the nearby LYMPH NODES examined via laparoscopy.

Cancer Treatment

Laparoscopy is sometimes used as part of a palliative cancer treatment to lessen uncomfortable symptoms. For example, cancer patients may need a feeding tube providing nutrition directly to the stomach if they are unable to eat normally; inserting the tube via laparoscopy saves the patient the ordeal of open surgery.

Procedure

Laparoscopy is a surgical procedure that is performed in the hospital. For diagnosis and biopsy, local anesthesia may be used, but during larger operations general anesthesia is required. For abdominal surgery, gas is pumped into the abdomen, using a hollow needle, to allow a surgeon a better view of the internal organs. The laparoscope is then inserted through the incision made by the needle. The image from the camera attached to the end of the laparoscope is seen on a video monitor. Sometimes, additional small incisions are made to insert other instruments that are used to lift the tubes and ovaries for examination or to perform surgical procedures.

There may be some slight pain or throbbing at the incision sites in the first day or so after the procedure, and the gas used to expand the abdomen may cause discomfort under the ribs or in the shoulder for a few days. Depending on the reason for the laparoscopy in gynecological procedures, some women may experience some vaginal bleeding. Many patients can return to work within a week of surgery, and most are back to work within two weeks.

Laparoscopy is a relatively safe procedure, especially if the physician is experienced; the risk of complication is approximately 1 percent.

laparotomy A surgical procedure in which the abdomen is opened. A laparotomy may be performed to diagnose or treat HODGKIN'S DISEASE, OVARIAN CANCER, PANCREATIC CANCER, and other gastrointestinal cancers.

See also LAPAROSCOPY.

laryngeal cancer Cancer of the larynx, which each year affects more than 12,000 people in the United States. The larynx (or voice box) is used to breathe, talk, or swallow, and is located at the top of the windpipe (the piece of cartilage that forms the front of the larynx is sometimes called the Adam's apple). The vocal cords form a *V* inside the larynx.

Cancer can develop in any region of the larynx, including the glottis (where the vocal cords are found), the supraglottis (the area above the cords), or the subglottis (the area that connects the larynx to the trachea). Almost all cancers of the larynx are squamous cell carcinomas that begin in the flat cells lining the epiglottis, vocal cords, and other parts of the larynx. If the cancer spreads outside the larynx (which it often does), it usually travels first to the lymph nodes in the neck, to the back of the tongue, to other parts of the throat and neck, or to the lungs. Sometimes it moves to other parts of the body.

Cancer of the larynx occurs most often in people over the age of 55. In the United States it is four times more common in men than in women and is more common among black Americans than among whites.

Cause

SMOKING and drinking ALCOHOL are two known risks for developing laryngeal cancer. Smokers are far more likely than nonsmokers to develop this disease, and the risk is even higher for smokers who drink alcohol heavily. People who stop smoking can greatly reduce their risk for cancer of the larynx (as well as cancer of the lung, mouth, pancreas, bladder, and esophagus). Even those smokers who already have cancer of the larynx can lower the risk of getting a second cancer of the larynx or a new cancer in another area by giving up smoking.

In addition to poor lifestyle choices, working with asbestos also can increase the risk of getting cancer of the larynx. Asbestos workers should follow work and safety rules to avoid inhaling asbestos fibers.

Symptoms

The symptoms of cancer of the larynx depend on the size and location of the tumor. Most cancers of the larynx begin on the vocal cords as painless growths that usually cause hoarseness or other voice changes. Tumors in the area above the vocal cords may cause a lump on the neck, a sore throat, or an earache. The rare tumors that begin in the area below the vocal cords can make it hard to breathe. A cough that does not go away or the feeling of a lump in the throat may also be warning signs of cancer of the larynx. As the tumor grows, it may cause pain, weight loss, bad breath, swallowing problems, and frequent choking on food.

Diagnosis

A complete physical exam will reveal general health and any lumps, swelling, tenderness, or other changes in the neck. If symptoms suggest a problem in the larynx, the doctor will look inside the larynx either by direct or indirect laryngoscopy.

In indirect laryngoscopy, the doctor looks down the throat with a small, long-handled mirror to check for abnormal areas and to see whether the vocal cords move as they should. This test is painless and can be performed in a doctor's office, although a local anesthetic may be sprayed in the throat to prevent gagging.

In direct laryngoscopy, the doctor inserts a device designed to allow viewing of the larynx (a laryngoscope) through the patient's nose or mouth to help the doctor visualize areas that cannot be seen with a simple mirror. A local anesthetic eases discomfort and prevents gagging. Patients may also be given a mild sedative to help them relax. Sometimes the doctor uses a general anesthetic to put the person to sleep. This exam may be done in a doctor's office, an outpatient clinic, or a hospital.

If any abnormal areas exist in the throat, a biopsy of the tissue is required to discover if there are malignant cells. For a biopsy, the patient is given a local or general anesthetic before tissue samples are removed through the laryngoscope.

Staging

If the tumor is malignant, it is important to know the stage of the disease so as to plan the best treatment. A tumor is staged by checking X-rays or scans. There are several different staging methods, but one of the most common uses to the letters *T*, *N*, and *M*. The letter *T* stands for tumor; the number following it describes the size and extent of the original tumor. For a tumor beginning in the vocal cords, the staging is as follows:

- T1 tumor: One site in the larynx
- T2 tumor: Two sites in the larynx
- T3 tumor: Tumor has caused one of the vocal cords to stop moving
- T4 tumor: Extends beyond the larynx

The letter *N* stands for node; it is followed by a number indicating whether any tumor has spread to the lymph nodes of the neck. There are four levels here as well, though they start at zero:

- N0: No evidence of any spread to the neck
- N1: One suspicious lymph node that is less than 3 cm in diameter
- N2: Suspicious nodes on both sides of the neck, or more than one suspicious node on one side, or a large node on one side, up to 6 cm
- N3: Suspicious node larger than 6 cm in diameter

The letter *M* stands for metastasis, spread of the cancer to other parts of the body. M0 indicates that the tumor has not spread, M1 indicates the tumor has spread.

The T, N, and M levels are combined as follows to produce the actual staging classification:

Stage I: T1, N0, and M0
Stage II: T2, N0, and M0
Stage III: T3, N0, and M0; also T1, T2, or T3, and N1, M0
Stage IV: T4, N0, or N1, M0; any T with N2 or N3 and M0; or M1 with any T or N level

The presence of any metastatic disease, or a tumor that invades adjacent structures, results in stage IV classification. Stage IV is also defined by a tumor that has spread extensively to the neck lymph nodes (N2 or N3).

Alternative Staging

Another popular staging method is described below:

Stage I: Cancer is very small and has not spread to lymph nodes in the area or to other parts of the body. The exact definition of stage I depends on where the cancer started, as follows:

- *supraglottis*—The cancer is only in one area of the supraglottis, and the vocal cords can move normally.
- *glottis*—The cancer is only in the vocal cords and the vocal cords can move normally.
- *subglottis*—The cancer has not spread outside of the subglottis.

Stage II: The cancer is only in the larynx and has not spread to lymph nodes in the area or to other parts of the body. The exact definition of stage II depends on where the cancer started, as follows:

- *supraglottis*—The cancer is in more than one area of the supraglottis, but the vocal cords can move normally.
- *glottis*—The cancer has spread to the supraglottis or the subglottis, or both. The vocal cords may or may not be able to move normally.
- *subglottis*—The cancer has spread to the vocal cords, which may or may not be able to move normally.

Stage III: Either of the following situations characterize a stage III cancer:

- The cancer has not spread outside of the larynx but the vocal cords cannot move normally, or the cancer has spread to tissues next to the larynx.
- The cancer has spread to one lymph node on the same side of the neck as the cancer, and the lymph node measures no more than 3 cm (just over an inch).

Stage IV: Any of the following may be true:

- The cancer has spread to tissues around the larynx, such as the pharynx or the tissues in the neck, and the lymph nodes may or may not contain cancer.
- The cancer has spread to more than one lymph node on the same side of the neck as the cancer to lymph nodes on one or both sides of the neck or to any lymph node that measures more than 6 cm (more than two inches).
- The cancer has spread to other parts of the body.

Recurrent: Recurrent disease means that the cancer has recurred after it has been treated, either in the larynx or in another part of the body.

Treatment

Treatment for cancer of the larynx depends on the exact location and size of the tumor and whether the cancer has spread, but it usually includes some combination of surgery, radiation, and CHEMOTHERAPY. The treatment choices need to be clearly understood because treatments for this disease may change the way a person looks, breathes, or talks. In many cases the patient meets with both the doctor and a speech pathologist to talk about treatment options and possible changes in voice and appearance.

Surgery   Surgery or surgery combined with radiation is suggested for some newly diagnosed patients. Surgery is also the treatment of choice if a tumor does not respond to radiation therapy or grows back after radiation therapy. When patients need surgery, the type of operation depends mainly on the size and exact location of the tumor. The following types of surgery may be performed for tumors in the larynx:

- *Cordectomy.* This surgery removes only the vocal cord.
- *Supraglottic laryngectomy.* This procedure removes only the supraglottis (the area above the vocal cords).
- *Partial (hemi-) laryngectomy.* This procedure removes only part of the larynx.
- *Total laryngectomy.* In this operation the entire larynx is removed. During this operation, a hole called a tracheostomy is made in the front of the neck to allow the patient to breathe.
- *Lymph node removal.* If cancer has spread to lymph nodes, the lymph nodes will be removed (lymph node dissection).
- *Laser surgery.* Lasers may be used to remove very early or very small cancers of the larynx. In this procedure, a narrow, intense beam of light is used to cut out the cancer.

Radiation   Radiation may be given either internally, by inserting radioisotopes through thin plastic tubes in the area where the cancer cells are found, or externally.

Chemotherapy   A wide variety of chemotherapy drugs may be given to help kill cancer cells that remain after surgery. These may include cisplatin, fluorouracil, hydroxyurea, bleomycin, doxorubicin, carboplatin, or mitomycin.

In the Future

Doctors are studying new types and schedules of RADIATION THERAPY, new drugs, new drug combinations, and new ways of combining various types of treatment. Scientists are trying to increase the effectiveness of radiation therapy by giving treatments twice a day instead of once, and studying drugs called radiosensitizers that make cancer cells more sensitive to radiation.

Because people who have had cancer of the larynx have an increased risk of getting a new cancer in the larynx or in the lungs, mouth, or throat, doctors are looking for ways to prevent these new cancers. Some research has shown that a drug related to vitamin A may protect people from new cancers.

laryngectomy   Surgery to remove part or all of the larynx, usually for the treatment of LARYNGEAL CANCER. Whether the procedure involves a partial or complete laryngectomy depends on the precise location of the tumor.

In this procedure, the surgeon first performs a tracheostomy, creating an opening (stoma) in the front of the neck that may be temporary or permanent. Air enters and leaves the trachea and lungs through this opening, and a tracheostomy tube keeps the new airway open.

A partial laryngectomy preserves the voice because the surgeon removes only part of the voice box (one vocal cord, part of a cord, or just the epiglottis) and the stoma is temporary. After a brief recovery period, the tracheostomy (trach) tube is removed; when the stoma closes within a week or so after surgery, most people can breathe and speak normally, although sometimes the voice may be hoarse or weak.

In a total laryngectomy, the entire voice box is removed, and the stoma is permanent. The patient (called a "laryngectomee") breathes through the stoma, and must learn to speak in a new way. A speech pathologist usually meets with the patient before surgery to explain the methods that can be used. In many cases, speech lessons can begin before the person leaves the hospital.

New Types of Speech

There are several ways a patient can learn to speak after removal of the voice box, such as using air forced into the esophagus to produce a voice (esophageal speech) or by using a mechanical larynx. Some people rely on a mechanical larynx only until they learn esophageal speech, some

decide to use this device instead of esophageal speech, and some use both. Even though esophageal speech may sound low-pitched and gruff, many people prefer this method because it sounds more like regular speech, there is nothing to carry around, and their hands are free.

Esophageal speech   With this method, a speech pathologist teaches the laryngectomee how to force air into the top of the esophagus and then push it out again. This creates a puff of air much like a burp that vibrates the walls of the throat, producing sound for the new voice. The tongue, lips, and teeth form words as the sound passes through the mouth.

For some laryngectomees, air for esophageal speech comes through a tracheoesophageal puncture. The surgeon creates a small opening between the trachea and the esophagus. A plastic or silicone valve is inserted into this opening through the stoma, which keeps food out of the trachea. When the stoma is covered, air from the lungs is forced into the esophagus through the valve. The air produces sound by making the walls of the throat vibrate. Words are formed in the mouth.

It takes practice and patience to learn esophageal speech, and not everyone is successful. How quickly a person learns, how natural the new voice sounds, and how understandable the speech is depend partly on the type and extent of the surgery. Other important factors are the patient's desire to learn and the help that is available.

Mechanical larynx   A mechanical larynx may be used until the person learns esophageal speech or if esophageal speech is too difficult. It may be powered by batteries (electrolarynx) or by air (pneumatic larynx).

One type of electrolarynx looks like a small flashlight and has a disk that produces a humming sound. When the device is held against the neck, the sound travels through the neck to the mouth. (This device may not be suitable for people who have had radiation therapy.) Another type of electrolarynx has a flexible plastic tube that carries sound to the person's mouth from a handheld device.

A pneumatic larynx is held over the stoma and produces vibrations by using air from the lungs. The sound it makes travels to the mouth through a plastic tube.

Prognosis

People who have been treated for cancer of the larynx have a higher-than-average risk of developing a new cancer in the mouth, throat, or other areas of the head and neck. This is especially true for smokers. Most doctors strongly urge their patients to stop smoking to cut down the risk of a new cancer and to reduce other problems, such as coughing.

Rehabilitation

Before leaving the hospital, the patient learns to remove and clean the trach tube or stoma button, suction the trach, and care for the area around the stoma, because the skin is less likely to become irritated if it is kept clean. Most people continue to use a stoma cover after the area heals. Stoma covers (such as scarves, neckties, ascots, and special bibs) help keep moisture in and around the stoma and help filter out dust and smoke. The cover also catches any discharge from the windpipe when the person coughs or sneezes. Whenever the air is too dry, as it may be in heated buildings in the winter, the tissues of the windpipe and lungs may react by producing extra mucus. Also, the skin around the stoma may get crusty and bleed. Using a humidifier at home or in the office can lessen these problems.

Those who have had neck surgery may find that their neck is somewhat smaller, and that it may not be as easy to move the neck, shoulder, and arm as well as before. Physical therapy may help.

After surgery, laryngectomees can do nearly all of the things they did before, but because they cannot hold their breath, straining and heavy lifting may be difficult. Laryngectomees must avoid swimming and water skiing unless they have special instruction and equipment, because it would be very dangerous if water entered the windpipe and lungs through the stoma. Wearing a special plastic stoma shield or holding a washcloth over the stoma keeps water out when showering or shaving.

larynx, cancer of the See LARYNGEAL CANCER.

lasers A treatment method that uses high-intensity light to destroy malignant cells. Lasers can treat cancer by shrinking or destroying a tumor with heat, or by activating a photosensitizing agent that destroys cancer cells. It is a common treatment for certain stages of vocal cord, cervical, skin, lung, vaginal, vulvar, and penile cancers. It is also used to ease the symptoms of cancer, such as bleeding or obstruction, especially when the cancer cannot be cured by other treatments. For example, lasers may be used to shrink or destroy a tumor that is blocking a patient's trachea, making it easier to breathe.

The term *laser* is an acronym for "light amplification by stimulated emission of radiation." While ordinary light occurs in many wavelengths and spreads in all directions, laser light is focused in a narrow high-energy beam. So powerful that it can cut through steel, lasers also can be used for very precise surgical work.

These high-powered light beams have several advantages over standard surgical tools. Because they are more precise than scalpels, the laser can make an incision while avoiding tissue around the wound. And because the heat they produce sterilizes the surgery site, lasers can reduce the risk of infection. The laser is so precise that only a small incision is needed, so the operation is faster and recovery is quicker because there is less bleeding, swelling, or scarring. The light from some lasers can be transmitted through a flexible endoscope fitted with fiber optics. This lets doctors see and work in parts of the body that could not otherwise be reached except by surgery. Lasers also may be used with low-power microscopes, giving the doctor a clear view of the site being treated. Used with other instruments, laser systems can produce a cutting area as small as 200 microns in diameter—less than the width of a very fine thread.

Although there are several different kinds of lasers, only three have gained wide use in medicine: carbon dioxide (CO_2) lasers, argon lasers, and neodymium:yttrium-aluminum-garnet (Nd:YAG) lasers. CO_2 and Nd:YAG lasers are used to shrink or destroy tumors.

Carbon Dioxide (CO_2) Laser

This type of laser can remove thin layers from the skin's surface without penetrating the deeper layers, which is especially useful for treating precancerous conditions and tumors that have not spread deeply into the skin. As an alternative to traditional scalpel surgery, the CO_2 laser is also able to cut the skin and can be used to remove skin cancers.

Argon Laser

Because this laser can pass through only superficial layers of tissue, it is useful in dermatology and in eye surgery. It is also used with photosensitizing dyes to destroy tumors in a procedure known as photodynamic therapy. Some of these dyes have a tendency to collect in cancer cells. When cancer cells treated with them are exposed to red light from a laser, the light is absorbed by the dye, which causes a chemical reaction that destroys the tumor. Photodynamic therapy is mainly used to treat tumors on or just under the skin or on the lining of internal organs. It can be directed through a bronchoscope into the lungs, through an endoscope into the esophagus and gastrointestinal tract, or through a cystoscope into the bladder.

Neodymium:Yttrium-Aluminum-Garnet (Nd:YAG) Laser

Light from this laser can penetrate deeper into tissue than other lasers and can cause blood to clot quickly. It also can be carried through optical fibers to reach less-accessible parts of the body. This type of laser is sometimes used to treat throat and ESOPHAGEAL CANCERS.

Laser-Induced Interstitial Thermotherapy

This new type of laser treatment uses heat to shrink tumors by damaging cancer cells or depriving them of substances they need to live. It is based on the same idea as a cancer treatment called hyperthermia.

latissimus dorsi (LATS) flaps A surgical procedure after a MASTECTOMY in which the latissimus dorsi, a broad, fan-shaped back muscle, and the overlying skin are used to create a breast during BREAST RECONSTRUCTION. The procedure may be used when there is not much skin or muscle at the mastectomy site. A saline implant is usually inserted as well.

LEEP See LOOP ELECTROSURGICAL EXCISION PROCEDURE.

leiomyomas A benign tumor in smooth muscle tissue, which can appear most often in the stomach, esophagus, small intestine, or uterus.

See also FIBROID.

leiomyosarcoma (LMS) A rare type of soft-tissue SARCOMA that begins in smooth muscle cells, most often of the uterus or abdomen. Smooth muscle cells make up the involuntary muscles, which are found in the uterus, stomach and intestines, blood vessel walls, and skin. *Involuntary* means a person cannot make these muscles move by thinking about them.

LMS appears most often in the uterus; it appears less often in the abdomen behind the intestines (retroperitoneal LMS) or in the skin (cutaneous LMS). GASTROINTESTINAL STROMAL TUMORS are a special kind of leiomyosarcoma. They first appear in a particular type of smooth muscle cell in the stomach or small intestine. They rarely arise from benign uterine FIBROIDS (LEIOMYOMAS) or leiomyomas of the stomach or intestine.

Treatment

LMS is a resistant cancer that is not very responsive to chemotherapy. Surgery, CHEMOTHERAPY, and radiation are all typical treatments. The prognosis is best when the cancer is surgically removed with wide margins, while it is small and contained.

Surgery Surgery is the most common treatment for adult soft tissue sarcoma, and if the tumor can be removed completely, it is the treatment of choice. A doctor may remove the cancer and some of the healthy tissue around the cancer, but sometimes all or part of an affected limb may need to be amputated to be sure all of the cancer is gone. If cancer has spread to the lymph nodes, they will be removed as well.

If the cancer cannot be completely removed, other methods might be used as well, depending on how many tumors there are and where they are located.

Radiation In situations where the tumor is inoperable, radiation can be used to shrink the growth so it can be surgically removed. Either internal or external RADIATION THERAPY is used to kill cancer cells and shrink tumors.

Chemotherapy Chemotherapy may be taken by mouth or injected. In soft tissue sarcoma, chemotherapy is sometimes injected directly into the blood vessels in the area where the cancer is found. This treatment is called "regional chemotherapy." Chemotherapy and/or radiation therapy may be used to shrink the cancer so it can be removed without amputating an entire arm or leg. Typical drugs include MAID (Mesna, Adriamyacin, Ifosfamide, DTIC), gemcitabine (Gemzar), or thalidomide. Some centers are studying the experimental drug Vitaxin for the treatment of LMS.

Prognosis

The prognosis for patients with LMS depends on the patient's age and the size, grade, and stage of the tumor. Patients over age 60, or tumors that are high grade or larger than 5 cm, are associated with a poorer prognosis.

leptomeningeal carcinoma Cancer that has spread from another part of the body to the tissue lining the brain and spinal cord. Many cancers can spread to this area, but the most common are LEUKEMIA, LYMPHOMA, BREAST CANCER, and LUNG CANCER. Other solid tumors that may spread to the leptomeninges include MELANOMA, cancers of the genitals and urinary tract, HEAD AND NECK CANCER, or ADENOCARCINOMA.

Signs that the cancer has spread include headache, mental changes, uncoordinated movements, facial distortions, seizures, nausea, and vomiting.

Diagnosis

This type of cancer is diagnosed by a CT scan, MRI, and lumbar puncture (spinal tap).

Treatment

Treatment may include any combination of CHEMOTHERAPY and RADIATION THERAPY. Typically, the chemotherapy drugs (Ara-C, methotrexate) are instilled into the spinal canal or into the cerebral ventricles through a special shunt called an ommaya reservoir.

leukapharesis A method of removing circulating stem cells from whole blood for infusion into patients undergoing high dose CHEMOTHERAPY, and STEM CELL transplant.

The technique is also used to remove the excess of white blood cells in a LEUKEMIA patient, which could otherwise clog small blood vessels. Once the white blood count climbs above 150,000 (which is 30 to 50 times the normal level), arteries can become blocked, leading to a stroke or heart attack.

An emergency leukapharesis can prevent this from happening by removing blood from the patient and filtering out excess white blood cells.

leukemia Cancer of the blood cells and BONE MARROW characterized by the uncontrollable buildup of blood cells. Each year nearly 30,000 adults and more than 2,000 children in the United States are diagnosed with one of many different forms of leukemia. The overall five-year survival rate has tripled in the past 40 years for patients with leukemia. In 1960 the overall five-year survival rate was 14 percent. By the 1970s it had reached 35 percent, and now the overall five-year survival rate is 46 percent.

Although leukemia can attack any of the different components that make up blood (including plasma, white blood cells, red blood cells, and platelets), most types of leukemia affect the white blood cells. White blood cells (leukocytes) help the body fight infections and other diseases. Red blood cells (erythrocytes) carry oxygen from the lungs to the body's tissues and carry carbon dioxide from the tissues back to the lungs; they give blood its color. Platelets (thrombocytes) help form blood clots that control bleeding.

Blood cells are produced in the bone marrow, the soft, spongy center of bones; once they are formed, new cells (called blasts) may remain in the marrow to mature, or they may travel to other parts of the body to mature. Normally, blood cells are produced in an orderly, controlled way, as the body needs them. When leukemia develops, the body produces large numbers of abnormal blood cells. In most types of leukemia, the abnormal cells are white blood cells. These leukemia cells usually look different from normal blood cells, and they do not function properly, crowding out other white blood cells, red blood cells, and platelets.

Leukemia makes up about 5 percent of all cancers in the United States; in 1999 there were 30,800 cases diagnosed, with about 22,100 deaths. Leukemia is the most common childhood cancer in the United States, but this type of cancer is actually far more common in adults. More than half of all leukemias occur in people over age 60, and men are affected about 30 percent more often than women. The disease also occurs slightly more often in whites than blacks.

Types of Leukemia

Leukemias are grouped into four categories, based on how quickly the disease develops and worsens, and by the type of blood cell that is affected.

Leukemia is either *acute* or *chronic.* In acute leukemia, the abnormal blood cells are blasts that remain very immature and cannot carry out their normal functions. The number of blasts rises rapidly, and the disease gets worse quickly as immature, functionless cells build up in the marrow and blood. The marrow often can no longer produce enough normal red blood cells, white blood cells, and platelets. ANEMIA (a lack of red cells) develops in virtually all leukemia patients. The lack of normal white cells impairs the body's ability to fight infections, and a shortage of platelets results in bruising and easy bleeding.

In chronic leukemia, some blast cells are present, but they do not multiply so quickly and they usually can carry out some of their normal functions. As a result, in the beginning patients with chronic leukemia do not have any symptoms. Only gradually their condition gets worse; as the number of abnormal cells increases, symptoms appear.

Leukemia can attack either of two main types of white blood cells—lymphoid cells or myeloid cells. When leukemia affects lymphoid cells, it is called lymphocytic leukemia. When myeloid cells are affected, the disease is called myeloid or myelogenous leukemia. Leukemia is thus divided into four categories: myelogenous or lymphocytic, each of which can be acute or chronic.

Acute lymphocytic leukemia (ALL)   This is the most common type of leukemia in young children, accounting for 45 percent of all leukemia cases in this age group. It is most likely to occur in children under age six. ALL is also common in adults aged 65 and older. During the period from 1992 to 1998, the relative survival rate for this type of leukemia was 63.5 percent (85 percent for children). It is also called acute lymphoblastic leukemia.

Acute myeloid leukemia (AML)   This type of leukemia is the second most common type of leukemia in children; it is more common in adults. It is sometimes called acute nonlymphocytic leukemia (ANLL) or acute myelogenous leukemia. Survival rate for this type is only 19 percent for adults, but 46 percent for children.

Chronic lymphocytic leukemia (CLL)   This most often affects adults over the age of 55, and although it sometimes occurs in younger adults, it almost never affects children. CLL accounts for about 7,000 new cases of leukemia each year, and the survival rates is 73 percent. CLL does not transform into ALL but can transform into an aggressive lymphoma.

Chronic myeloid leukemia (CML)   This occurs mainly in adults, although a very small number of children also develop this disease. CML accounts for about 4,400 new cases of leukemia each year; the survival rate is 34.5 percent. Most patients with CML develop AML.

Risk Factors

Experts do not know what causes leukemia, but several risk factors listed below have been identified.

Gender/race   The disease occurs in men more often than in women and is highest among Caucasians and lowest among Chinese, Japanese, and Koreans. The incidence in men is about 50 percent higher than in women for all racial/ethnic groups except Vietnamese, among whom the male rates are only slightly higher. Death rates are highest in Caucasians and African Americans and in Hawaiian men.

Radiation   The risk of getting leukemia is higher after exposure to large amounts of high-energy radiation, such as the radiation produced by atomic bomb explosions in Japan during World War II. Nuclear power plant accidents that release large amounts of radiation (such as Chernobyl in 1986) also can increase the risk of leukemia. It is suspected that many childhood leukemias may be linked to parental exposure to ionizing radiation before conception or during early fetal development.

Electromagnetic fields   Some research suggests that exposure to electromagnetic fields is a possible risk factor for leukemia, although no conclusive studies have proven this. (Electromagnetic fields are a type of low-energy radiation. They are generated by power lines and electric appliances.)

Genetic conditions   Certain genetic conditions, such as Down syndrome, can increase a child's risk of developing leukemia.

Toxic chemicals   Workers exposed to certain chemicals, such as benzene or FORMALDEHYDE, are at higher risk for leukemia. Chemotherapy drugs known as alkylating agents are associated with the development of leukemia many years later.

Viruses Scientists have identified the human T-cell leukemia virus-I (HTLV-I) as the cause of a rare type of chronic lymphocytic leukemia (human T-cell leukemia). The virus is not known to cause other, more common forms of the disease.

Blood disease People with MYELODYSPLASTIC SYNDROME (a condition in which the bone marrow malfunctions) are at increased risk of developing acute myeloid leukemia.

Symptoms

Because leukemia cells are abnormal, they cannot help the body fight infections; as a result, people with leukemia often get infections. In addition, people with leukemia often have too few healthy red blood cells and platelets, so they become weak and anemic, pale and tired. When there are not enough platelets, patients bleed and bruise easily.

People with acute leukemia develop symptoms suddenly, and typically are diagnosed when they go to their doctor because they feel sick. In chronic leukemia, symptoms may not appear for a long time; when symptoms do appear, they generally are mild at first and get worse gradually. Doctors often find chronic leukemia during a routine checkup—before there are any symptoms.

Some of the common symptoms of leukemia include

- fever, chills, and other flu-like symptoms
- weakness and fatigue
- infections
- loss of appetite and/or weight
- swollen or tender lymph nodes, liver, or spleen
- easy bleeding or bruising
- tiny red spots under the skin (petechiae)
- swollen or bleeding gums
- sweating, especially at night
- bone or joint pain

In acute leukemia, the abnormal cells may collect in the brain or spinal cord, causing headaches, vomiting, confusion, loss of muscle control, and seizures. Leukemia cells also can collect in the testicles and cause swelling. Some patients develop sores in the eyes or on the skin or notice problems with their gums, digestive tract, kidneys, or lungs. Chronic leukemia may affect the skin, central nervous system, digestive tract, kidneys, and testicles.

Diagnosis

In addition to general physical exams, the doctor feels for swelling in the liver, spleen, and LYMPH NODES under the arms, in the groin, and in the neck. Blood tests can help in the diagnosis, but while they may reveal that a patient has leukemia, they may not show what type of leukemia it is. To check further for leukemia cells or to find out what type of leukemia a patient has, a hematologist, oncologist, or pathologist examines a sample of bone marrow under a microscope. A spinal tap can identify leukemia cells in the fluid that fills the spaces in and around the brain and spinal cord. Chest X-rays can reveal signs of disease in the chest.

Treatment

Treatment for leukemia is complex and varies according to the type of leukemia, features of the leukemia cells, extent of the disease, whether the leukemia has been treated before, and the patient's age, symptoms, and general health.

Acute leukemia needs to be treated immediately to bring about a remission, followed by more therapy to prevent a relapse. Many people with acute leukemia can be cured.

Chronic leukemia patients who do not have symptoms may not require immediate treatment, but they need frequent checkups so the doctor can see whether the disease is progressing (called "watchful waiting"). When chronic leukemia begins to cause symptoms, treatment can often control the disease and its symptoms, but treatment can seldom cure it.

Chemotherapy Most patients with leukemia are treated with chemotherapy. Depending on the type of leukemia, patients may receive a single drug or a combination of two or more oral or IV drugs.

Some people with chronic myeloid leukemia receive a new type of treatment called targeted therapy, which blocks the production of leukemia cells but does not harm normal cells. Gleevec is the first targeted therapy approved for chronic myeloid leukemia.

Most common chemotherapy drugs are chosen according to the type of leukemia:

- ALL: asparaginase, daunorubicin, vincristine, prednisone, and methotrexate
- CLL: fludarbine, chlorambucil, cyclophosphamide, and prednisone
- Hairy cell: pentostatin and cladribine
- CML: alpha interferon or hydroxyurea

Radiation therapy   Some patients have radiation therapy in addition to chemotherapy. Radiation therapy for leukemia may be given either to the whole body or to one specific area of the body where there is a collection of leukemia cells, such as the spleen or testicles. Total-body irradiation usually is given before a bone marrow transplant.

Bone marrow transplants   Before undergoing a bone marrow transplant, the patient's leukemia-producing bone marrow is first destroyed by high doses of drugs and radiation. The affected marrow is then replaced by healthy bone marrow. The healthy marrow comes either from a donor or from the patient, whose marrow was removed, treated outside the body to remove leukemia cells, and stored before the drugs and radiation were given. Patients who have a bone marrow transplant usually stay in the hospital for several weeks. Until the transplanted bone marrow begins to produce enough white blood cells, patients have to be carefully protected from infection.

Biological therapy   Biological therapy involves treatment with substances that affect the immune system's response to cancer. INTERFERON is a form of biological therapy that can slow the growth of some types of leukemia, such as chronic myeloid leukemia. Some patients with chronic lymphocytic leukemia are given a type of biological therapy called MONOCLONAL ANTIBODIES, which bind to the leukemia cells and help the immune system kill leukemia cells in the blood and bone marrow.

Stem cell transplants   In this procedure a patient is treated with high doses of drugs, radiation, or both, which destroy leukemia cells and normal blood cells in the bone marrow. Later the patient can be given healthy stem cells. New blood cells develop from the transplanted stem cells.

Stem cells may come from the patient or from a donor. In an autologous stem cell transplantation, the patient's own stem cells are removed and treated to kill any leukemia cells. The stem cells are then frozen and stored. After the patient receives high-dose chemotherapy or radiation therapy, the stored stem cells are thawed and returned to the patient.

In an allogeneic stem cell transplantation, the patient is given healthy stem cells from a donor (such as a brother, sister, or parent), although sometimes the stem cells come from an unrelated donor. Doctors use blood tests to be sure the donor's cells match the patient's cells.

In a syngeneic stem cell transplantation, the patient is given stem cells from the patient's healthy identical twin. There are several types of stem cell transplantation:

- *Bone marrow transplantation.* The stem cells come from bone marrow.
- *Peripheral stem cell transplantation.* The stem cells come from peripheral blood.
- *Umbilical cord blood transplantation.* For a child with no donor, the doctor may use stem cells from the blood of an umbilical cord from a newborn baby. Sometimes umbilical cord blood is frozen for use later.

See also GRAFT-VS.-HOST DISEASE; LEUKEMIA AND LYMPHOMA SOCIETY.

Leukemia and Lymphoma Society   The world's largest voluntary health organization dedicated to funding blood cancer research, education, and patient services. The society's mission is to cure LEUKEMIA, LYMPHOMA, HODGKIN'S DISEASE, and MULTIPLE MYELOMA and to improve the quality of life of patients and their families. Since its founding in 1949, the society has provided more than $280 million for research specifically targeting blood-related cancers. For contact information, see Appendix I.

leukopenia   A condition in which there are too few white cells in a patient's blood, either as a result of LEUKEMIA or LYMPHOMA, or as a side effect of chemotherapy treatment.

Leydig cell tumors   Rare tumors of the testicle. While some of these tumors are malignant, pathologists are usually not able to determine if they are malignant simply by looking at them. Because of this, a radical orchiectomy, which can cure the potential cancer without the need for further treatment, is usually performed. (See TESTICULAR CANCER.)

lifestyle and cancer   Scientists have identified many factors that contribute to the development of cancer, including a number of lifestyle factors. Avoiding these risk factors whenever possible could have a significant effect on a person's chance of getting cancer. The main risk factors include the following.

Alcohol

Drinking ALCOHOL has been linked with an increased risk of cancer of the esophagus, oral cavity, pharynx and larynx, breast, and liver. Alcohol promotes several types of cancer by directly damaging cells in the mouth and larynx, or by indirectly affecting the liver and breast. The cancer risk from drinking alcohol is especially pronounced if it is combined with SMOKING cigarettes.

People who enjoy alcohol should drink moderately—for men, this means no more than two drinks a day. For women, just one drink a day is considered moderate.

Infections

A number of cancers have been linked to infectious agents, including parasites, viruses (such as the HUMAN PAPILLOMAVIRUS and the hepatitis virus), and the bacterium *Helicobacter pylori*, which causes stomach ulcers. Some cancers could be prevented with a hepatitis B vaccination and safe sex practices such as using a latex condom.

Diet

Researchers are sure that what we eat makes a difference in the chance of developing a variety of cancers. The content of each meal, as well as the way it is prepared, influences cancer risk. For example, meat grilled on a barbecue may be more risky than meat prepared by baking or boiling. Cured meats containing compounds such as nitrosamines have been linked to higher risk of cancers. Other evidence suggests that people with diets high in saturated fats have a higher cancer risk than those with lower-fat diets.

Studies do not provide clear evidence of an association between ARTIFICIAL SWEETENERS and human cancer, nor do they conclusively rule out a link. Early studies showed that cyclamate, one of several types of artificial sweeteners, caused BLADDER CANCER in laboratory animals.

ACRYLAMIDE, a probable human CARCINOGEN based on lab animal research, has been found in certain foods, with relatively high levels in potato chips and french fries, and lower levels in some breads and cereals. Scientists do not yet know whether acrylamide in food poses a health risk for humans, but the World Health Organization has concluded that further research is necessary to determine how acrylamide is formed during the cooking process and whether it is present in foods other than those already tested.

In some cases, not getting enough of certain foods can increase the risk of getting cancer. Eating a diet rich in fruits, vegetables, whole grains, and other plant-based foods is associated with a reduced chance of developing cancer.

Environmental Factors

There is evidence that many environmental factors may contribute to cancer development. For example, exposure to ASBESTOS in insulation materials causes two types of LUNG CANCER; combining smoking cigarettes with significant asbestos exposure raises the risk of lung cancer 90-fold.

Working with aromatic amines used in some industrial materials is associated with the development of bladder cancer, and BENZENE in varnish and glue increases the risk of LEUKEMIA.

Sedentary Lifestyle

Experts estimate that 32 percent of COLORECTAL CANCER may be linked to not getting enough exercise. Studies have shown that people who get regular exercise are less likely to develop colon or BREAST CANCER.

One theory suggests that exercise protects against colon cancer by stimulating intestinal contractions, which increase the speed at which stools move through the intestine and out of the body. This could reduce exposure of cells in the colon to potential carcinogens in the stools.

Obesity

Although study results have been conflicting, with some showing an increased cancer risk from obesity and others not showing such a risk, obesity does appear to be linked to some types of cancer. Obesity appears to increase the risk for cancers of the breast, colon, prostate, endometrium, cervix, ovary, kidney, gallbladder, liver, pancreas, rectum, and esophagus.

Smoking

Smoking is believed to play a role in approximately 30 percent of all cancer deaths in the United States, and 85 percent of lung cancer deaths. Other cancers that are strongly associated with smoking are bladder cancer, oral cavity cancers, cancers of the head and neck, esophageal cancer, and pancreatic cancer. Half of all bladder cancer patients are current or former smokers.

The only way to prevent cancers caused by cigarettes is not to smoke. A smoker's risk of developing cancer decreases dramatically after quitting and continues to decrease every year thereafter.

Sun Exposure

Exposure to the ultraviolet radiation in the Sun's rays is responsible for almost all cases of the skin cancer, BASAL CELL CARCINOMA and SQUAMOUS CELL CARCINOMA and is a major cause of malignant MELANOMA.

The best way to prevent skin cancer is to stay out of the sun as much as possible, wear protective clothing (including a hat that shields the back of the neck), and use a sunscreen with a sun protection factor (SPF) of 15 or higher. People also should avoid tanning booths (which increase the risk of cancer) and wear ultraviolet-light-filtering sunglasses.

Hormones

Increasing the amount of hormones in the body could increase the risk of certain cancers that need hormones to grow.

Birth control pills   Current or former use of oral contraceptives among women ages 35 to 64 did not significantly increase the risk of breast cancer, according to the Women's Contraceptive and Reproductive Experience study. Other studies have consistently shown that using these pills reduces the risk of OVARIAN CANCER, but there is some evidence that long-term use of these pills may increase the risk of CERVICAL CANCER and certain LIVER CANCERS.

Hormone replacement   The Women's Health Initiative concluded definitively in 2002 that postmenopausal women who take combined estrogen and progestin therapy increase the risk of invasive breast cancer. After an average of five years of follow-up for more than 16,000 women, the study found a 26 percent increase in breast cancer risk for those on the therapy as compared to women taking placebo. Observational studies also indicate an increase in risk among women taking estrogen alone. Estrogen (when used alone) increases the risk of UTERINE CANCER.

Fertility drugs   Some studies have found that certain fertility drugs increase a woman's risk for ovarian cancer, while others have not shown any increased risk from fertility drugs. These studies and other recent research raise questions about whether infertile women who take fertility drugs and do not become pregnant, or women who take certain fertility drugs for extended periods of time, may be at increased risk of developing ovarian cancer. However, these links have not been proven, and more research is needed.

Li-Fraumeni syndrome (LFS)   A rare condition in which at least three family members have cancer, and family members are at risk for developing certain cancers before age 45, including BREAST CANCER, soft tissue or bone SARCOMA, brain tumors, osteosarcoma, LEUKEMIA, or adrenocortical cancer. Although most hereditary cancer syndromes involve only one or two specific types of tumors, families with Li-Fraumeni syndrome are at risk for a wide range of malignancies. Each year, about five to 10 cases of soft tissue sarcoma occur per one million children younger than 15 years. Of children with soft tissue sarcomas, 5 percent to 10 percent have a family history of malignancy consistent with LFS.

Cause

An inherited inborn or spontaneous defect in the p53 gene causes this syndrome. The p53 mutations were reported first in 1990; subsequent studies have shown that more than two-thirds of LFS families have inherited mutations of one of the two copies of the p53 tumor suppressor gene; the second copy is normal. Mutations in certain areas of the gene cause more aggressive cancers than do mutations in others.

lip cancer   See ORAL CANCER.

liposarcoma   A cancer of the fatty tissue that occurs most often in middle-aged men. It is one of the least common soft tissue SARCOMAS (less than 5 percent of all soft tissue sarcomas are liposarcomas). They occur most often in the legs and the shoulder.

Fewer than 1,000 new cases of liposarcomas are diagnosed in the United States each year, and the average patient age at diagnosis is 50 years. The five-year survival rate ranges from 15 percent to 80 percent, with an average survival period of 7.4 years. These tumors commonly recur after surgery and often spread to the lung and liver. The overall five-year survival rate of patients with deep high-grade liposarcoma is less than 50 percent.

Symptoms
Typical symptoms vary but range from a painless slow-growing lesion to a painful rapidly growing mass. There may be weakness or limited motion, or (more rarely) generalized symptoms such as WEIGHT LOSS, lethargy, and FATIGUE.

Diagnosis
CT scans and BIOPSY are used to diagnose this condition. For small fatty tumors, excisional biopsy is recommended. For deeper tumors or those larger than 3 cm, diagnosis and treatment may involve open incisional biopsy and removal.

Treatment
Surgical removal is the treatment of choice for these tumors, although their location may make complete removal difficult. CHEMOTHERAPY and radiation may be effective.

liver cancer   Cancer of the liver is the most common solid tumor worldwide, with more than one million cases diagnosed each year. However, it is relatively rare in the United States and Europe, accounting for only 1.5 percent of all cancers (although the liver is a common site for cancer to spread to from other places in the body, such as the colon, lungs, or breast). When primary liver cancer spreads, the cancer cells tend to move into nearby lymph nodes and into the bones and lungs. Five-year survival rates for patients whose cancer has spread are very low in the United States, usually less than 10 percent. About 16,600 people in the United States will be diagnosed with liver cancer this year, and 14,100 will die of the disease.

Types of Liver Cancer
The several different types of cancer that can occur within the liver are discussed below.

Hepatocellular cancer   Most cancers that appear in the liver begin in the liver cells and are of an aggressive type called HEPATOCELLULAR CARCINOMA (or malignant hepatoma). This type of cancer is most clearly associated with hepatitis B and hepatitis C viral infections and cirrhosis. It accounts for about 84 percent of primary liver cancers in the United States, where five-year survival rates are 15 percent to 40 percent.

Bile duct cancer   Cancer of the bile ducts located within the liver (cholangiocarcinoma) accounts for about 13 percent of primary liver cancer in the United States. Several conditions increase the risk of developing BILE DUCT CANCER, including gallstones, gallbladder inflammation, and sometimes chronic ulcerative colitis. Certain liver parasites are recognized risk factors for this type of liver cancer, especially in parts of southeast Asia. Five-year survival rates are 15 percent to 40 percent.

Hepatoblastoma   Hepatoblastoma is a rare type of liver cancer usually found in children younger than age four. (Children also may develop childhood hepatocellular carcinoma.) Survival rates are 70 percent.

Angiosarcoma   Angiosarcoma (HEMANGIOSARCOMA) is a very rare form of liver cancer that begins in the liver's blood vessels. It accounts for only about one percent of primary liver cancers and has been associated with industrial exposures to vinyl chloride. Most people with angiosarcoma survive less than six months after diagnosis.

Risk Factors

Although doctors do not know the exact cause of liver cancer, they have identified certain risk factors. The more risk factors a person has, the greater the chance that liver cancer will develop, although many people with known risk factors for liver cancer do not develop the disease. Studies have identified the following risk factors:

Aflatoxin   Produced by certain types of mold, this harmful substance can cause liver cancer. AFLATOXIN can be found on peanuts, corn, and other nuts and grains, although the U.S. Food and Drug Administration does not allow the sale of foods that have high levels of aflatoxin.

Age   In the United States, liver cancer occurs more often in people over age 60 than in younger people.

Anabolic steroids   These male hormones are used to treat certain conditions and are sometimes used illegally by athletes to enhance performance. Long-term abuse may slightly increase the risk of liver cancer.

Arsenic   Exposure to ARSENIC has been linked to liver cancer. Arsenic is a chemical that can be used as a wood preservative, herbicide, insecticide, or in manufacturing some glass and metallic alloys. Arsenic is found in natural mineral deposits and occurs naturally in some drinking water.

Chronic liver infection (hepatitis)   Each of the six types of hepatitis (A, B, C, D, E, and G) is caused by a different virus; some of these viruses can invade the liver and cause a chronic infection. The most important risk factor for liver cancer is a chronic infection with either hepatitis B or C virus, which together account for more than 75 percent of chronic hepatitis cases worldwide and are responsible for the majority of the cases of hepatocellular carcinoma. These viruses can be passed from person to person through blood or, in the case of hepatitis B, sexual contact. Liver cancer may develop many years (generally 20 to 30) after infection with the virus. New research has found that people with active hepatitis B infections are 60 times more likely to develop liver cancer than those without evidence of the virus.

These infections may not cause symptoms, but blood tests can detect the virus. People who do not already have the hepatitis B virus can be protected with a hepatitis B vaccine. Researchers are now working to develop a vaccine to prevent hepatitis C infection.

Cirrhosis   This condition develops after liver cells are damaged and replaced with scar tissue. Cirrhosis may be caused by alcohol abuse, certain drugs and other chemicals, and certain viruses or parasites. About 5 percent of people with cirrhosis develop liver cancer, but between 50 percent and 70 percent of liver cancers in the United States are associated with cirrhosis.

Gender   Men are twice as likely as women to get liver cancer.

Family history   People who have family members with liver cancer may be more likely to get the disease.

Race   Caucasian men and women have the lowest rates for primary liver cancer; rates among African Americans and Hispanics are roughly twice as high as the rates in Caucasians. The highest incidence is among Vietnamese men (41.8 per 100,000), probably reflecting risks associated with the high prevalence of viral hepatitis infections in their homeland. Other Asian-American groups also have liver cancer incidence and mortality rates several times higher than the Caucasian population. Death rates among Chinese populations are the highest of all groups.

Polyvinyl chloride (PVC)   Direct contact with this chemical has been linked in some studies to hepatocellular carcinoma or angiosarcoma. It is used in manufacturing some types of plastics, such as PVC pipe.

Symptoms

Liver cancer is sometimes called a "silent disease" because in its early stage there may be no symptoms. Eventually, as the disease progresses, it may trigger symptoms such as:

- pain in the right upper abdomen extending to the back and shoulder
- swollen abdomen
- weight loss
- loss of appetite and feelings of fullness
- weakness
- fatigue

- nausea and vomiting
- jaundice
- fever

Diagnosis

The following procedures can help determine if a patient has liver cancer:

Physical exam   The doctor feels the abdomen to check the liver, spleen, and nearby organs for any lumps or changes in their shape or size. The doctor also checks for ASCITES, an abnormal buildup of fluid in the abdomen, and checks the skin and eyes for signs of jaundice.

Blood tests   Many blood tests, including ALPHA-FETOPROTEIN, may be used to check for liver problems.

CT/MRI and ultrasound scan   These scans can reveal tumors in the liver or abdomen.

Angiogram   In this test, a doctor injects dye into an artery to highlight blood vessels in the liver, revealing any existing tumors.

Biopsy   By removing a tissue sample, a doctor can detect cancer cells in the liver. The doctor may insert a thin needle into the liver to remove a small amount of tissue (fine-needle aspiration) or may sample tissue with a thick needle (core BIOPSY) or by inserting a laparoscope into a small incision in the abdomen.

Laparoscopy   With this technique, the surgeon inserts a thin, lighted tube through a small incision in the abdomen to view the liver (a biopsy can be done at the same time).

Staging

If liver cancer is diagnosed, the doctor needs to know the extent of the disease in order to plan the best treatment. The stage is based on the size of the tumor, the condition of the liver, and whether the cancer has spread. Careful staging shows whether the tumor can be removed with surgery (most liver cancers cannot be). "Localized resectable cancer" can be removed; "localized unresectable cancer" cannot be removed.

Localized resectable cancer   Early liver cancer in which there is no evidence that the cancer has spread to the nearby lymph nodes or to other parts of the body; the liver is still functioning well.

Localized unresectable cancer   This type of liver cancer cannot be removed by surgery even though it has not spread to the nearby lymph nodes or to distant parts of the body. Surgery to remove the tumor is not possible because of other conditions that cause poor liver function, because of where the tumor is located within the liver, or because of other health problems.

Advanced cancer   At this stage, liver cancer is found in both lobes of the liver or has spread to other parts of the body.

Recurrent cancer   Even when a tumor in the liver seems to have been completely removed or destroyed, the disease sometimes returns because undetected cancer cells remained somewhere in the body after treatment. Most recurrences occur within the first two years of treatment. If cancer returns, the patient may have surgery or a combination of treatments for recurrent liver cancer.

Treatment

Liver cancer can be cured only when it is found at an early stage and only if the patient is healthy enough to have surgery. Treatment for advanced liver cancer may involve chemotherapy, radiation therapy, or both. Because liver cancer is very hard to control with current treatments, many doctors encourage patients to consider taking part in research trials to test new treatments.

Surgery   Surgery to remove part of the liver is called partial hepatectomy, and the extent of surgery depends on the size, number, and location of the tumors, and how well the liver is working. The doctor may remove a piece of tissue that contains the liver tumor, an entire lobe of the liver, or an even larger portion of the liver. In a partial hepatectomy, the surgeon leaves a margin of normal liver tissue that will take over all the functions of the liver.

A liver transplant may be an option for some patients whose disease has not spread outside the liver but whose tumor cannot be removed because of poor liver function. After the transplant, the patient may need to stay in the hospital for several weeks to monitor whether the patient's body is accepting the new liver. The patient takes drugs, to prevent the body from rejecting the new liver, which may cause facial puffiness, high blood pressure, or an increase in body hair.

Localized unresectable Patients with this type of liver cancer cannot undergo surgery and may receive other treatments that control the disease by killing cancer cells with heat, such as with lasers or microwaves. In radiofrequency ablation, a special probe is used to kill cancer cells.

Hepatic arterial infusion In this procedure, CHEMOTHERAPY is injected into a tube inserted into the major artery that supplies blood to the liver, primarily affecting liver cells. Because only a small amount of the drug reaches other parts of the body, hepatic arterial infusion causes fewer side effects than standard chemotherapy. Side effects from hepatic arterial infusion may include infection and problems with the pump device, which may require removal.

Chemotherapy/radiation Either chemotherapy drugs (doxorubicin, cisplatin, or floxuridine), radiation, or a combination of both may be given to try to kill cancer cells.

Chemoembolization In this technique, a tiny catheter is directed into an artery in the leg and then moved into the hepatic artery; chemotherapy drugs are injected through the catheter into the liver. Tiny particles are used to block the flow of blood through the artery so that the drug stays in the liver longer. Depending on the type of particles used, the blockage may be temporary or permanent. Although the hepatic artery is blocked, healthy liver tissue continues to receive blood from the hepatic portal vein, which carries blood from the stomach and intestine.

Chemoembolization causes fewer side effects than chemotherapy because the drugs do not flow through the entire body. Still, chemoembolization sometimes causes nausea, vomiting, fever, and abdominal pain. The doctor can give medications to help lessen these problems. Some patients may feel very tired for several weeks after the treatment.

Alternative treatments People with cirrhosis, hepatitis, or multiple liver cancers in different locations usually are not candidates for surgery. For these people, alternative techniques may stop cancer growth temporarily and relieve symptoms, though they have not been proven to improve survival rates. These methods include percutaneous ethanol injection and cryosurgery.

In *percutaneous ethanol injection*, a doctor uses ultrasound guidance to inject alcohol directly into the liver tumor to kill cancer cells. The procedure may be performed once or twice a week. Local anesthesia is used unless the number of tumors requires general anesthesia. After this treatment patients may have fever and pain. These can be controlled with medication.

In *cryosurgery*, a metal probe is inserted through a small abdominal incision to freeze and kill cancer cells. The doctor may use ultrasound to help guide the probe. Because a smaller incision is needed for cryosurgery than for traditional surgery, recovery after cryosurgery is generally faster and less painful, and infection and bleeding are not as likely.

Pain

Pain is a common problem for people with liver cancer. The tumor can cause pain by pressing against nerves and other organs, and treatment for liver cancer may cause discomfort. There are several methods to reduce this pain:

- *Pain medicine.* Medicines often can relieve the pain of liver cancer.
- *Radiation.* Radiation can help relieve pain by shrinking the tumor.
- *Nerve block.* An alcohol injection into the area around certain nerves in the abdomen can block liver pain.

lobular carcinoma in situ See BREAST CANCER.

Look Good . . . Feel Better Program (LGFB) A free, nonmedical national public service program founded in 1989 and supported by corporate donors to help women offset appearance-related changes from cancer treatment. The Look Good . . . Feel Better program was developed by the CTFA Foundation, a charitable organization established by the Cosmetic, Toiletry, and Fragrance Association (CTFA), the AMERICAN CANCER SOCIETY (ACS), and the National Cosmetology Association. Today, LGFB group programs are held in every state and Puerto Rico, with products donated by 40 CTFA member companies. Teen and Spanish programs, self-help mailer kits, online programs, and a 24-

hour hotline are now offered—as well as numerous independent international LGFB programs across the globe:

- *Look Good . . . Feel Better.* This version includes programs and other services for women in English in all 50 states (International LGFB programs are also offered by sister organizations).

- *Luzca Bien . . . Siéntase Mejor.* This version offers bilingual (English and Spanish) group programs for Hispanic women in 14 locations: Albuquerque, Brownsville (Texas), Chicago, Dallas, Denver, Houston, Los Angeles, Miami, New York City, Phoenix, San Antonio, San Diego, San Francisco, and Washington, D.C. Spanish-language materials are available nationwide upon request.

- *Look Good . . . Feel Better for Teens.* This group offers programs for teen girls and boys in 13 cities—Boston, Columbus (Ohio), Denver, Durham (North Carolina), Houston, Memphis, New Haven, New York City, Palo Alto, Philadelphia, Rochester (Minnesota), Tampa, and Washington, D.C.—plus the 2bMe Web site with online demos.

Each two-hour hands-on workshop includes a 12-step skin care/makeup application lesson, demonstration of options for dealing with hair loss, and nail-care techniques. Held at comprehensive care clinics, hospitals, ACS offices, and community centers, local group programs are organized by the American Cancer Society, facilitated by LGFB-certified cosmetologists, and aided by volunteers. Patients in various stages of treatment receive makeover tips and personal attention from professionals trained to meet their needs. They also use and take home complimentary cosmetic kits with helpful instruction booklets. Professional advice is provided on wigs, scarves, and accessories. (Teen sessions also include social and health tips.) More than 40,000 individuals participate each year in small groups of five to 10, offering each patient a supportive circle, as well.

Self-help kits in English or Spanish with a 30-minute video and a makeover tips booklet are offered free to patients who cannot locally access LGFB. Call 1-800-395-LOOK to request a kit. For contact information, see Appendix I.

LOOP electrosurgical excision procedure (LEEP)
A simple surgical procedure that is used to treat abnormal changes of the cells lining the cervix (dysplasia). The procedure is also used occasionally to treat carefully chosen cases of CERVICAL CANCER.

In this technique, radio frequency current is used to remove abnormal tissues of the cervix. A chemical is applied afterward to prevent bleeding. LEEP has an advantage over other, more destructive, techniques (such as CO_2 laser or cryocautery): an intact tissue sample for analysis can be obtained. LEEP also is popular because it is inexpensive and simple.

Complications occur in about 1 to 2 percent of women undergoing LEEP and include bleeding or narrowing of the cervical opening.

lumpectomy   A surgical procedure in which only the cancerous tumor in the breast is removed, together with a rim of normal tissue. Any form of surgery that removes only part of the breast is considered "breast-conserving" or "breast preservation" surgery and goes by many names, including quadrantectomy or a wedge resection.

Technically, a lumpectomy is a partial MASTECTOMY, because part of the breast is removed—although exactly how much can vary a great deal from one woman to another. In a lumpectomy the surgeon removes not just the tumor but also an area of healthy tissue surrounding the tumor; if cancer cells are found in the margins of the breast tissue that was removed, the surgeon will perform a second surgery (called a re-excision) to try to remove the remaining cancer and obtain "clear margins." Some women need several such surgeries before clear margins are obtained.

After a successful lumpectomy, most women receive five to seven weeks of RADIATION THERAPY in order to eliminate any cancer cells that may be left in the remaining breast tissue. Evidence shows that for women with cancer in only one area of the breast, and whose tumor is smaller than 4 cm and removed with clear margins, lumpectomy followed by radiation is as effective as mastectomy.

While lumpectomy and radiation is an excellent option for many women with breast cancer, it is not the best treatment for everyone. A woman may choose mastectomy over lumpectomy if she already has had radiation to the same breast for an earlier breast cancer, has extensive cancer in the breast or two or more separate areas of cancer in the same breast, or has a small breast and a large tumor, so that removing the tumor would be extremely disfiguring. A woman also may choose mastectomy if multiple attempts to obtain clear margins have been unsuccessful, she has a connective tissue disease, or she is pregnant. Sometimes a woman may choose a mastectomy if she learns she carries the *BRCA* gene after discovering the lump. Other women cannot commit to the daily schedule of radiation therapy, or simply believe they would feel more comfortable with a mastectomy.

The risk of recurrence in the breast after lumpectomy (with clear margins) and radiation ranges between 5 percent and 15 percent; the average is about 10 percent. The larger the cancer, the closer the margins, and the more aggressive the cancer's personality, the higher the risk of recurrence.

lung cancer Cancer that begins in the lungs is less common today than a decade ago, but it is still the leading cause of cancer death in the United States for both men and women. In fact, lung cancer kills more people than COLORECTAL CANCER, BREAST CANCER, and PROSTATE CANCER combined. It is the second most common cancer among men and women (behind SKIN CANCER), with about 170,000 Americans diagnosed with the disease in 2003. Although the rate of lung cancer appears to be dropping among Caucasian and African-American men in the United States, it continues to rise among both these groups of women.

Types of Lung Cancer

Lung cancer is divided into two major types—non-small cell lung cancer and small cell lung cancer—depending on how the cells look under a microscope. Each type of lung cancer grows and spreads in different ways and is treated differently.

Non-small cell lung cancer Non-small cell lung cancer is more common than small cell lung cancer, and it generally grows and spreads more slowly. There are three main types of non-small cell lung cancer, which are named for the type of cells in which the cancer develops: squamous cell carcinoma (also called epidermoid carcinoma), adenocarcinoma, and large cell carcinoma.

Small cell lung cancer Small cell lung cancer, sometimes called oat cell cancer, is less common than non-small cell lung cancer and accounts for about 20 percent of all cases of lung cancer. This type of lung cancer grows more quickly and is more likely to spread to other organs in the body.

Causes

Lung cancer takes many years to develop, but changes in the lung can start almost as soon as a person is exposed to a CARCINOGEN. Soon after exposure begins, a few abnormal cells may appear in the lining of the bronchi. If a person continues to be exposed, more and more abnormal cells will appear, eventually becoming malignant and forming a tumor. The tumor grows, destroying nearby areas of the lung. Eventually, the tumor's abnormal cells can spread to nearby LYMPH NODES and to distant organs, such as the brain.

Eight out of 10 times, the carcinogens that trigger lung cancer are chemicals found in cigarette smoke. Cigarettes contain more than 4,000 different harmful chemicals and carcinogens that damage the cells in the lungs. The likelihood that a smoker will develop lung cancer is affected by the age at which smoking began, how long the person has smoked, the number of cigarettes smoked per day, and how deeply the smoker inhales. Stopping SMOKING greatly reduces a person's risk for developing lung cancer. Cigar and pipe smokers also have a higher risk of lung cancer than nonsmokers. The number of years a person smokes, the number of pipes or cigars smoked per day, and how deeply the person inhales all affect the risk of developing lung cancer. However, even cigar and pipe smokers who do not inhale are at increased risk for lung, mouth, and other types of cancer.

Other causes include:

Asbestos The name of a group of minerals that occur naturally as fibers and are used in certain industries. Asbestos fibers tend to break easily into particles that can float in the air and stick to clothes. When the particles are inhaled, they can lodge in the lungs, damaging cells and increasing the risk for lung cancer. Studies have shown that workers who have been exposed to large amounts of asbestos have a risk for developing lung cancer that is three to four times greater than that for workers who have not been exposed to asbestos. This exposure has been observed in such industries as shipbuilding, asbestos mining and manufacturing, insulation work, and brake repair. The risk of lung cancer is even higher among asbestos workers who also smoke. Asbestos workers should use the protective equipment provided by their employers and follow recommended work practices and safety procedures.

Gender   The rates of lung cancer among men are about two to three times higher than the rates among women in all races or ethnic groups.

Lung diseases   Certain lung diseases, such as tuberculosis (TB), increase a person's chance of developing lung cancer, which tends to develop in areas of the lung that are scarred from TB.

Pollution   Researchers have found a link between lung cancer and exposure to certain air pollutants, such as by-products of the combustion of diesel and other fossil fuels. However, this relationship has not been clearly defined, and more research is being done.

Race   Among men, the number of lung cancer cases per 100,000 ranges from a low of about 14 among American Indians to a high of 117 among African Americans. Between these two extremes, rates fall into two groups ranging from 42 to 53 for Hispanics, Japanese, Chinese, Filipinos, and Koreans, and from 71 to 89 for Vietnamese, Caucasians, Alaska Natives, and Hawaiians. The range among women is much narrower, from a rate of about 15 among Japanese to nearly 51 among Alaska Natives. Rates for the remaining female populations range from low rates of 16 to 25 for Koreans, Filipinos, Hispanics, and Chinese, to rates of 31 to 44 among Vietnamese, Caucasians, Hawaiians and African Americans.

Radon   RADON is an invisible, odorless, and tasteless radioactive gas that occurs naturally in soil and rocks, and that can seep into a building through gaps and cracks in the foundation or insulation, as well as through pipes, drains, walls or other openings. Radon damages the lungs and is the second leading cause of lung cancer in the United States today. Between 7,000 and 22,000 lung cancer deaths each year in the United States—12 percent of all lung cancer deaths—are linked to radon.

In some parts of the country, radon is found in houses, and people who work in mines also may be exposed. Smoking increases the risk for lung cancer even more for those already at risk because of exposure to radon.

A kit available at most hardware stores allows homeowners to measure radon levels in their homes. The home radon test is relatively easy to use and inexpensive, and radon problems can be corrected by venting basements where the gas collects.

Secondhand tobacco smoke   The chance of developing lung cancer is increased by exposure to environmental tobacco smoke (ETS)—the smoke in the air when someone else smokes. Exposure to ETS, or secondhand smoke, is called "involuntary" or "passive" smoking. Secondhand smoke is responsible for about 3,000 lung cancer deaths each year.

Toxins on the job   Asbestos is the best-known on-the-job carcinogen, but there are many others, including uranium, ARSENIC, and certain petroleum products. People in many different jobs may be exposed to carcinogens, such as those who work with certain types of insulation, in coke ovens, or who repair brakes. When exposure to job-related carcinogens is combined with smoking, the risk for getting lung cancer is sharply increased.

Personal history   A person who has had lung cancer once is more likely to develop a second lung cancer than is a person who has never had lung cancer. Quitting smoking after lung cancer is diagnosed may prevent the development of a second lung cancer.

Family history   Family history also appears to play a role in the development of lung cancer and other smoking-related cancers—even among family members who do not smoke. Studies have found that nonsmokers whose close family members have had lung cancer, cancers of the mouth and throat, or female breast cancer, are at greater risk of developing lung cancer themselves than are nonsmokers with no family history of cancer, according to a study by Yale Cancer Center researchers. Exposure to second-hand smoke from family members did not explain the greater prevalence of lung cancer in the nonsmokers with a family history of cancer as compared to the control group. A smoker's risk of developing cancer may be affected by genes that help detoxify the cancer-causing agents in tobacco smoke, as well as genes that affect the ability to repair genetic damage, and thus prevent the negative biological consequences of smoking.

Symptoms

Common signs and symptoms of lung cancer include

- a cough that does not go away and gets worse over time
- chest pain (constant)
- coughing up blood
- shortness of breath, wheezing, or hoarseness
- pneumonia or bronchitis (repeated episodes)
- swelling of the neck and face
- loss of appetite or WEIGHT LOSS
- FATIGUE
- rounding/curving of fingernails

Diagnosis

A lung cancer diagnosis begins with a person's medical history, smoking history, exposure to environmental and occupational substances, and family history of cancer. The doctor also performs a physical exam and may order a chest X-ray and other tests.

If lung cancer is suspected, sputum cytology (the microscopic examination of cells obtained from a deep-cough sample of mucus in the lungs) is a simple test that can detect lung cancer. However, to confirm a diagnosis of lung cancer, a doctor must examine tissue taken from the lung during a biopsy. A number of procedures may be used to obtain this tissue:

Bronchoscopy   To collect tissue samples, a doctor inserts a lighted bronchoscope into the patient's mouth or nose and down through the windpipe.

Needle aspiration   Tissue samples also may be obtained by using a needle inserted through the chest into the tumor.

Thoracentesis   Alternatively, a doctor can use a needle to remove a sample of the fluid surrounding the lungs to check for cancer cells.

Thoracotomy   Surgery to open the chest is sometimes needed to diagnose lung cancer, but this procedure is a major operation.

Lung Cancer Staging

Once a diagnosis has been made, a doctor will stage the disease to find out whether the cancer has spread and, if so, to what parts of the body. Lung cancer often spreads to the brain or bones, so knowing the stage of the disease helps the doctor plan treatment. Some tests used to determine whether the cancer has spread include:

CAT or MRI scan   These scans can provide detailed pictures of areas inside the body.

PET scanning   This type of scan can show whether cancer has spread to other organs, such as the liver. The patient swallows or receives an injection of a mildly radioactive substance, and a scanner records the level of radioactivity in certain organs, revealing abnormal areas.

Bone scan   This is one type of radionuclide scanning that can show whether cancer has spread to the bones. A small amount of radioactive substance is injected into a vein and will collect in areas of abnormal bone growth. A scanner measures the radioactivity levels in these areas and records them on X-ray film.

Mediastinoscopy/mediastinotomy   A mediastinoscopy can help show whether the cancer has spread to the lymph nodes in the chest by allowing a doctor to examine the center of the chest and nearby lymph nodes using a lighted scope. In mediastinoscopy, the scope is inserted through a small incision in the neck; in mediastinotomy, the incision is made in the chest. In either procedure, the scope is also used to remove a tissue sample. The patient receives a general anesthetic.

Staging Non-Small Cell Lung Cancer

The TNM staging system is used to describe the spread of non-small cell lung cancer. In this system, *T* stands for "tumor," and the numeral following it indicates its size and how far it has spread within the lung and to nearby organs. *N* stands for spread to lymph "nodes," and *M* is for "metastasis" (spread to distant organs). In TNM staging, information about the tumor, lymph nodes, and metastasis is combined and a stage is assigned to specific TNM groupings. The grouped stages are described using the number 0 and Roman numerals from I to IV.

T0: Cancer is found only in the layer of cells lining the air passages. It has not invaded other lung tissues. This stage is known also as carcinoma in situ.

TI: The cancer is no larger than 3 cm (slightly less than 1 $1/4$ inches), has not spread to the membranes that surround the lungs, and does not affect the main branches of the bronchi.

TII: The cancer meets at least one of these conditions: it is larger than 3 cm; involves a main bronchus but is not closer than 2 cm to the point where the trachea branches into the left and right main bronchi; has spread to the membranes that surround the lungs; or it may partially clog the airways but has not caused the entire lung to collapse or develop pneumonia.

TIII: The cancer has one or more of the following features:

- It has spread to the chest wall, the membranes surrounding the space between the two lungs, or membranes of the sac surrounding the heart.

- It has invaded a main bronchus and is closer than 2 cm to the point where the windpipe branches into the left and right main bronchi, but it does not affect this area.

- It has grown into the airways enough to cause an entire lung to collapse or to cause pneumonia in the entire lung.

TIV: The cancer has one or more of the following features:

- It has spread to the space behind the chest bone and in front of the heart, the trachea, the esophagus, the backbone, or the point where the windpipe branches into the left and right main bronchi.

- Two or more separate tumor nodules are present in the same lobe.

- There is a fluid containing cancer cells in the space surrounding the lung.

N0: No spread to lymph nodes

NI: Spread to lymph nodes within the lung and/or nodes located around the area where the bronchus enters the lung. Affected lymph nodes are on the same side as the cancerous lung.

NII: Spread to lymph nodes around the point where the windpipe branches into the left and right bronchi or to lymph nodes in the space behind the chest bone and in front of the heart. Affected lymph nodes are on the same side as the cancerous lung.

NIII: Spread to lymph nodes near the collarbone on either side or to lymph nodes on the side opposite the cancerous lung.

M0: No spread to distant organs or areas, such as other lobes of the lungs, lymph nodes further than those mentioned in N stages, and other organs or tissues such as the liver, bones, or brain.

MI: The cancer has spread distantly.

Staging Small Cell Lung Cancer

Although small cell lung cancers can be staged the same way as non-small cell lung cancer, most doctors prefer a two-stage system, involving either "limited stage" or "extensive stage."

Limited stage usually means that the cancer is only in one lung and in lymph nodes on the same side of the chest.

Spread of the cancer to the other lung, to lymph nodes on the other side of the chest, or to distant organs indicates "extensive" disease. Many doctors consider small cell lung cancer that has spread to the fluid around the lung an extensive stage.

"Recurrent stage" lung cancer means the cancer has returned to the lungs after treatment.

Small cell lung cancer is staged in this way because it helps separate patients who have a fair prognosis and may be cured from those who have a poor outlook with no chance of cure. About two-thirds of the people with small cell lung cancer have extensive disease when their cancer is first found.

Metastatic Lung Cancer

It is very common for a cancer that originates in some other part of the body to spread to the lungs, since all the blood from the heart flows through the lungs. The most common cancers that typically spread to the lungs include breast cancer, TESTICULAR

CANCER, colorectal cancer, MELANOMA, GERM CELL TUMORS, soft tissue SARCOMAS, and BONE CANCER.

Treatment

Treatment depends on a number of factors, including the type of lung cancer, the size, location, and extent of the tumor, and the patient's health. Many different treatments and combinations of treatments may be used to control lung cancer and to improve quality of life by reducing symptoms.

Surgery The type of surgery a doctor performs depends on the location of the tumor in the lung. An operation to remove only a small part of the lung is called a segmental or wedge resection. When the surgeon removes an entire lobe of the lung, the procedure is called a lobectomy; pneumonectomy is the removal of an entire lung. Some tumors are inoperable because of the size or location, and some patients cannot have surgery for other medical reasons.

Chemotherapy Even after cancer has been removed from the lung, cancer cells may still be present in nearby tissue or elsewhere in the body, so CHEMOTHERAPY may be used to control cancer growth or to relieve symptoms. Chemotherapy drugs typically given for all types of lung cancer include doxorubicin, cisplatin, cyclophosphamide, Taxol, taxotere, Gemzar, and carboplatin.

Radiation RADIATION THERAPY also may be used to relieve symptoms such as shortness of breath. Lung cancer is usually treated with external radiation, but it is also possible to treat this malignancy with an implant containing radioactive material placed directly into or near the tumor.

Laser treatment Photodynamic therapy is a type of LASER treatment in which a special chemical is injected into the bloodstream and absorbed by cells all over the body. The chemical rapidly leaves normal cells but remains in cancer cells for a longer time. A laser light aimed at the cancer activates the chemical, which then kills the cancer cells that have absorbed it. Photodynamic therapy may be used to reduce symptoms of lung cancer—for example, to control bleeding or to relieve breathing problems due to blocked airways when the cancer cannot be removed through surgery. It also may be used to treat very small tumors in patients for whom the usual treatments for lung cancer are not appropriate.

Non-small cell treatment The treatment for a patient with non-small cell lung cancer depends mainly on the size, location, and extent of the tumor. Surgery is the most common way to treat this type of lung cancer, but CRYOSURGERY (a treatment that freezes and destroys cancer tissue) may be used to control symptoms in the later stages. Chemotherapy drugs specific to non-small cell lung cancer include paclitaxel, cisplatin, taxotere, Gemzar, and carboplatin.

Small cell treatment Small cell lung cancer spreads quickly, so in many cases cancer cells have already spread to other parts of the body when the disease is diagnosed. Chemotherapy drugs specific to small cell lung cancer include etoposide, cisplatin, taxol, taxotere, vincristine, ifosfamide, and carboplatin.

Treatment may also include radiation therapy aimed at the tumor in the lung or tumors in other parts of the body (such as in the brain). Some patients have radiation therapy to the brain even though no cancer is found there. This treatment, called prophylactic cranial irradiation, is given to prevent tumors from forming in the brain. Surgery is part of the treatment plan for a small number of patients with small cell lung cancer.

Prognosis

The prognosis depends on the type of lung cancer, its stage, and the general health of the patient, but overall only 14 percent of patients with lung cancer survive for more than five years after diagnosis. However, five-year survival rates vary according to the type of lung cancer, including

- adenocarcinoma: 17 percent
- squamous cell carcinoma: 15 percent
- large cell carcinoma: 11 percent
- small cell carcinoma: 5 percent

Prevention

Never smoking is the best way to prevent lung cancer. If a smoker is able to stop smoking, the risk of lung cancer decreases each year as abnormal cells are replaced by normal cells. After 10 years, the risk drops to a third to a half of the risk for people who continue to smoke. However, it takes 20 to 25 years of not smoking for a former smoker's risk of lung cancer to return close to the level of those who have never smoked.

lutein   A plant chemical found most often in leafy green vegetables but also in other fruits and vegetables. Lutein belongs to a group of more than 600 PHYTOCHEMICALS called CAROTENOIDS, which are plant pigments that function as ANTIOXIDANTS. Evidence suggests that eating foods high in lutein may protect against BREAST CANCER.

See also DIET.

lycopene   One of more than 600 PHYTOCHEMICALS called carotenoids, with very powerful disease-fighting capabilities, particularly against PROSTATE CANCER, lycopene is associated with the red color in tomatoes. Tomato-based products, such as tomato sauce, tomato soup, and tomato juice, have the most concentrated source of lycopene. A number of studies have suggested that eating tomatoes and tomato products, such as sauce, paste, and soup, is associated with a lower prostate-cancer risk. Scientists proposed that lycopene gives the fruit its anti-cancer properties.

Cooked tomato sauces are associated with greater health benefits (compared to uncooked) because the heating process enables lycopene to be more easily absorbed by the body. Also, lycopene is fat-soluble, meaning that in order for the body to absorb it, it has to be eaten with at least a small amount of fat. Lycopene has been associated with a reduced risk for many cancers.

But while a tomato a day may help prevent prostate cancer, lycopene as a dietary supplement may not be enough—according to the first animal study comparing the cancer-preventing potential of tomato products to that of lycopene. Rats with prostate cancer survived longer when fed a diet that included whole tomato products but not when fed the same diet plus lycopene, according to Ohio State University Cancer Center scientists. The effect was most apparent when the animals' food intake was modestly restricted. The study, which was published in the November 4, 2003, issue of the *Journal of the National Cancer Institute,* strongly suggests that risks of poor dietary habits cannot be reversed simply by taking a pill. Instead, researchers recommend patients choose a variety of healthy foods, exercise, and weight control.

In the study, scientists first separated 194 rats with prostate cancer into three groups. A control group was fed a balanced diet containing no detectable lycopene; the second group received the control diet plus lycopene; and a third group received the control diet mixed with tomato powder made from tomato paste that included seeds and skins. Each group was subdivided into an energy-restricted group and an energy-unrestricted group. Animals in the unrestricted group received as much food as they wanted; energy-restricted animals received 20 percent less food than the unrestricted group. The experiment lasted about 14 months.

Rats in the tomato-fed, energy-unrestricted group showed a longer prostate-cancer-free survival compared to controls; their risk of dying from prostate cancer dropped by 26 percent. Animals in the tomato-fed, energy-restricted group fared even better, showing a 32 percent drop in risk. No benefit from lycopene alone was seen in either the energy-restricted or unrestricted groups. This does not mean that lycopene is useless, but it suggests that if men want the health benefits of tomatoes, they should eat tomatoes or tomato products and not rely on lycopene supplements alone.

lymphadenectomy   Removal and BIOPSY of LYMPH NODES to check for the extent of the spread of cancer. When cancer is being staged to determine whether or not it has spread, the surgeon will perform a biopsy of the lymph nodes to see if any malignant cells have spread there. The presence of cancer cells in the lymph nodes suggests that the cancer has spread from the primary site and is likely to spread to other parts of the body. Lymphadenectomy is also performed if a cancer recurrence is suspected.

See also SENTINEL NODE BIOPSY.

lymphangiography   An X-ray examination of a specific part of the body to check for enlarged lymph nodes. In this procedure, a dye is injected into the lymphatic vessels of the legs before X-rays are taken. Any enlarged lymph nodes will be revealed on the X-ray, which also may reveal an abnormal pattern of lymph drainage. This method can help diagnose LYMPHOMAS, HODGKIN'S DISEASE, certain women's reproductive cancers, or TESTICU-LAR CANCER.

lymphangiosarcoma   A rare type of soft tissue SARCOMA that begins in the lymphatic vessels in the arm. Lymphangiosarcoma is a rare but fatal complication of LYMPHEDEMA (buildup of lymph just under the skin after surgery to remove lymph nodes).

Lymphedema typically appears in BREAST CANCER patients; the average time between MASTECTOMY and the appearance of lymphangiosarcoma is about 10 years. After a patient develops lymphangiosarcoma, the average survival time is a little over one year. The exact cause is not known.

Lymphangiosarcoma first appears as one or more bluish red bumps on the affected arm or leg. The first slightly raised area in the skin of the arm or leg looks something like a bruise; later, more tumors appear and the bumps grow. Death usually results from tumor spread to the lungs.

lymphatic system   A network of capillaries, vessels, ducts, nodes, and organs that produce, filter, and carry lymph, a colorless liquid that bathes the body's tissues and contains cells that help the body fight infection. As lymph is slowly moved through larger and larger lymphatic vessels, it passes through LYMPH NODES that filter out substances harmful to the body; these nodes also contain lymphocytes and other cells that activate the immune system to fight disease. Eventually, lymph flows into one of two large ducts in the neck. The right lymphatic duct collects lymph from the right arm and the right side of the head and chest and empties into the large vein under the right collarbone. The left lymphatic duct collects lymph from both legs, the left arm, and the left side of the head and chest and empties into the large vein under the left collarbone.

The lymphatic system collects excess fluid and proteins from the tissues and carries them back to the bloodstream. Swelling (LYMPHEDEMA) may occur if there is an increase in the amount of fluid, proteins, and other substances in the body tissues because of problems in the blood capillaries and veins, or a blockage in the lymphatic system.

lymphedema   A fluid buildup that may collect in the arms or legs when lymph vessels or LYMPH NODES are blocked or removed. Although lymphedema is most often associated with BREAST CANCER, it can also develop after treatment for other types of cancer. Left untreated, this stagnant fluid interferes with wound healing and provides a culture medium for bacteria that can result in infection in the lymph nodes (lymphangitis).

If lymph nodes are removed, there is always a risk of developing lymphedema, either right after surgery, or weeks, months, even years later. Lymphedema also can develop if chemotherapy is unwisely administered to the side of the body on which surgery was performed. Patients who undergo repeated aspirations of fluid in the underarms, around a breast incision, or in the groin area often develop infection and, subsequently, lymphedema. Air travel has also been linked to the onset of lymphedema in patients after cancer surgery, probably as a result of the decreased cabin pressure. This is why cancer patients should always wear a compression garment (a special sleeve or stocking) when flying.

Lower-extremity lymphedema can be caused by the use of tamoxifen, commonly given after treatment for breast cancer. This medication can cause blood clots in the legs.

Risk Factors

There are a number of risk factors for the development of lymphedema:

- breast cancer, if patients have received radiation therapy or had lymph nodes removed. The more nodes removed, the higher the risk.

- surgical removal of lymph nodes in the underarm, groin, or pelvic regions

- RADIATION THERAPY to the underarm, groin, pelvic, or neck regions

- scar tissue in the lymphatic ducts or veins or under the collarbone caused by surgery or radiation therapy

- cancer that has spread to the lymph nodes in the neck, chest, underarm, pelvis, or abdomen

- tumors in the pelvis or abdomen that block lymph drainage

- being too thin or too heavy—these conditions may delay recovery and increase the risk for lymphedema.

Symptoms

Lymphedema can develop in any part of the body, causing symptoms such as a full sensation in the limb; tightened skin; decreased flexibility in the hand, wrist, or ankle; problems fitting into clothing; or tightness of a ring, wristwatch, or bracelet. A patient in the early stages of lymphedema will have swelling that indents with pressure, but remains soft. The swelling may easily improve by supporting the arm or leg in a raised position, gently exercising, and wearing elastic support garments.

However, continued problems with the lymphatic system cause the lymphatic vessels to expand. As lymph flows back into the body tissues, the condition worsens. This causes pain, heat, redness, and swelling as the body tries to get rid of the extra fluid. The skin becomes hard and stiff and no longer improves with raised support of the arm or leg, gentle exercise, or elastic support garments.

Stages

Lymphedema develops in a number of stages, from mild to severe.

Stage 1 (spontaneously reversible): In the initial stage of lymphedema, tissue will look pitted when pressed by fingertips. Typically, upon waking in the morning the affected area looks normal.

Stage 2 (spontaneously irreversible): In this intermediate stage, the tissue has a spongy consistency and will bounce back when pressed by fingertips, with no pitting. The area will begin to harden and get larger.

Stage 3 (lymphostatic elephantiasis): In this advanced stage, the swelling is irreversible and the affected area has usually grown quite large. The tissue is hard and unresponsive. Some patients consider undergoing reconstructive surgery (debulking) at this stage.

Acute Lymphedema

There are four types of acute lymphedema, which may be treated with different kinds of decongestive therapy, such as manual lymphatic drainage, bandaging, proper skin care and diet, compression garments (sleeves or stockings), or remedial exercises.

The first type of acute lymphedema is mild and lasts only a short time, appearing right after surgery to remove the lymph nodes. The affected limb may be warm and slightly red but is usually not painful. The problem improves within a week if the limb is supported in a raised position and if appropriate exercises are performed: for example, contracting the muscles in the affected limb (such as by making a fist and releasing it).

The second type of acute lymphedema occurs six to eight weeks after surgery or during radiation therapy. This type may be caused by inflammation of either lymphatic vessels or veins, producing a limb that is tender, warm, and red. It is treated by keeping the limb supported in a raised position and taking anti-inflammatory drugs.

The third type of acute lymphedema occurs after an insect bite, minor injury, or burn that causes an infection of the skin and the lymphatic vessels near the skin surface in an arm or leg that is chronically swollen. The affected area is red, very tender, and hot and is treated by supporting the affected arm or leg in a raised position and taking antibiotics. Using a compression pump or wrapping the affected area with elastic bandages should not be done during the early stages of infection. Mild redness may continue after the infection is healed.

The fourth and most common type of acute lymphedema develops very slowly and may become noticeable only two years or more after surgery—or not until many years after other cancer treatment. The patient may experience discomfort of the skin or aching in the neck, shoulders, spine, or hips caused by stretching of the soft tissues, overuse of muscles, or posture changes caused by increased weight of the arm or leg.

Temporary vs. Chronic Lymphedema

Temporary lymphedema lasts less than six months and does not involve hardening of the skin. A patient may be more likely to develop temporary lymphedema if there is

- a surgical drain that leaks protein into the surgical site
- inflammation
- inability to move the limb
- temporary loss of lymphatic function
- blockage of a vein by a blood clot or inflammation of a vein

Chronic (long-term) lymphedema is the most difficult of all types of swelling to treat; it occurs when the damaged lymphatic system of the affected area is not able to handle the increased need for fluid drainage from the body tissues. This may happen

- after a tumor recurs or spreads to the lymph nodes
- after an infection of the lymphatic vessels
- after periods of not being able to move the limbs
- after radiation therapy or surgery
- when early signs of lymphedema have not been controlled
- when a vein is blocked by a blood clot

Patients with chronic lymphedema are at increased risk of infection. No effective treatment is yet available for patients who have advanced chronic lymphedema. Once the body tissues have been repeatedly stretched, lymphedema may recur more easily.

Prevention

Poor drainage of the lymphatic system due to surgery to remove the lymph nodes or radiation therapy may make the affected arm or leg more susceptible to serious infection. Even a small infection may lead to serious lymphedema.

It is important that patients take precautions to prevent injury and infection in the affected arm or leg since lymphedema can occur 30 or more years after surgery. Breast cancer patients who follow instructions about skin care and proper exercise after mastectomy are less likely to experience lymphedema.

Exercise, which improves lymphatic drainage, can help prevent lymphedema. Breast cancer patients should do hand and arm exercises after mastectomy, and those who have surgery that affects pelvic lymph node drainage should do leg and foot exercises.

See also LYMPHANGIOSARCOMA.

lymph node dissection The removal of the LYMPH NODES from a specific area.

lymph nodes Small oval structures, ranging in size from a pinhead to a bean, that filter germs and for-

eign substances from lymph (the clear fluid that bathes many of the body's organs). When lymph nodes trap germs, they swell, which is why a swollen lymph gland is often a sign of infection or disease. A valuable part of the IMMUNE SYSTEM, lymph nodes are linked via lymphatic vessels throughout the body. Lymph nodes can be found under the arms, behind the knee and ears, in the groin, and in the abdominal cavity. (See also SENTINEL NODE BIOPSY, LYMPH NODE DISSECTION, and LYMPHEDEMA.)

lymphoblastic non-Hodgkin's lymphoma A type of NON-HODGKIN'S LYMPHOMA that usually occurs in children and young adults, usually arising in the chest.

See also LYMPHOMA.

lymphocytic lymphoma A type of NON-HODGKIN'S LYMPHOMA in which the cancer cells are quite small.

lymphoma A general term that refers to cancers that develop in the LYMPHATIC SYSTEM, which affects the immune system. Most lymphomas appear in the LYMPH NODES. Lymphomas, which include HODGKIN'S DISEASE and NON-HODGKIN'S LYMPHOMA, are the fifth most common type of cancer diagnosed and the sixth most common type to result in death in the United States. Lymphomas account for about 5 percent of all cases of cancer in this country. Of the two basic lymphoma types, non-Hodgkin's lymphoma is the more common.

Hodgkin's disease has unique characteristics that separate it from other types of lymphoma, such as the presence of giant abnormal cells called Reed-Sternberg cells. Hodgkin's also has a better prognosis than other types of lymphomas and is less likely to spread. Non-Hodgkin's disease is more likely to develop outside the lymph nodes (in bones or the liver).

See also LYMPHOMA RESEARCH FOUNDATION.

Lymphoma Research Foundation (LRF) A nonprofit foundation whose mission is to eradicate LYMPHOMA and serve those touched by the disease. In November 2001, the Cure for Lymphoma Foundation and the Lymphoma Research Foundation of America merged to become the Lymphoma Research Foundation.

With years of experience in developing programs for patients, caregivers, and professionals, and more than $7 million of research funded, the LRF provides comprehensive services and solutions for the lymphoma community. The LRF also advocates to make federal funding of lymphoma research a national priority. For contact information, see Appendix I.

lymphoplasmacytic disorders See LEUKEMIA.

lymphoproliferative disorders See LEUKEMIA.

lymphosarcoma An outdated name for a condition now known as LYMPHOBLASTIC NON-HODGKIN'S LYMPHOMA.

macrobiotic diet   Advocates of this semivegetarian diet believe that disease can be prevented by adjusting food, lifestyle, relationships, and environment. According to the macrobiotic philosophy, everything in the world (including cancer) has two opposite forces: yin and yang. Macrobiotic diet proponents believe that an imbalance of yin and yang may cause cancer, so the diet is planned to correct any imbalances of yin and yang that lead to ill health.

The modern macrobiotic diet contains 50 percent whole cereal and grains, 20 percent to 30 percent vegetables, 5 percent to 10 percent soups, and 5 percent to 10 percent beans and sea vegetables. Foods that may occasionally be eaten include fish, seafood, seasonal fruits, nuts, seeds, and other natural snacks. Sugar and meat are not allowed in a macrobiotic diet.

The American Medical Association, the U.S. Food and Drug Administration, and nutrition experts believe a macrobiotic diet can be harmful. The NATIONAL CANCER INSTITUTE (NCI) and the AMERICAN CANCER SOCIETY believe that a strict macrobiotic diet is not effective in treating or preventing cancer, and that there are risks associated with the diet.

Diet critics warn that the modern macrobiotic diet may not provide enough of certain nutrients, including protein, vitamins D and B_{12}, and the minerals zinc, calcium, and iron. An earlier version of the macrobiotic diet that included only grains has been associated with severe malnutrition and even death. According to the NCI, no clinical trials have been conducted showing the health benefits of the macrobiotic diet.

magnetic resonance imaging (MRI)   A diagnostic technique that uses a magnetic field rather than radiation (as used in X-rays and radionuclide scans) to produce pictures of structures inside the body. It is used to diagnose and evaluate the extent of cancer, and it can produce images of blood vessels, cerebrospinal fluid, cartilage, BONE MARROW, muscles, ligaments, and the spinal cord.

An MRI is more expensive than a CAT scan, but it produces pictures with greater clarity and definition. Because there are no dyes or radiation, it is considered to be safer than X-rays or CAT scans. However, patients with any metal in their body (such as pacemakers, joint pins, surgical clips, artificial heart valves, an IUD, or shrapnel) may not be given MRI scans.

MRI is the most effective diagnostic procedure for tumors in the neurological system and for HEAD AND NECK CANCER.

malignant fibrous histiocytoma (MFH)   A type of SARCOMA that usually occurs in the ends of long bones such as the arms or legs (especially in the knee). Most common in middle-aged men, MFH is usually treated with surgery and CHEMOTHERAPY.

malignant melanoma   See MELANOMA.

malt lymphoma   A type of NON-HODGKIN'S LYMPHOMA.

mammoplasty   Plastic surgery of the breast.
See also BREAST RECONSTRUCTION.

mammography   A special series of X-rays that show images of the soft tissues of the breast, designed to help find BREAST CANCER early, when it can still be cured. Yearly mammograms are recommended for women over 40 years old even if they have no signs of breast cancer, and for younger women who have symptoms of breast cancer or who have a high risk of getting breast cancer. The entire procedure for a screening mammogram takes about 20 minutes.

Only one or two mammograms out of every 1,000 lead to a diagnosis of cancer; about 10 percent of women will have a suspicious mammogram that requires further testing. Of women with these suspicious mammograms, only 8 percent to 10 percent will need a biopsy—and 80 percent of those biopsies will not be cancer.

The modern mammography machine is used only for breast X-rays to produce high-quality pictures with a low radiation dose (usually about 0.1 to 0.2 rads per picture). In the past there were concerns about radiation risks, but today's machines pose only a very small risk. For example, a woman who receives radiation as a treatment for breast cancer will receive several thousand rads, whereas a woman who has had a mammogram every year for 50 years will have received only 20 to 40 total rads. Moreover, mammograms use a different type of X-ray, which does not penetrate tissue as easily as the X-ray used for routine films of chest, arms, or legs.

When health-care professionals take a mammogram, the breast is squeezed between two plates to spread the tissue apart and to allow a lower dose of radiation. This procedure produces a black-and-white image of the breast tissue on a large sheet of film, which is interpreted by a radiologist. Reading mammograms is difficult because there is a wide range in what is considered normal, and the appearance of the breast on a mammogram varies a great deal from woman to woman. This is why it is extremely helpful for a radiologist to have previous X-ray films from the same woman for comparison.

Abnormal Findings

A mammogram may reveal tiny white spots on the film, which are tiny mineral deposits within the breast tissue called calcifications, or may highlight a suspicious mass.

Calcifications Macrocalcifications are large calcium deposits that appear in the breast as a result of aging, old injuries, or inflammation. These deposits are related to noncancerous conditions and do not require a biopsy. Macrocalcifications

occur in about half of all women over 50, and in one of 10 women under 50.

MICROCALCIFICATIONS are tiny specks of calcium in the breast that may appear alone or in clusters. The shape and location of microcalcifications can help a radiologist determine how likely it is that the areas are malignant. In some cases, microcalcifications do not require a BIOPSY, but only a follow-up mammogram within three to six months. In other cases, the microcalcifications are suspicious and a biopsy is recommended.

Mass A mass may occur with or without calcifications and can be caused by benign breast conditions or by breast cancer. Some masses can be monitored with periodic mammography, while others may need a biopsy. The size, shape, and margins of the mass help the radiologist to determine the likelihood of cancer. Many masses turn out to be cysts (a benign collection of fluid); to confirm that a mass is really a CYST, a doctor must either order a breast ultrasound or remove some fluid with a needle.

If a mass is not a cyst, then the patient may need more imaging tests. Prior mammograms may help show that a mass has not changed for many years, indicating a benign condition.

If a mass raises a significant suspicion of cancer, tissue must be removed for examination under the microscope to tell if it is cancer. This can be done with needle biopsy or open surgical biopsy.

The U.S. Food and Drug Administration (FDA) inspects and certifies all mammogram facilities in the United States.

Screening Mammograms

A screening mammogram is an X-ray of the breast in a woman who has no breast complaints. Screening mammography is designed to find cancer when it is still too small to be felt by a doctor or patient. Finding small breast cancers early by a screening mammogram greatly improves a woman's chance for successful treatment. A screening mammogram usually involves two X-rays of each breast.

The AMERICAN CANCER SOCIETY'S breast cancer detection guidelines call for yearly screening mammograms for all women 40 years of age and older, in part because results from a recent compilation of many studies found 17 percent fewer deaths from breast cancer among women in their 40s who had mammograms. The American Cancer Society believes that the benefits of a yearly mammogram for women 40 and older outweigh the effect of occasional false positive results that require a biopsy of benign conditions. While there is some risk of exposure to radiation, the low dose of radiation from modern mammography is not thought to pose a significant risk.

Because mammograms cannot find all breast cancers, the American Cancer Society recommends that in addition to regular mammograms, women without symptoms have yearly clinical breast exams by a health-care professional and perform monthly breast self-examinations. These guidelines apply only to women at usual risk for breast cancer, who have no symptoms of breast cancer. For these women, the society also recommends that women 20 to 39 have a physical examination of the breast every three years, performed by a health-care professional.

Women at high risk for breast cancer should discuss their situation with their doctor. In some cases, mammograms should be started before age 40, and a more frequent schedule of early detection tests may be appropriate. For example, doctors recommend that a baseline mammogram be done at age 25 for women whose genetic testing results show changes in breast cancer susceptibility genes (BRCA1/BRCA2).

Diagnostic Mammograms

A woman who either has a breast complaint (such as a breast mass) or whose screening mammogram has picked up an abnormality will be scheduled for a diagnostic mammogram. A diagnostic mammogram will involve more pictures to allow the radiologist to carefully study the breast condition. Special images known as cone views with magnification are used to make a small area of altered breast tissue easier to evaluate. As a result of the diagnostic mammogram, the doctor may suggest that a biopsy is needed to tell whether or not the lesion is cancer. About 80 percent of all breast lesions that are biopsied are found to be benign when evaluated under the microscope. If a biopsy is recommended, the woman should discuss the different types of biopsy with her doctor to determine which method of biopsy is best for her.

Breast Imaging Reporting and Data System

The American College of Radiology has developed a standard way of describing mammogram findings by giving the results a code numbered 0 through 5, called the Breast Imaging Reporting and Data System (BIRADS):

Category 0: Assessment is incomplete and additional imaging evaluation is needed. A possible abnormality may not be completely seen or defined and will need additional evaluation including the use of spot compression, magnification views, special mammographic views, or ultrasound.

Category 1: No significant abnormality to report. The breasts are symmetrical without masses, distortion, or suspicious calcifications.

Category 2: This is a negative mammogram that has found a benign lesion, such as benign calcifications, intramammary lymph nodes, and calcified fibroadenomas. Categorizing the mammogram this way ensures that other individuals viewing the mammogram will not misinterpret a benign finding as suspicious and documents the finding to use in future mammogram assessments.

Category 3: This is a "probably benign finding" that suggests the need for a short-term follow-up. Results in this category are probably benign, and the results are not expected to change. However, since it has not been proven benign, the doctor will want to see if the lesion changes over time. In this case, follow-up imaging is usually done every six months for a year, and then every year for two years. This helps avoid unnecessary biopsies but ensures that any malignancy will be detected within a short period of time.

Category 4: This result is a suspicious abnormality, requiring a biopsy. In this case, while the findings do not definitely look like cancer, there is a substantial probability of malignancy.

Category 5: These findings are characteristic of cancers, with a high probability of malignancy. Biopsy is very strongly recommended.

Mammogram Facility Certification

The MAMMOGRAPHY QUALITY STANDARDS ACT (MQSA) requires mammography facilities to adhere to strict quality standards. For example, mammography facilities must give women written results of their mammograms in easy-to-understand language within 30 days of the mammogram. Patients may also obtain their original mammogram (not a copy) from the facility so they may compare the results with previous mammograms.

Women do not need to be referred by a physician in order to have a mammogram at most facilities. Women who do not have a primary-care physician or do not wish to be referred by their physician may "self-refer" at most facilities. Self-referred patients with no doctor will receive both the simplified report and the report designated for the physician.

If an abnormality is found on the patient's mammogram, the facility is required to notify the patient and her physician (if appropriate) and recommend a suitable course of action. Women who do not receive their mammogram results within 30 days should contact the mammography facility and ask for the results. Women should not assume that their mammogram is normal if they do not receive the results. Facility certification can now be extended to include FDA-approved digital mammography units.

A woman can locate a nearby certified mammogram facility by visiting the Web site of the Center for Devices and Radiological Health of the FDA. This Web site (www.accessdata.fda.gov/scripts/cdrh/cfdocs/cfmqsa/search.cfm) includes an extensive mammography site database; women may search for a nearby mammography clinic by entering their state and zip code.

The following regulations govern every mammography facility in the United States:

- Physicians who interpret mammograms, radiologic technologists who perform mammography, and medical physicists who survey mammography equipment must have adequate training and experience.

- Each mammography facility must have an effective quality control program and maintain thorough records.

- Each facility must submit typical mammography images (X-rays) to the FDA for review. The FDA will evaluate the quality and amount of radia-

tion used to obtain the images (radiation levels are required to be low).

- Each mammography facility must develop systems for following up on mammograms that reveal abnormalities and for obtaining biopsy results.

- Each mammography facility must undergo yearly inspections by FDA or state-certified inspectors.

As of April 30, 2002, there were 9,433 MQSA-certified mammography facilities in the United States and its territories. Of these, 216 are in the process of becoming fully certified; the rest are already fully certified.

Mammography Quality Standards Act of 1992/1998   A federal law establishing requirements for the accreditation, certification, and inspection of MAMMOGRAPHY facilities to ensure that all women have access to high-quality mammography services. In the fall of 1998 Congress reauthorized MQSA, effective on May 7, 2002. Congress enacted the law because of the understanding that the effectiveness of mammography as a breast cancer detection technique is directly related to the quality of mammography procedures.

As a result of this legislation, facilities must be certified to lawfully perform mammography and to be reimbursed by MEDICARE and Medicaid for mammography services. In order to be certified, the equipment, personnel, and practice of the facility must be reviewed by an FDA-approved accreditation body. The facility must meet the following criteria:

- Each mammogram machine must be accredited.

- Certain personnel must meet strict standards, including radiologists, radiologic mammography technologists (the individuals who actually position women for the exam and take the mammogram pictures), and medical physicists (professionals who specialize in medical equipment and image production).

- Typical X-rays are reviewed for quality and information on radiation dose, which is required to be very low.

If the facility meets all of the appropriate standards, the FDA gives its certification. The FDA has a list of all of its certified mammography facilities by state and Zip code; it is also available at the FDA's Web site at www.fda.gov/cdrh/mammography/certified.html.

Reporting Results

Mammogram clinics are now required to notify women in writing about the results of their mammograms. The Mammography Quality Standards Act was recently changed in response to reports that some women were not learning soon enough that they had suspicious mammograms. Mammogram clinics are continuing to report mammogram results to the woman's doctor, who is responsible for ordering additional tests or treatments, but now clinics must mail women a separate, easy-to-understand report of their mammogram results within 30 days (sooner if the mammogram results suggest cancer is present) so that the woman knows the results even if her doctor has not yet called to inform her.

As of April 30, 2002, there were 9,433 MQSA-certified mammography facilities operating in the United States. Of these, 9,217 facilities are fully certified and the rest were in the process of becoming fully certified. Facilities that fail accreditation must stop providing mammography services. However, once the deficiencies have been corrected, a facility may apply for reinstatement to resume the accreditation process. FDA uses a state-of-the-art database, which tracks certification, inspections, and accreditation information, that allows it to assess facilities' compliance with MQSA.

marijuana (*Cannabis sativa L.*)   A member of the cannabis plant family that can relax the mind and body, ease NAUSEA, and heighten perception. One naturally occurring component of marijuana, delta-9-THC (dronabinol), is now available in synthetic form as the drug MARINOL, which is used to treat nausea and vomiting in CHEMOTHERAPY patients. Although marijuana use is illegal in the United States, the U.S. Food and Drug Administration in 1985 approved Marinol for cancer chemotherapy patients who failed to respond to conventional antinausea treatments.

Although research has shown that THC is more quickly absorbed from marijuana smoke than from an oral preparation, any antinausea effects of smoking marijuana may not be consistent because potency will vary depending on the source of the marijuana.

Eight states (Alaska, California, Colorado, Hawaii, Maine, Nevada, Oregon, and Washington) already allow seriously ill patients to use medical marijuana, usually through a doctor's recommendation and an independent board's certification. A similar bill that would have allowed medical marijuana in New Mexico was defeated in March 2003.

The Marinol patient assistance program is designed to help cover the costs of Marinol. For eligible patients with financial need, Marinol may be supplied free of charge. Information about the program is available at (800) 256-8918.

Marinol (dronabinol)   The synthetic version of medicinal MARIJUANA used to treat NAUSEA and vomiting in CHEMOTHERAPY patients who do not respond to any other antinausea medication.

mastectomy   Mastectomy is an operation to remove the breast (or as much of the breast as possible).

In *segmental mastectomy,* the surgeon removes the cancer and a larger area of normal breast tissue around it. Occasionally, some of the lining over the chest muscles below the tumor is removed as well. Some LYMPH NODES under the arm may also be removed.

In a *simple (or total) mastectomy,* the whole breast is removed; sometimes the lymph nodes under the arm are also removed.

In a *modified radical mastectomy,* the whole breast, most of the lymph nodes under the arm, and often the lining over the chest muscles are removed. The smaller of the two chest muscles is also taken out to help in removing the lymph nodes.

A *radical mastectomy* is the removal of the breast as well as the surrounding lymph nodes, muscles, fatty tissue, and skin. Formerly considered the standard surgery for women with breast cancer, this procedure is rarely used today. In rare cases, radical mastectomy may be suggested if the cancer has spread to the chest muscles.

To perform a simple mastectomy, a surgeon makes an incision along the perimeter of the breast closest to the tumor, leaving most of the skin intact. Typically, the nipple is not removed during a simple mastectomy, but the underlying tissue is gently cut free and removed. A drainage tube is inserted, and the wound is then closed with stitches, tape, or clips. A mastectomy with lymph node dissection usually lasts between two and three hours; immediate breast reconstruction will increase the length of surgery.

The drainage tube placed in the breast or under the arm removes blood and lymph node fluid that builds up during the healing process. Drainage tubes are usually removed within two weeks, when the drainage is reduced to less than 1 ounce a day.

Major soreness from mastectomy usually lasts two to three days, although many mastectomy patients do not experience soreness after surgery. Studies have shown that many women experience phantom breast sensations after mastectomy, including sensations of unpleasant itching, pins and needles, pressure, or throbbing. This pain probably occurs as the result of damage to nerves in the area. Women who experience breast pain prior to mastectomy are most likely to have sensations of pain in the breast area after surgery. Exercise or breast massage may help ease phantom breast pain; in more severe cases, drugs may be needed. Phantom breast pain does not indicate that cancer cells are still present in the breast area or that cancer may return.

Lymph Node Dissection

A radical mastectomy, modified radical mastectomy, or lumpectomy often includes the removal of lymph nodes from the underarm (axillary node dissection). After surgery, the lymph nodes are examined to determine whether the cancer has spread past the breast.

SENTINEL LYMPH NODE BIOPSY is a new form of lymph node dissection, in which only one to three sentinel lymph nodes (the first nodes in the lymphatic chain) are removed. In this procedure, blue dye is injected into the area near a tumor. The dye is then carried to the sentinel node (the lymph node most likely to harbor cancer cells if the disease has spread), where it can be identified visually by the surgery. If the sentinel node contains cancer, more lymph nodes are removed and examined, but if the sentinel node is cancer free, additional lymph node surgery may be avoided.

Research shows that sentinel lymph node biopsy may eliminate the need to remove many lymph nodes and may reduce the chances of lymphedema (chronic arm swelling).

Prophylactic Mastectomy

Preventive mastectomy is the surgical removal of one or both breasts in an effort to prevent or reduce the risk of breast cancer. The procedure of choice is a total mastectomy, in which the entire breast and nipple is removed. A subcutaneous mastectomy is recommended less often because this operation removes the breast tissue but spares the nipple, which increases the risk of leaving cancerous breast tissue behind.

A woman may consider preventive mastectomy on one side if she has already had one breast removed due to cancer. Preventive mastectomy may also be an option for women with the cancer-causing gene *BRCA1* or *BRCA2*, or who have a strong family history of breast cancer, especially if several close relatives developed the disease before age 50. In addition, preventive mastectomy is sometimes considered for women who have had lobular carcinoma in situ, a condition that increases their risk of developing breast cancer in the same or in the opposite breast. Rarely, preventive mastectomy may be considered for women with widespread breast microcalcifications or for women whose breast tissue is very dense. Dense breast tissue is linked to a higher risk of breast cancer and also makes it more difficult to diagnose breast problems.

Although having a preventive mastectomy can reduce a woman's risk, it cannot completely protect her from developing breast cancer. Because it is impossible for a surgeon to remove all breast tissue, breast cancer can still develop in the small amount of remaining tissue left behind.

The procedure should be considered in the context of each woman's unique risk factors and her level of concern. Women considering a preventive mastectomy should discuss with a doctor her risk of developing breast cancer, the surgical procedure and her feelings about it, alternatives to surgery, and possible complications.

Doctors do not always agree on the most effective way to manage the care of women with a strong family history of breast cancer or other risk factors. Some doctors recommend preventive mastectomy, while others may prescribe tamoxifen, a medication that can lessen the chance of getting breast cancer in women at high risk for the disease. Some doctors may advise periodic mammograms, regular checkups with a clinical breast examination, and monthly breast self-examinations to increase the chance of detecting breast cancer at an early stage. Although the effects are not proven, doctors may also encourage women at high risk to limit their consumption of alcohol, eat a low-fat diet, engage in regular exercise, and avoid hormone replacement therapy.

Breast Reconstruction

After mastectomy many women choose to have BREAST RECONSTRUCTION, in which either a saline implant or skin, fat, and muscle from a woman's abdomen, back, or buttocks are used to form a new breast. Before performing this type of procedure, the plastic surgeon carefully examines the breasts and discusses the appropriate types of reconstruction.

Women who have reconstructive surgery will be followed carefully to detect complications such as infection, movement of the implant, or contracture (the formation of a firm, fibrous shell around the implant). After surgery, patients will still need to be routinely screened for breast cancer because the risk of cancer cannot be completely eliminated.

Women who do not wish to have reconstruction surgery may be fitted with an artificial breast after healing from mastectomy. Most prostheses are made to resemble the body's own weight and touch. Several manufacturers also make special mastectomy bras with breast pockets.

maxillofacial prosthetic   A plastic or silicone replacement for a body part removed from the head because of cancer.

maxillofacial prosthodontist   A dental specialist who is an expert in restoring the oral area after cancer surgery, restructuring the face and head to improve speaking, eating, or swallowing.

mediastinoscopy   An examination of the space in the chest between the breastbone, lungs, and spine using a thin lighted instrument that is inserted through a small incision in the neck. The tube is passed behind the breastbone in front of the trachea so as to allow the surgeon to remove and examine the LYMPH NODES. This surgical procedure is performed under general anesthesia and can be used to diagnose or stage LUNG CANCER and LYMPHOMA.

medical oncologist   See ONCOLOGIST.

Medicare   A federally subsidized insurance program, established by Congress in 1965, for citizens over age 65. Medicare has two parts: Part A, which is free, pays all of the inpatient hospital care after a $876 deductible, and a variety of follow-up services. Part B, for which patients pay a monthly premium, pays 80 percent of doctors' services, outpatient hospital care, and other medical expenses. Some people also decide to buy "Medigap" insurance to cover the unpaid 20 percent of medical costs.

In addition to people over age 65, those who have permanent kidney failure or who have received Social Security Disability Income (SSDI) for 24 months are eligible to enroll.

Cancer patients whose disease has spread are usually considered permanently disabled and are therefore also eligible for Medicare, no matter what their age. Generally, if the cancer has spread to a major organ, such as the lung, liver, or brain, patients will be accepted into the program.

medullary cancer   A term used to describe cancer in the innermost part of an organ.

medullary carcinoma of the breast   A rare type of infiltrating ductal BREAST CANCER with a relatively well defined, distinct boundary between tumor tissue and normal breast tissue. It also has a number of other special features, including the large size of the cancer cells and the presence of immune system cells at the edges of the tumor.

Medullary carcinoma accounts for only about 5 percent of all breast cancers. It has a slightly better prognosis and a slightly lower chance of spreading than invasive lobular or invasive ductal cancers of the same size.

medulloblastoma See BRAIN CANCER.

melanin The pigment that gives skin, hair, and the iris of the eyes their color; the more melanin present, the darker the color. A person's level of melanin depends on race, heredity, and sun exposure. The amount of melanin in the skin is a major factor in the development of SKIN CANCER; dark-skinned people have a much lower rate of cancer of the skin.

melanoma The most deadly form of the three major types of SKIN CANCER. Melanoma is much more dangerous than other forms of skin cancer because of its tendency to spread rapidly to vital internal organs such as the lungs, liver, and brain. One in five patients afflicted with malignant melanoma dies of this cancer. It is the most often diagnosed cancer among women aged 25 to 29, and it ranks second in frequency only to BREAST CANCER among those women aged 30 to 34.

Symptoms

Melanoma usually begins as a pigmented growth on the skin, displaying many shades of color (including brown, black, pink, white, blue, and/or gray). It often has irregular outlines and may be larger than an ordinary mole. The spot may bleed, crust, or itch, and at times may develop within already existing moles. It is therefore important that any change in a mole be examined by a dermatologist.

Types of Melanoma

There are four types of melanoma, each with a characteristic growth pattern:

Superficial spreading melanoma This is the most common type, accounting for 70 percent of all cases. It typically begins from a preexisting mole and expands in a radial fashion before it enters a vertical growth phase.

Nodular melanoma A more aggressive tumor found more often in men, this accounts for about 15 to 30 percent of cases. It begins from normal skin and has no radial growth phase.

Lentigo maligna melanoma This type accounts for less than 10 percent of cases and is found more often on the face of a woman or an older person. The lesions, which are typically large and flat, are slow growing and rarely spread.

Acral lentiginous melanoma This type of melanoma, which occurs on the soles of the feet, accounts for less than 10 percent of lesions but occurs in a higher proportion of nonwhite patients (in whom it accounts for between 35 percent and 60 percent of lesions).

Causes/Risk Factors

In 1935, when few people habitually baked at the beach, melanoma was a rare disease, affecting only one in 1,500 Americans. Today the worldwide incidence of melanoma is increasing at a faster rate than any other type of cancer, with the exception of LUNG CANCER in women. In the United States alone, the incidence has tripled in the last 40 years and nearly doubled in the last decade. An estimated 40,300 Americans developed melanoma in 1997, and 7,300 died of the disease that year. Today, one in every 90 Caucasian Americans will eventually develop melanoma.

Those at higher risk have a family history of skin cancer, an abundance of moles (more than 100), fair skin, light hair, and blue-green or gray eyes. Recently scientists have identified a defective gene that appears to cause an inherited tendency to develop this type of deadly skin cancer, and that may also play a role in noninherited melanoma. About 10 percent of melanoma occurs in people with an inherited tendency, and it is unclear what percentage of inherited cases are due to this gene.

Normally, the gene acts as a brake on cancer, but those who inherit a defective version lose part of its protection, making them unusually susceptible to melanoma. The normal gene tells the body how to make a protein called p16, which helps regulate cell division. Studies have suggested that the p16 gene is a tumor suppressor cell that discourages development of tumors. These studies also indicated that defective versions play a role in cancer.

Defective versions of the gene also may be involved in many or even most cases of noninherited melanoma, according to research. In those cases, the gene would be inherited in normal form but would then mutate after exposure to sunlight. Researchers hope that studying this gene may someday lead to a screening test for those at risk, and for better treatments for the noninherited disease.

Other risk factors for developing melanoma are severe sunburns in childhood (even one raises the risk). Anyone with multiple moles may also suffer from DYSPLASTIC NEVUS SYNDROME and may be at increased risk for the development of melanoma.

All patients with a history of malignant melanoma have about a 5 percent risk of developing another, unrelated melanoma of the skin. This process is called multiple primary melanoma formation. If a second melanoma of the skin develops, it is important to determine whether it is a new skin melanoma (a second primary tumor) or a spreading of the original tumor. If the lesion has spread, the disease must be classified as Stage III, and the likelihood of death within five years increases significantly.

Although melanoma many times begins without the presence of a mole, it most often does start within such a growth.

Diagnosis

Because the skin can be so easily seen, malignant melanoma can be easier to spot than internal cancers. To make sure that people notice skin cancer, dermatologists recommend that everyone examine their skin twice a year, using a full-length and a handheld mirror. Any suspicious growths should be reported immediately to a dermatologist.

Treatment

Most skin cancers (even malignant melanoma) can be cured if discovered early enough, which is why attention to symptoms and regular self-exams are highly recommended. When cancers of the skin are discovered early, there are a variety of treatment possibilities, depending on the type of tumor, its size, location, and other factors affecting the patient's general health. A BIOPSY is often needed before a treatment option is chosen.

Surgical removal of the tumor, along with a margin of normal skin, is usually required, together with a SENTINEL NODE BIOPSY or possible surgical removal of nearby LYMPH NODES. A skin graft may be necessary after the tumor is removed.

CHEMOTHERAPY or radiation may be added to the treatment plan after the surgical removal of the tumor and surrounding skin. Radiation may be added to the treatment plan after the surgical removal of the tumor and surrounding skin, if residual tumor was present.

Prognosis

The thickness of the tumor is the single most important factor in determining prognosis. The cure rate approaches 100 percent if the melanoma is found early enough. However, if deep local spread has occurred, the number of people who live for at least five years is only 30 percent. With spread of cancer to distant sites, five-year survival is less than 10 percent.

melanoma, amelanotic   A type of SKIN CANCER in which the cells do not make melanin. Skin lesions are often irregular and may be pink, red, or have light brown, tan, or gray at the edges. (See also MELANOMA.)

meningeal carcinomatosis   Cancer that has spread from elsewhere in the body into the surface of the brain, causing confusion and a range of other neurological symptoms. This type of metastatic cancer is diagnosed with a spinal tap and biopsy. It is treated with CHEMOTHERAPY, injected into the spinal fluid but the prognosis is poor.

meningioma   See BRAIN CANCER.

menopause   The end of a woman's monthly menstrual cycle. Menopause usually occurs naturally in a woman's late 40s or early 50s, but it can also be surgically triggered with the removal of both ovaries (HYSTERO-OOPHORECTOMY) or by chemotherapy, which often destroys ovarian function.

Merkel cell carcinoma   A rare, aggressive type of SKIN CANCER in which malignant cells are found just under the skin, creating firm, painless, shiny lumps of skin that may be red, pink, or blue. Merkel cell carcinoma (also called neuroendocrine cancer of the skin) is usually found on the sun-exposed areas of the head, neck, arms, and legs, primarily in whites between 60 and 80 years of age. Only 5 percent of cases are diagnosed before age 50. In the United States, Merkel cell carcinoma is quite rare, accounting for far less than one percent of all skin cancers. Precise data on national incidence, however, are not available.

Merkel cell carcinoma grows quickly and often spreads to other parts of the body, first moving into the nearby lymph nodes and then on to the liver, bone, lungs, and brain.

Staging

After Merkel cell carcinoma has been diagnosed, more tests will be done to find out if cancer cells have spread to other parts of the body.

Stage I: Cancerous cells have not spread to lymph nodes or other parts of the body.

Stage II: The cancer has spread to nearby lymph nodes but has not spread to other parts of the body.

Stage III: The cancer has spread beyond nearby lymph nodes and to other parts of the body.

Recurrent: The cancer has recurred after initial treatment, either in the same location or in another part of the body.

Treatment

Treatment of Merkel cell carcinoma depends on the stage of the disease, and the patient's age and overall condition, but usually includes surgery to remove the tumor, followed by CHEMOTHERAPY and radiation. There are several different kinds of surgery to remove Merkel cell carcinoma, including wide surgical excision (removing the cancer and some surrounding skin), CRYOSURGERY to freeze and then remove the tumor, or tissue-sparing micrographic surgery to remove only the tumor.

Prognosis

The two-year survival rate for this cancer is 50 to 70 percent, because the lesions grow rapidly and often spread to other parts of the body. Even relatively small tumors are capable of spreading.

mesenchymoma, malignant A type of soft tissue SARCOMA that may appear in the arms, hands, legs, or feet. It is also known as mixed-cell sarcoma.

mesothelioma A rare form of cancer in which malignant cells grow in the mesothelium, the protective lining that covers most of the body's internal organs. Most people who develop mesothelioma have worked at jobs where they inhaled ASBESTOS particles.

The mesothelium has different names depending on the part of the body where it appears; it includes the pleura (lining of the chest), the pericardium (lining of the heart), and peritoneum (lining of the abdominal cavity). Although the number of reported cases has increased in the past 20 years, mesothelioma is still relatively rare. About 3,000 new cases are diagnosed in the United States each year, more often in men than in women, and more often among older people. By the year 2030, experts estimate there will be about 300,000 cases. Only about 20 percent of patients who find this deadly cancer early and treat it aggressively will reach the five-year-survival mark.

Cause

Working with asbestos is the major risk factor for mesothelioma; there is a link between asbestos and this disease in about 70 percent to 80 percent of all cases. However, mesothelioma also has been reported in some individuals without any known exposure to asbestos. (Although smoking does not seem to boost the risk of developing mesothelioma, the combination of smoking and asbestos exposure significantly increases a person's risk of developing cancer of the air passageways in the lung.)

The risk of mesothelioma rises with more extensive exposure to asbestos and longer exposure time. However, some individuals with only brief exposures have developed mesothelioma. On the other hand, not all workers who are heavily exposed develop asbestos-related diseases.

There is some evidence that people living with asbestos workers have an increased risk of developing mesothelioma, which may be caused by inhaling asbestos dust brought home on the clothing and hair of these workers.

Symptoms

Symptoms of mesothelioma, which may not appear until 50 years after exposure to asbestos, include

- shortness of breath and pain in the chest (pleural mesothelioma)
- weight loss
- abdominal pain and swelling
- bowel obstruction
- blood clotting abnormalities
- anemia
- fever
- If the cancer has spread beyond the mesothelium to other parts of the body, symptoms may include pain, trouble swallowing, or swelling of the neck or face.

Diagnosis

Mesothelioma is often confused with a number of other conditions. Diagnosis begins with a check for history of asbestos exposure together with a complete physical, including lung function tests and X-rays of the chest or abdomen. A CT or MRI scan may be used.

A biopsy can confirm the diagnosis: if the cancer is in the chest, the doctor may perform a thoracoscopy by making a small cut through the chest wall and inserting a thin, lighted tube into the chest between two ribs in order to obtain tissue samples. To biopsy suspected abdominal cancer, the doctor may perform a peritoneoscopy, making a small opening in the abdomen and inserting a peritoneoscope into the abdominal cavity. If these procedures do not yield enough tissue, more extensive diagnostic surgery may be necessary.

Staging

If the diagnosis is mesothelioma, the doctor will want to learn the stage of the disease to find out whether the cancer has spread and, if so, to which parts of the body. Knowing the stage of the disease helps the doctor plan treatment.

Mesothelioma is localized if the cancer is found only on the membrane surface where it originated. It is advanced if it has spread beyond the original membrane surface to other parts of the body, such as the lymph nodes, lungs, chest wall, or abdominal organs.

Treatment

Treatment may include some combination of surgery, CHEMOTHERAPY, and radiation. The doctor may remove part of the lining of the chest or abdomen and some of the tissue around it. For pleural mesothelioma, a lung may be removed in an operation called a pneumonectomy. Sometimes part of the diaphragm is also removed.

To ease symptoms and control pain, the doctor may use a needle or a thin tube to drain fluid that has built up in the chest (thoracentesis); fluid removal from the abdomen is called paracentesis. Drugs may be given through a tube in the chest to prevent more fluid from accumulating. Recently a new type of chemotherapy, Pemetrexed, in combination with cisplatin has been approved.

Prevention

The U.S. Occupational Safety and Health Administration sets limits for acceptable levels of asbestos exposure in the workplace. People who work with asbestos wear protective equipment to lower their risk of exposure. To reduce the chance of exposing family members to asbestos fibers, asbestos workers are usually required to shower and change their clothing before leaving the workplace.

metastasis   The spread of cancer cells to other areas of the body via the LYMPHATIC SYSTEM or the bloodstream.

microcalcifications   Tiny specks of calcium in the breast that may appear alone or in clusters and that may or may not signal BREAST CANCER. The shape and location of microcalcifications can help a radiologist determine how likely it is that the areas are malignant. In some cases, microcalcifications do not require a biopsy but only a follow-up mammogram within three to six months. In other cases, the microcalcifications are suspicious and a biopsy is recommended.

mistletoe   A semiparasitic plant that has been used for centuries to treat numerous human ailments; recently mistletoe extracts have been shown to kill cancer cells in the laboratory and to stimulate the immune system. Mistletoe for humans is used primarily in Europe, where a variety of different extracts are marketed as injectable prescription drugs. These extracts are not available commercially in the United States.

Although mistletoe plants and berries are considered poisonous to humans, few serious side effects have been associated with mistletoe extract use.

The use of mistletoe as a treatment for cancer has been investigated in more than 30 clinical studies. Reports of improved survival, better quality of life, or stimulation of the immune system have been common, but nearly all of the studies had major weaknesses that raise doubts about the reliability of the findings, according to federal researchers. Also, no evidence exists that stimulating the immune system can improve the ability to fight cancer. At present, the U.S. government does not recommend the use of mistletoe for the general public.

Meanwhile, experts are investigating two components of mistletoe, viscotoxins and lectins, that they think may be responsible for certain anticancer effects. Viscotoxins are small proteins that can kill cells and possibly stimulate the immune system. Lectins are complex molecules of protein and carbohydrates that can trigger biochemical changes.

Because of mistletoe's ability to stimulate the immune system, it has been classified as a type of BIOLOGICAL RESPONSE MODIFIER (a diverse group of biological molecules that have been used to treat cancer or to lessen the side effects of anticancer drugs).

Commercially available extracts of mistletoe are marketed in Europe under a variety of brand names, including Iscador, Eurixor, Helixor, Isorel, Iscucin, Plenosol, and ABNOBAviscum. Some extracts are marketed under more than one name. For example, Iscador, Isorel, and Plenosol are also sold as Iscar, Vysorel, and Lektinol, respectively. All of these products are prepared from *Viscum album Loranthacea* (*Viscum album L.* or European mistletoe).

Mistletoe grows on several types of trees, and the chemical composition of extracts derived from it depends on the species of the host tree (such as apple, elm, oak, pine, poplar, and spruce), the time of year harvested, how the extracts are prepared, and the commercial producer.

At present, at least one U.S. investigator has approval to study mistletoe as a treatment for cancer.

Side Effects

Reported side effects have generally been mild, including soreness and inflammation at injection sites, headache, fever, and chills. A few cases of severe allergic reactions, including anaphylactic shock, have been reported.

However, mistletoe plants and berries are considered poisonous, causing seizures, vomiting, and death after ingestion. The severity of the toxic effects associated with mistletoe ingestion may depend on the amount consumed and the type of mistletoe plant.

mixed germ cell tumor A tumor containing more than one type of GERM CELL CANCER (for example, teratoma and seminoma).

monoclonal antibodies (MOABs) Synthetic antibodies produced by a single type of cell that are specific for a particular antigen. Researchers are examining ways to create MOABs specific to the antigens found on the surface of cancer cells.

MOABs are made by injecting human cancer cells into mice so that their immune systems will make antibodies against these cancer cells. The mouse cells producing the antibodies are then removed and fused with lab-grown cells to create "hybrid" cells (hybridomas) that can produce large quantities of pure antibodies. These antibodies may be used in cancer treatment in a number of ways:

- They can be programmed to act against cell growth factors, interfering with the growth of cancer cells.
- They may be linked to anticancer drugs, radioisotopes (radioactive substances), or other toxins. When the antibodies latch onto cancer cells, they deliver these poisons directly to the tumor, helping to destroy it.
- They may help destroy cancer cells in bone marrow that has been removed from a patient in preparation for a bone marrow transplant.
- MOABs carrying radioisotopes may also prove useful in diagnosing certain cancers, such as colorectal, ovarian, and prostate.

Rituxan (rituximab) and Herceptin (trastuzumab) are monoclonal antibodies that have been approved by the FDA. Rituxan is used for the initial treatment of B-cell NON-HODGKIN'S LYMPHOMA or when it has returned after a period of improvement or has not responded to chemotherapy. Herceptin is used to treat metastatic BREAST CANCER in patients with tumors that produce excess amounts of a protein called HER-2. (About 25 percent of breast cancer tumors produce excess amounts of HER-2.) Researchers also are testing MOABs in clinical trials to treat LYMPHOMA, LEUKEMIA, COLORECTAL CANCER, LUNG CANCER, BRAIN CANCER, PROSTATE CANCER, and other types of cancer.

mouth cancer   See ORAL CANCER.

mucinous carcinoma   A rare type of invasive ductal BREAST CANCER (also called colloid carcinoma) that is formed by mucus-producing cancer cells. This type of breast cancer has a slightly better prognosis and a slightly lower chance of spreading than does invasive lobular or invasive ductal cancers of the same size.

multiple myeloma   An incurable type of cancer that affects certain BONE MARROW white blood cells called plasma cells, which produce antibodies that move through the bloodstream to help fight harmful substances. Each type of plasma cell responds to only one specific substance by making a large amount of one kind of antibody. The antibody finds and acts against that one substance. Because the body has many types of plasma cells, it can respond to many substances. When cancer involves plasma cells, the body keeps producing more and more of these cells. The unneeded plasma cells—all abnormal and all exactly alike—are called myeloma cells.

Myeloma cells tend to collect in the bone marrow and in the hard, outer part of bones. Sometimes they collect in only one bone and form a single tumor called a plasmacytoma. In most cases, however, the myeloma cells collect in many bones, often forming many tumors and causing other problems. When this happens, the disease is called multiple myeloma. Although multiple myeloma affects the bones, it begins in cells of the immune system. These cancers are different from bone cancer, which actually begins in cells that form the hard, outer part of the bone.

Each year nearly 13,000 people in the United States are diagnosed with multiple myeloma. Half of these patients will die within five years of diagnosis. Because people with multiple myeloma have an abnormally large number of identical plasma cells, they also have too much of one type of antibody. These myeloma cells and antibodies can cause a number of serious medical problems: as myeloma cells increase in number, they damage and weaken bones, causing pain and sometimes fractures. Bone pain can make it difficult for patients to move.

When bones are damaged, calcium is released into the blood. This may lead to hypercalcemia—too much calcium in the blood. Hypercalcemia can cause loss of appetite, abdominal pain, nausea, thirst, fatigue, muscle weakness, restlessness, and confusion.

Because myeloma cells prevent the bone marrow from forming normal plasma cells and other white blood cells that are important to the immune system, myeloma patients may not be able to fight infection and disease. The cancer cells also may prevent the growth of new red blood cells, causing anemia. Patients may have serious problems with their kidneys, because excess antibody proteins and calcium can prevent the kidneys from filtering and cleaning the blood properly and eventually leading to kidney failure.

Symptoms

In the earliest stage of the disease, there may be no symptoms. When symptoms do occur, patients commonly have bone pain, often in the back or ribs. Patients also may have broken bones, weakness, fatigue, weight loss, or repeated infections. When the disease progresses, symptoms may include nausea, vomiting, constipation, problems with urination, and weakness or numbness in the legs.

Diagnosis

Multiple myeloma may be found as part of a routine physical exam before patients have symptoms of the disease. If a patient has bone pain, X-rays can show whether any bones are damaged or broken. Samples of the patient's blood and urine are checked to see whether they contain high levels of antibody proteins (M proteins).

A bone marrow aspiration or a bone marrow BIOPSY can check for myeloma cells. In an aspiration, the doctor inserts a needle into the hip bone or breast bone to withdraw a sample of fluid and cells from the bone marrow. To do a biopsy, the doctor uses a larger needle to remove a sample of solid tissue from the marrow. A pathologist examines the samples under a microscope to see whether there are any myeloma cells.

Treatment

Treatment decisions for multiple myeloma are complex, and both plasmacytoma and multiple myeloma are very hard to cure. Although patients who have a plasmacytoma may be free of symptoms for a long time after treatment, many eventually develop multiple myeloma. For those who have multiple myeloma, treatment can improve their quality of life by controlling the symptoms and complications of the disease. People who have multiple myeloma but do not have symptoms of the disease usually do not receive treatment (smoldering myeloma). For these patients, the risks and side effects of treatment are likely to outweigh the possible benefits. However, these patients are watched closely, and they begin treatment when symptoms appear.

Chemotherapy Patients who need treatment for multiple myeloma usually receive CHEMOTHERAPY and sometimes RADIATION THERAPY. Doctors may prescribe two or more drugs that work together to kill myeloma cells. In May 2003 a novel cancer treatment was approved by the government—the first anticancer PROTEASOME INHIBITOR, which targets an enzyme key to cell growth (uncontrolled cell growth is the hallmark of cancer). Scientists hope that if they interfere with proteasome action, cancer cells will die. The drug THALIDOMIDE has become a first-line treatment in multiple myeloma especially when combined with steroids (dexamethasone).

RADIATION THERAPY five times a week for four to five weeks is the standard treatment for people who have a single plasmacytoma. People who have multiple myeloma sometimes receive radiation therapy in addition to chemotherapy. The purpose of the radiation therapy is to help control the growth of tumors in the bones and relieve the pain that these tumors cause.

Patients with multiple myeloma frequently have pain caused by bone damage or by tumors pressing on nerves. Doctors often suggest that patients take pain medicine and/or wear a back or neck brace to help relieve their pain. Some patients find that techniques such as relaxation and imagery can reduce their pain.

Preventing or treating bone fractures is another important part of supportive care. Because EXERCISE can reduce the loss of calcium from the bones, doctors and nurses encourage patients to be active, if possible.

Because multiple myeloma weakens the IMMUNE SYSTEM, patients must be very careful to protect themselves from infection. It is important that they stay out of crowds and away from people with colds or other infectious diseases. Any sign of infection (fever, sore throat, cough) should be reported to the doctor right away. Patients who develop infections are treated with antibiotics or other drugs. Patients who have anemia may have transfusions of red blood cells or erythropoeitin. Transfusions can help reduce the shortness of breath and fatigue that can be caused by anemia.

Cause

At this time, doctors do not know what causes this disease or how to prevent it. Although scientists cannot explain why one person gets multiple myeloma and another does not, we do know that most multiple myeloma patients are between 50 and 70 years old. This disease affects blacks more often than whites and men more often than women.

A person's family background also appears to affect the risk of developing multiple myeloma; children and brothers and sisters of patients who have this disease have a slightly increased risk. Farmers and petroleum workers exposed to certain chemicals also seem to have a higher-than-average chance of getting multiple myeloma. In addition, people exposed to large amounts of radiation (such as survivors of the atomic bomb explosions in Japan) have an increased risk for this disease.

Scientists have some concern that smaller amounts of radiation (such as the amounts that radiologists and workers in nuclear power plants are exposed to) also may increase the risk. Scientists do not have clear evidence that large numbers of medical X-rays increase the risk for multiple myeloma. In fact, most people receive a fairly small number of X-rays, and scientists believe that the benefits of medical X-rays far outweigh the possible risk for multiple myeloma. In most cases, people who develop multiple myeloma have no clear risk factors. The disease may be the result of several factors (known and/or unknown) acting together.

Multiple Myeloma Research Foundation (MMRF)

A nonprofit organization that provides research funding in the field of MULTIPLE MYELOMA, and information to people with cancer and their family members. Services include a quarterly newsletter, research roundtables, seminars, advocacy, fundraising events, referrals to support groups, and financial assistance. MMRF has raised more than $15 million, funding more than 36 research institutions around the globe and supporting the most promising areas of multiple myeloma research. By building interdisciplinary collaborations among researchers, pharmaceutical companies, biotech firms, and the NATIONAL CANCER INSTITUTE, the MMRF is expanding therapeutic treatments for myeloma and extending the lives of multiple myeloma patients worldwide.

The MMRF was established in 1998 and founded by twin sisters Karen Andrews and Kathy Giusti, after Kathy was diagnosed with multiple myeloma. Today the MMRF is the largest nonprofit foundation dedicated to the single mission of accelerating the search for a cure for this disease. For contact information, see Appendix I.

myelodysplasia (MDS)

A puzzling, life-threatening group of conditions in which the BONE MARROW produces abnormal white cells, red cells, and platelets. It is also called pre-leukemia, since some patients with this disease later develop acute myeloid LEUKEMIA.

Normally, bone marrow cells called blasts develop and mature into several different types of blood cells that have specific jobs in the body; red cells carry oxygen, white cells fight infection, and

platelets stop bleeding. In myelodysplasia (MDS), these blast cells fail to respond to normal control signals, so they do not mature and are unable to function properly. When too many of these blasts remain in the bone marrow, levels of the circulating, mature blood cells fall. In addition they may not function properly due to being misshapen.

The risk of developing MDS rises dramatically with age. Rare under the age of 40, MDS affects about three people per 100,000 over the age of 50; MDS also is slightly more common in men than in women. Fewer than 100 new cases of MDS are reported in the United States each year in children.

Because the process is gradual and because most patients are over age 65, it is not necessarily a terminal disease. However, some patients do succumb to the direct effects of the disease through loss of the ability to fight infections and control bleeding. In addition, within six months to 10 years, about 30 percent of MDS patients develop acute myeloid leukemia (AML), a type of bone marrow cancer that does not respond well to chemotherapy.

While a total of between 70 to 75 percent of patients diagnosed with MDS eventually succumb to the direct effects of MDS or to AML, a group of patients with MDS will still live a normal life span.

Cause

In most cases, no cause can be identified. Some evidence suggests that certain people are born with a tendency to develop MDS that can be triggered by an external factor. If the external factor cannot be identified, then the disease is referred to as primary MDS. In some cases, the trigger is exposure to radiation, BENZENE, or CHEMOTHERAPY drugs. Patients taking chemotherapy drugs for other cancers (such as HODGKIN'S DISEASE and LYMPHOMA) are at risk of developing MDS for up to 10 years after treatment. This type of secondary MDS is usually associated with multiple chromosome abnormalities in the bone marrow that often can develop quickly into AML.

Patients whose disease is known to have been caused by exposure to radiation, benzene, or previous chemotherapy have a particularly poor outlook.

There are no known food or agricultural products that cause MDS. While daily alcohol consumption may lower red blood cell and platelet counts, alcohol does not cause MDS. There is not enough data to determine if smoking increases the risk of developing MDS, although the risk of developing AML is 1.6 times greater for smokers than for nonsmokers.

Symptoms

Most problems arise from low levels of normal blood cells. Symptoms depend on the degree of low counts and abnormal function of the white cells, red cells, and/or platelets. In some patients, only one of the cell types is affected, whereas in others all three may be abnormal.

Low levels of red blood cells lead to anemia, with pale skin, shortness of breath, and palpitations. Severe anemia reduces blood flow to the heart, which may trigger chest pains (angina) or heart attack in older patients.

Low levels of white cells (NEUTROPENIA) may increase risk of bacterial infections, such as skin infections, sinus infections (with nasal congestion), lung infections (with cough and shortness or breath), or urinary tract infections (with painful and frequent urination). Fever may accompany these infections.

Low levels of platelets (THROMBOCYTOPENIA) may cause bleeding and easy bruising even after a very minor scrape. Nosebleeds are common and patients often experience bleeding gums, especially after dental work.

Some patients develop abdominal swelling due to enlargement of the liver or spleen; more rarely, lymph glands are enlarged.

Diagnosis

A simple blood test may suggest DMS, but a bone marrow test can confirm the diagnosis. Chromosomal analysis of the bone marrow cells can provide clues as to the prognosis. A scoring system called the International Prognostic Index can identify the number of blasts (immature blood cells) present in the marrow. That information plus the number of the three blood cells types that are affected can provide important prognostic information.

Aggressiveness and Prognosis

Currently, two scoring systems are used to describe the type or aggressiveness of MDS and the prognosis for the patient: the International Prognostic Scoring System (IPSS) and the French-American-British (FAB) classification system.

International Prognostic Scoring System (IPSS)

This newer system for grading the severity of MDS involves scoring the patient's risk from the disease—that is, the chance of a shortened life expectancy and the transformation into AML. The IPSS Score is a function of the percentage of blasts appearing in the bone marrow, the identification of chromosomal abnormalities in bone marrow blood cells, and the blood cell counts and other blood test findings.

- *Low-risk group:* About half of these patients will survive 5.7 years and 25 percent will develop AML within 9.4 years.

- *Intermediate-risk group 1:* About half of these patients will survive 3.5 years, and 25 percent of patients will develop AML within 3.3 years.

- *Intermediate-risk group II:* About half of patients will survive a year, and 25 percent of patients will develop AML within a year.

- *High-risk group:* About half of patients will survive 4.5 months, and 75 percent will develop AML.

French-American-British (FAB) classification system

This scoring method was developed in the early 1980s by a group of physicians from France, the United States, and Great Britain. The most important criterion for classification in the FAB system is the percentage of blast cells in the marrow, with less than 2 percent blasts considered normal for healthy bone marrow. There are five categories of MDS in this system:

- *Refractory anemia (RA):* Patients do not respond (that is, they are refractory) to iron or vitamins. There may be mild to moderate low platelets or white counts, with fewer than 5 percent blasts in the bone marrow. Less than 10 percent of patients having refractory anemia develop AML. Median survival of patients with refractory anemia is about four years.

- *Refractory anemia with ringed sideroblasts (RARS):* Sideroblasts are red blood cells containing granules of iron; ringed sideroblasts are abnormal. In patients with this disorder, less than 5 percent of marrow cells are blasts; less than 5 percent of the patients having RARS develop AML. The median survival of this group of patients is 55 months.

- *Refractory anemia with excess blasts (RAEB):* Five to 20 percent of the marrow cells are blasts, and the circulating blood also contains 1 to 5 percent blasts. Between 20 to 30 percent of patients with RAEB develop AML. Median survival for patients in this group is about two years.

- *Refractory anemia with excess blasts in transformation (RAEB-T):* Twenty to 30 percent of the marrow cells are blasts, and more than 5 percent blasts are found in the bloodstream; 75 percent of these patients develop AML. Some experts believe that patients in this group should be classified as having a form of AML, since these patients would have access to treatments approved for AML but not yet approved for treating MDS. Median survival for patients having refractory anemia with excess blasts in transformation is about six months.

- *Chronic myelomonocytic leukemia (CML):* The marrow contains 1 to 20 percent blasts with an increase in blood and marrow white blood cells (monocytes) that remove dead, injured, or cancerous cells. This type of leukemia is different from chronic granulocyte leukemia. Median survival of patients having CMML is about three years.

Treatment

There are no specific proven treatments for myelodysplasia. Patients whose only problem is anemia are usually treated with regular blood transfusions. About 30 percent of low-risk patients may benefit from injections of the red cell growth factor ERYTHROPOIETIN. Similar results are obtained using immunosuppressive agents such as anti-thymocyte globulin or cyclosporin. Thalidomide also may be useful.

If the bone marrow stain shows deposits of iron in the red cells, indicating sideroblastic ANEMIA, then the patient may take 100 mg of pyridoxine twice a day. Pyridoxine therapy can relieve sideroblastic anemia through increases in red cell counts for about 5 percent of MDS patients; however, pyridoxine doses about 100 mg twice daily

can produce side effects such as tingling of the fingers.

Patients with low white cell counts who have experienced at least one infection may benefit from white cell growth factors such as a GRANULO-CYTE COLONY-STIMULATING FACTOR (G-CSF), like Neupogen or filgrastim, or a granulocyte macrophage colony-stimulating factor (GM-CSF), like Leukine or sargramostim. Seventy-five percent of the patients who use G-CSF or GM-CSF experience increased white cell production that may help to reduce the likelihood of additional infection. Neupogen and Leukine do not cause serious side effects, but these medications have not been shown to prolong survival.

There is no growth-factor medication for patients with low platelet counts, but research suggests that treatment with growth factor medications, such as interleukin-11, interleukin-6, and, in particular, thrombopoietin, may help. Platelet transfusions are rarely given unless the platelet count is below 10,000 per microliter of blood (normal counts range from 150,000 to 450,000). Patients eventually become resistant to the transfused platelets, so transfusions of new platelets would periodically be necessary.

Patients with high-risk MDS may benefit from chemotherapy using cytosine arabinoside or melphalan, but the chance of controlling MDS with chemotherapy is only about 30 percent. Even in successful cases, the disease often returns within a year, which is why aggressive chemotherapy is given to only a few MDS patients.

Bone marrow transplantation is a potential very effective treatment—and perhaps even a cure—but it carries a great deal of risk and requires donation of matched marrow. The objective of the procedure is to replace all myelodysplastic cells with donated normal cells. First, patients are given chemotherapy that kills the patient's marrow and blood cells, including the myelodysplastic cells; injected donated marrow then travels to the patient's bones, where it reproduces. If there are no complications, the donated marrow will take over the functions of the original marrow. Patients who survive the complications have a good chance of being cured. To match, the marrow must be donated by a sibling (or, on a very rare occasion, by a matched unrelated donor) and must be of the same transplantation type. Matching of transplantation type, which is determined through a blood test, should not be confused with matching of blood type. Unfortunately, transplantation type between children and parents are not similar enough to qualify as a match.

Besides the risk of rejection from insufficiently-matched transplantation type, there are other risks. The patient's liver or lungs may be damaged and there is the ever-present risk of infection. In addition, the transplanted bone marrow (graft) could reject the patient (host), which is known as graft-versus-host disease. In this case, the white blood cells from the donated marrow would attack the patient's tissues. Complications associated with standard bone marrow transplantation kill between 30 to 50 percent of treated patients within a year after the procedure.

Any potential gain in survival time is usually not considered worth the risk for most MDS patients, since this is a disease that typically develops late in life. Therefore, patients over age 60 usually do not undergo bone marrow transplants. The decision for younger patients, especially those with additional medical issues, is more difficult. About 500 MDS patients have undergone bone marrow transplantation and almost all have been under age 40.

Scientists are now investigating the possibility of providing a "mini" bone marrow transplant as an option for the older patient with access to matching marrow. Mini-transplants utilize a lower dose of chemotherapy to destroy most or all of the myelodysplastic cells. The lower dose is better tolerated by older patients, thus the patient will suffer fewer side effects of the chemotherapy and, being stronger, may have a greater chance of surviving the transplant. (Younger patients, who generally are more vigorous, receive the standard dose of chemotherapy to ensure that all myelodysplastic cells have been killed.) Studies of mini-transplants for patients 55 to 70 years old are in progress.

MDS is very rare in young people, and teens are often treated differently for MDS than older adults. The most common treatment for teens with MDS includes chemotherapy and bone marrow transplant. Chemotherapy treatment for MDS often resembles that for acute myelogenous leukemia. Bone marrow transplantation, using high doses of chemotherapy and radiation, is also used for teens with MDS if there is a suitable donor.

myelodysplastic syndrome   A blood disease in which the BONE MARROW does not function normally. People with this disease are at increased risk of developing acute myeloid LEUKEMIA. Myelodysplastic syndrome is also called preleukemia or smoldering leukemia.

myomectomy   The removal of fibroids (noncancerous tumors) from the wall of the uterus. Myomectomy is the preferred treatment for symptomatic fibroids in a woman who wants to keep her uterus. Larger fibroids must be removed with an abdominal incision, but small fibroids can be taken out using laparoscopy or hysteroscopy. A myomectomy is an alternative to hysterectomy that can relieve fibroid-induced menstrual symptoms that have not responded to medication.

Usually, fibroids are buried in the outer wall of the uterus and abdominal surgery is required. If they are on the inner wall of the uterus, uterine fibroids can be removed using hysteroscopy. Fibroids on a stalk (pedunculated) on the outer surface of the uterus can be removed with LAPAROSCOPY. Removing fibroids through abdominal surgery is a more difficult and slightly more risky operation than a hysterectomy because the uterus bleeds from the sites where the fibroids were, and it may be difficult or impossible to stop the bleeding. This surgery is usually performed under general anesthesia, although some patients may be given a spinal or epidural anesthesia. The incision may be horizontal (the "bikini" incision) or a vertical incision from the navel downward.

After separating the muscle layers underneath the skin, the surgeon makes an opening in the abdominal wall. Next, the surgeon makes an incision over each fibroid, grasping and pulling out each growth. Each opening in the uterine wall is then stitched with sutures. The uterus must be meticulously repaired in order to eliminate potential sites of bleeding or infection. Then, the surgeon sutures the abdominal wall and muscle layers above it with absorbable stitches and closes the skin with clips or nonabsorbable stitches.

When appropriate, a laparoscopic myomectomy may be performed. In this procedure the surgeon removes fibroids with the help of a laparoscope inserted into the pelvic cavity through an incision in the navel. The fibroids are removed through a tiny incision under the navel that is much smaller than the 4- or 5-inch opening required for a standard myomectomy.

If the fibroids are small and located on the inner surface of the uterus, they can be removed with a thin telescope-like device called a hysteroscope, which is inserted into the vagina, through the cervix, and into the uterus. This procedure does not require any abdominal incision, so hospitalization is shorter.

Surgeons often recommend hormone treatment with a drug called leuprolide (Lupron) two to six months before surgery in order to shrink the fibroids so they are easier to remove. In addition, Lupron stops menstruation, so women who are anemic have an opportunity to build up their blood count. While the drug treatment may reduce the risk of excess blood loss during surgery, there is a small risk that temporarily smaller fibroids might be missed during myomectomy, only to enlarge later after the surgery is completed.

Patients may need four to six weeks of recovery following a standard myomectomy before they can return to normal activities, but women who have had laparoscopic or hysteroscopic myomectomies can leave the hospital the same day.

There is a risk that removal of the fibroids may lead to such severe bleeding that the uterus itself will have to be removed. Because of the risk of blood loss during a myomectomy, patients may want to consider banking their own blood before surgery.

nasopharyngeal cancer See HEAD AND NECK CANCER.

National Alliance of Breast Cancer Organizations
A network of BREAST CANCER organizations that provides information, assistance, and referrals to anyone with questions about breast cancer and acts as a voice for the interests and concerns of breast cancer survivors and women at risk. Services include information referrals, job-discrimination-related advocacy, and professional education. For contact information, see Appendix I.

National Asian Women's Health Organization (NAWHO) A nonprofit organization founded in 1993 to achieve health equity for Asian Americans. NAWHO's goals are to raise awareness about the health needs of Asian Americans through research and education and to support Asian Americans as decision makers through leadership development and advocacy. Through its innovative programs, NAWHO is increasing knowledge of BREAST CANCER and CERVICAL CANCER, training violence-prevention advocates, expanding access to immunizations, changing attitudes about reproductive health care, and breaking the stigma around depression and mental health. For contact information, see Appendix I.

National Bone Marrow Transplant Link A national clearinghouse that provides information about a variety of BONE MARROW TRANSPLANT issues. Services include patient advocacy, research funding, referrals, and a resource guide. For contact information, see Appendix I.

National Brain Tumor Foundation Nonprofit foundation that offers resources and support, and funds research into the treatment of BRAIN CANCER. Affected patients can receive referrals to a network of support groups. For contact information, see Appendix I.

National Breast and Cervical Cancer Early Detection Program A government program that works in states, U.S. territories, and tribal organizations to ensure that women who have little or no insurance have access to lifesaving cancer screening, diagnostic services, and treatment. As of 2002, the program had provided BREAST CANCER and CERVICAL CANCER screening services to more than 1.5 million uninsured and underinsured women. For contact information, see Appendix I.

National Breast Cancer Coalition (NBCC) The nation's largest breast-cancer grassroots advocacy group, composed of more than 600 member organizations and 70,000 individual members. The group fights BREAST CANCER through action, advocacy, and public education. NBCC and its sister organization, the National Breast Cancer Coalition Fund, work to educate and train people to be effective activists. Services include referrals, education and training, advocacy, and volunteer services. For contact information, see Appendix I.

National Cancer Institute (NCI) A component of the National Institutes of Health, the NCI was established under the National Cancer Act of 1937 as the federal government's principal agency for cancer research and training. The National Cancer Act of 1971 broadened the scope and responsibilities of the NCI and created the National Cancer Program, which conducts and supports research, training, health information dissemination, and other programs concerning the cause, diagnosis, prevention, and treatment of cancer; rehabilitation from cancer; and the continuing care of cancer patients and their families. The NCI is responsible for coordinating the National Cancer Program.

Services include the NCI's comprehensive database, which contains peer-reviewed summaries and the most current information on cancer treatment, screening, prevention, genetics, and supportive care. The NCI also maintains a registry of cancer clinical trials being conducted worldwide and directories of physicians, professionals who provide genetic counseling services, and organizations that provide care to people with cancer. For contact information, see Appendix I.

National Cancer Institute (NCI) Cancer Centers Program A program through which the NCI designates and supports more than 50 cancer centers engaged in multidisciplinary research to reduce cancer incidence, morbidity, and mortality. NCI grants under the program support three types of centers: COMPREHENSIVE CANCER CENTERS, CLINICAL CANCER CENTERS, and CANCER CENTERS.

Several cancer centers existed in the late 1960s, and the National Cancer Act of 1971 strengthened the program by authorizing the establishment of 15 new cancer centers and the continued support for existing ones. The passage of the act also dramatically transformed the centers' structure and broadened the scope of their mission to include all aspects of basic, clinical, and cancer control research. In 1990 there were 19 Comprehensive Cancer Centers in the nation. Today, more than 40 cancer centers meet the NCI criteria for "comprehensive" status. Each type of cancer center has special capabilities for conducting new research that can exploit important new findings and address timely questions. All NCI-designated cancer centers are reevaluated each time their Cancer Center Support Grant comes up for renewal (generally every three to five years).

Since the passage of the National Cancer Act of 1971, the Cancer Centers Program has continued to expand. Today NCI-designated cancer centers continue to work toward creating new and innovative approaches to cancer research. Through interdisciplinary efforts, cancer centers can effectively move this research from the laboratory into

clinical trials and into clinical practice. Patients seeking clinical oncology services (screening, diagnosis, or treatment) can obtain those services at Clinical Cancer Centers or Comprehensive Cancer Centers. They can also participate in clinical trials (research studies involving human subjects) at these types of cancer centers. Most Cancer Centers are engaged almost entirely in basic research and do not provide patient care. Information about referral procedures, treatment costs, and services available to patients can be obtained from the individual cancer centers; for contact information, see Appendix II.

NCI-designated cancer centers are defined as follows:

Comprehensive Cancer Center

To attain recognition from NCI as a Comprehensive Cancer Center, an institution must pass rigorous peer review. Under guidelines revised in 1997, a Comprehensive Cancer Center must perform research in three major areas: basic research; clinical research; and cancer prevention, control, and population-based research. It must also have a strong body of interactive research that bridges these research areas. In addition, a Comprehensive Cancer Center must conduct outreach and education, directed toward and accessible to both healthcare professionals and the lay community.

Clinical Cancer Centers

These centers must have active programs in clinical research, and may also have programs in another area (such as basic research; or prevention, control, and population-based research). Clinical Cancer Centers focus on both laboratory research and clinical research within the same institutional framework.

Cancer Center

The general term "Cancer Center" refers to an organization with scientific disciplines outside the specific qualifications of a comprehensive or clinical center. Such centers may, for example, concentrate on basic research, epidemiology and cancer control research, or other areas of research.

National Cervical Cancer Coalition (NCCC) A coalition of cervical cancer patients and their family members and caregivers, women's groups, scientists, labs, corporations, hospitals, and other organizations interested in educating the public about CERVICAL CANCER prevention, screening and treatment options, and follow-up programs. The NCCC emphasizes outreach support to women and family members battling cancer. The NCCC places a personal focus on providing outreach support to women and family members.

The NCCC developed the nation's first hotline for women with cervical cancer and their family members and developed the cervical cancer quilts project that travels the country and helps to place a personal face on the battle against cervical cancer. The NCCC also began the nation's free "Pap smear day," the second Friday of January, for women who have not had a Pap smear for three years. For contact information, see Appendix I.

National Childhood Cancer Foundation The foundation supports the work of the most prestigious childhood cancer treatment and research center in North America, the Children's Oncology Group (COG). COG was formed by the merger of four national pediatric cancer research organizations: the Children's Cancer Group, the Intergroup Rhabdomyosarcoma Study Group, the National Wilm's Tumor Study Group, and the Pediatric Oncology Group. The organization conducts clinical trials of new therapies for childhood cancer. For contact information, see Appendix I.

National Children's Cancer Society (NCCS) A nonprofit organization that provides children from birth to 18 years who have cancer, and their families, with emotional support and direct financial support for cancer-related expenses. The NCCS works with more than 200 pediatric oncology hospitals and cancer centers to identify and help any family able to demonstrate financial need regardless of socioeconomic status prior to diagnosis. Services include financial and in-kind assistance, advocacy, support services, education, and prevention programs. Since its inception in 1987, the NCCS has distributed in excess of $25,000,000 in direct financial assistance to help more than 10,000 children and their families. For contact information, see Appendix I.

National Children's Leukemia Foundation (NCLF) One of the leading nonprofit organizations in the fight against LEUKEMIA and cancer in children and adults. The NCLF was established to support the unfortunate in various programs, to provide the cure for children and adults, and to ease the family's burden during their hospital stay. The foundation's 24-hour hotline (800-448-3467) offers comprehensive information to any caller and provides referrals for initial testing, physicians, hospital admissions, and treatment options. For contact information, see Appendix I.

National Coalition for Cancer Survivorship (NCCS) The only patient-led advocacy organization working to ensure quality cancer care on behalf of 8.9 million U.S. survivors of all types of cancer and those who care for them. Founded in 1986, the NCCS continues to lead the cancer survivorship movement. By educating all those affected by cancer and speaking out on issues related to quality cancer care, the NCCS hopes to empower every survivor. The NCCS serves a key role in policymaking in Washington, D.C., as well as a source of support for thousands of survivors and their families. Services include referrals, information, education, and advocacy. For contact information, see Appendix I.

National Comprehensive Cancer Network (NCCN) A nonprofit alliance of the world's leading CANCER CENTERS established in 1995 to support member institutions in the evolving managed care environment. The NCCN tries to strengthen the mission of member institutions by providing state-of-the-art cancer care, advance cancer prevention, screening, diagnosis, and treatment through excellence in basic and clinical research, and enhance the effectiveness and efficiency of cancer care delivery.

The NCCN develops programs and products that, in partnerships with managed care companies, employers, and unions, offer people greater access to leading doctors, superior treatment, programs that continuously improve the effectiveness of treatment, and management that enhances the efficiency of cancer care delivery. For contact information, see Appendix I.

National Family Caregivers Association   A non-profit association that provides educational and emotional support for family caregivers. Services include advocacy; individual, family, group, peer, and bereavement counseling; and education. For contact information, see Appendix I.

National Hospice and Palliative Care Organization   The largest nonprofit membership organization representing HOSPICE and PALLIATIVE TREATMENT programs and professionals in the United States. The organization is committed to improving end-of-life care and expanding access to hospice care with the goal of enhancing quality of life for people who are dying and their loved ones.

Considered to be the model for quality, compassionate care at the end of life, hospice involves a team-oriented approach to medical care, pain management, and emotional and spiritual support expressly tailored to the patient's wishes. Support also is extended to the family and loved ones. Generally, care is provided in the patient's home or in a homelike setting operated by a hospice program. MEDICARE, private health insurance, and Medicaid in most states cover hospice care for patients who meet certain criteria.

In recent years, many hospice care programs have added "palliative care" to their names to reflect the range of care and services they provide as hospice care and palliative care share the same core values and philosophies.

Those offering palliative care seek to address not only physical pain, but also emotional, social, and spiritual pain in individuals with advanced or terminal illness, to achieve the best possible quality of life for patients and their families. Palliative care extends the principles of hospice care to a broader population that could benefit from receiving this type of care earlier in an illness or disease process.

To better serve individuals who have advanced illness or are terminally ill and their families, many hospice programs encourage access to care earlier in the illness or disease process. Health-care professionals who specialize in hospice and palliative care work closely with staff and volunteers to address all of the symptoms of illness, with the aim of promoting comfort and dignity.

The National Hospice and Palliative Care Organization, founded in 1978 as the National Hospice Organization, changed to its current name in February 2000. With headquarters in Alexandria, Virginia, the organization advocates for the terminally ill and their families. It also develops public and professional educational programs and materials to enhance understanding and availability of hospice and palliative care; convenes frequent meetings and symposia on emerging issues; provides technical informational resources to its membership; conducts research; monitors congressional and regulatory activities; and works closely with other organizations that share an interest in end-of-life care. For contact information, see Appendix I.

National Lymphedema Network (NLN)   A non-profit organization that provides support, education, and information on LYMPHEDEMA. This internationally recognized organization was founded in 1988 by Saskia R. J. Thiadens, R.N. It is supported by tax-deductible donations and is a driving force behind the movement in the United States to standardize quality treatment for lymphedema patients nationwide. In addition, the NLN supports research into the causes and possible alternative treatments for this often incapacitating, long-neglected condition. The NLN provides a toll-free recorded information line (1-800-541-3259); referrals to lymphedema treatment centers, health-care professionals, training programs, and support groups; a quarterly newsletter with information about medical and scientific developments, support groups, pen pals/Internet pals; educational courses; a biennial national conference on lymphedema; and an extensive computer database. For contact information, see Appendix I.

National Marrow Donor Program   A national group that maintains a registry of BONE MARROW donors, provides information on how to become a donor, and organizes donor recruitment drives. For contact information, see Appendix I.

National Ovarian Cancer Coalition (NOCC)   The leading OVARIAN CANCER public information and education organization in the United States. The NOCC initiated the first toll-free ovarian cancer information line (1-888-OVARIAN), maintains the most comprehensive Web site for ovarian cancer support in the world (www.ovarian.org), and has built a network of many state chapters across the United States. For contact information, see Appendix I.

National Patient Advocate Foundation A national network for health-care reform that supports legislation to enable cancer survivors to obtain insurance funding for medical care and participation in clinical trials. The foundation provides referrals, information, education, advocacy, benefits, and health insurance assistance. For contact information, see Appendix I.

National Patient Air Transport Hotline A clearinghouse used to find air transportation for patients who cannot afford travel for medical care. For contact information, see Appendix I.

National Surgical Adjuvant Breast and Bowel Project (NSABP) A cooperative group supported by the NATIONAL CANCER INSTITUTE (NCI) that for more than 40 years has designed and conducted clinical trials that have changed the way BREAST CANCER is treated and, more recently, prevented. It was the NSABP's breast cancer studies that led to the establishment of lumpectomy-plus-radiation, rather than radical mastectomy, as the standard surgical treatment for breast cancer. The group was also the first to demonstrate that adjuvant therapy could increase survival rates, and the first to demonstrate on a large scale the preventive effects of the drug tamoxifen in breast cancer.

Since its inception, the NSABP has enrolled more than 60,000 women and men in clinical trials in breast and COLORECTAL CANCER. Headquartered in Pittsburgh, the group has research sites at nearly 200 major medical centers, university hospitals, large oncology practice groups, and health maintenance organizations in the United States, Canada, Puerto Rico, and Australia. At those sites and their satellites, more than 5,000 physicians, nurses, and other medical professionals conduct NSABP treatment and prevention trials. Their presence at local hospitals and medical facilities means

that state-of-the-art clinical trials can be provided to patients near their homes.

The NSABP was one of the first organizations to undertake large-scale studies in the prevention of breast cancer, and its Breast Cancer Prevention Trial, which included more than 13,000 women at increased risk for breast cancer, demonstrated the value of the drug tamoxifen in reducing the incidence of the disease in this population. A second prevention trial, currently under way, the Study of Tamoxifen and Raloxifene (STAR), compares the effect of these two drugs in reducing the incidence of breast cancer.

Native Americans and cancer See AMERICAN INDIANS/ALASKA NATIVES AND CANCER.

natural killer cells (NK cells) A type of white blood cell that can kill tumor cells and infected body cells. NK cells kill on contact by binding to the target cell and releasing a burst of toxic chemicals. Normal cells are not affected by NK cells, which play a major role in cancer prevention by destroying abnormal cells before they can become dangerous.

nausea Feelings of nausea may start within one to four hours after receiving chemotherapy for cancer; the worst nausea occurs during the first 12 to 24 hours. After that, there may be occasional or unexpected episodes of mild nausea or vomiting. Fortunately, since the mid-1990s several very strong nausea medicines have become available that reduce or eliminate this side effect.

A few chemotherapy drugs—vincristine, carboplatin, bleomycin, 5-FU, METHOTREXATE, and VP 16—do not usually cause NAUSEA. However, if a patient's particular drug regimen is likely to cause significant nausea, IV drugs are given with chemotherapy to prevent this side effect.

Preventing Nausea

Patients should eat lightly before and for one to two days after chemotherapy, avoiding fried food, fruit juice, spicy foods, and items such as hamburger, steak, or hot dogs.

Patients who will receive chemotherapy that is likely to cause nausea will be given medicine to prevent nausea before chemotherapy is administered. They also will be given prescriptions for medicines to prevent nausea at home. Typical antinausea medications include prochlorperazine (Compazine), lorazapam (Ativan), dexamethasone (Decadron), ondansatron (Zofran), granisetron (Kytril), and dolasetron (Anzemet). All of these medications work well for nausea, but certain drugs may work better for one person than another.

Tips to Ease Nausea

Certain dietary choices can help ease nausea. These include crackers, toast, oatmeal, soft bland vegetables and fruits, clear liquids, and skinned baked chicken. Foods to be avoided include fatty, greasy, or fried foods, sweets, and hot or spicy foods. Patients should not force themselves to eat during periods of nausea, because this may trigger aversions to favorite foods.

Patients with nausea should drink liquids between meals, not during meals. It also may help to eat in a room other than the kitchen if cooking smells make nausea worse.

neutropenia A blood condition in which there are too few neutrophils, a type of white blood cell. About 60 percent of all white blood cells are neutrophils. Because neutrophils are important in helping the body fight infections, low levels of neutrophils mean a person is much more likely to get infections.

Neutropenia can be caused by CHEMOTHERAPY or RADIATION THERAPY, or by cancer cells that directly infiltrate the BONE MARROW, interfering with the production of blood cells. Neutropenia also may be caused by a BONE MARROW TRANSPLANT.

People with neutropenia get infections easily and often, usually in the lungs, mouth and throat, sinuses, and skin. Painful mouth ulcers, gum infections, ear infections, and periodontal disease are common. Severe, life-threatening infections may occur.

In general, the blood of healthy adults contains about 1,500 to 7,000 neutrophils per mm^3 (children under six may have a lower neutrophil count). The severity of neutropenia generally depends on the absolute neutrophil count (ANC) and is described as follows:

- Mild neutropenia an ANC between 1,000 per mm^3 and 1,500 per mm^3
- Moderate neutropenia an ANC between 500 per mm^3 and 1,000 per mm^3
- Severe neutropenia an ANC below 500 per mm^3.

Treatment

Often the patient must be hospitalized and receive intravenous antibiotics. Neutropenia caused by chemotherapy is treated by stopping the drugs until the white blood cell count increases (usually within a week).

nicotine See SMOKING.

non-Hodgkin's lymphoma Cancerous growth of the lymphocytes within the lymph tissues other than HODGKIN'S DISEASE. Non-Hodgkin's LYMPHOMA occurs frequently between the ages of 60 and 70, and affects adult men more than adult women, and whites more often than people of other races. The disorder affects about 16 in every 100,000 people (about 45,000 Americans), and its incidence is growing for unknown reasons.

Chances of survival depend on the grade and stage of cancer, overall health, and response to treatment, but from 50 to 80 percent of patients survive five years or more. Ironically, the higher-grade aggressive types are more likely to be cured with CHEMOTHERAPY, but lower-grade lymphoma patients often can have longer average survival times, with mean survival reaching 10 years in some cases. Most children respond well to treatment, even though children tend to have the higher-grade, aggressive types of non-Hodgkin's lymphoma. As many as 70 to 90 percent of children survive five years or more.

Types of Non-Hodgkin's Lymphoma

Non-Hodgkin's lymphoma is categorized by the appearance of the lymphocytes under a microscope and by the results of specialized testing. Different types of lymphoma occur in different age groups.

Adult non-Hodgkin's lymphoma is classified by the appearance of cells taken during a biopsy, taking into account the size, type, and distribution of cancer cells in the lymph node. The three types are low grade (slower-growing), intermediate grade, and high grade (aggressive). Low-grade lymphomas include small lymphocytic lymphoma, follicular small cleaved-cell lymphoma, and follicular mixed-cell lymphoma. Intermediate-grade lymphomas include follicular large-cell lymphoma, diffuse small cleaved-cell lymphoma, diffuse mixed lymphoma, and diffuse large-cell lymphoma. High-grade lymphomas include immunoblastic lymphoma, lymphoblastic lymphoma, and small noncleaved (Burkitt's and non-Burkitt's) lymphoma.

Childhood non-Hodgkin's lymphomas include lymphoblastic lymphoma, large cell lymphoma, and small noncleaved cell lymphoma (including Burkitt's and non-Burkitt's lymphomas). Note that high-grade (aggressive) non-Hodgkin's lymphomas usually affect children and young adults.

In addition, non-Hodgkin's lymphoma may be either B cell or T cell; most, however, are B cell.

Causes

Several risk factors may contribute to the development of lymphoma:

Environmental factors   Recent studies show a possible link between lymphoma and exposure to certain chemicals, herbicides, and insecticides. Further study is needed.

Gender   Non-Hodgkin's lymphoma is more common among men than women in every racial and ethnic group except Koreans, in which there is a slightly higher risk among women.

Genetic factors   Studies indicate that patients with certain inherited immunodeficiency disorders, such as Wiskott-Aldrich syndrome, may have an increased risk of lymphoma.

Race   Incidence is highest among Caucasians (19.1 and 12.0 per 100,000 men and women, respectively) and lowest among Koreans (5.8 and 6.0 per 100,000). Vietnamese men have the second highest rates, followed by Caucasian Hispanic, African-American, Filipino, Hawaiian, Chinese, and Japanese men. Among women, Caucasian Hispanics accounted for the second highest rates, followed by Filipino, Japanese, African-American, and Chinese women.

Death rates are highest for Hawaiian men (8.8 per 100,000), even though their incidence is considerably lower than that of Caucasian men.

Viral infections   Research suggests links between lymphoma and certain viruses, such as the EPSTEIN-BARR VIRUS and the human immunodeficiency virus (AIDS virus). For example, one study found that Burkitt's disease was related to Epstein-Barr virus in nearly all African cases and in 15 percent of U.S. cases. AIDS patients also are more susceptible to both Hodgkin's and non-Hodgkin's lymphomas but primarily non-Hodgkins.

Symptoms

The main symptom of non-Hodgkin's lymphoma is swelling of LYMPH NODES in the neck, under the arms, or in the groin. Other symptoms can include fever, night sweats, fatigue, abdominal pain, unexplained weight loss, and itchy skin.

Because lymph-node swelling in lymphoma is usually painless, nodes may slowly enlarge over a long period before the patient notices. The fever commonly associated with lymphoma may mysteriously appear and disappear for several weeks before the patient sees a doctor. Even the unexplained weight loss caused by lymphoma—usually at least a 10 percent loss of body weight in six months or less—may progress for months before the patient seeks medical help.

Diagnosis

If lymphoma is suspected based on medical history and physical examination, the doctor will order blood tests and a lymph node biopsy. In the biopsy, a doctor injects a local anesthetic above a swollen lymph node and removes a small sample of tissue with a sterile needle. Occasionally, an entire lymph node is surgically removed for biopsy, because this can provide a better sample for a definitive diagnosis. Other diagnostic procedures may include X-rays to evaluate the chest, bones, liver, and spleen; a bone marrow biopsy; PET scan; and a computed tomography (CT) scan of the abdomen.

Staging

Once the diagnosis of lymphoma has been made, the next step is staging to determine the extent of cancer spread. The same staging system is used for both Hodgkin's and non-Hodgkin's lymphomas. Staging ranges from Stage I (limited spread, such as cancer in only one lymph node) to Stage IV (extensive spread outside the lymph system, possibly with bone marrow or other organ involvement).

Occasionally, laparoscopic surgery is performed to ensure proper staging. In this procedure, a small incision is made in the abdomen, and a laparoscope is used to see if cancer has spread to any of the internal organs. During the procedure, small pieces of tissue also may be removed and examined microscopically for signs of cancer.

Treatment

Treatment for non-Hodgkin's lymphoma depends on whether it is a low-, intermediate-, or high-grade lymphoma, the stage of the disease, and the age and health of the patient.

Early stage, low grade   This slow-growing lymphoma can be treated with radiation therapy if the patient has symptoms or if the disease spreads significantly. Sometimes, simple observation can be the best course.

Advanced stage, low grade   This type of lymphoma may be treated in a variety of ways, ranging from chemotherapy with or without radiation therapy to bone marrow transplantation.

Intermediate grade   This may be treated with combination chemotherapy. More advanced stages may require higher-dose chemotherapy and possibly bone marrow or stem-cell transplantation.

High grade   This aggressive lymphoma requires high-dose combination chemotherapy and possibly a BONE MARROW TRANSPLANT or stem cell transplant. In recent clinical trials, radioimmunotherapy has been used to treat advanced, or recurrent lymphomas. In this technique, the doctor injects antibodies with radioactive iodine into the patient's bloodstream to attack and destroy cancer cells. Researchers are studying other biological therapies that use the immune system to fight cancer.

All grades of B-cell lymphomas may benefit from the addition of the monoclonal antibody Rituxan.

nonspecific immunomodulating agents   Substances that stimulate or indirectly augment the immune system. Often these agents target key immune system cells. Two nonspecific immunomodulating agents used in cancer treatment are bacillus Calmette-Guérin (BCG) and levamisole.

BCG, which has been widely used as a tuberculosis vaccine, is used in the treatment of superficial BLADDER CANCER after surgery. BCG may work by stimulating an inflammatory (and possibly an immune) response. A solution of BCG is instilled in the bladder, where it remains for about two hours before the bladder is emptied. This treatment is usually performed once a week for six weeks.

Levamisole is used along with fluorouracil (5-FU) chemotherapy in the treatment of stage III (Dukes' C) COLORECTAL CANCER following surgery. Levamisole may act to restore depressed immune function. Levamisole, however, is not as widely used today because leucoverin (folinic acid) in combination with 5-FU has been found to be as effective with fewer side effects.

Nurses' Health Study (NHS)   A project at Brigham and Women's Hospital in Boston that tracks health information of female nurses across the country. It is among the largest prospective investigations into the risk factors for major chronic diseases in women.

The Nurses' Health Study was established in 1976 by Dr. Frank Speizer, and a second study of younger nurses—the Nurses' Health Study II—was established in 1989 by Dr. Walter Willett. The studies have grown to include a team of clinicians, epidemiologists, and statisticians at the Channing Laboratory along with collaborating investigators and consultants in the surrounding medical community composed of the Harvard Medical School, Harvard School of Public Health, Brigham and Women's Hospital, Dana-Farber Cancer Institute, Boston Children's Hospital, and Beth Israel Hospital.

The primary motivation for starting the first NHS was to investigate the potential long-term consequences of the use of birth control pills, a potent drug that was being prescribed to hundreds of millions of healthy women. Registered nurses were selected to be followed prospectively because experts believed their nursing education would allow them to respond accurately to brief, technically worded questionnaires. The first study includes 122,000 nurses who are contacted every two years to answer a follow-up questionnaire that asks about diseases and health-related topics including smoking, hormone use, and menopausal status.

Because researchers recognized that diet and nutrition would play important roles in the development of chronic diseases, in 1980 they added a diet questionnaire. Subsequent diet questionnaires were collected in 1984, 1986, and every four years since. Questions related to quality of life were added in 1992 and repeated every four years. Because certain aspects of diet cannot be measured by questionnaire (for example, the mineral content of food, which varies with the soil in which it is grown), the nurses submitted 68,000 sets of toenail samples between the 1982 and 1984 questionnaires.

To identify potential biomarkers, such as hormone levels and genetic markers, researchers collected 33,000 blood samples in 1989. A second blood collection from those who previously gave a sample was conducted in 2000/2001.

Nurses' Health Study II

The primary motivation for developing the Nurses' Health Study II was to study oral contraceptives, diet, and lifestyle risk factors in a population younger than the original Nurses' Health Study. This younger generation included women who started using oral contraceptives during adolescence, and who were therefore exposed to these hormones during their early reproductive life. Several case-control studies suggesting such exposures might be associated with substantial increases in risk of BREAST CANCER provided a particularly strong justification for investment in this large cohort. In addition, researchers planned to collect detailed information on type of oral contraceptive used, which was not obtained in the earlier Nurses Health Study.

The initial target population included women between the ages of 25 and 42 years in 1989; the upper age was to correspond with the youngest age group in the first Nurses' Health Study. A total of 116,686 women remain in the second Nurses Health Study.

Every two years, nurses receive a follow-up questionnaire with questions about diseases and health-related topics including smoking, hormone use, pregnancy history, and menopausal status. In 1991 the first food-frequency questionnaire was collected, and subsequent food-frequency questionnaires are administered at four-year intervals. A two-page quality-of-life supplement was included in the first mailing of the 1993 and 1997 questionnaires. Blood and urine samples from approximately 30,000 nurses were collected in the late 1990s.

nutrition and cancer treatment   While good nutrition may not cure cancer, dietary factors do play an important role in cancer treatment. A patient battling a serious disease needs adequate nutrition to maintain strength and overall well-being, keep the immune system functioning, prevent the breakdown of body tissue, and help the body heal. A well-nourished person is better able to tolerate treatment side effects and may be able to handle more aggressive treatments.

Good nutrition also may increase the odds of survival for people battling cancer. In one study of people with HEAD AND NECK CANCER, the two-year survival rate was six times higher among those who were well nourished than those with poor nutrition. In general, a cancer patient should get the best possible mix of nutrients without too much fat.

Nutrition can be a problem for people with cancer for several reasons. The cancer itself may interfere with eating and digestion because of problems chewing and swallowing, gastrointestinal tract blockages, or interference with digestive enzymes and hormones. Cancer treatment such as radiation and chemotherapy can cause nausea, vomiting, swallowing problems, painful mouth sores and sore throat, and dry mouth. Surgery also can make it difficult to eat. Treatment may alter a patient's ability to taste or smell. Depression and lack of energy may make a person not want to eat, and appetite and metabolism may change.

Loss of appetite can be caused by the cancer itself, cancer treatment, or depression. CACHEXIA is the medical term for the wasting and dramatic weight loss seen in many cancer patients. Body organs starve and waste along with muscle and fat. About two-thirds of all cancer patients, and nearly all patients with cancer that has spread, experience weight loss due to decreased appetite or cachexia. While these may not be preventable, attention to eating and good nutrition will allow a better quality of life, help the body tolerate treatment, and can contribute to better resistance to infection.

Improving Nutrition

There are a number of lifestyle changes that cancer patients can make to try to improve their nutrition. These include

- *Relaxation.* Patients should choose a quiet place to eat, listening to soothing music and trying to lessen distractions.
- *Presentation.* Patients can try to make eating a more pleasurable experience by trying to prepare and present food in appetizing, attractive ways.
- *No set mealtimes.* Patients should eat when they are hungry and not wait for mealtime. Because nausea or lack of appetite may come and go, patients should eat whenever they feel they can.
- *Small meals.* It is often better to eat many small meals throughout the day instead of loading the stomach with three big meals.
- *Snack.* Patients should keep snacks nearby and eat between meals.
- *Favorite foods.* Cancer patients should concentrate on having favorite foods available, which will sometimes help improve appetite.
- *Change diet.* Sometimes eating a different type of food can stimulate the appetite.
- *Watch temperature.* Cancer patients should pay attention to the temperature of the foods they eat. Some patients find that warm or room-temperature food is better tolerated; others find that cold foods are more soothing. In general, hot and spicy foods are not well tolerated by most patients.
- *Avoid strong smells.* Patients should avoid cooking foods with unpleasant smells. It may be better to eat food with little or no smell, such as cottage cheese or crackers.
- *Load calories.* Patients can get extra calories by adding dry milk, honey, jam, or brown sugar to food whenever possible.

Nausea Tips

Patients who feel nauseated should call the doctor for antinausea medication. Taken as directed, it is often quite effective. Patients who are vomiting should not try to eat or drink until the vomiting has stopped. Good diet choices for nausea include crackers, toast, oatmeal, soft, bland vegetables and fruits, clear liquids, and skinned baked chicken. Foods to be avoided are fatty, greasy, or fried foods, sweets, and hot or spicy foods. Patients should not force themselves to eat during periods of nausea, because this may trigger aversions to favorite foods.

Patients with nausea should drink liquids between meals, not during meals. It also may help to eat in a room other than the kitchen if cooking smells make nausea worse.

Physical Eating Problems

Some patients may have trouble with eating due to physical problems related to cancer or treatment. If this is the case, patients should

- avoid foods that may irritate the mouth, such as spicy, acidic, citrus, or salty foods.
- take very small bites of food at a time instead of full mouthfuls.
- cook foods until they are very tender.
- puree foods in a blender or food processor.
- mix foods with broth, sauces, or thin gravies to make them easier to swallow.
- drink through a straw.

obesity Different from simply being overweight, obesity increases a person's chance of developing cancer. People who are overweight weigh too much because of fat, muscle, bone, and/or water retention. People who are obese have an abnormally high and unhealthy proportion of body fat.

More than 65 percent of all American adults are overweight to some extent, and almost 25 percent are obese; moreover, the number of obese people has increased steadily since the 1970s and 1980s. The obesity epidemic continued into the 1990s; from 1991 to 1998 obesity increased in every state of the United States, in both sexes, among smokers and nonsmokers, and across race/ethnicity, age, and educational levels. Because of this dramatic rise, even a minor link between risk and obesity is cause for concern.

Researchers have found a consistent relationship between obesity and a number of diseases, including diabetes, heart disease, high blood pressure, and stroke. Although study results related to cancer have been conflicting, with some showing an increased risk and others not showing such an association, obesity does appear to be linked to some types of cancer. Obesity appears to increase the risk of cancers of the breast, colon, prostate, uterine lining, cervix, ovary, kidney, and gallbladder. Studies have also found an increased risk for cancers of the liver, pancreas, rectum, and esophagus.

Although there are many theories about how obesity increases cancer risk, the exact mechanisms are not known. They may be different for different types of cancer. Also, because obesity develops through a complex interaction of heredity and lifestyle factors, it is not easy to tell whether the obesity or something else led to the development of cancer.

Drawing conclusions from studies of obesity is made more difficult by the fact that definitions and measurements of *overweight* and *obese* vary from study to study. This problem affected early study results and made it difficult to compare data across studies.

Most researchers currently use a formula based on weight and height, known as body mass index (BMI), to study obesity as a risk factor for cancer. According to a U.S. government panel, which is consistent with the recommendations of many other countries and the World Health Organization, *overweight* is defined as a BMI of 25 to 30, and *obese* is a BMI of 30 or more. Health risks increase gradually with increasing BMI. BMI is useful in tracking trends in the population because it provides a more accurate measure of overweight and obesity than does weight alone. By itself, however, this measurement cannot give direct or specific information about a person's health.

To figure out BMI:

1. Square one's height (multiply one's height in inches times the same number).
2. Divide one's weight in pounds by one's height squared.
3. Multiply this answer by 703.
4. The result is one's BMI.

For example, a woman who is 65 inches tall and weighs 130 pounds would perform the following calculations:

1. 65 inches × 65 inches = 4225.
2. 130 ÷ 4225 = .0307692
3. .0307692 × 703 = 21.6

Alternatively, to find out a person's BMI without doing the math, it is possible to use a BMI calculator online at the Web site of the Centers for Disease Control and Prevention, and plug in numbers for height and weight. The Web address is: http://www.cdc.gov/nccdphp/dnpa/bmi/calc-bmi.htm.

A Swedish study published in the January 2001 issue of *Cancer Causes and Control* found 33 percent more cases of cancer among obese subjects than in the general population (25 percent more among men and 37 percent more among women). The obese patients had an increased risk for HODGKIN'S DISEASE (among men) and cancers of the endometrium, kidney, gallbladder, colon, pancreas, bladder, cervix, ovary, and brain. An association between obesity and LIVER CANCER was also found, but that may be explained by the presence of diabetes and alcoholism in these patients. The researchers also found some cancers associated with obesity that were not found by previous researchers, including NON-HODGKIN'S LYMPHOMA (among women) and cancers of the small intestine and larynx.

More studies are needed to evaluate the combined effects of diet, body weight, and physical activity. For some types of cancer, such as colon and breast, it is not clear whether the increased cancer risk is due to extra weight, inadequate consumption of fruits and vegetables, or a high-fat, high-calorie diet. Lack of physical activity also contributes to obesity and appears to be associated with increased risk of cancers of the breast and colon. Physical inactivity may also be associated with other types of cancer, such as prostate cancer. However, because physical activity level is difficult to measure, its impact on cancer may be underestimated due to misclassification.

In the future, researchers may measure physical fitness, rather than level of physical activity. Physical fitness appears to predict heart disease better than measures of physical activity; the same may be true for cancer. The complex relationship between physical activity and obesity makes it important that researchers include both factors in future epidemiological investigations.

A panel of experts who met at the International Agency for Research on Cancer (IARC) in Lyon, France, concluded that being overweight and having a sedentary lifestyle are associated with several diseases, including cancer. The panel recommended that prevention of obesity begin early in life, based on healthy eating habits and regular physical activity. The panel advised people who are overweight or obese to avoid gaining additional weight, and to lose weight through dietary changes and exercise. The IARC, which is part of the World Health Organization, coordinates and conducts research on the causes of cancer and develops scientific strategies for cancer control.

oncogenes Genes that may trigger cancer or allow it to grow. Normally these genes—when not damaged—are responsible for helping normal cells to grow and develop. When damaged in some way, these genes can cause cells to become malignant. Cancer-susceptibility genes include:

APC: COLORECTAL CANCER
ATM: BREAST CANCER, NON-HODGKIN'S LYMPHOMA, LEUKEMIA, and LIVER CANCER
BRCA1 and BRCA2: Breast cancer, OVARIAN CANCER, PROSTATE CANCER, PANCREATIC CANCER, and MELANOMA.
CDH1: STOMACH CANCER
CDK4: This gene, also known as p15, INK4b, and MTS2, has been linked to higher rates of MELANOMA.
CDKN2: Also known as p16, INK4a, or MTS1, this gene has been linked to higher rates of melanoma.
EXT2: Chondrosarcoma
KIT: GASTROINTESTINAL STROMAL TUMORS
LKB1: This gene, also known as STK11, is linked to colon, breast, pancreatic, testicular, and ovarian cancer.
MEN1: Endocrine (pituitary, pancreas, parathyroid) tumors.
MET: KIDNEY CANCER
MLH1 and MSH2: These genes have each been implicated in colon, ovarian, endometrial, and stomach cancers.
MSH6: Also known as GTBP, this gene has been linked to colon, endometrial, and stomach cancers.
NF-1: BRAIN CANCER and SARCOMA

NF-2: BRAIN CANCER, among others

p53: Breast cancer, SARCOMA, and brain cancer

PMS 1 and 2: These genes, discovered in 1994, have both been linked to colon, ovarian, endometrial, and stomach cancers.

PTCH: SKIN CANCER and brain cancer in children

PTEN: Breast and THYROID CANCER

RB1: This gene, the first of the oncogenes to be discovered (1986), has been linked to the development of retinoblastoma, sarcoma, and other cancers.

RET: Thyroid cancer

SMAD4: Also known as DPC4, this gene is linked to colon cancer.

TGFBR2: Colon cancer

TSC1 and 2: Kidney cancer and brain cancer

VHL: Kidney cancer and brain cancer

WT1: WILM'S TUMOR

oncogenic virus A virus that can help stimulate cancer to grow. There are more than 100 of these viruses known to exist. Many are "slow viruses" that live in the body for many years. The HUMAN PAPILLOMAVIRUS is one type of oncogenic virus. It is linked to almost all cases of CERVICAL CANCER.

oncologist Physician whose primary interest is cancer. Clinical oncologists are the physicians who treat cancer patients. In most cases, when a person is diagnosed with cancer, a clinical oncologist takes charge of the patient's overall care through all phases of the disease. Within the field of clinical oncology there are three primary disciplines: medical oncology, surgical oncology, and radiation oncology.

- *Medical oncologists* are physicians who specialize in treating cancer with medicine/CHEMOTHERAPY.

- *Surgical oncologists* are physicians who specialize in surgical aspects of cancer including biopsy, staging, and surgical resection of tumors.

- *Radiation oncologists* are physicians who specialize in treating cancer with therapeutic radiation.

- *Pediatric oncologists* are recognized by the American Society of Clinical Oncology (ASCO) as constituting a fourth separate and distinct specialty within the field of oncology. Pediatric oncologists

specialize in the treatment of children with cancer and incorporate all three primary oncology disciplines in the care of their patients.

Education and Training

Clinical oncologists complete between four and seven years of postgraduate medical education, depending on their primary discipline. In the United States, medical, radiation, and pediatric oncology are recognized as medical specialties by the American Board of Medical Specialties.

In order to become practicing cancer specialists, medical oncologists usually take board exams administered by the American Board of Internal Medicine (ABIM), and radiation oncologists usually take board exams administered by the American Board of Radiology. Surgical oncologists do not have an equivalent specialty board, but general surgeons are certified by the American Board of Surgery; those surgeons who choose to specialize further in oncology receive a "certificate of special competence" once they have completed their oncology training program.

Pediatric oncologists are separately certified by the ABIM after passing a joint exam in hematology/oncology. They are also specifically trained in one of the three primary oncologic disciplines. These cancer specialists require a unique subset of skills because children with cancer have unique problems that require specialized care across the entire spectrum of treatment.

Regardless of their own particular discipline, medical, radiation, and surgical oncologists are broadly trained in all three areas of oncology and are knowledgeable about the appropriate use of each treatment approach. Within the three disciplines, oncologists may further specialize in specific types of cancer such as BREAST CANCER, LUNG CANCER, PROSTATE CANCER, LEUKEMIA, LYMPHOMA, and so on.

oncology The branch of medicine that deals with the study of cancerous tumors.

oncology clinical nurse specialist (CNS) An advanced practice nurse with a master's degree who has received extensive education in the needs of cancer patients. These nurses specialize in oncology work, primarily in hospitals, to provide and supervise care for cancer patients who are either chronically or critically ill. They monitor their patients' physical conditions, prescribe medication, and manage symptoms. They are trained to apply nursing theory and research to clinical practice and may function as researchers, administrators, consultants, and educators in this field.

The oncology CNS can help patients who are trying to deal with their diagnosis and/or treatment regimen. Symptom management, maintaining health and wellness during treatment, and coping with information about cancer and its treatment are all areas where the clinical nurse specialist can help patients and families. The oncology CNS works closely with the entire health-care team to ensure that a patient's plan of care is comprehensive, is tailored to the patient's needs, and is clear and manageable for the patient and family. The CNS can help the patient and family understand and cope with a cancer diagnosis.

oral cancer A type of cancer that may affect the lip, tongue, salivary glands, gum, mouth, pharynx, oropharynx, and hypopharynx. Oral cavity cancer occurs when cells divide abnormally in the lip or mouth. The oral cavity includes the gums, lips, inside of the cheeks, teeth, roof and floor of the mouth, and underside and front two-thirds of the tongue.

Risk Factors

There are a number of risk factors that may influence the onset of oral cancer.

Gender Oral cancer is far more common among men; out of 30,100 new cases a year, fewer than 10,000 of them will be in women.

Tobacco use Oral cavity cancer is strongly associated with SMOKING or chewing tobacco. About 90 percent of people with oral cavity cancers use tobacco; risk increases with the amount and duration of tobacco use.

Alcohol ALCOHOL use and exposure to sunlight also increase the risk of oral cavity cancer.

Race Among men, the highest rates are in African Americans, followed by Caucasians (especially non-Hispanic Caucasians), Vietnamese, and native Hawaiians. Less variation occurs in women,

among whom high rates occur in non-Hispanic Caucasians, African Americans, and Filipinos. Although reasons for these racial/ethnic and sex differences have not been established, differences in the extent of exposure to risk factors for oral cavity cancer are presumably largely responsible.

Age Incidence of oral cavity cancer increases with age in all groups except the oldest age group of black men and women. The greatest increase in rates occurs between the 30- to 54-year-old group and the 55- to 69-year-old group

Betel nut use Chewing of betel nut is not a common practice in the United States, but it is a widespread habit in some parts of the world. Chewing betel nuts is also a known cause of oral cancer.

Symptoms

Most of the symptoms of oral cavity cancers can be caused by other, less serious disorders. But if any symptoms persist for two weeks or longer, they deserve immediate attention. The most common symptom of oral cavity cancer is a mouth sore that doesn't heal. Other common symptoms of oral cavity cancer, as described by the AMERICAN CANCER SOCIETY, include

- a lump or mass in the neck
- a persistent feeling that something is caught in the throat
- a persistent discoloration in the mouth
- a persistent lump or thickening in the cheek
- a persistent sore throat
- voice changes
- difficulty chewing or swallowing
- difficulty moving your jaw or tongue
- loosening teeth
- numbness of the tongue or other area of the mouth
- pain around the teeth or jaw
- pain or irritation in the mouth that does not go away
- sudden unexplained WEIGHT LOSS
- jaw swelling (this may cause dentures to fit poorly or become uncomfortable)

Diagnosis

Every routine visit to a doctor or dentist should include an oral exam, with careful observation of the tissues of the mouth for abnormalities. The doctor may feel with gloved fingers for any lumps or masses. If the doctor suspects anything abnormal, further examinations will be performed. The next step may be a referral to an oral surgery specialist or an ear, nose, and throat surgeon. Usually procedures are performed in the office or as same-day procedures in a hospital operating room. Small mirrors or a fiberoptic scope (a thin tube with a tiny camera) may be used to get a closer look at structures in the back of the throat, the voice box, or the nose. To confirm or rule out cancer, the surgeon will perform a biopsy, extracting a small piece of tissue from the abnormal area.

Because oral cavity cancer is closely related to other cancers, diagnosis is commonly followed by close examination of the larynx, esophagus, and lungs using a fiberoptic scope.

Staging

Doctors identify a cancer's development by giving it a numerical "stage." A stage 0 or stage I or II tumor has not invaded very far into surrounding tissues, while a stage III or IV tumor may be spreading throughout and beyond surrounding tissues.

Treatment

The type of treatment recommended varies depending on the cancer's origin and its stage of development. The most common treatments for oral cavity cancer are surgery, RADIATION THERAPY, and CHEMOTHERAPY.

If cancer is discovered at an earlier stage, the chances for successful treatment are much improved. In early stage I and II tumors, usually surgery or radiation therapy is required. One treatment might be favored over the other because of side effects. For example, depending on the location of the cancer, surgery might be preferred as a way of avoiding radiation's effect on surrounding healthy tissue. In other cases, surgery might significantly alter the ability to speak or eat, which would make radiation more desirable. Later stage III and IV tumors usually require more extensive surgery.

After oral cavity cancer treatments a patient may need rehabilitation to recover the ability to speak and eat, or cosmetic surgery (if extensive surgery was performed).

Surgery   This is the most common treatment, and it involves removing the tumor and some surrounding tissue. In many cases, surgery can be performed directly through the mouth, but sometimes a tumor can be reached only through the neck or jaw.

When cancer cells have spread into the lymph nodes, the surgeon will perform a "neck dissection" to remove the cancer-containing lymph nodes in hopes of containing the cancer before it spreads throughout the body.

Radiation therapy   This is the primary treatment for some small tumors. It may also be used after surgery to ensure that all cancer cells are destroyed. When a cure is not possible, radiation may be used to alleviate symptoms such as pain, bleeding, or difficulty swallowing.

Chemotherapy   Drug treatments may help shrink tumors before surgery is performed. Researchers are currently studying whether chemotherapy combined with radiation therapy, instead of surgery, can be effective in treating large cancers confined to the head and neck.

Prognosis

The earlier oral cavity cancer is discovered, the better the prognosis; up to 90 percent of people with early-stage oral cancer survive at least five years after diagnosis. For later-stage cancers, the survival rate to at least five years ranges from 20 percent to 50 percent. However, even after successful treatment, up to 40 percent of people with oral cancer later develop another cancer, so follow-up examinations are crucial.

Other Cancers

People with oral cavity cancer have an increased risk for developing cancer of the throat, esophagus, or lung. In fact, 15 percent of people diagnosed with oral cavity cancer are simultaneously diagnosed with cancer of the larynx, esophagus, or lung. From 10 percent to 40 percent of those with oral cavity cancer will later develop one of these cancers or a new oral cavity cancer.

Prevention

The greatest risk factors for oral cancer are smoking and smokeless tobacco. Drinking alcohol is another significant risk factor. People who use tobacco and drink alcohol have an even higher risk. Therefore, stopping smoking and not using smokeless tobacco can have a big impact on oral cancer risk.

Cancer of the lip is associated with sunlight exposure. Patients who are exposed to sunlight (especially on the job) should try to avoid the sun during the peak midday hours, wear a wide-brimmed hat, and use sunscreen and lip balm that protect against ultraviolet light.

Some evidence suggests that diets high in fruits and vegetables reduce the risk of developing this cancer.

organochlorines　A group of chlorinated hydrocarbons that include the banned pesticide DDT, which has been linked to BREAST CANCER in the United States. DDT was once widely used in agriculture and malarial control programs around the world. It was effectively banned for use as a pesticide in the United States in 1972 (almost 30 years after it was introduced), although it can remain active in tissues for up to 50 years. It was banned because of its toxicity and because it does not disperse in the environment but instead builds up in biological systems. The meat of animals that have consumed DDT—or of animals that have eaten animals tainted with DDT—is poisonous to eat.

Although its link with cancer is controversial, women with breast cancer were five times as likely to have DDT pesticide residues in their blood, according to a recent British study published in the spring of 2003. DDT is considered to be an environmental source of ESTROGEN. The authors say that their new study adds to the growing body of evidence for an association between environmental estrogens and the rising incidence of breast cancer. The study included 600 women referred for breast lumps to one hospital in Liege, Belgium, between September 1999 and February 2000. Before surgery or drug treatment, the women were tested for total levels of organochlorines and hexachlorobenzene (HCB) in their blood.

The results showed significant differences between healthy women and those with breast cancer: The breast cancer patients were over five times as likely to have detectable levels of DDT above 0.5 parts per billion as the healthy women, and more than nine times as likely to have detectable levels of HCB in their blood. The highest levels detected were 20 parts per billion.

While this research does not prove a definitive link between estrogenic pesticide residues and breast cancer, there is extensive published evidence on the ability of hormones to promote animal and human cancers.

organ transplants and cancer　Occasionally, patients who have received organ transplants have developed cancer from cells contaminating the transplant. Recently a team of Italian researchers found that five patients who developed a rare type of SKIN CANCER (KAPOSI'S SARCOMA) after an organ transplant may have received cancer seed cells from the donor. Kaposi's sarcoma is one of the most frequent transplant-related tumors. It appears in about one out of every 200 transplant recipients—400 to 500 times the rate of the general population. In 2004, Scottish doctors reported two cases of patients developing malignant MELANOMA from transplanted kidneys, although the donor was successfully treated for the cancer many years earlier.

However, transfer of cancer from a donated organ to a transplant patient is rare, and the chances of it happening long after the donor was treated were thought to be extremely unlikely. In the cases involving Kaposi's sarcoma, researchers studied eight patients—six women and two men—who received kidneys from male donors and who developed Kaposi's sarcoma nine months to 40 months later. In analyzing the cancer cells from the women, the researchers detected Y-chromosome DNA in four cases. DNA is the molecule that determines a human's development. Women have two X chromosomes while men have one X and one Y chromosome. Thus, the presence of the Y-chromosome DNA in the women's cancer indicates that the cells originated with a man. There was no evidence of Y chromosomes in the cancer in the other two women or in normal cells from any of the women. Using DNA analysis of the cancer cells in the men, the researchers found that in one case the cancer DNA was related to that of the donor.

Kaposi's sarcoma can be treated by reducing or ending the suppression of the patient's IMMUNE SYSTEM, allowing it to battle the cancer, but that also can mean the immune system attacks the transplanted organ, causing it to be rejected. Researchers noted that the organ donors had no symptoms of Kaposi's sarcoma, which suggests they are infected with the cancer-causing virus but that their bodies destroy the cancer cells when they form. Once the infected organ is transplanted into someone with a weakened immune system, however, the cancer cells can grow and cause disease.

ostomy A surgical opening (stoma) in the body to allow for the release of urine from the bladder, or feces from the bowel, often as a treatment for COLORECTAL CANCER.

A colostomy is created when a portion of the colon or the rectum is removed and the remaining colon is brought to the abdominal wall. It may further be defined by the portion of the colon involved and/or its permanence. An ileostomy is a surgically created opening in the small intestine so that the intestine is brought through the abdominal wall to form a stoma. Ileostomies may be temporary or permanent and may involve removal of all or part of the colon. A device is attached to the stoma as soon after surgery as possible.

Each time the device is changed, the skin around the stoma is washed with soap and water, rinsed, and patted dry. A sticky substance may be used to seal the device, and deodorant drops are added to the ostomy bag.

Some colostomates can "irrigate," using a procedure much like an enema to clean stool directly out of the colon through the stoma. This requires a special irrigation system, including an irrigation bag with a connecting tube, a stoma cone, and an irrigation sleeve. After irrigation, some colostomates can use a stoma cap to cover and protect the stoma. This procedure is usually done to avoid the need to wear a pouch.

An ostomy should not limit a patient's activities, including participation in sports. Many physicians do not allow contact sports because of possible injury to the stoma from a severe blow or because the pouching system may slip, but these problems can be overcome with special ostomy supplies. However, weight lifting may cause a hernia at the stoma. Many people with ostomies are distance runners, skiers, swimmers, and participants in many other types of athletics.

Patients may bathe with or without a pouching system in place. Normal exposure to air or contact with soap and water will not harm the stoma, and water does not enter the opening.

After an ostomy, the patient's diet must be adjusted to include foods the body can easily digest and absorb. Foods should be gradually reintroduced into the diet so that the effect of each food on the ostomy function can be monitored. Some less digestible or high-roughage foods are more likely to create blockage problems (such as corn, coconut, mushrooms, nuts, and raw fruits and vegetables).

ovarian cancer A type of cancer that begins in the ovaries, the fifth most common cancer in women. Each year it is diagnosed in about 25,500 American women, and almost 16,090 women die of the disease annually.

Ovarian cancer cells can break away from the ovary and spread to other tissues and organs in a process called shedding. When ovarian cancer sheds, it tends to form new tumors on the peritoneum (the large membrane that lines the abdomen) and on the diaphragm (the thin muscle that separates the chest from the abdomen).

Types of Tumors

There are three basic types of ovarian tumors, which are designated by where they form. Ovarian cancer that begins on the surface of the ovary, epithelial carcinoma, is the most common. About 90 percent of ovarian cancers develop in the thin layer of tissue that covers the ovaries. This form of ovarian cancer generally occurs in postmenopausal women.

Ovarian cancer that begins in the egg-producing cells is called a germ cell tumor and generally occurs in younger women. Cancer that begins in the supportive estrogen- and progesterone-producing tissue holding the ovaries together is called a stromal tumor. Both germ cell and stromal tumors are rare and are usually benign.

Causes

The exact causes of ovarian cancer are not known, but studies show that a number of factors may increase the chance of developing this disease.

Heredity Ovarian cancer, like all cancers, is caused by a combination of genetic and environmental factors. A woman's risk of developing ovarian cancer is often related to her personal and family history of cancer. In the United States a woman has a 1.8 percent chance of developing ovarian cancer in her lifetime, but a woman with an affected first-degree relative (such as her mother or sister) is believed to have a 4 percent to 7 percent lifetime chance of developing this cancer. In families where the pattern of ovarian, breast, and other cancers suggests the cancers are inherited, a woman's chance of developing ovarian cancer may be as high as 45 percent.

A woman can inherit an increased risk for ovarian cancer from either her mother or father's side of her family. She has a greater probability of developing this cancer if a first-degree relative (mother, sister, or daughter) has, or has had, ovarian cancer, BREAST CANCER, or COLORECTAL CANCER. The likelihood is especially high if two or more first-degree relatives have had the disease. The risk is somewhat lower, but still above average, if other relatives (grandmother, aunt, cousin) have had ovarian cancer. Furthermore, women with a strong family history of ovarian cancer are more likely to develop the disease at an early age (younger than 50). Women of Ashkenazi (Eastern European) Jewish descent are at even greater risk if they have an affected family member.

Studies show that inheriting a defect in either of two breast cancer genes (*BRCA1* or *BRCA2*) can increase a woman's risk of developing ovarian cancer by about 13 percent to 50 percent. Normally, these genes help to prevent cancer, but if a woman has inherited a mutated *BRCA1* or *BRCA2* gene, her ovaries and breasts are more susceptible to the development of cancer.

Although many women have a family history of ovarian or breast cancer, only about five percent to 10 percent of ovarian cancers are thought to be the result of inherited cancer susceptibility genes. A family history of ovarian and/or breast cancer may or may not indicate that one has inherited an increased likelihood of developing cancer. Most cases of ovarian cancer are sporadic, meaning they occur in women who do not have a family history of ovarian cancer.

Taking a detailed three-generation family history, or pedigree, is an essential element in the assessment of a woman's chances of developing ovarian or other cancers. Evidence of a hereditary susceptibility to cancer within a family includes

- Two or more women with ovarian and/or breast cancer, especially if the diagnoses occur before menopause.
- A woman who has had separate diagnoses of breast and ovarian cancer.
- A woman who has had breast cancer in both breasts.
- A man with breast cancer in addition to a female relative with breast or ovarian cancer.
- A woman with ovarian cancer at any age who is of Ashkenazi Jewish ancestry.

Members of families with many cases of these diseases may consider having a special blood test to see if they have a genetic change in *BRCA1* or *BRCA2*. Although having such a genetic change does not mean that a woman is sure to develop ovarian or breast cancer, those who have the genetic change may want to discuss their options with a doctor.

Age The likelihood of developing ovarian cancer increases as a woman gets older. Most ovarian cancers occur in women over the age of 50, with the highest risk in women over 60.

Childbearing Women who have never had children are more likely to develop ovarian cancer than women who have had children. In fact, the more children a woman has had, the less likely she is to develop ovarian cancer.

Personal history Women who have had breast or colon cancer may have a greater chance of developing ovarian cancer than women who have not had breast or colon cancer.

Fertility drugs Drugs that cause a woman to ovulate may slightly increase a woman's chance of developing ovarian cancer. Researchers are studying this possible association.

Talc Some studies suggest that women who have used talc in the genital area for many years may be at increased risk of developing ovarian cancer.

Hormone replacement therapy (HRT) Some evidence suggests that women who use HRT after menopause may have a slightly increased risk of developing ovarian cancer.

Race Incidence is highest among American Indian women, followed by Caucasian, Vietnamese, Caucasian Hispanic, and Hawaiian women. Rates are lowest among Korean and Chinese women. Death rate is highest among Caucasian women, followed by Hawaiian women and African-American women. Caucasian women have the highest ovarian cancer mortality rate.

Preventive Factors

Some studies have shown that breast-feeding and taking birth control pills may lower a woman's chance of developing ovarian cancer. These two factors both decrease the number of times a woman ovulates, and studies suggest that reducing the number of ovulations during a woman's lifetime may lower her risk for ovarian cancer. Women who have had tubal ligation to prevent pregnancy or who have had a hysterectomy also have a lower risk of developing ovarian cancer. In addition, some evidence suggests that reducing the amount of fat in the diet may lower the risk of developing ovarian cancer.

Women who are at high risk for ovarian cancer due to a family history of the disease may consider having their ovaries removed before cancer develops (prophylactic oophorectomy). This procedure almost always protects women from developing ovarian cancer. However, they still have a slight chance of developing peritoneal cancer in the area where the ovaries were removed.

Symptoms

Ovarian cancer often shows no obvious signs or symptoms until late in its development. As a tumor grows in an ovary, it may press on the bowel, bladder, or other organs in the abdominal cavity, causing vague symptoms that are easily confused with those of other conditions. Fluid may collect in the abdomen, causing a condition known as ASCITES, which may make a woman feel bloated, or her abdomen may look swollen.

When symptoms do appear, they may include

- general abdominal discomfort and/or pain (gas, indigestion, pressure, swelling, bloating, cramps)
- nausea, diarrhea, constipation, or frequent urination
- appetite loss
- feeling full even after a light meal
- pelvic pressure
- weight gain or loss with no known reason
- abnormal bleeding from the vagina

Diagnosis

The sooner ovarian cancer is found and treated, the better a woman's chance for recovery. But because the disease is difficult to detect in its early stage, only 25 percent of ovarian cancers are found before tumor growth has spread into tissues and organs beyond the ovaries. If symptoms do appear, a doctor will evaluate a woman's medical history, perform a physical exam, and order diagnostic tests, including:

- *Pelvic exam.* To find any abnormality in the shape or size of ovaries. (Although a PAP SMEAR is often done along with the pelvic exam, it is not a reliable way to find or diagnose ovarian cancer.)
- *Ultrasound or CAT scans.* To check the ovaries for any growths. A CAT scan is a series of detailed pictures of areas inside the body created by a computer linked to an X-ray machine.
- *CA 125 assay.* A blood test used to measure the level of CA-125, a tumor marker that is often found in higher-than-normal amounts in the blood of women with ovarian cancer.
- *Lower GI series.* A series of X-rays of the colon and rectum to make tumors or other abnormal areas easier to see. A CAT scan may be used.
- *Biopsy.* To remove tissue for examination under a microscope. To obtain the tissue, the surgeon performs a laparotomy (an operation to open the abdomen). If cancer is suspected, the surgeon removes the entire ovary (oophorectomy). (Removing just a sample of tissue by cutting

through the outer layer of the ovary could allow cancer cells to escape and cause the disease to spread.)

Staging

If the diagnosis is ovarian cancer, the doctor will want to learn the stage of disease to find out whether the cancer has spread and, if so, to what parts of the body. The stages of the tumor, which can be determined during surgery, are as follows:

Stage I: Growth of the cancer is limited to the ovary or ovaries.

Stage IA: Growth is limited to one ovary, and the tumor is confined to the inside of the ovary. There is no cancer on the outer surface of the ovary, there are no ascites containing malignant cells, and the covering of the ovary is intact.

Stage IB: Growth is limited to both ovaries, without any tumor on their outer surfaces. There are no ascites present containing malignant cells, and the capsule is intact.

Stage IC: The tumor is classified as either Stage IA or IB, and one or more of the following are present:

- Tumor is present on the outer surface of one or both ovaries.
- The capsule has ruptured.
- There are ascites containing malignant cells or with positive peritoneal washings.

Stage II: Growth of the cancer involves one or both ovaries with pelvic extension.

Stage IIA: The cancer has extended to and/or involves the uterus or the fallopian tubes, or both.

Stage IIB: The cancer has extended to other pelvic organs.

Stage IIC: The tumor is classified as either Stage IIA or IIB, and one or more of the following are present:

- Tumor is present on the outer surface of one or both ovaries.
- The capsule has ruptured.
- There are ascites containing malignant cells or with positive peritoneal washings.

Stage III: Growth of the cancer involves one or both ovaries, and one or both of the following are present:

- The cancer has spread beyond the pelvis to the lining of the abdomen.
- The cancer has spread to lymph nodes. The tumor is limited to the true pelvis but with histologically proven malignant extension to the small bowel or omentum.

Stage IIIA: During the staging operation, the practitioner can see cancer involving one or both of the ovaries, but no cancer is grossly visible in the abdomen and it has not spread to lymph nodes. However, when biopsies are checked under a microscope, very small deposits of cancer are found in the abdominal peritoneal surfaces.

Stage IIIB: The tumor is in one or both ovaries, and deposits of cancer are present in the abdomen that are large enough for the surgeon to see but do not exceed 2 cm in diameter. The cancer has not spread to the lymph nodes.

Stage IIIC: The tumor is in one or both ovaries, and one or both of the following are present:

- The cancer has spread to lymph nodes.
- The deposits of cancer exceed 2 cm in diameter and are found in the abdomen.

Stage IV: This is the most advanced stage of ovarian cancer. Growth of the cancer involves one or both ovaries, and distant metastases have occurred. The presence of ovarian cancer cells in the cavity that surrounds the lungs is also evidence of Stage IV disease.

Treatment

Many different treatments and combinations of treatments are used with ovarian cancer.

Surgery   Surgery is the usual initial treatment for women diagnosed with ovarian cancer, with the removal of the ovaries, fallopian tubes, uterus, and the cervix. This operation is called a HYSTERECTOMY with bilateral SALPINGO-OOPHORECTOMY. Often, the surgeon also removes the thin tissue covering the stomach and large intestine, and abdominal lymph nodes. If the cancer has spread, the surgeon usually removes as much of the cancer as possible in a procedure called tumor debulking. This procedure reduces the amount of cancer that will have to be treated later with CHEMOTHERAPY or RADIATION THERAPY.

Chemotherapy Chemotherapy may be given to destroy any cancerous cells that may remain in the body after surgery, to control tumor growth, or to relieve symptoms of the disease. Most drugs used to treat ovarian cancer are given intravenously, although some oral medications are also available. Another method is to instill the drug directly into the abdomen through a catheter (intraperitoneal chemotherapy). Certain drugs used in the treatment of ovarian cancer can cause some hearing loss or kidney damage. To help protect the kidneys while taking these drugs, patients may receive extra fluid intravenously.

After chemotherapy is completed, "second-look surgery" may be performed to examine the abdomen directly, allowing the surgeon to remove fluid and tissue samples to see whether the drugs have been successful.

Radiation therapy This treatment affects the cancer cells only in the treated area and may be given either externally or internally. In intraperitoneal radiation, radioactive liquid is instilled directly into the abdomen through a catheter.

Ovarian Cancer National Alliance A patient-led umbrella organization uniting OVARIAN CANCER activists, women's health advocates, and health-care professionals in an effort to increase public and professional understanding of ovarian cancer and to work toward more effective diagnostics, treatments, and a cure. The group was formed in September 1997, when leaders from seven ovarian cancer groups joined forces. The primary goal was to establish a coordinated national effort to place ovarian cancer education, policy, and research issues prominently on the agendas of national policy makers and women's health-care leaders. The group supports research and provides information and patient support. For contact information, see Appendix I.

ovarian cysts Small, fluid-filled sacs or pockets located within or on the surface of an ovary that are not usually malignant. Some time during their lifetime many women develop harmless ovarian cysts, which present little or no discomfort. However, some cysts produce severe symptoms that can be life threatening.

The normal ovary produces a normal cyst with each menstrual cycle during a woman's reproductive years. The normal cyst (follicle) contains the egg and usually is less than 3 cm. After ovulation this cyst remains behind but is rarely bigger than 5 cm and disappears with each menstrual cycle. Cysts are considered to be abnormal if they persist throughout multiple cycles, are 6 cm or larger, or are formed during childhood or after menopause. The vast majority of these abnormal cysts are still benign.

Although cyst formation is a normal part of ovulation in premenopausal women, cysts that do not go away or that occur after menopause need to be evaluated. Doctors do not know if these benign ovarian cysts will develop into OVARIAN CANCER, but to be sure, experts usually recommend that they be removed.

Types of Ovarian Cysts

There are two types of functional cysts—follicular cysts or corpus luteum cysts. The follicle releases an egg when the pituitary gland sends a burst of hormone called luteinizing hormone (LH). A follicular cyst begins when LH does not surge, and the chain reaction does not start. The result is a follicle that does not rupture or release its egg; instead it grows until it becomes a cyst. Follicular cysts are usually harmless, rarely cause pain, and often disappear on their own within two or three menstrual cycles.

If the LH does surge and an egg is released, the follicle responds to LH by producing large quantities of estrogen and progesterone in preparation for conception. This change in the follicle is called the corpus luteum. However, sometimes after the egg's release, its escape hole seals off and tissues accumulate inside, causing the corpus luteum to expand into a cyst. Although this cyst usually disappears on its own in a few weeks, it can grow to almost four inches in diameter and has the potential to bleed into itself or twist the ovary, causing pelvic or abdominal pain. If it fills with blood, the cyst may rupture, causing internal bleeding and sudden, sharp pain.

Benign cysts do not invade neighboring tissue the way malignant tumors do, but if a benign ovarian cyst is large, it can cause abdominal discomfort and may interfere with the production of ovarian hormones, causing irregular vaginal bleeding or an increase in body hair. If a large tumor or cyst presses on the bladder, a woman may need to urinate more frequently.

Some women develop less common types of cysts that in rare cases can become cancerous. These cysts, which raise cancer risk when they develop in women between the ages of 50 and 70, include the following types:

Dermoid cysts These are actually benign tumors called teratomas that may contain hair, skin, or teeth. They form from cells that produce human eggs. Although they are rarely malignant, they can become large and cause painful twisting of the ovary and fallopian tube.

Endometriomas These form in women who have endometriosis, a condition in which uterine cells grow outside the uterus. Occasionally, some endometrial tissue may attach to the ovary and form a cyst.

Cystadenomas These develop from ovarian tissue and may be filled with a watery liquid or mucus. They can grow up to 12 inches or more, twisting the ovary and fallopian tube.

Symptoms

An ovarian cyst may not cause any symptoms at all, or it may trigger the following symptoms:

- menstrual irregularities
- pelvic pain—constant or intermittent dull ache that may radiate to the back and thighs
- pelvic pain shortly before a menstrual period begins or ends
- pelvic pain during sex
- nausea, vomiting, or breast tenderness similar to the discomfort experienced during pregnancy
- abdominal fullness or heaviness
- rectal or bladder pressure
- difficulty emptying the bladder completely

A woman who experiences severe or spasmodic pain in the lower abdomen, accompanied by fever and vomiting, should see a doctor. These symptoms, or symptoms of shock (cold, clammy skin; rapid breathing; light-headedness; or weakness), require immediate emergency medical attention.

Diagnosis

A cyst on an ovary may be found when a doctor feels the ovaries during a pelvic exam. If a cyst is suspected, doctors often advise further testing to determine its type and whether treatment is necessary. To identify the type, a doctor may perform a pelvic ultrasound. In this painless procedure, a transducer is inserted into the vagina to create a video screen image of the uterus and ovaries. This image can then be photographed and analyzed by the doctor to confirm the presence of a cyst, help identify its location, and determine whether it is solid or filled with fluid. Fluid-filled cysts tend to be benign, but solid material in cysts may indicate the need for further evaluation.

Alternatively, a doctor may insert a laparoscope into the abdomen through a small incision to view the ovaries, drain fluid from a cyst, or take a sample for biopsy.

The following factors indicate that a cyst might be cancerous:

Size About 5 percent of growths smaller than about two inches are cancerous, but the likelihood of cancer increases to 10 to 20 percent when the growth is between two and four inches, and increases again to 40 to 65 percent when the tumor is bigger than four inches.

Age The chance that a cyst is malignant is about 25 percent at age 50. The risk gradually increases with age, so that by 80 it reaches about 60 percent.

Postmenopause Only about 10 percent of postmenopausal ovarian cysts are functional cysts; the other 90 percent are tumors with cysts that can be either benign or malignant. Doctors do not know why ovarian cysts form after menopause, but they do know that the number of years a woman has been postmenopausal or whether she takes hormone replacement therapy has nothing to do with the development of ovarian cysts.

Treatment

Treatment depends on a woman's age, the type and size of the cyst, and symptoms.

Functional ovarian cysts typically disappear within 60 days without any treatment. Oral contraceptive pills may be prescribed to help establish normal cycles and decrease the development of functional ovarian cysts. Ovarian cysts that do not seem normal may require surgical removal by laparoscopy or exploratory laparotomy. Surgical removal is often necessary if a cyst is larger than 6 cm or lasts longer than six weeks. Treatment may include:

Watchful waiting A woman can wait and be reexamined in four to six weeks if she is not yet menopausal, ovulates, has no symptoms, and an ultrasound reveals a simple, fluid-filled cyst. Follow-up pelvic ultrasounds at periodic intervals are usually recommended to see if the cyst has changed in size. Watchful waiting, including regular monitoring with ultrasound, also is a common treatment option recommended for post-menopausal women if a cyst is fluid filled and less than two inches in diameter.

Birth control pills If a woman has a benign cyst that is large and causes considerable symptoms, birth control pills may help shrink it. Taking birth control pills may also reduce the chances of cysts growing. Women who have been on birth control pills for more than three years may also cut the chance of developing ovarian cancer in half.

Surgery A doctor may recommend removing a cyst that is bigger than two inches in diameter, or is solid, filled with debris, growing, or persisting through two or three menstrual cycles. Cysts also may be removed if they are irregularly shaped, cause pain or other symptoms, and can be found on both ovaries. If a cyst is not cancerous, it can be removed and the ovaries left intact in a procedure known as CYSTECTOMY. It's also possible to remove the one affected ovary and leave the other intact in a procedure known as HYSTERO-OOPHORECTOMY.

Leaving at least one ovary intact will enable the body to keep producing estrogen. However, if a cyst is cancerous, the doctor may advise a hysterectomy to remove both ovaries and uterus. Because the risk of ovarian cancer increases after menopause, doctors more often recommend surgery when a cystic mass develops on the ovaries after menopause.

Prevention

There is no way to prevent the growth of ovarian cysts, but regular pelvic examinations can ensure that ovarian changes are diagnosed as early as possible. In addition, women should note any changes in their monthly cycle, including atypical symptoms that may accompany menstruation or that persist over more than a few cycles.

ovaries, removal of See HYSTERO-OOPHORECTOMY.

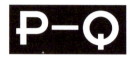

pain control Controlling cancer pain is a key component of any overall treatment plan; the most successful methods combine multiple therapies to prevent pain. When pain does break through, the proper dose of pain reliever should be taken immediately. Many patients have a tendency to wait until the pain is excruciating before seeking relief, but waiting too long often results in more pills and less effective pain control.

Estimates of persistent pain among cancer patients range from about 14 percent to almost 100 percent. The most common estimates found that pain was poorly controlled in 26 to 41 percent of all cancer patients. One obstacle to measuring the scope of the problem is that patients, themselves, often give their doctors poor insight into their pain; some believe that pain is just part of the cancer experience and must be tolerated. Other patients have an unrealistic fear of opiates and often choose to suffer instead of asking for the drugs.

The best pain treatment depends on the level of pain and its cause. Mild pain often can be treated with acetaminophen, aspirin, or a nonsteroidal anti-inflammatory drug (NSAID). Ibuprofen and naproxen are two NSAIDs frequently suggested for mild cancer pain. Moderate to severe pain generally requires an opioid, usually beginning with codeine and progressing to other options, such as oxycodone, morphine, and hydromorphone.

Long-acting narcotics such as methadone and sustained-release morphine sulfate are used when breakthrough pain is a problem. For patients who have trouble swallowing pills, options include liquid morphine and a fentanyl skin patch.

Although pain is not always a prominent feature of cancer, it is one of the most feared symptoms, but today there is no reason why most patients with cancer pain cannot be made comfortable.

The first step in managing cancer pain is proper evaluation. There are various types of pain in cancer, including pain caused by injury to tissues around the tumor (nociceptive pain), the tumor's stimulation of nerves (neuropathic pain), and by individual mental responses to sensation from the tumor (psychogenic pain). Not surprisingly, self-reporting by the patient is the most important way to assess the pain. A full history, physical exam, and appropriate lab and imaging studies (X-ray, CT, MRI) should reveal how the disease process is producing pain. The pain's intensity, features, and what affects it are all important in helping to decide the best strategy for treatment.

Acute Pain

Certain procedures involved in cancer diagnosis or treatment can sometimes produce acute pain, including LUMBAR PUNCTURE (spinal tap), BONE MARROW BIOPSY, pleural tap, CHEMOTHERAPY (especially by injection), immunotherapy (pain in the joints or muscles), and radiation (inflammation of the mucous membranes). Such attacks can usually be managed with adequate doses of nonmorphine painkillers.

Chronic Pain

Chronic cancer pain is most commonly related to bone discomfort. Experts do not known why some bone metastases are painless and others are painful. If the spine is involved, there may be damage to the spinal cord or nerve roots.

Other types of chronic pain conditions are due to nerve pain, such as the POSTMASTECTOMY PAIN SYNDROME due to nerve damage from surgery or radiation. Chemotherapy can sometimes cause persistent nerve pain, which stops when the drug is discontinued.

Opioid Drugs

The most typical way to ease pain in cancer patients are the derivatives of morphine, called opioid derivatives. The choice of drug will depend on the patient's age, the presence of liver or kidney disease, and possible interactions with other medications. While taking drugs by mouth is usually preferred, other methods (such as the transdermal skin patch) can be used if there is difficulty in swallowing or any severe gastrointestinal upset.

For continuous or frequently recurring pain, it is usually best to have a fixed schedule for dosing (such as every four hours) rather than giving the drug "as needed." Starting at a low dose, the dosage is increased until pain stops or side effects prevent an increase. If pain "breaks through" the schedule, a "rescue dose" can be added immediately; rescue dose levels are typically 5 to 15 percent of the total daily dose of the drug.

Oral doses can be given more often, if necessary, with as little as two hours between doses; the minimum interval between intravenous (IV) administrations can be as short as 10 to 15 minutes. There is no "correct" or "maximum" dose for cancer patients—the correct dose is simply whatever prevents pain.

In many cases, the development of side effects does not prevent further increase in doses; the treating physician can prescribe medications or other therapies to counteract the most common problems seen with opioids, such as nausea, vomiting, and constipation.

Non-Opioid Analgesics

Acetaminophen and nonsteroidal anti-inflammatory drugs (NSAIDs) are good painkillers, but they have a maximum dose level above which no more benefit can be expected. These medications are most useful in people with bone pain, or inflammatory pain in which the affected area is warm, red, and swollen. The newer COX-2 inhibitors may be superior types of NSAIDs in avoiding possible stomach or kidney toxicity.

In addition, certain types of cancer pain may respond well to a particular drug directed at the tissue involved. Bone pain, for instance, can be treated with bisphosphonates (Fosamax) or calcitonin.

Adjuvant Drugs

Adjuvant medications are drugs that help analgesics work more effectively. Some drugs that are not primarily painkillers may still have pain-relieving activity. For instance, steroids, antidepressants, some anesthetics, antiepilepsy drugs, and major tranquilizers may each be helpful in various cases of nerve pain. They are usually given after opioid therapy has been stabilized. Adjuvant drugs include

- *Tricyclic antidepressants* such as amitriptyline and doxepin can improve the action of opioids.
- *Benzodiazepines* such as lorazepam and diazepam control anxiety, which can allow reduction in the dosage of pain pills.
- *SSRIs (selective serotonin reuptake inhibitors)* and other antidepressants improve mood.
- *Nerve-pain modulators* such as gabapentin control pain other than by affecting opioid brain receptors.

Radiation and Chemotherapy

In addition to its main use as a way of destroying cancer cells, radiation therapy is often used to control pain, chiefly in managing the spread of cancer to the bone from the lung, breast, or prostate. Chemotherapy can provide pain relief in pancreas and prostate cancer by shrinking a tumor, but often there is the problem of balancing this sort of improvement against the toxic effects that chemotherapy can produce.

Nondrug Therapy

There are many alternative treatments for cancer patients whose pain is not adequately controlled by medication, primarily provided by specialists in hospital settings. A cancer treatment center or pain clinic is the best place for getting information and advice on these therapeutic approaches, if the patient's cancer management team does not offer them. The most common include

- acupuncture
- exercise
- heat or cold treatment
- massage
- breathing exercises

- relaxation techniques
- hypnosis
- individual, group, or family psychological therapy

palliative treatment   Medical treatment used to treat pain and symptoms of cancer patients, and to improve their quality of life when a cure is not possible. This can be achieved by using medications, radiation, or surgery. For example, irradiating bone may not cure BONE CANCER but can ease the pain.

See also HOSPICE.

pancreatic cancer   A type of cancer that affects the pancreas, a gland located deep in the abdomen between the stomach and the spine that makes insulin, other hormones, and pancreatic juices containing enzymes that help digest food. Cancer of the pancreas is extremely deadly, with the poorest likelihood of survival among all of the major malignancies. Although pancreatic cancer accounts for only 2 percent of all newly diagnosed cancers in the United States each year, it accounts for 5 percent of all cancer deaths.

In the United States pancreatic cancer is diagnosed in more than 29,000 people every year and an equal number die; it is the fifth leading cause of cancer death. Pancreatic cancer typically is highly aggressive and is one of the least curable malignancies. Only 4 percent of the people with pancreatic cancer are alive five years after diagnosis.

Most pancreatic cancers are ADENOCARCINOMAS that begin in the ducts that carry pancreatic juices. When this cancer spreads outside the pancreas, malignant cells are often found in nearby LYMPH NODES. If the cancer has reached these nodes, it means that cancer cells may have spread to other lymph nodes or other tissues, such as the liver or lungs. Sometimes cancer of the pancreas spreads to the peritoneum, the tissue that lines the abdomen.

Cause

No one knows the exact causes of pancreatic cancer, although research has shown that people with certain risk factors are more likely than others to develop it. However, most people with known risk factors do not get pancreatic cancer, and many who do get the disease have none of these factors.

The following risk factors have been linked to pancreatic cancer:

Age   The likelihood of developing pancreatic cancer increases with age. Most pancreatic cancers occur in people over the age of 60.

Smoking   Cigarette smokers are two or three times more likely than nonsmokers to develop pancreatic cancer; SMOKING is the only proven risk factor.

Gender   More men than women are diagnosed with, and die from, pancreatic cancer.

Race   African-American men and women have incidence and mortality rates that are about 50 percent higher than the rates for Caucasians. Rates for native Hawaiians are somewhat higher than the rates for Caucasians, whereas rates for Hispanics and the Asian-American groups are generally lower.

Family history   The risk for developing pancreatic cancer triples if a person's mother, father, sister, or brother had the disease. Also, a family history of COLORECTAL CANCER or OVARIAN CANCER increases slightly the risk of pancreatic cancer.

Chronic pancreatitis   Chronic pancreatitis is a painful condition of the pancreas that may increase the risk of pancreatic cancer.

Diet   A diet high in starchy foods such as potatoes, rice, and white bread may increase the risk of pancreatic cancer in women who are overweight and sedentary, according to a study by researchers at the Dana-Farber Cancer Institute, Brigham and Women's Hospital, and the Harvard School of Public Health. The study suggests that excess insulin (a substance used by the body to process the sugar in foods) can promote the development of pancreatic cancer. Other dietary risk factors that have been suggested but not confirmed include coffee drinking and high-fat diets.

Diabetes   Pancreatic cancer occurs more often in people who have diabetes than in people who do not. Studies have demonstrated that insulin encourages the growth of pancreatic cancer cells, and people who are obese, physically inactive, or have adult-onset diabetes mellitus tend to be "insulin resistant," causing them to produce larger-than-normal amounts of insulin to compensate and putting themselves at greater risk for pancreatic cancer.

Toxins   Some studies suggest that exposure to certain chemicals in the workplace may cause pancreatic cancer.

Symptoms

Pancreatic cancer is sometimes called a "silent disease" because symptoms rarely appear in the early stages. As the cancer grows, symptoms may include:

- pain in the upper abdomen or upper back
- jaundice, often painless
- weakness
- loss of appetite
- nausea and vomiting
- weight loss

Diagnosis

If a patient has symptoms that suggest pancreatic cancer, the doctor will take a careful medical history and may perform a number of procedures, including one or more of the following:

Physical exam   The exam includes checks for signs of jaundice; changes near the pancreas, liver, and gallbladder; and ASCITES (an abnormal buildup of fluid in the abdomen).

Lab tests   Samples of blood, urine, and stool will be checked for bilirubin and other substances. Bilirubin is a substance that is passed from the liver to the gallbladder and then the intestine. If the bile duct is blocked by a tumor, the bilirubin cannot pass through normally, which will increase the level of bilirubin in the blood and or urine. High bilirubin levels can be caused by both cancer and noncancerous conditions.

CT scan   This scan searches for abnormalities in the pancreas and other abdominal organs and blood vessels.

Ultrasound   In addition to the more familiar exterior ultrasound device, a doctor may choose to use internal ultrasound (endoscopic ultrasound). In this test, a thin, lighted tube is passed through the patient's mouth and stomach, down into the first part of the small intestine. The doctor slowly withdraws the endoscope from the intestine toward the stomach to make images of the pancreas and surrounding organs and tissues. In an ERCP test (endoscopic retrograde cholangiopancreatography) the doctor passes an endoscope through the patient's mouth and stomach, down into the first part of the small intestine and then slips a smaller tube through the endoscope into the bile ducts and pancreatic ducts. After injecting dye through the catheter into the ducts, the doctor takes X-rays to see whether the ducts are narrowed or blocked by a tumor or other condition. A brushing may be taken to collect cells for a pathology reading.

PTC (percutaneous transhepatic cholangiography)   In this test, a dye is injected through a thin needle into the liver, highlighting the bile ducts. Unless there is a blockage, the dye should move freely through the bile ducts. The dye illuminates the bile ducts on X-rays.

Biopsy   In some cases, pancreatic tissue may be removed and inspected under a microscope for cancer cells. Tissue may be obtained with FINE-NEEDLE ASPIRATION by inserting a needle, guided by X-ray or ultrasound, into the pancreas to remove cells. Alternatively, a sample of tissue may be obtained during endoscopic ultrasound or ERCP. The least common method is to obtain the tissue through an abdominal incision during surgery.

Treatment

Because pancreatic cancer is very hard to control, many doctors encourage patients to consider taking part in a clinical trial, an important option for people in all stages of the disease. Treatments offered in trials may be able to control the disease and help patients live longer and feel better. When a cure or control of the disease is not possible, some patients and their doctors choose PALLIATIVE TREATMENT, which tries to improve quality of life by diminishing pain and other problems caused by this disease.

At present, pancreatic cancer can be cured only when it is found at an early stage, before it has spread. Depending on the type and stage, pancreatic cancer may be treated with surgery, radiation therapy, chemotherapy, or a combination of these options.

Surgery   The surgeon may remove all or part of the pancreas, depending on the location and size of the tumor, the stage of the disease, and the patient's general health.

- *Whipple procedure*. If the tumor is in the widest part of the pancreas, the surgeon removes this part of the pancreas together with part of the small intestine, bile duct, and stomach. Nearby tissues also may be removed.

- *Distal pancreatectomy.* The surgeon removes the body and tail of the pancreas if the tumor is in either of these parts; the spleen is also removed.
- *Total pancreatectomy.* The entire pancreas, part of the small intestine, a portion of the stomach, the common bile duct, the gallbladder, the spleen, and nearby lymph nodes are removed. Sometimes the cancer cannot be completely removed, but if the tumor is blocking the common bile duct or duodenum, the surgeon can create a bypass to allow fluids to flow through the digestive tract. This can relieve jaundice and pain caused by a blockage. Alternatively, blockage may be relieved without bypass surgery by placing a stent (a tiny plastic or metal mesh tube that helps keep the duct or duodenum open in the blocked area).

Removal of part or all of the pancreas may make it hard for a patient to digest foods. A specific diet plan together with medications can help relieve diarrhea, pain, cramping, or feelings of fullness. During recovery from surgery, the doctor will carefully monitor the patient's diet and weight. At first, a patient can eat only liquids and may receive extra nourishment intravenously or by an abdominal feeding tube. Solid foods are added to the diet gradually.

Some patients may not produce enough pancreatic enzymes or hormones after surgery; those who do not have enough insulin may develop diabetes. Needed insulin, other hormones, and enzymes all can be replaced.

Radiation therapy   Radiation therapy may be given alone, or with surgery, chemotherapy, or both. Doctors may use radiation to destroy cancer cells that remain in the area after surgery, or to relieve pain and other problems caused by the cancer.

Chemotherapy   Drugs may be given to kill cancer cells, or to help reduce pain and other problems caused by pancreatic cancer. They may be given alone, with radiation, or with surgery and radiation.

See also PANCREATIC CANCER ACTION NETWORK.

Pancreatic Cancer Action Network (Pan CAN) A nonprofit advocacy organization that educates health professionals and the general public about PANCREATIC CANCER to increase awareness of the disease. PanCAN also advocates for increased funding of pancreatic cancer research and promotes access to and awareness of the latest medical advances, support networks, clinical trials, and reimbursement for care. For contact information, see Appendix I.

Pap test (Papanicolaou smear)   A painless laboratory examination that is used to detect CERVICAL CANCER in women. Cervical cancer strikes about 10,520 American women; 3,900 women will die of this disease each year. Because this type of cancer usually grows slowly, regular Pap smears can identify it early, when cells are just beginning to become malignant. This can help doctors cure or even prevent cervical cancer.

However, Pap smears are not perfect. More than two million a year are inconclusive—some cells appear abnormal, but it is unclear if this is because of a benign condition or a precancerous situation.

In spring 2003, the U.S. government approved a test for HUMAN PAPILLOMAVIRUS (HPV), the virus that causes most cases of cervical cancer, to be included in every regular Pap smear for women over age 30. However, the new addition to the Pap smear is not automatic—women will have to choose if they want to add the HPV test, which costs about $50. Automatic HPV screening is not recommended for women younger than 30 because they are the most likely to have transient, harmless, HPV infections.

The new test will require some patient education, because millions of women could learn they have HPV even though their Pap results are negative. However, most of those infections are harmless, and these women will become infection free within the year. Women whose Pap smear shows no signs of cancer and who are free of HPV can safely wait three years to be rechecked, according to new physician guidelines distributed in the wake of the U.S. Food and Drug Administration ruling. Women who do not choose HPV testing, or who show signs of the infection, will need more frequent Paps.

HPV is a sexually transmitted virus believed to infect some 40 million Americans at any one time. Most people's bodies quickly eliminate the infection, and most HPV strains are harmless and cause no symptoms, but a few types of HPV can cause cervical cancer if the infection lingers. While there is no treatment for HPV, women diagnosed with the condition should get another Pap within six to 12 months to spot any problems early.

Experts do not know how many cases of cervical cancer the new HPV test will help catch or prevent, but it should help detect rare fast-growing cervical cancer that appears between regular Paps.

Patient Advocate Foundation   A national network for health-care reform that supports legislation to enable cancer survivors to obtain insurance funding for medical care and participation in clinical trials. The group serves as an active liaison between patients and their insurer, employer, and/or creditors to resolve insurance, job retention, and/or debt crisis matters relative to their diagnosis through case managers, doctors, and attorneys. The Patient Advocate Foundation seeks to safeguard patients through effective mediation, ensuring access to care, maintenance of employment, and preservation of their financial stability. Services include referrals, information, advocacy, benefits, and health insurance assistance. For contact information, see Appendix I.

penile cancer   Cancer of the tissues in the penis, a rare kind of cancer in the United States. About 1,400 new cases of penile cancer will be diagnosed in the United States each year, and an estimated 200 men will die. Penile cancer occurs in about one American man in 100,000, accounting for just about 0.2 percent of cancers in men and 0.1 percent of cancer deaths in men in the United States.

Penile cancer is much more common in some parts of Africa and South America, where it accounts for up to 10 percent of cancers in men. Many scientists currently believe that some penile tumors are caused by cancer-producing effects of substances that get trapped within the foreskin if they are not washed away on a regular basis. This could be why this particular malignancy is extremely common in Third World countries, with lower standards for public health and personal hygiene. The low incidence in North America and Europe could be due to better sanitary and hygienic conditions along with commonly practiced circumcision.

Types of Penile Cancer
The penis contains several types of cells, and different types of penile cancer can develop in each kind of cell. These include epidermoid carcinoma, verrucous carcinoma, squamous cell carcinoma, ADENOCARCINOMA, MELANOMA, BASAL CELL CARCINOMA, and SARCOMA.

Epidermoid carcinoma   Epidermoid carcinoma is a type of cancer in which cells tend to develop much like the cells of the outer layer of the skin (epidermis). About 95 percent of penile cancers develop from flat skin cells that tend to grow slowly; when found early, these tumors usually can be cured. This type of cancer can appear anywhere on the penis, but most develop on the glans, or on the foreskin in men who have not been circumcised.

Verrucous carcinoma   This uncommon benign but aggressive tumor resembles a benign genital wart; when it appears on the genitals, it is sometimes also called a Buschke-Lowenstein tumor. It can spread deeply into surrounding tissue but rarely spreads to other parts of the body.

Adenocarcinoma   This very rare type of penile cancer can develop from sweat glands in the skin of the penis. Paget's disease of the penis is a condition in which ADENOCARCINOMA cells are found in the penile skin. Although the cancer cells at first spread within the skin, they may eventually invade underneath the skin and spread to lymph nodes. Paget's disease can affect skin anywhere in the body, but it most often affects skin around the anus. (This condition should not be confused with Paget's disease of the bone, an entirely different disease.)

The earliest stage of squamous cell cancer is called squamous cell carcinoma in situ (CIS). Penile CIS is contained entirely within the skin of the penis and has not yet spread to deeper tissues of the penis. CIS of the glans is sometimes called erythroplasia of Queyrat. The same condition, when found on the shaft of the penis, is called BOWEN'S DISEASE.

Melanomas   About 2 percent of penile cancers are melanomas, which develop from pigment-producing skin cells called melanocytes. This type of cancer is more dangerous because it spreads more quickly. Melanomas usually develop from sun-exposed areas of skin, but some of these cancers can develop on the penis or other areas not likely to become sunburned.

Basal cell carcinoma   This slow-growing cancer represents less than 2 percent of penile cancers. It rarely spreads to other parts of the body.

Sarcoma   The remaining 1 percent of penile cancers are sarcomas—cancers that develop from the blood vessels, smooth muscle, and other connective tissue cells of the penis.

Benign and Precancerous Conditions

Sometimes abnormal but benign growths develop on the penis, some of which may eventually evolve into invasive cancer if they are not treated. These precancerous conditions can resemble warts or irritated patches of skin and may develop on the glans, the foreskin, or along the shaft. Some of these benign conditions include condylomas—wartlike growths that look like tiny cauliflowers, ranging from microscopic to more than an inch or more in diameter.

Symptoms

In most cases, the first sign of penile cancer is a painless ulcer on the glans, foreskin, or the shaft of the penis. Other symptoms include changes in color, skin thickening, or a tissue buildup. Most penile cancers are not painful, although there may be some bleeding. Penile cancers may look red, blue, or brown, and appear as small velvety or crusty bumps, or flat. Swelling at the end of the penis (especially when the foreskin is constricted) is a common sign of penile cancer. There may be a persistent foul-smelling discharge beneath the foreskin. If cancer has progressed to a more advanced stage, the lymph nodes in the groin may be swollen.

Most lesions on the penis are caused by viral, bacterial, or fungal infections, or allergic reactions, all of which will respond readily to antibacterial or antifungal ointments and creams. Growths or areas that do not heal should be considered malignant until proven otherwise.

Risk Factors

The exact cause of most penile cancers is not known, but the disease is associated with a number of risk factors.

Human papillomavirus   Many researchers believe that infection by HUMAN PAPILLOMAVIRUS (HPV) is the most important avoidable risk factor for penile cancer. HPVs are a group of more than 100 types of viruses called papillomaviruses because they can cause warts (papillomas). Different HPV types cause different types of warts; some types cause common warts on the hands and feet, others cause warts on the lips or tongue.

Other HPV types, which are transferred sexually, can infect the genital organs and the anal area. A person's risk of sexually transmitted HPV infection increases with sex at an early age, having many sexual partners or having sex with a partner who has had many other partners, and having unprotected sex. When HPV infects the skin of the external genital organs and anal area (around the opening of the intestinal tract), it often causes raised, bumpy warts. HPV types HPV 6 and HPV 11 cause most genital warts, but these warts rarely develop into cancer. However, other sexually transmitted HPVs have been linked with genital or anal cancers in both men and women. These are called "high-risk" HPV types and include HPV 16, HPV 18, HPV 33, HPV 35, HPV 45, among some others.

HPVs can also cause flat warts on the penis that are not visible and cause no symptoms. Flat warts caused by low-risk HPV types have little or no effect on cancer risk, but flat warts caused by high-risk HPV types can become malignant.

There is currently no cure for HPV infection, but the warts and abnormal cell growth these viruses cause can be effectively treated. These treatments can destroy warts and prevent them from developing into cancers.

New tests are now available that can identify the type of DNA in an HPV and identify the exact HPV type that is causing an infection. At this time, it is not clear how treatment will be affected by this information. HPV testing and typing are not presently routinely recommended, and most health-care professionals do not use this testing. However, scientists are studying ways to find out how this test can help prevent genital cancers.

Smoking People who smoke are exposing themselves to many cancer-causing chemicals that affect more than the lungs. These harmful substances are absorbed into the bloodstream and circulate throughout the body, especially in men who also have HPV infections.

Smegma Oily secretions from the skin, dead skin cells, and bacteria can accumulate under the foreskin, creating a thick, odorous substance called smegma. Some studies suggested that smegma may contain cancer-causing substances, but most recent studies disagree. Smegma is unlikely to have a significant impact on the risk of developing penile cancer. However, if uncircumcised men do not retract the foreskin and thoroughly wash the entire penis, the presence of smegma may irritate and inflame the penis.

Phimosis A condition that makes the foreskin hard to retract, so that men are less likely to clean the penis routinely and effectively. This can lead to a buildup of smegma.

Psoriasis treatment Men who have a skin disease called psoriasis and who have received a combination treatment involving a drug called psoralen and exposure to ultraviolet light have a higher rate of penile cancer.

Age Most cases of the disease are diagnosed in men over age 50, but about 20 percent occur in men younger than 40.

AIDS Men with AIDS may have a higher risk of penile cancer, which could be due to lowered immune response.

Circumcision Some experts have suggested that removing part or the entire foreskin provides some protection against cancer of the penis by helping to improve hygiene. Whether circumcision is a risk factor is a controversial issue. However, penile cancer risk is low in some uncircumcised populations, and circumcision is strongly associated with other socioethnic practices associated with lower risk. Most studies have concluded that circumcision alone is not the major factor preventing cancer of the penis.

Diagnosis

When penile cancer is detected early, treatment is simplest, more likely to result in a cure, and less likely to cause significant side effects or complications. Unfortunately, early diagnosis of penile cancer is often missed because it is so rare in the United States that many physicians may only see two or three cases in a lifetime.

Because several harmless conditions (such as genital warts) may produce similar symptoms, a doctor should visually examine any suspicious signs on the penile surface. If cancer is suspected, a biopsy and other tests may be recommended.

Biopsy In this procedure, a small piece of the skin tissue is removed so a pathologist can check it under a microscope for cancer cells.

An incision BIOPSY removes only a portion of the affected tissue and is performed on lesions that are larger, ulcerated, or that appear to grow deeply into the tissue. These biopsies are usually done in a doctor's office, clinic, or outpatient surgical center with the patient under local anesthesia. Results are usually available within three to four days.

Fine-needle biopsy (FNA) In this procedure, the biopsy can be done in a doctor's office with only local anesthesia. A doctor places a thin needle directly into the mass for about 10 seconds, withdrawing cells and a few drops of fluid to be viewed under a microscope. If the mass is an enlarged lymph node deep inside the body and the doctor cannot feel it, imaging methods such as ultrasound or a CT scan can be used to guide the needle into it. FNA may sometimes be used instead of a lymph node dissection for some patients.

Sentinel node biopsy This is an alternative to total LYMPH NODE DISSECTION that has been used successfully for some patients with BREAST CANCER or malignant MELANOMA; some doctors recommend its use for some men with penile cancer.

In this procedure, a radioactive tracer and/or a blue dye is injected into the region of the tumor, where it is carried to a sentinel node (the first lymph node receiving lymph from the tumor and the one most likely to contain a metastasis if the cancer has spread). The surgeon finds this node during the operation either visually (by the blue dye) or with a Geiger counter (radioactive tracer) and removes it. If the sentinel node contains cancer, more LYMPH NODES are removed. If the sentinel node does not have cancer cells, additional lymph node surgery may be avoided. Using this approach, fewer patients will need to have many lymph nodes removed.

Removing lymph nodes carries a risk of side effects such as LYMPHEDEMA (fluid accumulation in tissues) and problems with wound healing.

Computed tomography (CT) This test can help tell if penile cancer has spread into the liver, lungs, or other organs. CT scans can also be used to guide a biopsy needle precisely into a suspected metastasis.

Chest x-ray This may be taken to determine whether penile cancer has spread to the lungs.

Staging

Stage 0: The cancer has not invaded below the superficial layer of skin and has not spread to lymph nodes or distant sites.

Stage I: Cancer cells are found only on the surface of the glans (the head of the penis) and on the foreskin (the loose skin that covers the head of the penis). It has not spread to lymph nodes or distant sites.

Stage II: Cancer cells are found in the deeper tissues of the glans and have spread to the shaft of the penis (the long, slender cylinders of tissue inside the penis that contain spongy tissue and expand to produce erections).

Stage III: The cancer has

- invaded the penis, but not the urethra or prostate, and has spread to many superficial groin lymph nodes but not to distant sites OR

- invaded the urethra or prostate and may or may not have spread to single or multiple superficial groin lymph nodes, but has not spread to distant sites.

Stage IV: The cancer has

- invaded nearby tissues and may or may not have spread to groin lymph nodes, but has not spread to distant sites OR

- invaded and spread to lymph nodes deep in the groin, but not to distant sites OR

- invaded tissue, may or may not have spread to lymph nodes, and has spread to distant sites.

Recurrent: The cancer has returned after treatment has ended. Recurrent penile cancer may return to the same location, or to any other part of the body.

Treatment

Treatment of cancer of the penis depends on the stage of the disease, the type of disease, and the patient's age and overall condition. Standard treatment may be considered because of its effectiveness in patients in past studies, or participation in a clinical trial may be considered. Not all patients are cured with standard therapy, and some standard treatments may have more side effects than are desired. Men treated with conservative techniques (such as topical CHEMOTHERAPY and LASER surgery) and some men treated with a partial penectomy retain enough of the penis to achieve an erection sufficient for penetration during sexual intercourse.

Treatments for patients with cancer of the penis include surgery, RADIATION THERAPY, chemotherapy, and BIOLOGICAL THERAPY.

Surgery This is the most common treatment for all stages of penile cancer. If the lesion is limited, a doctor may recommend small local excision or Moh's surgery (a procedure in which layers of abnormal tissue are shaved off until normal tissue is reached). These procedures are not very disfiguring, but careful follow-up is critical to identify early recurrence. When lesions are small, it is very unlikely that cancer has spread to lymph and, therefore, removal of the lymph nodes is usually not necessary.

If the lesion is larger, more tissue must be removed, along with lymph nodes in the groin. In these circumstances, combinations of surgery, radiation, and chemotherapy may be necessary.

Wide local excision removes only the cancer and some normal tissue on either side. If the cancer is limited to the foreskin, treatment will probably be wide local excision and circumcision. Microsurgery is an operation that removes the cancer and as little normal tissue as possible, with the aid of a microscope to make sure all the cancer cells are removed. If the cancer begins in the glans and does not involve other tissues, treatment may involve microsurgery plus topical chemotherapy (Fluorouracil cream). Laser surgery also can be used to remove cancer cells.

Amputation of the penis (either partial or total) is the most common and effective treatment. Lymph nodes in the groin may be taken out during surgery.

Radiation/chemotherapy Radiation may be used alone or after surgery. Topical chemotherapy with Fluorouracil cream is sometimes used for very small surface cancers, but otherwise chemotherapy is not a common treatment for penile cancer.

Biological therapy This prompts the immune system to fight cancer. It uses material made by the body or a lab to boost, direct, or restore the body's natural defenses against disease. Biological treatment is sometimes called biological response modifier (BRM) therapy.

Prognosis

About 67 percent of men are likely to live five years or longer after the diagnosis and treatment of penile cancer. The sooner the cancer is detected and the earlier its stage, the better the chances are for a complete cure and long-term survival. About 80 percent of men with Stage I or Stage II cancers that have not spread to lymph nodes can expect to live at least five years, but the five-year survival rate drops to 50 percent in men with Stage III disease and 20 percent in men with Stage IV penile cancer.

Prevention

Experts believe that the large variations in penile cancer rates around the world strongly suggest that it is a preventable disease. The best way to reduce the risk of penile cancer is to avoid known risk factors whenever possible. Of course, some men with penile cancer have no known risk factors, so it is not possible to completely prevent this disease.

Circumcision In the past, many experts believed that circumcision was a good way to prevent penile cancer because studies reported much lower penile cancer rates among circumcised men. However, most researchers now believe those studies were flawed because they failed to consider other factors that are now known to affect penile cancer risk.

For example, some studies suggest that circumcised men tend to have other lifestyle factors associated with lower penile cancer risk—they are less likely to smoke or have multiple sexual partners, and more likely to have better personal hygiene. Most researchers believe that the penile cancer risk among uncircumcised men without known risk factors living in the United States is extremely low.

The current consensus of most experts is that circumcision should not be recommended as a prevention strategy for penile cancer.

Sexual practices On the other hand, avoiding sexual practices likely to result in HPV infection might lower penile cancer risk (and will certainly have an even more significant impact on CERVICAL CANCER risk). Until recently, experts thought that the use of condoms could prevent HPV infection, but research now shows that condoms do not protect against HPV infection very well. That is because the virus can be transmitted by skin contact with any HPV-infected area of the body, such as skin of the genital or anal area not covered by the condom.

Moreover, HPV can be passed on to another person even when warts or other symptoms are not visible and can be present for years with no symptoms. The longer a person remains infected with any type of HPV that can cause cancer, the greater the risk that infection will lead to cancer. For these reasons, postponing the beginning of sexual activity and limiting the number of sexual partners are two ways to reduce the chances of developing penile cancer.

Quit smoking Quitting smoking or never starting in the first place is an excellent recommendation for preventing many diseases, including penile cancer.

Good hygiene Because some studies suggest that smegma underneath the foreskin may contain cancer-causing substances, many public health experts recommend that uncircumcised men should retract the foreskin to clean the entire penis.

personality and cancer Although the idea has been popular for a long time, there is no scientific evidence for the belief that there is such a thing as a "cancer personality." It is certainly possible that people who have been diagnosed with cancer are anxious and depressed, but this does not mean that these uncomfortable emotions caused the malignancy.

A June 2003 Japanese study found that personality type does not appear to be associated with the risk of cancer. Researchers examined the incidence of cancer among 30,000 people in Japan who had completed personality questionnaire with four personality subscales: extroversion (sociability, liveliness), neuroticism (emotional instability, anxiousness), psychoticism (tough-mindedness, aggressiveness, coldness), and social naiveté or conformity. During seven years of follow-up, there were 986 cases of cancer but no association between any personality subscales and risk of total cancer, or of stomach, colorectal, lung, or BREAST CANCER. Although higher levels of neuroticism were associated with cancers diagnosed in the first three years of follow-up, the authors suggest that neuroticism may be a consequence of cancer rather than a cause.

pesticides   See ENVIRONMENTAL FACTORS.

pharynx cancer   See LARYNGEAL CANCER.

phenolics   A very large category of more than 2,000 PHYTOCHEMICALS. The term *phenol* comes from the chemical structure of these phytochemicals, which vary from having one to several phenol groups with the ability to mop up many FREE RADICALS as they circulate through the bloodstream. Phenolics are considered to be some of the most powerful antioxidants and are studied for their ability to interfere with tumors.

phenoxodiol   A synthetic experimental anticancer drug that in studies has killed 100 percent of ovarian cancer cells, including those cells resistant to "gold standard" CHEMOTHERAPY drugs such as paclitaxel and carboplatin. The tests were conducted on human cell lines at Yale University School of Medicine.

The drug induces OVARIAN CANCER cell death by changing a signal pathway in cancerous cells that otherwise does not allow unhealthy cells to die. The findings indicate that the drug could be successful at treating other cancer types as well, according to the study published in the May 1, 2003, issue of *Oncogene*. The researchers also tested phenoxodiol in mice and found there was a three fold reduction in the size of tumors compared with a control group. No side effects were noted.

A phase II trial using phenoxodiol for women with chemo-resistant ovarian cancer is under way at Yale University. Five phase I human trials with phenoxodiol are complete and have shown few side effects. Preliminary results of a trial conducted at the Cleveland Clinic found that more than half of the 10 patients tested on the experimental drug showed some response. Each of these patients had different types of advanced cancer that did not respond to chemotherapy.

Ovarian cancer is the most lethal gynecologic malignancy and is the fifth leading cause of all cancer deaths in women. Although the initial response to chemotherapy is better than 80 percent, most ovarian cancer recurs because of chemotherapy resistance.

Phenoxodiol may solve the problem of how to promote a cancer cell to die when for some reason it has been programmed to live. Cells constantly die in the human body, and that is important, because all cells must eventually die and be replaced. When cancer cells do not die, problems occur. A key objective in cancer therapy is to find a way to trigger natural cell death (called APOPTOSIS) in cancer cells.

Under U.S. law, a new drug cannot be marketed until it has been investigated in clinical trials. After the safe and successful results of these trials are submitted in a new drug application to the U.S. Food and Drug Administration (FDA), the FDA must approve the drug as safe and effective before it can be marketed.

pheochromocytoma   See ADRENAL CANCER.

Physician's Data Query (PDQ)   A comprehensive cancer database maintained by the National Cancer Institute. It has been distributed since 1984 to physicians and the public, and it is now available by fax, e-mail, conventional mail, and the Internet, in both English and Spanish. The PDQ contains peer-reviewed information summaries on cancer treatment, screening, prevention, genetics, and supportive care, and directories of physicians, professionals who provide genetics services, and organizations that provide cancer care.

The PDQ also contains the world's most comprehensive cancer clinical trials database, with about 1,800 abstracts of trials that are open and accepting patients, including trials for cancer treatment, genetics, diagnosis, supportive care, screening, and prevention. In addition, there is access to about 12,000 abstracts of closed clinical trials that have been completed or are no longer accepting patients.

The PDQ cancer information summaries are updated monthly by six editorial boards composed of specialists in adult treatment, pediatric treatment, complementary and alternative medicine, supportive care, screening and prevention, and genetics. The boards review current literature from more than 70 biomedical journals, evaluate its relevance, and synthesize it into clear summaries.

phytochemicals Substances found only in plants that provide health benefits in addition to those provided by vitamins and minerals alone. Phytochemicals are natural compounds that protect plants from the ravages of sunlight and other environmental threats. Many of these compounds are currently under investigation for their roles in blocking the formation of some cancers. They may also protect against some forms of heart disease, arthritis, and other degenerative diseases.

While phytochemicals can be found in varying amounts in all fruits, vegetables, grains, oils, nuts, and seeds, some of these have higher levels of phytochemicals, which makes them a better choice in a healthful DIET. Among the thousands of different phytochemicals in plants, each one could potentially have some benefit to humans. Some of these phytochemicals are currently being studied for their potential to prevent certain cancers. Many studies already have provided evidence that eating more fruits and vegetables decreases the risk of several different types of cancer, including cancer of the mouth and throat, lungs, stomach, colon and rectum, pancreas, breast, and bladder. In fact, phytochemical research helped prompt the NATIONAL CANCER INSTITUTE to initiate its "5-a-Day" program for healthy eating, in which consumers are urged to eat more foods such as GARLIC, broccoli, onions, and SOY PRODUCTS.

Phytochemicals, which represent thousands of different components in plant foods, differ from vitamins and minerals in that they are not considered "essential" nutrients. A diet including phytochemicals from a wide range of fruits and vegetables has been associated with the prevention and treatment of cancer. Since different phyto-chemicals are present in different foods, eating a varied diet is important to ensuring that a person gets all the cancer protection possible. The specific phytochemical content of different fruits and vegetables tends to vary by color, and each phytochemical has unique functions. Some phytochemicals act as ANTIOXIDANTS, some protect and regenerate essential nutrients, and others work to deactivate cancer-causing substances. Some beneficial phytochemicals are as follows:

- *Allium compounds* such as allyl sulfides may help detoxify and rid the body of some carcinogenic compounds. Food sources include onions, garlic, scallions, and chives.

- *Carotenoids* such as alpha-carotene, beta-carotene, cryptoxanthin, lycopene, and LUTEIN work as antioxidants, helping to offset harm caused by environmental pollutants such as pesticides and smoking. Food sources include dark green, orange, or red fruits and vegetables, especially carrots, sweet potatoes, tomatoes, spinach, broccoli, cantaloupe, and apricots.

- *Glucosinolates* such as glucobrassicin are metabolized to produce two other phytochemicals, isothiocyanates and INDOLES, which trigger production of enzymes that block cell damage due to carcinogens. Food sources include cruciferous vegetables such as broccoli, broccoli sprouts, cabbage, and Brussels sprouts.

- *Polyphenols* such as ellagic acid and ferulic acid are thought to prevent conversion of substances into carcinogens and inhibit mutations. Food sources include oats, soy beans, and fruits and nuts—especially strawberries, raspberries, blackberries, walnuts, and pecans.

- *Flavonoids* include more than 2,000 powerful antioxidants from sources such as coffee, tea, cola, berries, tomatoes, potatoes, broad beans, broccoli, Italian squash, onions, and citrus fruits.

In the Future

Some day, scientists may succeed in developing "super" breeds of certain foods with an extra dose of beneficial phytochemicals. Seed catalogs already offer home gardeners the opportunity to buy seeds for several especially powerful vegetables, such as broccoli sprouts. They contain sulforaphane, a potent inducer of detoxifying enzymes. In fact, three-day-old broccoli sprouts have between 20 and 50 times more sulforaphane than does mature broccoli. In one study, rats fed sulforaphane developed fewer malignant tumors, and their tumors developed at a slower rate.

In addition to high-sulforaphane broccoli sprouts, consumers also can now buy HIGH-LYCOPENE tomatoes and high-beta-carotene cauliflower. Soon, some package labels may even list the amounts of dominant protective substances, just as food labels today list the amount of calories or carbohydrates.

See also PHYTOESTROGENS.

phytoestrogens ESTROGEN-like compounds found in plants. Many different plants produce compounds that may mimic or interact with human estrogen hormones. At least 20 such compounds have been identified in at least 300 plants from more than 16 different plant families. These compounds are weaker than human estrogens and can be found in herbs and seasonings such as GARLIC or parsley, as well as in soybeans, wheat, vegetables, fruits, and coffee. Most consumers are exposed to many of these plant compounds when they eat fruits and vegetables.

Because scientists have found phytoestrogens in human urine and blood samples, they know that these compounds can be absorbed into the human body. After being consumed, phytoestrogens can be excreted, absorbed into the body, or broken down into other potent phytoestrogen compounds.

Phytoestrogens differ remarkably from synthetic ENVIRONMENTAL ESTROGENS in that they are easily broken down, are not stored in tissue, and are quickly excreted.

Scientists do not agree on the role that phytoestrogens play in human health. When consumed as part of an ordinary diet, phytoestrogens are probably safe and may even help protect against certain cancers of the breast, uterus, and prostate.

However, eating too many phytoestrogens may cause some health problems. Laboratory animals, farm animals, and wildlife whose entire diet was made up of phytoestrogen-rich plants developed reproductive problems. While humans almost never have an exclusive diet of phytoestrogen-rich

foods, those who eat uncooked soy or take phytoestrogen pills may be exposing themselves to some health risks. Many natural compounds, especially hormones, can be potent and can have both good and bad health effects, depending on how much of them are in the body. These substances should always be used in moderation to avoid any unintentional health consequences.

Cancer Prevention

Phytoestrogens have been investigated as possible cancer preventives. One study found that Asians who eat large amounts of SOY PRODUCTS containing high levels of phytoestrogens have lower rates of hormone-dependent cancers than do Westerners, who do not traditionally eat these products. Asian immigrants to the West increase their risks of cancer as they include more protein and fat and reduce fiber and soy.

Scientists suggest that even short-term exposure to phytoestrogens may offer some long-term protection against some cancers, including breast, colon, prostate, liver, and LEUKEMIA. According to some animal studies, soy-based compounds can protect against some types of cancer and may even slow down tumor growth.

The health effects of phytoestrogens may depend on the kind and amount of phytoestrogens eaten, and the age, sex and health of the diner. There is strong evidence that a high lifetime exposure to human estrogens, such as estradiol, increases the risk of certain kinds of cancer, such as UTERINE CANCER. Phytoestrogens may help reduce that risk because they may lower a person's lifetime exposure to human estrogens by competing for estrogen receptor sites in the body, or changing the way human estrogens are broken down.

Health Risks

The most likely risks associated with phytoestrogens are linked to infertility and developmental problems, although very large amounts of dietary phytoestrogens would probably be needed to create these risks.

Humans have used plants for medicinal and contraceptive purposes for hundreds of years. Many plants historically used to prevent pregnancies or cause abortions contain phytoestrogens and other hormonally active substances. For instance, during the fourth century B.C., Hippocrates noted that Queen Anne's lace prevented pregnancies. Modern scientists know that its seeds contain a chemical that blocks progesterone, a hormone that is necessary for establishing and maintaining pregnancy.

Phytoestrogens behave like hormones, and as with any hormone, too much or too little can alter hormone-dependent tissue functions. Taking too much of any hormone may not be good for anyone. Similarly, too many phytoestrogens, at the wrong time, may have some adverse health effects. (See also ENVIRONMENTAL ESTROGENS; PHYTOCHEMICALS.)

placental alkaline phosphatase   A tumor marker sometimes occasionally used to detect for GERM CELL CANCERS, particularly seminoma. However, it is not used very often, and it is more likely to be used by a pathologist examining a specimen than in a blood test.

pleural effusion, malignant   A buildup of fluid in the space between the lungs and the interior walls of the chest (the pleural cavity) caused by cancer. About 12 percent of patients with LUNG CANCER also have malignant pleural effusion. This condition could also be caused by BREAST CANCER, STOMACH CANCER, PANCREATIC CANCER, or OVARIAN CANCER—or by the spread of malignant cells into the lung from other areas.

polio vaccine and cancer   See SIMIAN VIRUS 40.

polycyclic aromatic hydrocarbons (PAHs)   A group of chemicals formed during the incomplete burning of coal, oil, gas, wood, garbage, or other organic substances, such as tobacco and charbroiled meat. There are more than 100 different PAHs, but they usually occur as complex mixtures (for example, as part of combustion products such as soot), not as single compounds.

PAHs usually occur naturally, but they can be manufactured as individual compounds for research purposes. A few PAHs are used in medicines and to make dyes, plastics, and pesticides; others are contained in asphalt used in road construction. They can also be found in substances such as crude oil, coal, coal tar pitch, creosote, and roofing tar. They are found throughout the environment in the air, water, and soil.

Although the health effects of individual PAHs are not exactly alike, the following 17 PAHs are more harmful than others:

- acenaphthene
- acenaphthylene
- anthracene
- benz[a]anthracene
- benzo[a]pyrene
- benzo[e]pyrene
- benzo[b]fluoranthene
- benzo[g,h,i]perylene
- benzo[j]fluoranthene
- benzo[k]fluoranthene
- chrysene
- dibenz[a,h]anthracene
- fluoranthene
- fluorene
- indeno[1,2,3-c,d]pyrene
- phenanthrene
- pyrene

PAHs usually enter the environment in the air, from volcanoes, forest fires, residential wood burning, and auto exhaust. They can enter surface water through discharges from industrial plants and wastewater treatment plants, or the soil at hazardous waste sites if they escape from storage containers. PAHs in general do not easily dissolve in water; instead, they are more likely to be found in air or on the surfaces of small solid particles. They can travel long distances before they return to Earth in rainfall or particle settling. The PAH content of plants and animals living on the land or in water can be many times higher than the content of PAHs in soil or water. PAHs can break down to longer-lasting products by reacting with sunlight and other chemicals in the air, generally over a period of days to weeks. Breakdown in soil and water generally takes weeks to months and is caused primarily by the actions of microorganisms.

Because PAHs are found throughout the environment, it is possible to be exposed to them at home or on the job, via cigarette smoke, exhaust, asphalt roads, coal or coal tar, wildfires, agricultural burning, residential wood burning, municipal and industrial waste incineration, and hazardous waste sites. PAHs have been found in some drinking water supplies in the United States. PAHs are present in creosote-treated wood products, cereals, grains, flour, bread, vegetables, fruits, meat, processed or pickled foods, and contaminated cow's milk or human breast milk. Cooking meat or other food at high temperatures, which happens during grilling or charring, increases the amount of PAHs in the food.

PAHs are stored primarily in the kidneys, liver, and fatty tissue; smaller amounts are stored in the spleen, adrenal glands, and ovaries, although they are probably excreted within a few days.

Several PAHs (benz[a]anthracene, benzo[a]-pyrene, benzo[b]fluoranthene, benzo[j]fluoranthene, benzo[k]fluoranthene, chrysene, dibenz[a,h]anthracene, and indeno[1,2,3-c,d]pyrene) have caused tumors in lab animals. Human studies have shown that breathing or having skin contact with PAH mixtures for long periods can cause cancer.

The Department of Health and Human Services (DHHS) has determined that benz[a]anthracene, benzo[b]fluoranthene, benzo[j]fluoranthene, benzo[k]fluoranthene, benzo[a]pyrene, dibenz[a,h]-anthracene, and indeno[1,2,3-c,d]pyrene are known animal carcinogens. The International Agency for Research on Cancer (IARC) has determined that benz[a]anthracene and benzo[a]pyrene are probably carcinogenic to humans; benzo[b]fluoranthene, benzo[j]fluoranthene, benzo[k]fluoranthene, and indeno[1,2,3-c,d]pyrene are possibly carcinogenic to humans; and anthracene, benzo[g,h,i]perylene, benzo[e]pyrene, chrysene, fluoranthene, fluorene, phenanthrene, and pyrene are not classifiable as to their carcinogenicity to humans.

The U.S. Environmental Protection Agency or (EPA) has determined that benz[a]anthracene, benzo[a]pyrene, benzo[b]fluoranthene, benzo[k]-fluoranthene, chrysene, dibenz[a,h]anthracene, and indeno[1,2,3-c,d]pyrene are probable human carcinogens and that acenaphthylene, anthracene, benzo[g,h,i]perylene, fluoranthene, fluorene, phen-

anthrene, and pyrene are not classifiable as to human carcinogenicity. Acenaphthene has not been classified for carcinogenic effects by the DHHS, IARC or EPA.

Measuring PAH Exposure

PAHs can be measured in blood, urine, or body tissues. Although tests can show that a person has been exposed to PAHs, they cannot be used to predict whether any health effects will occur or to determine the extent or source of the exposure. However, these tests are not routinely available at a doctor's office because special equipment is required to detect these chemicals.

Federal Regulations

The EPA has suggested that exposure to the following daily amounts of individual PAHs is not likely to cause any harmful health effects:

0.3 milligrams (mg) of anthracene
0.06 mg of acenaphthene
0.04 mg of fluoranthene
0.04 mg of fluorine
0.03 mg of pyrene per kilogram of body weight
    (one kilogram is equal to 2.2 pounds)

From what is currently known about benzo[a]-pyrene, the federal government has developed regulatory standards and guidelines to protect people from the potential health effects of PAHs in drinking water. The EPA has provided estimates of levels of total cancer-causing PAHs in lakes and streams.

The National Institute for Occupational Safety and Health concluded that occupational exposure to coal products can increase the risk of lung and skin cancer in workers.

poverty and cancer   Research confirms that the poor are more likely to die from cancer, which is a reversal from the 1950s, when the rates were nearly 50 percent higher among those who were economically advantaged. Researchers explained that the trend matched the socioeconomic patterns of cigarette SMOKING: in the 1990s, richer people were less likely to smoke than poor people.

Between 1950 and 1960, the male cancer death rate was about 50 percent higher in the richest counties than in the poorest counties. The gap between the groups narrowed in the 1970s, and by 1998, the cancer death rates were 19 percent higher in the poorest counties than in the richest counties.

Because many years elapse between the time someone starts smoking and when they die of lung cancer, experts expect the difference in men's death rates from cancer between the rich and the poor to continue to widen in the near future.

progestin   The hormonal ingredient in oral contraceptive pills that provides the highest level of protection against OVARIAN CANCER. The cancer risk was cut in half in all women taking pills containing the hormones ESTROGEN and PROGESTIN, according to analysis by the Duke Comprehensive Cancer Center. Moreover, women who took a version of the pills containing higher levels of progestin had a reduced risk of ovarian cancer of an additional 50 percent.

The pills used by women in the study 20 years ago are not now commonly available, since birth control pill formulas have changed over the years as research showed that pills with lower hormone levels were effective contraceptives. Pills with lower levels of hormone generally have fewer side effects.

prostate cancer   The leading cancer diagnosed among men in the United States, striking about one out of every 11 Caucasian men and one out of every nine African-American men, with diagnosis usually occurring at age 70 or older. Many older men, however, will develop "silent" prostate cancer that produces few (if any) symptoms and does not affect life expectancy.

Prostate cancer incidence has been increasing rapidly in recent years, probably because of the greater use of prostate cancer screening—especially the widespread introduction of the PROSTATE-SPECIFIC ANTIGEN (PSA) TEST. As yet, however, there is little medical consensus about prostate cancer's etiology, recommendations for screening, or usefulness of early detection and treatment.

Prostate cancer is the most common solid tumor among American men, and the second leading cause of cancer deaths in this country. About 220,000 new cases of prostate cancer are diagnosed each year in the United States. Because most prostate cancers are tiny, have not spread, and don't cause symptoms, another 9 million American men may have prostate cancer without knowing it.

The incidence rates for prostate cancer, which is rare before age 50, have been particularly high in the developed areas of the world, such as North America, Europe, Australia, and New Zealand. These high incidence rates may, in part, reflect better cancer detection strategies.

Prostate cancer develops from cells inside the prostate gland, found near the neck of the bladder, that produces part of the fluid of semen. When cells in the prostate become malignant, they remain within the gland in about a third of all men as they grow older. In many cases, it takes decades for this limited type of cancer to spread beyond the prostate gland's tough outer shell. Before they spread, up to 90 percent of these cancers can be cured with local treatment, such as radical prostatectomy (surgical removal of the prostate gland) or radiation therapy.

However, If cancer grows beyond the prostate gland, it may invade surrounding parts of the bladder and urethra, causing urinary problems. The cancer also may spread to nearby lymph nodes, or to the bones, liver, or rectum. Cancers that have spread to lymph nodes or other organs generally are not curable, although they often can be kept under control for a number of years with proper treatment.

Cause

Experts do not know what causes prostate cancer, but theoretically all men are at risk for developing this disease. Experts do know that this type of cancer—like breast cancer—is stimulated by hormones. Prostate cancer is stimulated by the male hormones TESTOSTERONE and dihydrotestosterone (a chemical that the body makes from testosterone).

Another chemical called transferrin, which is stored in the bones, also appears to stimulate the growth of prostate cancer cells. As prostate cancer develops, it secretes chemicals that make blood vessels grow into the cancer and bring nutrients to nourish the malignant cells.

The prevalence of prostate cancer rises with age, and the increase with age is more significant with prostate cancer than with any other type of cancer.

A number of risk factors are known to be linked to the development of prostate cancer, including:

Age   The remarkably sharp increase in incidence with age is a hallmark of this type of cancer. A man's risk of developing prostate cancer before age 39 is only one out of 100,000; this drops to one out of 103 between age 40 and 59, and plummets to one out of eight for men between 60 and 79. Microscopic traces of prostate cancer can be identified in about 30 percent of men at age 60, and 50 percent to 70 percent at age 80. For every 10 years after age 40, the incidence of prostate cancer doubles.

Sixty percent of all newly diagnosed prostate cancer cases and almost 80 percent of all deaths occur in men 70 years of age and older. In most older men, the prostate cancer does not grow, and many die of other causes and are not identified as having prostate cancer before they die. Mortality rates for prostate cancer are much lower than the incidence rates because survival for men with this cancer is generally quite high.

Race   Prostate cancer is directly related to a man's race. African-American men are 60 percent more likely to develop prostate cancer than other men, and they are twice as likely to die of the disease than are Caucasian men, perhaps because they also tend to have prostate cancers that are more advanced at the time of diagnosis. Only 66 percent of African-American men with prostate cancer survive at least five years after diagnosis, versus 81 percent of Caucasian men. In addition, U.S. black men have the highest rates of this cancer in the world. Elevated rates of prostate cancer have been observed in temperate and tropical South America (especially Brazil), where substantial numbers of men of African descent live. Among African countries, those with higher incidences of prostate cancer also have relatively higher per capita incomes and life expectancies.

Although the incidence of prostate cancer among Caucasians is quite high, it is distinctly lower than among African Americans; Asian and Native American men have the lowest rates. The incidence rate among African-American men (180.6 per 100,000) is more than seven times that among Koreans (24.2). While men of Asian descent living in the United States have lower rates of prostate cancer than do Caucasian Americans, they have higher rates than Asian men in their native countries. Japan has the lowest prostate cancer death rate in the world, compared to Switzerland, which has the highest.

Researchers suspect that genetic differences, diet, or lifestyle factors may help to explain the higher rates of prostate cancer among African-American men, who also are more likely to develop an aggressive form of prostate cancer. This is particularly interesting in light of the fact that blacks in Africa have one of the lowest rates of prostate cancer in the world.

In addition to having higher rates of prostate cancer, African-American men may be less likely to seek or receive treatment and so are more likely to die of this disease. When they do receive adequate treatment, African-American men with prostate cancer appear to live as long as Caucasian men after diagnosis.

Family history   Men with a family history of prostate cancer are also at increased risk. Whether this is genetic or due to shared environmental influences (or both) is unclear. Between 5 percent to 10 percent of all cases of prostate cancers are considered to be hereditary. A man whose father or brother has been diagnosed with prostate cancer has double the risk of getting prostate cancer; having more than one first-degree relative with this type of cancer increases the risk even further. Genetic factors may be responsible for about half the rare early-onset prostate cancers that develop in men under the age of 55. The younger the family member is when diagnosed with prostate cancer, the higher the risk for other male relatives of being diagnosed at a younger age as well. The risk also increases with the number of relatives affected with prostate cancer. However, sons of a man diagnosed with prostate cancer after age 70 probably have no higher risk than does any other man in the general population.

Prostate cancer genes   Some genes do appear to increase the risk of prostate cancer. These include the HPC1 gene, the *BRCA1/BRCA2* genes, and the P53 chromosome. HPC1 appears to cause about a third of all inherited cases of prostate cancer. The *BRCA1* and *BRCA2* genes are primarily linked to breast cancer; however, there is a suggestion that *BRCA1* and possibly *BRCA2* are also linked to prostate cancer risk in men. Men who have inherited an abnormal *BRCA1* gene have a threefold higher risk of developing prostate cancer than other men.

Changes in the p53 chromosome are associated with high-grade aggressive prostate cancer.

Hormones   The development of prostate cancer is related to hormones, because men who have had their testicles removed (castrated) rarely develop this malignancy. There is also a link between prostate cancer and high levels of testosterone.

Diet   There is a growing body of evidence that suggests diet may be related to prostate cancer. A high-fat diet (especially animal fat and high-fat dairy products) is associated with an increased risk for prostate cancer, and a diet low in selenium and vitamin E may contribute to the risk. Research has shown that tumors grown in the lab grow faster when the amount of fat in the diet was 40.5 percent and grew more slowly with a 21 percent fat content. The average North American diet contains 40 percent fat, which is significantly higher than Asian countries. There is also current interest in the possibility that the low risk of prostate cancer in certain Asian populations may result from their high intake of soy products.

Obesity   While there does not seem to be a clear link between body size and prostate cancer risk, men who gained weight in early adulthood and who then develop prostate cancer seem to have more aggressive cancers.

Smoking   While smoking does not seem to trigger the development of prostate cancer, smokers tend to have more aggressive forms of prostate cancer than do nonsmokers.

Vasectomy   The effects of vasectomy on the risk of prostate cancer is not clear, but at present most experts believe that having a vasectomy does not increase a man's risk of prostate cancer. While some studies suggest that there may be a higher risk among men with vasectomies, these men tend to have lower grade, earlier stage prostate cancer associated with a better prognosis. Other studies have not found any link between the procedure and prostate cancer.

Symptoms

In early stages, prostate cancer rarely causes symptoms. Typically it grows very slowly, and some of the symptoms linked to enlargement of the prostate are also the same as for benign prostatic hyperplasia (BPH). If the prostate cancer spreads into the urethra or bladder neck, it can cause the following problems:

- urinary problems
- decreased force of the urine stream
- frequent urination and an intense need to urinate
- inability to urinate
- repeated urinary tract infections
- blood in the urine or semen
- fatigue
- weight loss
- aches and pains

If prostate cancer spreads to the bones, it may cause a continual or intermittent bone pain that may be located in just one area or moves around the body. More common sites for spread of prostate cancer to the bones include the ribs, hips, back, and shoulder. Because some of these sites are also common areas for the development of arthritis, it can be hard to tell the difference. Significant weakening of the bones may lead to fractures.

Prostate cancer also may spread to the lymph nodes or other organs, it can cause swollen glands, weight loss, anemia, and shortness of breath. Cancer that has spread to the spine may cause paralysis if the nerves become compressed. If the cancer grows into the bladder or affects most of the pelvic lymph nodes, it may obstruct one or both of the ureters, which drain urine from the kidneys into the bladder. This obstruction may cause a drop in urine volume (or total absence of urine if both ureters are blocked), back pain, nausea and vomiting, and, sometimes, fevers.

Screening

The goal of prostate cancer screening is to find this malignancy while it is still at the early, curable stage. However, experts disagree about whether all men should be screened routinely for prostate cancer, since prostate abnormalities are so common and because in many cases prostate cancer never threatens a man's life. Nevertheless, regular screening does greatly increase the chances that prostate cancer will be detected at an early stage; for this reason, many experts recommend that prostate screening should be performed once a year for all men except those who had a very low baseline PSA (under 2 [see below]), who may want to consider screening every other year. The AMERICAN CANCER SOCIETY recommends that all men be offered routine screening for prostate cancer starting at age 50 and that African-American men consider screening at age 45.

The best way to screen for prostate cancer is a combination of a digital rectal exam (DRE) of the prostate and a blood test known as the PROSTATE SPECIFIC ANTIGEN TEST (PSA test). PSA is a protein produced by the prostate and normally secreted into the semen; in prostate cancer (and some other prostate disorders) large amounts of PSA can leak out of the prostate, raising PSA levels in the blood. In the DRE test, a doctor inserts an index finger into the rectum and gently feels the surface of the prostate through the rectal wall to check for lumps, hardness, and enlargement.

The combination PSA-DRE is important because men with a normal PSA may still have prostate cancer; if a rectal exam reveals a firm area, a biopsy should be performed. Only about one quarter of prostate cancers are found by a DRE (more are detected by an abnormal PSA). Most health care providers and Medicare cover annual DREs and PSAs for qualified Medicare patients over age 50.

Patients should tell the doctor if they are taking any prescription or over-the-counter medication to treat an enlarged prostate. Certain prostate medications, such as finasteride (Proscar) or saw palmetto, can affect the results of the PSA test.

In addition, a doctor will usually take a personal medical history, including a history of any noncancerous condition of the prostate, such as inflammation of the prostate or enlarged prostate, and any history of prostate cancer in first degree relatives.

Diagnosis

If a man's PSA level is high or the digital rectal exam (DRE) is abnormal, the doctor will order a biopsy of the prostate, usually performed while guided by a transrectal ultrasound. In the biopsy, tissue is removed from the top, middle, and bottom of the gland on both sides, or from any suspicious areas identified by DRE or ultrasound.

Depending on the biopsy results, PSA level, physical findings, and family history of prostate cancer, a doctor may order additional tests to determine whether the cancer has spread to the lymph nodes, bones or other sites. These tests may include a computed tomography scan, magnetic resonance imagining scan, or bone scan.

Sometimes, prostate cancer may be discovered when a pathologist examines tissue removed during a transurethral prostatectomy (TURP) for an enlarged prostate (BENIGN PROSTATE HYPERPLASIA). This happens about 10 to 15 percent of the time.

Staging

The most common way to determine how likely the prostate cancer is to grow and spread quickly is to "stage" the cancer using a Gleason score. If prostate cancer is diagnosed, the laboratory will assess how abnormal the cancer cells look, and assign a Gleason score to the tumor; the score ranges from 1 (low grade) to 5 (high grade).

The grade of prostate cancer cells describes how those cells look, whether or not they are aggressive and very abnormal (high grade), or not aggressive or barely abnormal (low grade). The grade of the cancer is an important factor in predicting long-term results of treatment and survival.

Prostate cancer may have cells of different grades, so the pathologist assigns numbers to the two most common types present, ranging from 1 to 5. A Gleason score is the total of these two numbers; for example, a man with a Gleason grade of 3 and 4 would have a Gleason score of 7. Low-score cancers are those with a Gleason score of 2, 3, or 4; intermediate-score cancers are those with a Gleason score of 5, 6, or 7; high-score cancers have a Gleason score of 8, 9, or 10.

Prevention

The American Cancer Society recommends that men limit intake of high-fat foods from animal sources and eat five or more servings of fruits and vegetables each day. Several things may help prevent the development of prostate cancer, including eating a low-fat diet, getting lots of exercise, and taking certain medications. A man may be able to decrease the risk for prostate cancer by eating a low-fat diet high in vitamin E and selenium, and natural antioxidants such as LYCOPENE may help to protect men from prostate cancer. These helpful foods include tofu and soy milk, tomatoes, green tea, strawberries, raspberries, blueberries, red grapes, peas, watermelon, rosemary, garlic, and citrus fruits.

Vitamin E may reduce the risk, according to a recent study among more than 29,000 men in Finland. About half of the men took 50 mg of vitamin E daily, and this group experienced 32 percent fewer cases of prostate cancer than among men who did not take Vitamin E supplements. Foods rich in vitamin E include vegetable oils, particularly those from safflower, sunflower, and cotton seeds; wheat germ and whole grains; and whole nuts, such as almonds. Currently, however, doctors do not recommend vitamin E or selenium supplements to decrease prostate cancer risk.

Getting lots of exercise appears to lower the risk of developing prostate cancer.

The drug finasteride (Proscar) reduced the risk of prostate cancer by nearly 25 percent, according to a June 2003 report representing the culmination of three decades of research that began in the early 1970s at University of Texas Southwestern Medical Center. The study in *The New England Journal of Medicine* showed that finasteride, which is already proven effective as a therapy for enlarged prostate, also delays or prevents prostate cancer and reduces the risk of urinary problems. However, the drug has significant sexual side effects and may increase the risk of high-grade prostate cancer in some patients, the study reports.

Finasteride inhibits the conversion of testosterone to dihydrotestosterone by the enzyme 5-alpha reductase. By doing so, it reduces by 90 percent the level of dihydrotestosterone (the primary androgen in the prostate that is involved in the development of prostate cancer). The findings are the result of the Prostate Cancer Prevention Trial, a seven-year study involving 9,457 men.

Treatment

Prostate cancer is the most frequently diagnosed cancer (not including skin cancer) in men, but 80 to 90 percent of untreated prostate cancers would not decrease survival or quality of life. However, most cases of prostate cancer are treated because a few men clearly do benefit from early diagnosis and aggressive treatment of the cancer and, in fact, may die without it. For this reason, treatment is usually recommended for most men with prostate cancer, even though many men experience negative side effects as a result of treatment and most of them would not have been harmed if their cancer was untreated.

Treatment for prostate cancer varies a great deal depending on the extent of cancer, its chances of spreading, and the man's age, life expectancy, willingness to risk side effects, and underlying health conditions.

If the cancer is confined to the prostate gland and has spread, there are at least three treatment options: watchful waiting, radiation treatment, and surgery to remove the prostate (prostatectomy).

Watchful waiting In this type of treatment, the patient receives no immediate medical or surgical treatment, but a doctor monitors regular PSA testing and DREs. This strategy generally is reserved for men with a low-grade tumor as evidenced by the Gleason score, or elderly men who are too weak to tolerate radiation or surgery, or who also suffer from other serious medical conditions that limit life expectancy.

Radiation therapy External beam radiation involves five to seven weeks of treatments given by machine aimed at the prostate. Alternatively, the radiation can be given internally (BRACHYTHERAPY) by implanting radioactive seeds or pellets directly inside the prostate with a sterile needle guided by either ultrasound or magnetic resonance imaging (MRI). Side effects of RADIATION THERAPY may include impotence (up to 50 percent of patients), diarrhea, rectal bleeding, and incontinence. In general, more men experience side effects from external-beam radiation than from brachytherapy.

Surgery A radical prostatectomy involves the removal of the prostate gland, seminal vesicles, and sometimes the nearby pelvic LYMPH NODES. Side effects from this procedure can include incontinence and impotence, both of which are more common after radical prostatectomy than after radiation therapy. Recently, a new "nerve-sparing" surgical technique has helped preserve sexual potency in many men who undergo radical prostatectomy.

Hormonal/radiation treatment For men whose prostate cancer has grown beyond the prostate capsule but has not spread to other locations in the body, radiation therapy combined with hormonal therapy is usually the preferred treatment.

Androgen deprivation For men whose prostate cancer has spread to other areas of the body, doctors usually prescribe androgen-deprivation therapy. Androgens are male sex hormones (such as testosterone); androgen-deprivation therapy reduces levels of testosterone and other androgens that stimulate the prostate cancer to grow. Today, doctors most commonly use drugs to either block the effects of testosterone or stop its production by the testicles.

An alternative way of blocking the androgens is to surgically remove the testicles (orchiectomy).

Side effects of androgen-deprivation therapy include impotence, weight gain, decreased sex drive, and osteoporosis. Some men experience hot flashes, which often can be controlled by medication.

Side Effects of Treatment

Men who undergo treatment for prostate cancer must be prepared for the possibility of urinary incontinence or a decline in their ability to have an erection. Urinary problems may result after damage to the urethra during treatment for prostate cancer because the urethra runs through the prostate. This incontinence may be temporary or permanent.

Impotence may be caused by damage to the bundle of nerves responsible for erection that run along each side of the prostate. Eventually, a man's sexual potency may return to normal, depending on his health and age. Fortunately there are several treatments from which to choose that may help restore erections, including medications such as VIAGRA, vacuum devices, and PENILE PROSTHETIC IMPLANTS.

prostate-specific antigen blood test   A screening test that measures the amount of PSA (prostate-specific antigen) in a man's blood. A PSA blood test is part of routine prostate cancer screening for most men over 50. If the test result shows a moderately elevated PSA level, a referral for a BIOPSY is usually recommended. However, there is now evidence that suggests biopsy should not be performed until the test is repeated because PSA levels commonly fluctuate above and below the normal range.

PSA is a chemical made by the prostate gland. The PSA is a sensitive but not flawless test for prostate cancer, since high PSA levels can be caused by other conditions in addition to malignancy. The test often flags a high number of men who do not have prostate cancer, yet recent studies have found that prostate cancer screening has increased survival. The American Urologic Association and the American College of Surgeons recommend that most men start prostate cancer screening at the age of 50. African-American men with a family history of prostate cancer should start screening at age 40.

PSA is produced in both normal and malignant prostate glands, but it is not found in significant amounts elsewhere in the body. Normally, only a small amount of PSA can be detected in a man's blood. However, when the prostate gland becomes damaged or inflamed for a variety of reasons, PSA leaks into the blood more easily, which raises the blood level of this chemical.

Normal Ranges

A man's normal PSA level should range between 1 and 4, although some experts suspect that the level changes depending on a man's race and age. The baseline measurement of a man's PSA is less important than tracking the change over time. Age-adjusted normal ranges for a man between age 40 and 49 is 0 to 2.5. For men between ages 50 and 59, the upper level increases to 3.5; for men between 60 and 69, the upper level increases to 4.5; for men 70 to 79, the upper level increases to 6.5.

PSA can occur in two forms in the blood, either as bound PSA (in which the PSA is attached to proteins) or free PSA (in which it is not attached). The amount of both bound and free PSA is measured and the total is then calculated. In cases of a mildly elevated PSA (between 4 and 10), the free-to-bound PSA ratio may help a doctor decide whether or not to perform a biopsy. The higher this ratio number, the less likely that there is prostate cancer. A free PSA value above 14 to 25 percent suggests that prostate cancer is less likely.

High PSA Levels

A number of things can increase the PSA level, including anything that might irritate the prostate gland. This could include a urinary tract infection, a recent urinary catheter, prostate stones, a recent prostate biopsy, a vigorous rectal exam, prostatic massage, or prostate surgery. Even sexual intercourse can increase the level up to 10 percent.

Benign enlargement of the prostate (BPH) may increase the PSA level because a larger prostate means more prostate cells are available to produce more PSA. However, the condition of BPH tends to produce lower levels of PSA than does prostate cancer. And because the prostate continues to grow as men age, the PSA may continue to increase slightly from year to year. However, some experts do believe that normal enlargement with aging should still not increase a man's PSA by more than 0.7 percent a year or by more than 20 percent of the previous level.

Fluctuating Levels

The PSA test is very sensitive, and because any inflammation or irritation of the prostate can affect PSA levels, the PSA test may fluctuate in men without prostate cancer. In a 2003 study published in the *Journal of the American Medical Association*, researchers from Memorial Sloan-Kettering Cancer Center and colleagues studied nearly 1,000 men who had five consecutive PSA tests over a four-year period. Up to one-third of these men had elevated PSA levels; a finding which usually results in a referral for a prostate biopsy. However, subsequent testing of the same men a year or more later indicated that the PSA levels for half of the men had returned to normal. Had a biopsy been performed, it may have been unnecessary.

Researchers concluded that a single elevated PSA level does not automatically warrant a prostate biopsy. Instead, experts recommend having the findings confirmed by repeating the PSA test after waiting at least six weeks. Even if the repeat test shows an elevated level, prostate cancer will only be discovered in about one-quarter of men who undergo biopsy. A policy of confirming newly elevated PSA levels several weeks later may reduce the number of unnecessary procedures as well as the number of men diagnosed with a small incidental tumor that poses no threat to life or health. Waiting to confirm the diagnosis will not have a negative effect on those men who actually have prostate cancer, experts note, because a delay in diagnosis of a few weeks or months is unlikely to alter treatment outcome.

Drugs and PSA Levels

Any drug that affects the size of the prostate or the amount of testosterone produced by the testicles will affect PSA levels. Finasteride (Proscar), a medication used to help shrink a prostate enlarged as a result of BPH, will decrease the PSA level by up to 50 percent. This decrease will occur when taking this drug no matter what the baseline PSA had been. Any steady increase of PSA while taking this medication needs to be evaluated immediately. Moreover, the amount of free PSA should not decrease while taking this drug.

Medications that decrease the testosterone levels may cause prostate tissue to shrink and will, therefore, also lower PSA levels. Alternatively, boosting the testosterone levels may stimulate the growth of both normal and malignant prostate cells. Although testosterone therapy has not been shown to trigger the development of prostate cancer, it is true that prostate cancer is composed of cells, some of which are and some are not sensitive to hormones. The cells not sensitive to hormones will grow no matter how much testosterone is present, but the hormone-sensitive cells may be affected by testosterone levels.

Therefore, men on testosterone therapy have a theoretical risk that the testosterone may cause an undetected prostate cancer to grow. For this reason, men taking this drug treatment should have a digital rectal exam and a PSA level every six months (instead of yearly). Any significant increase in PSA level or a change in the rectal exam results during testosterone therapy needs to be evaluated.

Having the Test

A PSA test should ideally be performed by the same lab each time, since different labs may use different forms of PSA tests.

proteasome inhibitor A type of chemotherapy drug that works by targeting an enzyme key to cell growth. Since uncontrolled cell growth is the hallmark of a cancer cell, scientists hope that if they interfere with this enzyme, cancer cells will die.

The first PROTEASOME INHIBITOR to be approved in the United States was Velcade (bortezomib), approved for the treatment of MULTIPLE MYELOMA, a type of cancer that is treatable but not curable. Because normal cells also contain proteasome, they too are vulnerable to the drug. Side effects include many typical of chemotherapy, such as nausea, fatigue, diarrhea, constipation, headache, decreased appetite, decreased blood cell production, and nerve damage.

Velcade maker Millennium Pharmaceuticals is studying whether Velcade also could treat advanced colon or LUNG CANCER.

5Q minus syndrome   A rare disorder, caused by loss of part of the long "Q arm" of chromosome 5, that affects bone marrow cells, causing treatment-resistant ANEMIA that may lead to acute myelogenous LEUKEMIA.

R. A. Bloch Cancer Foundation, Inc. Nonprofit foundation that offers a cancer hotline, support groups, and educational presentations. The foundation's toll-free hotline matches newly diagnosed patients with someone who has survived the same cancer. For contact information, see Appendix I.

rad An outdated term to indicate a unit of radiation dose, replaced by the term *gray*. One gray equals 100 rads.

radiation therapy A method of treating cancer using radiation directed at the body by a machine, or from radioactive material placed directly in the body (BRACHYTHERAPY). External radiation is usually given daily for several weeks on an outpatient basis. Implants usually require a hospital stay. Radiation therapy is also sometimes used before surgery to destroy cancer cells, especially if the tumor is large or not easily removed.

radiation oncologist See ONCOLOGIST.

radionuclide scan An imaging technique that uses a small dose of a radioactive chemical (isotope) called a tracer to identify areas of the body where the radioactivity accumulates.

radon A naturally occurring, odorless, tasteless, and colorless radioactive gas produced by the breakdown of radium in soil, rock, and water. Studies have shown that Iowa has the highest average radon concentrations in the United States. The high concentrations in Iowa and the upper Midwest are due primarily to glacial deposits left more than 10,000 years ago.

Long-term exposure to radon gas in the home is associated with increased LUNG CANCER incidence and presents a significant environmental health hazard. The health risk posed by residential radon exposure may have been substantially underestimated in studies, according to investigators at the University of Iowa College of Public Health.

While radon concentrations tend to be highest in basements, people typically spend limited time there. A more accurate assessment of risk can be formulated by linking multiple radon measurements taken within a home to how much time someone spends in various part of the home.

Although the majority of lung cancer deaths are attributable to the voluntary habit of SMOKING, researchers estimate that residential radon exposure accounts for approximately 19,000 of the 160,000 lung cancer deaths that occur each year in the United States. Smoking increases the risk of lung cancer even more for those already at risk because of exposure to radon.

Because of the magnitude of lung cancer incidence and its poor survival rate, even secondary causes of lung cancer, such as prolonged residential radon exposure, are important.

A kit available at most hardware stores allows homeowners to measure radon levels in their homes. The home radon test is relatively easy to use and inexpensive, and radon problems can be corrected by venting basements where the gas collects.

Reach to Recovery A program sponsored by the AMERICAN CANCER SOCIETY in which volunteers who have survived BREAST CANCER and gone on to live normal, productive lives offer understanding, support, and hope to newly diagnosed patients and their families. Through face-to-face visits or by phone, Reach to Recovery volunteers provide support for anyone newly diagnosed or facing recurrence.

Volunteers are trained to provide support and up-to-date information, including literature for spouses, children, friends, and other loved ones. Volunteers can also, when appropriate, provide breast cancer patients with a temporary artificial breast, information on types of permanent prostheses, and lists of places to purchase those items.

Reach to Recovery works with carefully selected and trained volunteers who have fully adjusted to their breast cancer treatment. All volunteers complete an initial training and participate in ongoing continuing education sessions. For contact information, see Appendix I.

reconstructive surgeon   A physician (also called a "plastic and reconstructive surgeon") who uses special techniques to repair visible skin defects and problems in underlying tissue, caused by surgery or by the cancer itself. A reconstructive surgeon can use grafts of the skin, bone, and cartilage to repair defects and can transfer tissue from one part of the body to another. In these techniques, the surgeon carefully prepares the patient's skin and tissues using precise cutting and suturing techniques to minimize scarring. Recent advances in the development of miniaturized instruments, new materials for artificial limbs and body parts, and improved surgical techniques have expanded the range of reconstructive operations that can be performed. Most reconstructive surgery involves a stay in the hospital and general anesthesia.

The risks associated with reconstructive surgery include the postoperative complications that can occur with any surgical operation under anesthesia, such as infection, internal bleeding, pneumonia, and reactions to the anesthesia. In addition to these general risks, reconstructive surgery carries specific risks

- undesirable scar tissue
- persistent pain, redness, or swelling
- infection related to inserting a prosthesis, which can be caused by contamination at the time of surgery or from bacteria migrating into the area around the prosthesis at a later time
- anemia or fat embolisms from liposuction
- rejection of skin grafts or tissue transplants
- loss of normal feeling or function in the area of the operation

- complications resulting from unforeseen technological problems (such as the discovery in the mid-1990s that breast implants made with silicone gel could leak into the patient's body)

rectal exam   A physical examination in which the doctor inserts a lubricated, gloved finger into the rectum (the last few inches of the digestive tract) to feel for abnormal areas. This is one diagnostic test for COLORECTAL CANCER.

See also PROSTATE CANCER.

recurrence   The return of cancer after treatment, which may occur either at the original site of the disease or at another location (metastasis).

red blood cells   A type of blood cell that carries oxygen from the lungs to other parts of the body. Red blood cells contain hemoglobin, an iron-rich protein that is responsible for absorbing oxygen in the lungs and later releasing it to the body's tissues. CHEMOTHERAPY drugs kill rapidly dividing cells, including red blood cells. This is why more than 60 percent of chemotherapy patients eventually develop a deficiency of red blood cells called ANEMIA, leading to FATIGUE, dizziness, headaches, and shortness of breath.

During chemotherapy treatment patients have regular blood tests to check the number of red cells in the blood; the next chemotherapy treatment may be postponed, and a blood transfusion given, if the counts are very low. Other treatments for anemia include injections of erythropoietin (EPO), which can boost red blood cell count.

Erythropoietin is a major blood growth factor that encourages the bone marrow to produce more red blood cells. Although it is a naturally occurring substance, it can now be made in the laboratory in much larger quantities than patients normally produce on their own. EPO is often given near the end of chemotherapy treatment for patients who are anemic, very tired, or breathless. Occasionally, EPO can cause side effects, including flu symptoms, rashes, or high blood pressure.

relapse   See RECURRENCE.

Relief Band Explorer   A patented, watchlike electronic medical device that provides drug-free, noninvasive relief from NAUSEA and vomiting. It relieves symptoms by gently stimulating nerves on the underside of the wrist. When activated, the device emits a low-level electrical current across two small electrodes on its underside. It is available by prescription for the treatment of nausea and vomiting caused by CHEMOTHERAPY. The band is the only medical device to be approved by the U.S. Food and Drug Administration for use in hospitals and doctors' offices for the treatment of severe forms of nausea and vomiting from chemotherapy.

Report on Carcinogens A biennial federal report on cancer-causing substances. The report, mandated by the Public Health Services Act, contains a list of chemicals and exposure circumstances that are known to be human CARCINOGENS or that may reasonably be anticipated to be human carcinogens. The report also contains information received from federal agencies relating to estimated exposures and exposure standards or guidelines.

The evaluation of substances is performed by National Toxicology Program scientists and by other federal health research and regulatory agencies.

Information provided includes dose response, route of exposure, chemical structure, metabolism, pharmacokinetics, sensitive subpopulations, and genetic effects.

resveratrol An organic compound that is produced by many plants during times of environmental stress, such as adverse weather or insect, animal, or pathogenic attack, and that may protect against cancer.

Resveratrol has been identified in more than 70 species of plants, including mulberries and peanuts, but grapes and wine are particularly good sources. Research indicates this chemical acts as an antioxidant and damps down the cellular processes involved in the promotion and growth of cancerous cells.

Resveratrol is found in the skin (not the flesh) of grapes; fresh grape skin contains about 50 to 100 micrograms of resveratrol per gram, while red wine concentrations range from 1.5 to 3 milligrams per liter. The concentrations of resveratrol in fruits vary considerably. One large study found about five parts per million of resveratrol in French red

wines; muscadine grapes and products contain even higher levels of resveratrol. In 1996 muscadine wines made in North Carolina were found by researchers at the Campbell School of Pharmacy to average 50 parts per million.

Researchers at the University of Illinois found that resveratrol inhibited the development of lesions and reduced the number of skin tumors in cancer-prone mice by up to 90 percent. Scientists at the University of California at Davis found that similar cancer-prone mice fed a diet that included resveratrol avoided cancerous tumors 40 percent longer than sibling mice with no resveratrol in their diets.

This compound is also thought to be partly responsible for the cholesterol-lowering effects of red wine and may explain the "French paradox"—that is, why those consuming a Mediterranean-type diet with a lot of fat and plenty of red wine appear to have a low risk of heart disease.

retinoblastoma See EYE CANCER.

rhabdomyosarcoma A type of cancer growing from striated muscle cells in the voluntary muscles (muscles, such as triceps or biceps, a person can use by conscious intention). (See also SARCOMA.)

RhoGD12 A newly discovered gene that may be responsible for stopping the spread of some cancer cells. This gene is missing (or present in low levels) in invasive, metastatic cancer. The discovery of this gene could lead to new tests to help doctors determine the best way to treat individual cancers and eventually could lead to gene therapy to treat aggressive forms of cancer.

To isolate the gene responsible for metastasis, researchers compared two types of BLADDER CANCER—one aggressive and invasive, the other a localized, nonspreading cancer. The aggressive form of cancer had low levels of RhoGD12.

Cancer can develop only when the body's functions go awry. Normally, human cells grow to replace old, dying cells. If new cells form when the body does not need them and older cells do not die off, a tumor may develop from all those extra cells. Some tumors are benign and generally do not cause problems, but others are malignant, invading and damaging other cells and moving to other parts of the body via the bloodstream. For that malignant process to occur, many genes must be altered or destroyed. Replacing the function of even one of those damaged genes may stop the process that lets tumors spread.

Researchers have found reduced levels of RhoGD12 in 105 tumors from prostate, lung, breast, colorectal, gastroesophageal, kidney, liver, ovarian, and pancreatic cancers.

One day, researchers may develop a test to assess levels of RhoGD12 in tumors, which would help doctors treat their patients more accurately and effectively. For example, someone with low levels of RhoGD12 might be a good candidate for chemotherapy, since it is likely their tumor would be more aggressive. After more research, it might be possible to replace RhoGD12 in cancer patients so their cancer does not spread.

The gene does not appear to affect tumor growth but inhibits the spread of existing tumors. That means cancer patients would still need to have surgery to have tumors removed but might not need chemotherapy afterward because the cancer cells would not spread to other sites in the body.

Ronald McDonald Houses A group of special houses around the world that provide a "home away from home" for families who need a place to stay while a sick child in the family is cared for at a nearby hospital. To date, more than 10 million families with sick children have stayed at a Ronald McDonald House, saving more than $120 million in housing and meal costs.

Dedicated administrative and volunteer staff focus on the family so the family can focus on the needs of their sick child. Families support and coach each other, and children, often self-conscious and embarrassed about their illnesses, feel at home in the warm and nurturing environment.

The first Ronald McDonald House opened in Philadelphia in 1974 thanks to the efforts of Fred Hill, a Philadelphia Eagles football player. When his daughter Kim was diagnosed with LEUKEMIA, Hill and his wife camped out on hospital chairs and benches, eating food from vending machines. They noticed other families, many who had traveled great distances, suffering the same fate.

Hill was introduced to Dr. Audrey Evans, a pediatric ONCOLOGIST at Children's Hospital in Philadelphia who had dreamed of providing temporary housing for families like the Hills. With considerable help from local McDonald's franchisees and Hill's teammates, Hill and Dr. Evans soon founded the first Ronald McDonald House. For contact information, see Appendix I.

saccharin See ARTIFICIAL SWEETENERS.

St. John's wort An herb widely used as an over-the-counter remedy for mild depression. It may interfere with Camptosar, a common CHEMOTHERAPY drug, reducing Camptosar's effectiveness for weeks after people stop taking the herbal supplement. In a small study, doctors showed that St. John's wort decreases blood levels of one chemotherapy drug by about 40 percent. This effect lingered for more than three weeks after people stopped taking the supplement. Despite the small size of the study, experts said the findings are compelling because they fit with earlier reports showing that St. John's wort can disrupt drug treatment.

In 2000 the U.S. Food and Drug Administration warned that the herb can interfere with protease inhibitors (drugs that are widely used to treat AIDS). St. John's wort interferes with an enzyme, called P450, that the body uses to break down many drugs. Because of this, St. John's wort is believed to inhibit many of the most widely prescribed medicines. Among others are digoxin and beta-blockers (both used for heart disease), seizure medicines, and drugs used to prevent organ rejection after transplants.

salpingectomy The removal of one or both of a woman's fallopian tubes. A bilateral salpingectomy (removal of both the tubes) is usually done if the ovaries and uterus are also going to be removed. If the fallopian tubes and the ovaries are both removed at the same time, this is called a SALPINGO-OOPHORECTOMY. A salpingo-oophorectomy is necessary when treating ovarian and ENDOMETRIAL CANCER because the fallopian tubes and ovaries are the most common sites to which cancer may spread.

Regional or general anesthesia may be used. Often a laparoscope (a hollow tube with a light on one end) is used in this type of operation, which means that the incision can be much smaller and the recovery time much shorter. In this procedure, the surgeon makes a small incision just beneath the navel. The surgeon inserts a short, hollow tube into the abdomen and, if necessary, pumps in carbon dioxide gas in order to move the intestines out of the way and better view the organs. After a wider double tube is inserted on one side for the laparoscope, another small incision is made on the other side through which other instruments can be inserted. After the operation is completed, the tubes and instruments are withdrawn. The tiny incisions are sutured and there is very little scarring.

Most women are out of bed and walking around within three days. Within a month (or longer, if the woman had open abdominal surgery), a woman can slowly return to normal activities such as driving, exercising, and working.

salpingo-oophorectomy The surgical removal of a fallopian tube and an ovary to treat OVARIAN CANCER or other gynecologic cancers. If only one tube and ovary are removed, the woman may still be able to conceive and carry a pregnancy to term.

If the procedure is performed through a laparoscope, the surgeon can avoid a large abdominal incision and can shorten recovery to about three or four weeks. With this technique, the surgeon makes a small cut through the abdominal wall just below the navel. The patient can be given either regional or general anesthesia; if there are no complications, the patient can leave the hospital in a day or two.

If a laparoscope is not used, the surgery involves an incision four to six inches long into the abdomen either extending vertically up from the pubic bone toward the navel, or horizontally (the "bikini incision") across the pubic hairline. The scar from a bikini incision is less noticeable, but some surgeons prefer the vertical incision because it provides greater visibility while operating.

If performed through an abdominal incision, salpingo-oophorectomy is major surgery that requires three to six weeks for full recovery. There may be some discomfort around the incision for the first few days after surgery, but most women are walking around by the third day. Within a month or so, patients can gradually resume normal activities such as driving, exercising, and working. Immediately following the operation, the patient should avoid sharply flexing the thighs or the knees. Persistent back pain or bloody or scanty urine indicates that a ureter may have been injured during surgery.

If both ovaries are removed in a premenopausal woman as part of the operation, the sudden loss of ESTROGEN will trigger an abrupt premature menopause that may involve severe symptoms of hot flashes, vaginal dryness, painful intercourse, and loss of sex drive (surgical menopause). In addition to these symptoms, women who lose both ovaries also lose the protection these hormones provide against heart disease and osteoporosis many years earlier than if they had experienced natural menopause. Women who have had their ovaries removed are seven times more likely to develop coronary heart disease and much more likely to develop bone problems at an early age than are premenopausal women whose ovaries are intact.

Reaction to the removal of fallopian tubes and ovaries depends on a wide variety of factors, including the woman's age, the condition that required the surgery, her reproductive history, how much social support she has, and any previous history of depression. Women who have had many gynecologic surgeries or chronic pelvic pain seem to have a higher tendency to develop psychological problems after the surgery.

sarcoma A type of cancer that usually begins as a painless swelling in the soft tissues of the body, including fat, blood vessels, nerves, muscles, skin, and cartilage. About 40 percent of sarcomas begin in the legs and feet, 20 percent begin in the hands and arms, and 20 percent first appear in the trunk. The rest originate in the head or neck.

sarcomas, soft tissue Malignant tumors that develop in soft tissue, such as fat, muscles, nerves, tendons, and blood and lymph vessels. Sarcomas are unusual in that they can occur in any site of the human body, although about half of them are found in the arms and legs.

There are more than 50 different types of these sarcomas and sarcoma-like growths, grouped together by their shared microscopic characteristics, similar symptoms, and treatment similarities. (Bone tumors, or osteosarcomas, also are called sarcomas, but they are in a separate category because they have different clinical and microscopic characteristics and are treated differently.)

Sarcomas can invade surrounding tissue and can spread to other organs, forming secondary tumors. The cells of secondary tumors are similar to those of the original (primary) cancer; these secondary tumors are called "metastatic soft tissue sarcoma" because they are part of the same cancer and are not a new disease. High-grade soft tissue sarcomas of the arms and legs most often spread to the lungs; soft tissue sarcomas inside the abdomen often spread to the liver.

Soft tissue sarcomas are relatively uncommon, accounting for less than 1 percent of all new cancer cases each year, or about 8,100 new cases a year. They are found in all ages and in both sexes; about 850 to 900 of these growths will occur among children and adolescents under age 20. Most patients with this type of cancer can be cured. In fact, the five-year survival rate for people with early stage soft tissue sarcomas is about 90 percent.

If a soft tissue sarcoma recurs, in about 70 percent of patients this happens in the first two years. However, patients with sarcoma are usually followed for a minimum of 10 years, because some patients can have a very late recurrence of their tumor. Such late recurrences often respond well to treatment, however, and can be readily and effectively treated.

Types of Adult Soft Tissue Sarcomas

Fibrosarcoma: Cancer appearing in the fibrous tissue of the arms, legs, or trunk.

Malignant fibrous hystiocytoma: Cancer appearing in the fibrous tissue of the legs.

Dermatofibrosarcoma: Cancer appearing in the fibrous tissue of the arms, legs, or trunk.

LIPOSARCOMA: Cancer appearing in the fat of the arms, legs, and trunk.

Rhabdomyosarcoma: Cancer appearing in the striated muscles of the arms and legs.

Leimyosarcoma: Cancer appearing in the lymph vessels of the arms.

Synovial sarcoma: Cancer appearing in the synovial tissue (linings of joint cavities and tendon sheaths) of the legs.

Neurofibrosarcoma: Cancer appearing in the peripheral nerves of the arms, legs and trunk.

Extraskeletal chondrosarcoma: Cancer appearing in the cartilage and bone-forming tissue of the legs.

Extraskeletal osteosarcoma: Cancer appearing in the cartilage and bone-forming tissue of the legs and trunk not involving the bone.

Soft Tissue Sarcomas in Children

Rhabdomyosarcoma: Cancer appearing in the striated muscle. Embryonal forms affect the head and neck and the genitourinary tract, appearing between infancy and age 4. Alveolar forms appear in the arms, legs, and head and neck from infancy through age 19.

Leiomyosarcoma: Cancer appears in the smooth muscle of the trunk, between ages 15 and 19.

Fibrosarcoma: Cancer appears in the fibrous tissue of the arms and legs, between ages 15 and 19.

Malignant fibrous histiocytoma: Cancer appears in the fibrous tissue of the legs, between ages 15 and 19.

Dermatofibrosarcoma: Cancer appears in the fibrous tissue of the trunk, between ages 15 and 19.

Liposarcoma: Cancer that originates in the fat tissue of the arms and legs, between ages 15 and 19.

Infantile hemangiopericytoma: Cancer that originates in the blood vessels in the arms, legs, trunk, head and neck, primarily in children from infancy through age four.

Synovial sarcoma: Cancer that originates in the linings of the joint cavities and tendon sheaths of the legs, arms, and trunk, primarily in teens aged 15 through 19.

Malignant peripheral nerve sheath tumors: Also called neurofibrosarcomas, malignant schwannomas, or neurogenic sarcomas, these cancers originate in the peripheral nerves of the arms, legs, and trunk, primarily in teens between ages 15 and 19.

Alveolar soft part sarcoma: Cancer originating in the muscular nerves of the arms and legs, primarily in children from infancy through age 19.

Extraskeletal myxoid chondrosarcoma: Cancer originating in the cartilage and bone-forming tissue of the legs, primarily in children aged 10 through 14.

Extraskeletal mesenchymal: Cancer originating in the cartilage and bone-forming tissue of the legs, primarily in children aged 10 through 14.

Cause

Scientists do not fully understand why some people develop sarcomas while most others do not. However, by identifying common characteristics in groups with unusually high occurrence rates, researchers have been able to single out some factors that may play a role in causing soft tissue sarcomas, including the following:

- *On-the-job exposure.* Studies suggest that workers exposed to phenoxyacetic acid in herbicides and chlorophenols in wood preservatives may have an increased risk of developing soft tissue sarcomas. An unusual percentage of patients with a rare blood vessel tumor (angiosarcoma of the liver) have been exposed to vinyl chloride, used to manufacture certain plastics.

- *Radiation.* In the early 1900s, radiation was used to treat many conditions, such as enlarged tonsils, adenoids, and thymus gland. Later, researchers found that high doses of radiation caused soft tissue sarcomas in some patients. Because of this risk, radiation treatment for cancer is now planned to ensure that the maximum dosage of radiation is delivered to diseased tissue while surrounding healthy tissue is protected as much as possible.

- *Retroviruses.* Researchers believe that a herpesvirus plays an indirect role in the development of KAPOSI'S SARCOMA, a rare cancer of the cells that line blood vessels in the skin and mucus membranes. Kaposi's sarcoma often occurs in patients with AIDS, but this form of Kaposi's sarcoma has different characteristics and is treated differently than typical soft tissue sarcomas.

- *Genetics.* Inherited mutations may trigger the development of soft tissue sarcomas. A few families have more than one member in the same generation who has developed sarcoma or other forms of cancer at an unusually high rate. Sarcomas in these family clusters, which represent a very small fraction of all cases, may be related to a rare inherited genetic alteration.

- *Inherited diseases.* Certain inherited diseases are associated with an increased risk of developing soft tissue sarcomas. For example, people with Li-Fraumeni syndrome (associated with alterations in the p53 gene) or von Recklinghausen's disease (also called neurofibromatosis, and associated with alterations in the NF1 gene) are at an increased risk of developing soft tissue sarcomas.

Symptoms

Soft tissue sarcomas can appear almost anywhere in the body; about half occur in the arms, legs, hands, or feet; 40 percent occur in the chest, back, hips, shoulders, and abdomen; and 10 percent occur in the head and neck.

In the early stages, soft tissue sarcomas usually do not cause symptoms because soft tissue is relatively elastic, so tumors can grow fairly large before they cause any problems. The first noticeable symptom is usually a painless lump or swelling. As the tumor grows, it may cause other symptoms, such as pain or soreness, as it presses against nearby nerves and muscles.

Diagnosis

Imaging studies can help identify suspicious masses, using ultrasound, magnetic resonance imaging (MRI), and computed tomography (CT) scans. Because sound waves are reflected differently off tumors than normal tissues, ultrasound can sometimes identify a mass for biopsy. With a CT scan, X-ray images are taken from different angles and then combined by a computer, producing a cross-section picture of the suspicious area. For surveillance during follow-up, CT/PET (computed tomography and positron-emittance tomography) is now often used in combination to show both location and activity if a tumor should arise. If the CT/PET study indicates a

recurrence, the doctor may order a separate CT study for precise information about the location of the tumor.

MRI is similar to a CT scan but uses large magnets and radio waves to produce images. MRI is better than a CT scan at showing blood vessels in greater detail and to picture cross-sections from multiple angles.

Biopsy In some situations, imaging study results are so clear they can indicate surgery without doing a BIOPSY. Even in these situations, a biopsy is performed to be sure the tumor is a sarcoma and not another type of cancer or a noncancerous disease. During this procedure, a surgeon makes an incision or uses a special needle to remove a tumor sample, which is then examined under a microscope. If it is malignant, the pathologist can usually determine the type of cancer and its grade.

The grade of the tumor is determined by how abnormal the cancer cells look under a microscope; this predicts the probable growth rate of the tumor and its tendency to spread. Low-grade sarcomas are unlikely to spread, but high-grade sarcomas are more likely to spread to other parts of the body.

Treatment

In general, treatment for soft tissue sarcomas depends on the stage of the cancer, which is based on the size and grade of the tumor, and whether the cancer has spread to the lymph nodes or other parts of the body. Treatment options for soft tissue sarcomas include surgery, radiation therapy, and chemotherapy.

Surgery Surgery is the most common treatment for soft tissue sarcomas. If possible, the doctor may remove the cancer and a safe margin (about 2 to 3 centimeters) of the healthy tissue around it.

Although amputation of an arm or leg was once a standard treatment for soft-tissue sarcomas, today amputations are performed in only between 5 and 15 percent of cases nationwide. In most cases, limb-sparing surgery is an option to avoid amputation. In this procedure, as much of the tumor is removed as possible, and RADIATION THERAPY or chemotherapy is given either before the surgery to shrink the tumor or after surgery to kill the remaining cancer cells.

Radiation Radiation therapy is commonly given to limit the risk of a local recurrence at the same place where the sarcoma was removed; it may be used either before surgery to shrink tumors or after surgery to kill any cancer cells that may have been left behind. Although small sarcomas can be treated by surgery alone, most sarcomas are bigger than 5 centimeters and so are routinely managed by a combination of surgery and radiation therapy.

Compared to other tumors, a larger margin of normal tissue is subjected to radiation in surgery for soft-tissue sarcoma because sarcoma can spread along muscles and between them in ways that sometimes cannot be seen or felt. Microscopically, sarcoma cells can trickle out and be left behind after surgery. For this reason, radiation oncologists typically irradiate tissue 5 to 10 centimeters (approximately 2 inches) beyond where the tumor was confined.

BRACHYTHERAPY, which involves delivering radiation therapy locally, can be administered in two different ways to treat soft-tissue sarcoma. In one approach, during surgery after the tumor is removed, catheters are inserted into the tumor bed. After the surgical wound heals for five to six days, radiotherapeutic seeds are inserted into each of the catheters. The seeds stay in place for several days, delivering a high dose of radiotherapy. After the treatment is completed, the radiotherapeutic seeds and the catheters are removed. In some situations, brachytherapy may be administered for two to three days plus five weeks of external radiation.

A second form of brachytherapy (high-dose-rate intraoperative radiation therapy) is delivered entirely during surgery, followed by a course of external beam radiation therapy. This approach is most useful for the retroperitoneum and chest, where it is not feasible to leave catheters in place.

External-beam radiation therapy uses doses of radiation delivered from outside the body, focusing on the region of the tumor and surrounding tissues. It typically takes between seven and eight weeks of five-day-a-week treatments, before or after surgery.

Soft-tissue sarcoma is a treatable cancer, even when it recurs locally. Local recurrence does not necessarily mean that the first treatment was inadequate and it does not mean that the person with the recurrence cannot be cured. Many patients with local recurrence also receive adjuvant radiation therapy with surgery, depending on the method and extent of previous surgery and radiotherapy. Even after a local recurrence, amputation is usually not necessary to treat sarcoma of the extremities.

Chemotherapy When a patient's tumor is a type that might spread, chemotherapy may be used as an additional therapy, either before or after surgery. In addition to destroying microscopic areas of cancer cells, this treatment can reduce the size of the primary sarcoma before the operation.

Surgical removal of a primary sarcoma, sometimes followed by radiation therapy, will cure many patients, but in some patients, sarcoma spreads through the blood to distant sites, such as the lungs or liver. Today, fewer than 20 percent of all soft-tissue sarcomas have spread before they are diagnosed.

Even patients who appear to have a primary sarcoma may have a few cells that spread but that cannot be detected, even with modern imaging techniques. Doctors can estimate the chances that a tumor has spread, based on the size of a sarcoma and its appearance under the microscope.

Today, doctors often give chemotherapy before surgery to patients with large, fast-growing sarcomas. The terms "neoadjuvant chemotherapy" and "preoperative chemotherapy" are used to describe this strategy. In addition to destroying microscopic cancer cells, this approach often reduces the size of the primary sarcoma, which may allow the surgeon to perform a less radical operation and save some patients from an amputation. Preoperative chemotherapy may also contribute to better chances of survival.

Doxorubicin and ifosfamide are the chemotherapy drugs most widely used to treat sarcoma. In certain patients, chemotherapy that includes both doxorubicin and ifosfamide almost doubles the likelihood of shrinking a sarcoma, compared with older treatments.

Chemotherapy may be used in combination with radiation therapy either before or after surgery to try to shrink the tumor or kill any remaining cancer cells. If the cancer has spread to other areas of the body, chemotherapy may be used to shrink tumors and reduce the pain and discomfort they cause, but is unlikely to eradicate the disease. The use of chemotherapy to prevent the spread of soft tissue sarcomas has not been proven to be effective.

selective estrogen-receptor modulators (SERMS)

A group of drugs that cause ESTROGEN-like responses in certain tissues while preventing estrogen-like responses in other parts of the body. Specifically, SERMs block the actions of estrogen in breast tissues and certain other tissues by occupying the estrogen receptors on cells. With a SERM in the estrogen receptor, there is no place for the real estrogen to attach. SERMs are helpful in treating breast cancer because unlike natural estrogen, they do not send messages to the cell nucleus to grow and divide. Three of the best-known SERMs are tamoxifen (Nolvadex), raloxifene (Evista), and toremifene (Fareston).

SERMs do send estrogen-like signals when they attach to receptors on bone cells, liver cells, and elsewhere in the body. The result is that SERMs seem to help prevent or slow osteoporosis in postmenopausal women and may help lower cholesterol (produced in the liver). This dual effect—blocking estrogen in some places and imitating estrogen in other places—allows SERMs to have multiple beneficial effects in many women with BREAST CANCER.

Tamoxifen

Tamoxifen, in use for more than 20 years, was the first SERM to become available. In appropriate women, it is a powerful weapon against breast cancer. Many large studies show that tamoxifen can reduce the chances of cancer returning, progressing, or starting in the first place (in cases in which a woman has many risk factors). Side effects include hot flashes, vaginal dryness or discharge, irregular periods, nausea, and cataracts. Rare side effects include blood clots and an increased risk of ENDOMETRIAL CANCER. Tamoxifen may be recommended for both pre- and postmenopausal women with all stages of disease.

Toremifene

This is a relatively new SERM with properties and side effects similar to those of tamoxifen, but unlike tamoxifen, toremifene does not seem to increase the risk of endometrial cancer. Based on research available to date, the U.S. Food and Drug Administration (FDA) has restricted the use of toremifene to postmenopausal women whose breast cancer has spread.

Raloxifene

This SERM medication strengthens bones and is FDA approved for treating osteoporosis in postmenopausal women. Raloxifene was found to lower the risk of breast cancer in postmenopausal women with osteoporosis, but testing has not been completed on women with breast cancer. The STAR (Study of Tamoxifen and Raloxifene) study is now comparing tamoxifen to raloxifene in their ability to decrease breast cancer incidence in high-risk women.

Side effects are similar to those of tamoxifen, including hot flashes, vaginal changes, and rarely, blood clots, stroke, and pulmonary embolism. Raloxifene does not seem to increase the risk of endometrial cancer.

sentinel node biopsy A new surgical technique in BREAST CANCER treatment that is an alternative to standard LYMPH NODE DISSECTION, sparing many women more invasive surgery and side effects. However, the sentinel node procedure is not appropriate for everyone. It has its own limitations and drawbacks, and must be done by a surgeon who has significant experience with the technique.

The "sentinel" LYMPH NODE is the first node that filters fluid draining from the area of the breast. If cancer cells are breaking away from the tumor and traveling away from the breast, the sentinel node is more likely than other lymph nodes to contain cancerous cells.

Instead of removing 10 or more lymph nodes and analyzing all of them to look for cancer, the sentinel node biopsy procedure removes only the single node most likely to have malignant cells. If this node is clean, chances are the other nodes have not been affected. In practice, the surgeon usually removes a cluster of two or three nodes—the sentinel node and those closest to it—during a sentinel node biopsy.

Sentinel node dissection is a good option for women with early-stage, invasive breast cancer who have a low to moderate risk of lymph node involvement. In these women, it is critical to find out if the cancer has moved beyond the breast.

However, a sentinel node biopsy is not warranted if the surgeon has good reason to believe that a woman's lymph nodes are involved; in this case, a standard axillary lymph node dissection with multiple nodes removed makes the most sense. This is because the surgeon does not want to miss a significant amount of cancer that may be in the nodes. It is also important to know how many nodes are involved, because researchers have found that the more nodes that are involved, the more serious the disease and the more aggressive treatment should be.

In general, sentinel node dissection is *not* appropriate for the following women:

- anyone who is likely to have cancer in the lymph nodes;
- women with any prior surgery or treatment that could have altered the normal pattern of lymph drainage;
- women over the age of 50 whose lymphatic flow may be altered by the wear and tear of the aging process;
- women who had chemotherapy before surgery to reduce the size of a large cancer, or to treat many involved lymph nodes (lymphatic flow may be altered by the inflammation and scar tissue that occur as the body and the chemotherapy battle the tumor).

In the operating room, the surgeon injects a radioactive liquid, a blue dye, or both into the area around the tumor, and then watches to see where the dye travels and concentrates. A special instrument is used to track the radioactive liquid. This process illuminates the pathway by which the lymph travels when it drains away from the part of the breast with the tumor, indicating which lymph node is the "sentinel node" for a particular tumor.

After the sentinel node and one or two nodes closest to it are removed, the surgeon will look at them and feel them in the operating room to see if they seem to be affected by cancer. Next, the nodes are sent to the pathology lab for analysis under a microscope.

If the sentinel node does not show any cancer, it is likely that no other axillary lymph nodes contain cancer, which means it is also likely that the cancer has not spread beyond the breast. Treatment decisions can be made with this important information in mind.

If the sentinel node does contain cancer, another treatment step may be needed. During surgery, if a surgeon suspects that the sentinel node just removed is affected by cancer, he or she may decide to remove more nodes for evaluation (an axillary dissection) during the same operation. If the laboratory finds significant cancer present in the sentinel node (or nodes) after surgery, the surgeon may recommend an axillary dissection to remove and analyze more lymph nodes from the armpit.

Alternatively, the medical team may recommend that radiation treatment of surrounding lymph nodes is the best way to treat cancer that may have spread there. The need for additional treatment (surgery, radiation, or both) if the sentinel node turns out to be involved represents a key limitation of the sentinel lymph node approach. For this reason, many doctors favor the traditional lymph node approach.

On the other hand, when a surgeon has to remove only one lymph node, or a small cluster of two or three nodes to know whether or not breast cancer has spread, it leaves the other lymph nodes intact. This avoids uncomfortable temporary side effects, such as lymph backup in the armpit, that often occur after traditional lymph node removal. Traditional surgery also can cause other lingering side effects, including mild discomfort, numbness and heightened sensitivity in the armpit and the upper arm, and swelling of the arm on the side of the affected breast (LYMPHEDEMA). The more surgery a woman has in the breast/armpit area, the more potential for numbness and discomfort.

Sertoli cell tumors   Rare tumors of the testicle. While some of these tumors are malignant, doctors are usually not able to determine if the tumor is malignant simply by visual inspection. Sertoli cells are responsible for nurturing the immature sperm, trapping male hormones necessary for sperm production. They also form tight junctions with other Sertoli cells to form a blood-testis barrier, preventing any sperm proteins from leaving the testes to provoke an immune response that would sterilize the male. This barrier is one reason why CHEMOTHERAPY does not kill all the GERM CELLS in the testes and is also why a cancerous testicle must always be removed. When a Sertoli cell tumor is suspected, a radical orchiectomy is usually done and will cure the cancer without the need for further treatment.

See also LEYDIG CELL TUMORS; TESTICULAR CANCER.

shark cartilage   See CARTILAGE (SHARK AND BOVINE).

sigmoidoscopy   An examination of the last third of the large intestine, including the rectum and the last part of the colon.

silicone breast implants and cancer   There is no association between breast implants and the subsequent risk of BREAST CANCER, according to one of the largest studies on the long-term health effects of silicone breast implants. Breast implants first appeared on the market in 1962, but since the beginning there have been a number of reports of connective tissue disorders and cancers among implant patients caused by silicone leaking from ruptured implants. In 1992, because of a lack of sufficient evidence on the long-term safety of implants, the U.S. Food and Drug Administration restricted the use of silicone breast implants to women seeking breast reconstruction in controlled clinical trials, and Congress directed the National Institutes of Health to undertake a large follow-up study to evaluate the long-term health effects of the implants.

Researchers from the NATIONAL CANCER INSTITUTE found no change in breast cancer risk for women with silicone implants who were followed for more than 10 years. However, the results did not confirm the findings from several other studies that implants reduce a woman's risk for breast cancer. This may be because of the longer follow-up times in this study as compared with most others.

This study did not assess women undergoing breast reconstruction after breast cancer surgery, so it is not possible to predict whether similar results would be found for this population. The majority of the previous studies had also focused on women who received implants for cosmetic reasons. It is estimated that between 1.5 million and 2 million U.S. women have had breast implants since they first appeared on the market in 1962. Future analyses of the data will evaluate the risk of other cancers, connective tissue disorders, and causes of death.

simian virus 40 (SV40)   A virus that infects several species of monkeys without causing symptoms or disease. The virus was discovered in 1960 in rhesus macaque monkey kidney cells used to produce the original Salk and Sabin polio vaccines. The virus has been shown to cause tumors in mice when injected in high amounts and has been detected in some human tumors, particularly pleural mesothelioma—a rare cancer of the membrane covering the lungs. Suspicions about a link between the vaccine and SV40 arose as rates of pleural mesothelioma increased between 1975 and 1997.

Because the mass immunization program for polio began in 1955, before the discovery of the virus, contaminated vaccine lots were inadvertently used for the first few years of the program. When reports appeared in 1961 that injection of SV40 into hamsters triggered tumors, the U.S. government began a screening program requiring that all new lots of poliovirus vaccine be free of SV40 because of concerns about possible adverse effects on human health. (However, earlier lots were not withdrawn from the mass immunization program.)

No SV40 has been found in the polio vaccine lots tested after 1963, and the polio vaccine currently used in the United States is produced under carefully regulated conditions designed to ensure that contamination with SV40 does not occur. As a result of the earlier contamination, however, it is estimated that 10 million to 30 million people vaccinated in the United States from 1955 through early 1963 were inadvertently exposed to live SV40. Over the last 40 years, scientists have been trying to discover whether SV40 has caused health problems, including cancer, in people.

Concern about SV40 increased in the last few years when more and more labs, using an extremely sensitive molecular biology technique, found traces of the virus in some rare human tumors, including:

- pleural mesothelioma (a cancer of the lining of the lung)

- osteosarcoma (a type of bone cancer)
- ependymoma brain tumors
- choroid plexus tumors of the brain
- NON-HODGKIN'S LYMPHOMA

Other studies reported that SV40 T-antigen, a viral protein, binds to human tumor suppressor proteins such as p53 and RB, suggesting this might be how it triggers the onset of cancer.

In 2002 researchers established a link between SV40 and non-Hodgkin's lymphoma. After examining nearly 400 tumors and control tissues, scientists found the viral footprint for SV40 in the tumors of 43 percent of non-Hodgkin's lymphoma patients and nine percent of Hodgkin's lymphoma cases. The percentage of SV40-positive findings among healthy subjects and patients with other types of adult and pediatric cancers (other than bone tumors) was zero to 6 percent.

Researchers say the findings confirm earlier research on hamsters that associated SV40 with brain and bone tumors, mesotheliomas, and B-cell lymphomas. SV40 previously had been associated in humans with brain and BONE CANCER and mesothelioma, but the human LYMPHOMA connection is new. Researchers have been looking for a viral connection with lymphoma for several decades, and EPSTEIN-BARR VIRUS sequences have been found in some lymphomas of Hodgkin's and non-Hodgkin's types. Scientists know that SV40 activates a protein that interacts with and deactivates the proteins that control the normal cellular life cycle, creating immortal malignant cells.

Not all studies, however, have found that SV40 plays a significant role in human cancer. Epidemiology studies involving decades of observations in the United States and Europe have failed to detect an increased cancer risk in those likely to have been exposed to the virus. These include a long-term Swedish study, which followed 700,000 people who received SV40-contaminated vaccine, a 22-year German study of 886,000 people who received the contaminated vaccine as infants, a 20-year study of 1,000 people in the United States inoculated as infants with contaminated vaccines, and a 30-year follow-up of 10 percent of the entire U.S. population (using data from the National Can-

cer Institute's Surveillance, Epidemiology, and End Results registry). The Centers for Disease Control and Prevention has found no evidence that SV40-contaminated vaccine lots cause cancer.

A recent study compared vaccine exposure and subsequent rates of pleural mesotheliomas in the United States. Using cancer data from the National Cancer Institute's Surveillance, Epidemiology, and End Results Program, researchers with the Albert Einstein College of Medicine in New York City analyzed age- and sex-specific rates of pleural mesothelioma from 1975 through 1997 and compared the data with information on exposure to the SV40-contaminated poliovirus vaccine.

The researchers discovered that the increase in pleural mesothelioma cases occurred primarily among men over age 75—the age group least likely to have been exposed to the contaminated vaccine. Cases of the cancer among men in the age group that *had* been exposed to the vaccine remained either stable or decreased. The patterns among women were similar.

Sisters Network The first national BREAST CANCER survivors support group organized for African-American women. Services include community education and awareness programs, person-to-person support, a speakers' bureau, and national newsletter. Sisters Network is committed to increasing local and national attention to the devastating impact that breast cancer has in the African-American community. Sisters Network has expanded through 35 affiliate chapters in Dallas; Austin; Atlanta; Baton Rouge; Jacksonville, Florida; Rochester, New York; St. Louis; Newark; Chicago; and Los Angeles. The group has more than 2,000 members. For contact information, see Appendix I.

skin cancer The most common type of cancer, affecting more than one million Americans each year—a number that is increasing quickly. About 80 percent are basal cell, 16 percent squamous cell, and 4 percent are melanoma, the most serious form of skin cancer. Prolonged exposure or intermittent overexposure to sunlight is the primary cause of skin cancer. About 90 percent of all skin cancer is related to sun exposure, and most skin cancers are found on parts of the body exposed to sunlight.

Because ultraviolet light can damage DNA, exposing the skin to sunlight increases the risk that an individual will develop skin cancer. Skin type is a very important factor in the development of skin cancer. Fair-skinned people who tend to burn easily and tan poorly are at greatest risk; darker skinned people are at a lower risk.

Scientists have found they can determine a person's skin cancer risk by measuring a specific mutation in a tumor-suppressor gene called p53. They found specific changes in the building blocks for this gene in three quarters of samples taken from the sun-exposed skin of cancer patients. Almost no DNA from the nonexposed skin of these patients—or the skin of those who spend less time outdoors—had this mutation.

There are three basic types of skin cancer: BASAL CELL CARCINOMA, squamous cell carcinoma, and MELANOMA. Basal cell carcinoma usually appears as a small, shiny bump on sun-exposed areas, such as the face, neck, chest, upper back, and hands, primarily in fair-skinned people (especially those who burn easily). The lesions gradually grow and may crust, bleed, or ulcerate, although they do not usually spread. Local destruction of the skin and underlying tissues may be considerable if this type of cancer is left untreated.

Squamous cell carcinoma also usually occurs on exposed skin. Tumors typically appear as a red, scaly patch that grows slowly, occasionally becoming a nodule and often getting crusted or eroded. Bleeding is common. Basal cell and squamous cell cancers are almost certainly related to cumulative sun exposure. Unlike basal cell carcinoma, squamous cell cancers tend to grow more often and may spread.

Basal cell and squamous cell cancers account for about a half million new cases each year; cure rates are excellent if these lesions are discovered and effectively treated early.

Malignant melanoma is the most deadly skin cancer. Melanomas are usually small brown, black, or multicolored patches, plaques, or nodules with an irregular outline. They may crust on the surface or bleed, and many of them appear in existing moles. Melanoma is much more dangerous than other forms of skin cancer because of its tendency

to spread quickly to vital internal organs such as the lungs, liver, and brain.

Warning Signs

The most obvious skin sign is a change in any spot or sore that

- changes color
- gets bigger in size or thickness
- changes in texture
- is irregular in outline
- is bigger than the size of a pencil eraser
- appears after age 21
- continually itches, hurts, crusts, scabs, erodes, or bleeds
- does not heal
- appears pearl-colored, translucent, tan, brown, black, or multicolored and is growing

Diagnosis

Because the skin can so easily be seen, skin cancer is easier to spot than cancer inside the body. To make sure that skin cancer is recognized early, dermatologists recommend that everyone examine the skin twice yearly, using a full-length mirror and a handheld mirror. When doing a self-exam, people should look for the early warning signs (see above) but also look at any changes in the skin. Coupled with yearly skin exams by a physician, self-exams are the best way to ensure early detection and treatment of skin cancer.

Treatment

Most skin cancers (even malignant melanoma) can be cured if discovered early enough, which is why attention to symptoms and regular self-exams is highly recommended. When cancers of the skin are discovered early, there are a variety of treatments, depending on the tumor size, location, and other factors affecting the person's general health. A biopsy is often studied before a treatment plan is prepared.

Prevention

In addition to the issue of avoiding excess sun exposure, scientists have found that some foods and nutrients may counteract the development of melanoma. They say best choices are omega-3 fatty acids and ANTIOXIDANTS (including vitamin E, vitamin C, and BETA-CAROTENE).

The AMERICAN CANCER SOCIETY estimates that about 80 percent of skin cancers could be prevented if people protected themselves from the sun. It recommends the following ways to avoid skin cancer:

- Because ultraviolet rays are strongest between 10 A.M. and 4 P.M., people should limit exposure during those hours—winter and summer. UV rays can penetrate water and clouds, so even on cloudy days people should protect themselves.

- Sunscreen with a skin protection factor of 15 or higher should be applied 15 to 20 minutes before going outdoors and reapplied after swimming, sweating, or toweling off. Although it is important to avoid sunburn, especially during childhood and adolescence, sunscreen is not recommended for children younger than six months of age. Infants should be kept in the shade.

- People should wear protective clothing, including a wide-brimmed hat to shade the face, neck, and ears.

- Sunglasses are vital to protect the eyes—even for small children. UV rays are very damaging to eyes.

- It is important to avoid sunlamps and tanning booths, which are as harmful to the skin as the sun.

- Some prescription drugs (such as antibiotics) can greatly increase the skin's sensitivity to the sun.

See also SKIN CANCER FOUNDATION.

Skin Cancer Foundation   The only international organization concerned solely with the world's most common malignancy—SKIN CANCER. This nonprofit organization conducts public and medical education programs and provides support for medical training and research to help reduce the incidence and death rate. More than 6,000 specialists are affiliated with the foundation through its honorary fellows program. The foundation has created teaching materials for distribution to schools, community education seminars, and consumer awareness programs in pharmacies and department stores.

smokeless tobacco   There are two types of smokeless tobacco: snuff and chewing tobacco. Smokeless tobacco users have a high risk of ORAL CANCER, THROAT CANCER, and cancers of the larynx and esophagus. (Oral cancer can include cancer of the lip, tongue, cheeks, gums, and the floor and roof of the mouth.) People who use snuff for a long time have a much greater risk for cancer of the cheek and gum than people who do not use tobacco. The possible increased risk for other types of cancer from smokeless tobacco is being studied.

Snuff is finely ground tobacco packaged dry, moist, or in pouches resembling tea bags. The user places a pinch between the cheek and gum. Inhaling dry snuff through the nose is more common in European countries than in the United States.

Chewing tobacco is available in loose leaf, plug, or twist forms; the user puts a wad inside the cheek. Smokeless tobacco is sometimes called "spit" or "spitting tobacco" because people spit out the tobacco juices and saliva that build up in the mouth.

Chewing tobacco and snuff contain 28 carcinogens, including the tobacco-specific nitrosamines (TSNAs) formed during the curing, fermenting, and aging process. TSNAs have been detected in smokeless tobacco at levels 100 times higher than the levels of other nitrosamines allowed in bacon, beer, and other foods. Other cancer-causing substances in smokeless tobacco include formaldehyde, acetaldehyde, crotonaldehyde, hydrazine, arsenic, nickel, cadmium, benzopyrene, and polonium (that gives off radiation).

Nicotine is also found in smokeless tobacco at levels two to three times higher than the amount found in cigarette tobacco. People who consume eight to 10 dips or chews a day receive the same amount of nicotine as those who smoke 30 to 40 cigarettes a day. Nicotine is absorbed more slowly from smokeless tobacco than from cigarettes, but more nicotine per dose is absorbed from snuff and chewing tobacco than from cigarettes—and the nicotine stays in the bloodstream for a longer time.

Because of the addictive properties and documented health risks associated with smokeless tobacco, it should not be used for the purpose of quitting cigarette smoking. Smokeless tobacco can cause addiction to nicotine, oral leukoplakia (white mouth lesions that can become cancerous), gum disease, gum recession, loss of bone in the jaw, tooth decay, tooth loss, tooth abrasion, yellowing of teeth, chronic bad breath, high blood pressure, and increased risk for heart disease.

The use of moist snuff and other types of smokeless tobacco almost tripled from 1972 through 1991 in the United States.

smoking   The single greatest cause or correlate of cancer is smoking. The linkage between smoking and cancer has existed since 1950 and has been confirmed by hundreds of studies. Smoking greatly increases LUNG CANCER risk, it is directly related to MOUTH CANCER and ESOPHAGEAL CANCER, and has been shown to increase risk for cancers of the pancreas, stomach, and bladder. Smoking has also been associated with LEUKEMIA and cancers of the cervix, liver, breast, and colon. Chewing tobacco, far from being a safe alternative, is associated with an increased risk of cancers of the mouth and throat. Smoking pipes or cigars has been shown to cause cancer of the mouth, throat, and lungs. Tobacco use accompanied by heavy alcohol consumption has been identified as an important risk factor for head, neck, and esophageal cancer.

In addition to its direct cancer-causing effects, cigarette smoking also enhances the cancer-causing abilities of other factors. For example, people who work with ASBESTOS are five times as likely to develop lung cancer as those who do not work with asbestos, but those who work with asbestos and smoke have a risk 90 times greater than those who are not exposed to asbestos and do not smoke.

Smoking is estimated to be a factor in about 30 percent of all cancer deaths in the United States, and about 85 percent of lung cancer deaths. Moreover, the more extensive the exposure to cigarette smoke, the greater the risk of developing cancer, although there is no safe dose for tobacco exposure. The age at which smoking began, how long smoking has continued, and the number of cigarettes smoked per day all play a part in determining the specific risk for an individual.

Women who as teenagers started smoking regularly within five years of their first menstrual period were 70 percent more likely to develop breast cancer before age 50 than nonsmokers, according to a recent Canadian study. Even if they quit in their early 20s, the damage may already have been done. Although there is never a good time to start smoking, for women, the five years after they have their first menstrual period is the most dangerous time. The theory is that during puberty, breast cells are developing so rapidly that they are more susceptible to damage caused by the carcinogens in tobacco smoke.

Smokers Who Quit

The only preventive measure is not to smoke. A smoker's risk of developing cancer decreases dramatically immediately after quitting and continues to decrease every year thereafter, although that drop varies from disease to disease. (It can take up to 20 or 25 years after a person stops smoking, for example, before the risk of lung cancer equals the risk of a nonsmoker.) Data suggest that quitting smoking may halt the early stages of cancer, although it may have little effect on the late stages of cancer. How much preventive effect a person gets from quitting depends on the duration and quantity of smoking.

How to Quit

Nicotine is one of the most addictive substances there is, and it can be difficult to quit the habit without help. Prescription and over-the-counter medications and skin patches can help smokers quit. Others find that hypnosis and other types of behavioral therapy are also effective.

Social Security Disability Insurance (SSDI)   A government social program that pays benefits to a person who is "insured," meaning the person worked long enough and paid Social Security taxes. If a person expects to be disabled for at least six months, he or she may be eligible for SSDI. Often the government accepts as a disability cancer that has spread (such as metastatic breast cancer).

Society of Gynecologic Oncology   A nonprofit international organization made up of obstetricians and gynecologists specializing in gynecologic ONCOLOGY. Its purpose is to improve the care of women with gynecologic cancer, to raise standards of practice in gynecologic oncology, and to encourage ongoing research. For contact information, see Appendix I.

soy products   Foods (such as tofu and miso) that contain proteins and substances called ISOFLAVONES that may have health benefits, including relief from symptoms of menopause and reduced risk of heart disease and bone loss. In addition, soy isoflavones may help prevent some kinds of cancer; scientists are currently studying the effect of soy on BREAST CANCER, PROSTATE CANCER, and COLORECTAL CANCER.

Isoflavones are a type of PHYTOESTROGEN, which is a naturally occurring plant estrogen that may offer some of the benefits of ESTROGEN in women without increasing the risk of breast cancer.

Studies have not been done on the effects of soy on a healthy human prostate, but men with prostate cancer are routinely advised to eat soy foods because soy isoflavones have been shown to reduce the growth of prostate cancer cells in test tubes.

However, the effects of soy on cancer, especially on cancer fueled by estrogen, are not fully understood. Current advice for eating soy ranges from eating none to eating soy foods (not soy pills and powder) several times a week as a low-fat replacement for animal protein. Patients should seek medical advice regarding soy for their individual needs. Soy can be obtained by eating

- tofu (a curd made from cooked, pureed soybeans)
- miso (a mixture of fermented soybean paste and a grain such as rice or barley)
- dried soybeans
- roasted soybeans or nuts (soybeans that are soaked in water and baked)
- edamame and natto (steamed whole green beans, and fermented, cooked whole beans)
- tempeh (a combination of whole, cooked soybeans and grains cultured with an edible mold)
- soy milk (the liquid expressed from cooked, pureed soybeans)

The ability of the body to use the nutrients in soy foods varies with the food and how it was made. In general, soy that has been processed the least (such as tofu, tempeh, and mature, green, and roasted soybeans) contains the most protein and naturally occurring isoflavones. Soy germ is the source highest in isoflavones.

spermatocytoma   Also called "spermatocytic seminoma," this is a unique type of benign tumor, distinct from other GERM CELL CANCERS, that occurs only in men and never outside the gonads. It is not found in conjunction with any other germ cell tumor and occurs almost exclusively in men over the age of 50. It represents only 2 to 3 percent of all testicular tumors; in 10 percent of patients it occurs in both testicles. (See also TESTICULAR CANCER.)

spinal cord tumor   A benign or cancerous growth in the spinal cord, between the membranes covering the spinal cord, or in the spinal canal. A tumor in this location can compress the spinal cord or its nerve roots, so even a noncancerous growth can be disabling unless properly treated.

The spinal cord contains bundles of nerves that carry messages between the brain and the body. Because the spinal cord is rigidly encased in bone, any tumor that grows on or near it can compress the nerves and interfere in this communication. Because the spinal cord is such a small structure, tumors within it usually cause symptoms involving both sides of the body. This distinguishes them from BRAIN TUMORS, which usually cause symptoms only on one side of the body. Also, most spinal cord tumors appear below the neck after nerves to the arms have branched off the spinal cord, so that only leg function is affected.

About 10,000 Americans develop spinal cord tumors each year, and about 40 percent of these are cancerous. Like brain tumors, spinal cord growths are rare, and newly formed tumors that begin within the spinal cord are unusual, especially among children and the elderly. More typically, tumors originate elsewhere in the body and move through the bloodstream to the spinal cord. Scientists do not know what causes these tumors, although the noncancerous growths may be hereditary or present since birth.

Symptoms
A tumor in the top of the spinal column can cause pain radiating from the arms or neck; a tumor in

the lower spine may cause leg or back pain. If there are several tumors in different areas of the spinal cord at the same time, they may cause symptoms in a variety of spots on the body. When the tumor presses on the spinal cord, it causes symptoms including:

- back pain
- severe or burning pain in other parts of the body
- numbness or cold
- progressive loss of muscle strength or sensation in the legs
- loss of bladder or bowel control

Diagnosis

A tumor that compresses the spinal cord is a medical emergency, but prompt intervention may prevent paralysis. If a neurological exam and review of symptoms suggest a spinal cord tumor, the doctor may order additional tests, such as an MRI or CT scan, blood and spinal fluid studies, biopsy, bone scan, or myelography (an X-ray of the spinal cord highlighted by a contrast dye).

Treatment

Surgery is usually the first step in treating benign and malignant tumors outside the spinal cord, but tumors inside the spinal cord may not be able to be completely removed with surgery. In this case, a lamenectomy (a surgical procedure to relieve pressure on the cord) with radiation and chemotherapy treatments may be effective. Treatment also may include pain relievers and cortisone drugs to lessen swelling around the tumor and ease pressure on the spinal cord.

Early diagnosis and treatment may be effective, but long-term survival also depends on the tumor's type, location, and size. Surgery to remove the bone around the cord can ease pressure on the spinal nerves and nerve pathways (lamenectomy), which will usually ease pain and other symptoms; however, it may make walking more difficult. Physical therapy and rehabilitation may help.

Prevention

Since spinal cord tumors usually are the result of a cancer that has first appeared elsewhere in the body, early detection of cancer in other organs may prevent spinal cord tumors. Changes in unhealthy lifestyles (such as quitting SMOKING) can lower the risk of the development of other types of cancer, which may help.

squamous cell carcinoma of the skin   The second most common type of SKIN CANCER (after BASAL CELL CARCINOMA), which affects more than 100,000 Americans each year. The number of cases has risen dramatically since the 1980s, increasing at a rate of about 10 percent a year. At especially high risk of developing squamous cell cancer are people with weakened immune systems, including people who are HIV-positive, organ transplant recipients, or those who take immune-suppressing drugs. Squamous cell carcinoma is also the cell type found in most HEAD AND NECK CANCER, ESOPHAGEAL CANCER, and ANAL CANCER.

This type of cancer begins in the squamous cells that make up most of the upper layer of skin. Squamous cell cancers may be found on all areas of the body, including the mucous membranes, but they are most often found on areas exposed to the Sun. Although squamous cell carcinomas start in the top layer of skin, they can eventually spread to underlying tissues if untreated. Rarely, they spread to distant tissues and organs, which can be fatal. Squamous cell carcinomas that spread most often begin from chronic inflammatory skin conditions or on the mucous membranes, lips, ears, scrotum, or vulva.

Causes

Chronic exposure to sunlight causes most cases of squamous cell cancer, which is why tumors are usually found on areas of the body that are exposed to sunlight. The rim of the ear and the lower lip are particularly prone to this type of cancer.

Squamous cell cancers also may appear on skin that has been injured by burns, scars, long-standing sores, exposure to X-rays, or chemicals (such as arsenic and petroleum by-products). In addition, chronic skin inflammation or medical conditions that suppress the immune system for long periods of time may encourage squamous cell carcinoma. Sometimes, however, squamous cell carcinoma begins spontaneously on what seems to be normal, healthy skin. Some researchers believe this type of cancer may be hereditary.

Anyone with a long history of sun exposure can develop squamous cell cancer, but those with fair skin, light hair, and blue, green, or gray eyes are at highest risk. Dark-skinned people are far less likely to develop any form of skin cancer, but more than two-thirds of skin cancers in African Americans are squamous cell carcinomas, found most often on sites where the skin has been inflamed or burned.

Some skin conditions, such as ACTINIC KERATOSIS, actinic cheilitis, leukoplakia, and BOWEN'S DISEASE, are associated with eventual development of squamous cell carcinoma. These precursor conditions, if properly treated, can be prevented from developing into a squamous cell carcinoma.

Symptoms

Squamous cell carcinomas may feature a small, flat, persistent, scaly red patch with irregular borders that sometimes crust or bleed, an elevated growth with a central depression that sometimes bleeds, a wartlike crusting growth that may bleed, or an open, persistent sore that bleeds and crusts.

Diagnosis

The diagnosis is confirmed with a skin examination and biopsy. The doctor may shave away only a small piece of abnormal skin or may remove the entire abnormal area and send it to the lab for examination. In the lab a pathologist will assign a grade or stage for the cancer, on a scale from 1 to 4, based on the number and appearance of abnormal cells, and how deeply they have invaded the skin. In general, the higher the grade or stage of a squamous cell carcinoma, the greater are its chances for spreading. If the lab reports a high risk that the cancer may spread, further tests may be used to check for cancer spread.

Treatment

If tumor cells are found, the doctor will outline possible treatment based on type, size, and location of the tumor and on the patient's age and health. It is usually performed on an outpatient basis. Local anesthetics are used to prevent pain during the procedure. Once treatment is completed, follow-up skin examinations are required every three months for a few years, then every six months thereafter.

Excision The most common way to remove a skin cancer is by excising the entire growth together with an additional border of normal skin as a safety margin. The site is then stitched closed, and the tissue is sent to the lab to determine if all malignant cells have been removed.

Electrosurgery A doctor may scrape the tumor from the skin with a curette while using an electric needle to burn a safety margin of normal skin around the tumor at the base of the scraped area. This technique is repeated several times to make sure the tumor has been completely removed.

Cryosurgery With CRYOSURGERY, the doctor does not cut the growth but instead freezes the lesion by applying liquid nitrogen with a special spray; this method does not require anesthesia and produces no bleeding. It is easy to administer and is the treatment of choice for those who have bleeding disorders or who are intolerant to anesthesia. After this treatment, patients experience redness, swelling, blistering, and crusting.

Lasers In laser surgery a beam of light is focused onto the lesion, either to remove it or destroy it by vaporization. The major advantage of this technique is that it seals blood vessels as it cuts.

Radiation In radiation therapy, X-rays are directed at the malignant cells. Treatments are given several times a week for a few weeks. Radiation therapy is most often used with older patients or with those in poor health, because it may be less traumatic.

Mohs' surgery Using microscopically controlled surgery, the doctor removes successive thin layers of the malignant tumor, checking each layer thoroughly under a microscope. This is repeated until the tissue is free of tumor. This technique saves the most healthy tissue and has the highest cure rate. It is often used for tumors that have recurred, for large tumors, or for areas where recurrences are most common (the nose, ears, and around the eyes).

Other treatments These include topical 5-fluorouracil, an anticancer drug applied directly to the skin, or interferon alfa injected directly into the tumor.

Prognosis

When removed early, squamous cell carcinomas are easily treated, but the larger the growth, the more extensive the treatment must be. While squamous cell carcinoma does not spread to vital organs very often, if it does, it can be fatal. Typically, an untreated squamous cell carcinoma that has reached a diameter of more than 2 cm (about three-quarters of an inch) is three times more likely to spread than a smaller cancer.

If a patient is diagnosed with one squamous cell carcinoma, there is also a greater chance of developing other squamous cell carcinomas in the future. Having had a BASAL CELL CARCINOMA also makes it more likely that a squamous cell cancer will develop. No matter how carefully a tumor is removed, another can develop in the same place, usually within the first two years of treatment. It is therefore important to examine the surgical site periodically. If the cancer recurs, the doctor may recommend a different type of treatment the second time.

Prevention

Because squamous cell cancer is caused by unprotected exposure to sunlight, protecting skin from the Sun can help prevent these tumors. This includes:

• using sunscreen with an SPF of 15 or above, with a broad spectrum of protection against both ultraviolet-A and ultraviolet-B rays

• avoiding sun exposure during peak intensity (in most parts of the United States, from about 10 A.M. to 3 P.M.)

• using sunglasses with ultraviolet light protection

• wearing long pants, a shirt with long sleeves, and a hat with a wide brim

• limiting sun exposure when taking certain drugs, including some antibiotics and certain drugs used to treat psychiatric illness, high blood pressure, heart failure, acne, or allergies

• limiting sun exposure when using nonprescription skin-care products containing alpha hydroxy acids, which can make skin more vulnerable to damage from sunlight.

Skin self-examinations should be performed every one to two months, using a mirror to check for abnormalities on less visible areas (back, shoulders, upper arms, buttocks, and the soles of the feet).

staging   A medical attempt to find out whether a patient's cancer has spread and, if so, to what parts of the body. A doctor stages cancer by studying information obtained during surgery, X-rays and other imaging procedures, and lab tests. Knowing the stage of the disease helps the doctor plan treatment.

Typically, cancer stages are numbered from I through IV; for some types of cancer, scientists have subdivided those Roman numerals into "a" and "b" subcategories. In general, the higher the stage, the more extensive the disease and the farther the spread.

Starbright Foundation   A nonprofit foundation dedicated to the development of projects that help seriously ill children combat the medical and emotional challenges they face. Starbright projects address a child's pain, fear, loneliness, and depression, which can be as damaging as the sickness itself. Through the efforts of Starbright Chairmen Steven Spielberg and General H. Norman Schwarzkopf, leaders in technology, medicine, and entertainment work together to ensure that no child need sacrifice quality of life to an illness. The organization supports research and provides a number of special projects, such as:

• *Starbright World,* a private online community connecting more than 30,000 children with chronic illness so they can chat, e-mail, read bulletin boards, find friends, learn about health-care conditions, surf Web sites and play games. Starbright World can be accessed by registered users from hundreds of homes and 97 children's hospitals across North America.

• *Starbright Hospital Pals,* an intervention for health-care professionals that uses the well-known purple dinosaur Barney to provide companionship and a sense of support for preschoolers undergoing radiation for cancer. For radiation to be effectively administered, a child must be alone in a treatment room and remain perfectly still for long periods of time. In many cases, anesthesia is necessary in order for a child to remain still; although anesthesia is safe, receiving it on a daily basis is not healthy. The program is designed to educate children about radiation, lessen anxiety, provide support, and decrease the need for anesthesia for children undergoing radiation therapy. Prior to treatment, children sit with an animated Barney doll and watch a video that helps them understand what to expect during radiation therapy. Barney interacts in real time with the child and video, and reinforces important topics. During treatment, Barney tells stories to the children and offers words of encouragement to help them remain still and calm throughout the procedure. Starbright Hospital Pals is offered free of charge to radiation therapy programs that provide services for children.

- *Starbright Videos with Attitude,* in which teens and preteens discuss creative strategies and solutions for coping with the challenges of serious medical conditions. These programs are designed for children aged 10 to 18 and health-care professionals who work with adolescents.

For contact information, see Appendix I.

statistics in cancer   Cancer is second only to heart disease as the leading cause of death in the United States. Each year about 1.3 million new cases of cancer are diagnosed in this country, and about 550,000 Americans will die of this disease. From birth to death, men have a 43 percent chance of developing some form of cancer (including non-fatal cancers such as SKIN CANCER), and women have a 38 percent chance. However, in the past few decades, new cancer cases and cancer death rates are decreasing overall. Today more than 60 percent of those diagnosed with cancer will not die of the disease within five years—which means they are living longer than ever before.

The usefulness of cancer statistics depends on how they are interpreted and used. While cancer statistics are often cited in medical stories, and they can be helpful for a broad perspective, they are less helpful when it comes to understanding one person's specific outlook. For example, most people have heard that a woman's lifetime risk of developing BREAST CANCER is one in eight. These are frightening odds for women who misinterpret that statistic to mean that at any time, at any moment, they have a one in eight chance of having breast cancer. In fact, the *actual* chance of developing

breast cancer changes throughout a woman's life, so that a 20-year-old woman has a *current* risk of only one in 2,500 of developing the disease within the next 10 years; a 50-year-old woman has a current risk of about one in 39. Moreover, heredity, ethnicity, reproductive history, lifestyle, and other risk factors all contribute to a person's overall cancer risk.

Most Common Types of Cancer

LUNG CANCER is the leading cause of cancer-related death in both men and women. Although PROSTATE CANCER and breast cancer occur more commonly than lung cancer, early detection and treatment have led to lower death rates. However, death rates for prostate cancer are still high in African-American men. African-American men are two to three times more likely to die of prostate cancer than are white men. According to the AMERICAN CANCER SOCIETY, the most common types of cancer in the United States are

- BASAL CELL CARCINOMA and squamous cell carcinoma: 1 million new cases a year
- prostate cancer: 220,900 new cases a year, with 28,900 yearly deaths
- breast cancer (women and men): 212,600 new cases a year, with 40,200 yearly deaths
- lung cancer: 171,900 cases a year, with 157,200 yearly deaths
- COLORECTAL CANCER: 147,500 cases a year, with 57,100 yearly deaths

Incidence

"Incidence" is the number of new cases of cancer developed in a population group for a specific period of time—usually one year. For example, the total 2001 incidence of TESTICULAR CANCER in the United States was about 7,200 men. Incidence rate is the number of new cases per population segment. The incidence rate usually is expressed in terms of the number of cases per 100,000 people. For example, the *incidence rate* for testicular cancer in the United States is about four new cases per 100,000 men.

Prevalence

"Prevalence" refers to the total number of people with cancer or with a particular risk factor for cancer at a particular moment in time in the entire population. For large groups of people, prevalence is estimated by collecting information from a smaller subset of people and then extrapolating that information to the general population.

For example, by collecting DNA information from breast cancer patients, scientists have estimated that the prevalence of the *BRCA-1* breast cancer susceptibility gene in the total population is between 0.04 percent and 0.2 percent meaning that many fewer women than 1 percent of the total population have this.

Morbidity/Mortality

"Morbidity" is a term that means "a state of illness." For instance, experts may comment that smoking is a major cause of morbidity in the United States. "Mortality" pertains to death. The "mortality rate" is the number of people in a population group who die of cancer within a set period of time (usually one year). A cancer mortality rate usually is expressed in terms of deaths per 100,000 people. For example, the mortality rate for STOMACH CANCER in the United States in 1930 was 28 (28 deaths per 100,000 people) but by 1992 had dropped to 4 (4 deaths for every 100,000).

Prognosis

"Prognosis" is the prediction of the outcome of a disease, usually including the chances for recovery. While physicians may base a prognosis on statistical precedents, each patient's prognosis is affected by many factors, including the patient's age and general health, the type and stage of cancer, and the effectiveness of the particular treatment used. Therefore, while a prognosis may help explain the seriousness of a disorder or guide treatment decisions, it cannot be used to predict disease outcomes for an individual.

Survival Rate

"Survival rate" refers to the number of people who develop cancer and survive over a period of time. Scientists commonly use five-year survival as the standard statistical basis for defining when a cancer has been successfully treated.

The five-year survival rate includes anyone who is living five years after a cancer diagnosis, including those who are cured, those in remission, and those who still have cancer and are undergoing treatment. For example, when colorectal cancers are detected early, the five-year survival rate is 92 percent, meaning that 92 percent of all colorectal cancer patients live at least five years after diagnosis if the cancer is detected early.

The overall five-year survival rate measures everyone who has ever been diagnosed with a particular cancer equally, which may lead to distorted statistics. For example, a 90-year-old man and a 30-year-old man who have the same cancer will be grouped together. The 90-year-old may die of other causes within the five-year period due to normal life expectancy, and this can skew the data. A more statistically accurate view of survival is the relative five-year survival rate, which compares a cancer patient's survival rate with the survival rate of the general population, taking into account differences in age, gender, race, and other factors. In this case, the 30-year-old and the 90-year-old would be treated as statistically different.

Risk

"Risk" refers to the chance that an individual will contract a disease. "High risk" is a term used when the chance of developing cancer is higher than the chance for the general population. For example, people who smoke have a high risk of developing lung cancer compared with people who do not smoke.

Risk factor is anything that has been identified as increasing a person's chance of getting a disease. It can be controllable or uncontrollable, personal or environmental. For example, risk factors for developing colon cancer include having a hereditary predisposition to the disease (uncontrollable) and eating a high-fat diet (controllable). Relative risk is a measure of how much a particular factor increases the risk for a specific cancer. For example, the risk for developing ovarian cancer increases by 300 percent for a woman with a close-family history of the disease compared with a woman without a family history. In this example, the relative risk of developing ovarian cancer is three for those with a family history, meaning they have three times the risk.

Attributable risk is a measure of how much of the total incidence of disease is caused by a particular risk factor. For example, even though the relative risk of developing breast cancer for a woman with the *BRCA-1* gene is high, most cases of breast cancer are not caused by the *BRCA-1* gene since the prevalence of the *BRCA-1* gene is low.

Lifetime risk is the probability of developing or dying of cancer during one's lifetime. A person has a lifetime risk of two in five of developing cancer, meaning that for every five people in the population, two eventually will develop cancer. The lifetime risk of dying of cancer is one in five. (See also individual cancers for more information on specific cancer statistics.)

stem cells A type of cell that is able to produce other cells when it divides. Usually stem cells refer to blood cells. Most stem cells are found in the bone marrow, but some stem cells, called peripheral blood stem cells, can be found in the bloodstream. Umbilical cord blood also contains stem cells. Stem cells can divide to form more stem cells, or they can mature into white blood cells, red blood cells, or platelets.

Stem Cell Transplant

High-dose CHEMOTHERAPY can severely damage or destroy a patient's BONE MARROW so that the patient is no longer able to produce needed blood cells. Destroying the marrow may be a part of treatment for diseases that affect the bone marrow (such as LEUKEMIA) or, as in the case of TESTICULAR CANCER, it may simply be a side effect of treatment.

A stem cell transplant allows stem cells that were damaged by treatment to be replaced with healthy stem cells that can produce the blood cells the patient needs. A stem cell transplant allows a patient with leukemia to be treated with high doses of drugs, radiation, or both. The high doses destroy both leukemia cells and normal blood cells in the bone marrow. Later the patient can be given healthy stem cells, and new blood cells develop from these transplanted cells.

Stem cells may come from the patient (autologous transplant) or from a donor (allogeneic transplant). In an autologous stem cell transplantation, the patient's own stem cells are removed, and the cells treated to kill any leukemia cells. The stem cells are then frozen and stored. After the patient receives high-dose chemotherapy or radiation therapy, the stored stem cells are thawed and returned to the patient. In an allogeneic stem cell transplantation, the patient is given healthy stem cells from a donor (such as a brother, sister, or parent), although sometimes the stem cells come from an unrelated donor. Doctors use blood tests (HLA testing) to be sure the donor's cells match the patient's cells. In a syngeneic stem cell transplantation, the patient is given stem cells from the patient's healthy identical twin.

Types of Stem Cell Transplants

There are several types of stem cell transplantation:

- *Bone marrow transplantation.* The stem cells come from bone marrow.

- *Peripheral stem cell transplantation.* The stem cells come from peripheral blood.

- *Umbilical cord blood transplantation.* For a child with no donor, the doctor may use stem cells from the blood of an umbilical cord from a newborn baby. Sometimes umbilical cord blood is frozen for later use.

stereotactic radiosurgery This new technique focuses high doses of radiation at a tumor while minimizing radiation delivered to normal tissue. After the location of the tumor is precisely measured by CT or MRI scans, radiation beams are aimed from several directions to meet at the tumor. Photon beams from a linear accelerator or X-rays from cobalt-60 are often used, although proton beams can also be used. This treatment may be useful when tumors are in locations where conventional surgery would damage essential tissues or when the patient's condition does not permit conventional surgery.

stomach cancer Cancer of the stomach (also known as "gastric cancer") affects 24,000 Americans every year. It is more common among men, with incidence peaking between age 50 and 59. Nearly 13,000 Americans die of stomach cancer each year, making it the seventh leading cause of cancer deaths in the United States.

Only about a fourth as common today in the United States as it was just 70 years ago, the lower rate is probably due to changes in diet and advances in food refrigeration. Stomach cancer incidence and mortality rates have been declining for several decades in most areas of the world. Nevertheless, worldwide, stomach cancer was the most common form of cancer in the 1970s and early 1980s. Stomach cancer incidence shows substantial variation internationally. Rates are highest in Japan and eastern Asia and are also high in eastern Europe and parts of Latin America. Incidence is generally lower in western Europe and the United States.

Stomach cancer is still a significant problem because it is hard to diagnose in its early stages when successful treatment is possible. If it is detected in its earliest stages, the five-year survival rate is 90 percent. Unfortunately, most Americans are not diagnosed until stomach cancer is more advanced. For the most advanced stage of stomach cancer, the five-year survival rate is only 3 percent.

Stomach cancer can develop in any part of the stomach and may spread throughout the stomach and to other organs. It may grow along the stomach wall into the esophagus or small intestine, and it also may extend through the stomach wall and spread to nearby LYMPH NODES and to organs such as the liver, pancreas, and colon. Stomach cancer also may spread to distant organs, such as the lungs, the lymph nodes above the collarbone, and the ovaries.

Types of Stomach Cancer

The most common type of stomach cancer is gastric ADENOCARCINOMA (cancer of the glandular tissue in the stomach). Other, rarer forms of stomach cancer include non-Hodgkin's LYMPHOMA (cancer involving the lymphatic system) and SARCOMA (cancer of the connective tissue, such as muscle, fat, or blood vessels).

Cause

At this time, doctors do not know what causes stomach cancer, although they have been able to pinpoint some risk factors. These risk factors include the following.

Age   Stomach cancer is found most often in people over age 55, and it usually occurs between ages 50 and 70. It is rare before age 40.

Gender   Stomach cancer affects men twice as often as women.

Race   Stomach cancer is more common in African Americans than in Caucasians. It occurs often among Koreans, Vietnamese, Japanese, Alaska Natives, and Hawaiians. Those groups at

intermediate risk include Hispanic, Chinese, and African American populations. Filipinos and non-Hispanic Caucasians have substantially lower incidence than the other groups.

Although stomach cancer is much more common in some countries, such as Japan, Korea, parts of Eastern Europe, and Latin America, people of Japanese ancestry who live in the United States have a much lower incidence of stomach cancer, suggesting environmental influences such as diet.

Diet   People in countries with high rates of stomach cancer typically have diets filled with foods that are preserved by drying, smoking, salting, or pickling. Food preserved in these ways has a higher amount of nitrates and nitrites, which may play a role in the development of stomach cancer. On the other hand, fresh foods (especially fresh fruits and vegetables and properly frozen or refrigerated fresh foods) may protect against this disease. Studies have suggested that eating foods that contain BETA-CAROTENE and vitamin C may decrease the risk of gastric cancer.

Helicobacter pylori   Some studies suggest that the bacterium *Helicobacter pylori,* which may cause stomach inflammation and ulcers, may be an important risk factor for this disease. According to the World Health Organization, at least 335,000 out of 800,000 new cases of gastric cancer annually can be attributed to *H. pylori* infection. Although most people with *H. pylori* never develop stomach cancer, people with *H. pylori* infection nevertheless have a three to eight times greater risk of developing gastric cancer than those not infected.

Toxins   Exposure to certain dusts and fumes in the workplace has been linked to a higher than average risk of stomach cancer.

Smoking/alcohol   Some scientists believe SMOKING or ALCOHOL abuse may increase stomach cancer risk. The irritation caused by these habits particularly increases the risk of cancer of the upper part of the stomach, the portion closest to the esophagus.

Previous stomach surgery   Surgery here may result in higher levels of nitrite-producing bacteria and bile in the stomach, which increases the risk for stomach cancer.

Genetics   Stomach cancers are two to four times more common for immediate family members of people who have had the disease. However, more than 90 percent of people with stomach cancer have no family members with stomach cancer.

Preexisting conditions People who already have chronic gastritis, intestinal metaplasia, pernicious ANEMIA, or GASTRIC POLYPS may have a higher-than-average risk of developing stomach cancer.

Symptoms

Stomach cancer can be hard to diagnose early because there are often no symptoms in the initial stages. In many cases, the cancer has spread before it is found. When symptoms do occur, they are often so vague that the person ignores them.

Microscopic bleeding, which can be detected only by examining the stool for blood, is the most common early sign of both malignant and benign stomach tumors. Stomach cancer can cause the following:

- heartburn or indigestion
- abdominal discomfort or pain
- nausea and vomiting after meals
- diarrhea or constipation
- stomach bloating after meals
- appetite loss
- weakness
- fatigue
- blood in vomit or stool
- persistent low fever

Any of these symptoms may be caused by cancer or by other, less serious health problems, such as a stomach virus. People who have any of these symptoms should see a gastroenterologist (a doctor who specializes in diagnosing and treating digestive problems).

Diagnosis

To find the cause of symptoms, the doctor asks about the patient's medical history, does a physical exam, and may order laboratory studies. The patient may also have one or all of the following exams:

- *Fecal occult blood test.* A test for hidden (occult) blood in the stool, done by placing a small

amount of stool on a plastic slide or on special paper and having it tested in a lab. Since both noncancerous and malignant conditions may cause bleeding, having blood in the stool does not necessarily mean that a person has cancer.

- *Upper GI series.* X-rays of the esophagus and stomach (the upper gastrointestinal tract) taken after the patient drinks a barium solution (sometimes called a barium swallow). The barium outlines the stomach on the X-rays, helping the doctor find tumors or other abnormal areas. During the test, the doctor may pump air into the stomach to make small tumors easier to see.

- *Endoscopy.* An exam of the esophagus and stomach using a thin, lighted tube called a gastroscope, which is passed through the mouth and esophagus to the stomach. The patient's throat is first sprayed with a local anesthetic to reduce discomfort and gagging. Through the gastroscope, the doctor can look directly at the inside of the stomach. If an abnormal area is found, the doctor can remove some tissue through the gastroscope. Another doctor, a pathologist, examines the tissue under a microscope to check for cancer cells. This procedure—removing tissue and examining it under a microscope—is called a biopsy. A biopsy is the only sure way to know whether cancer cells are present.

Staging

If there are cancer cells in the tissue sample, it is important to know the stage of the disease. Knowing whether and how far the cancer has spread helps determine treatment and prognosis. Because stomach cancer can spread to the liver, the pancreas, and other organs near the stomach as well as to the lungs, the doctor may order scans or other tests to check these areas. Staging may not be complete until after surgery, when the nearby lymph nodes and abdominal tissue samples are removed.

The system most often used to stage stomach cancer in the United States is the American Joint Commission on Cancer TNM system. T stands for the "tumor" itself (a numeral following indicates how far it has spread within the stomach and into nearby organs), N stands for spread to lymph "nodes," and M refers to "metastasis" to distant organs.

T Stages of Stomach Cancer

The stomach is made of five layers. The innermost layer is the mucosa, where stomach acid and digestive enzymes are produced. Next is a supporting layer called the submucosa, which is surrounded by the muscularis, a layer of muscle that moves and mixes the stomach contents. The next two layers are the subserosa and the outermost serosa, which act as wrapping layers for the stomach.

Tis (carcinoma in situ): Cancer cells are limited to the stomach lining (mucosa) and have not invaded deeper layers of the stomach

T1: Tumor invades underneath the mucosa, into the submucosa.

T2a: Tumor invades the muscle layer below the mucosa and lamina propria (the thin layer of connective tissue beneath the epithelium of an organ)

T2b: Tumor invades subserosa (the layer between the muscle layer and the serosa).

T3: Tumor perforates the serosa but does not invade any adjacent organ.

T4: Tumor perforates the serosa and invades an adjacent organ or other structures such as major blood vessels.

N Stages of Stomach Cancer

N0: No spread to nearby (regional) lymph nodes.

N1: The cancer has spread to one to six nearby lymph nodes.

N2: The cancer has spread to seven to 15 nearby lymph nodes.

N3: The cancer has spread to more than 15 nearby lymph nodes.

M Stages of Stomach Cancer

M0: No distant spread

M1: Spread of the cancer to tissues or organs far away from the stomach

TNM Stage Grouping

After the T, N, and M stages of the patient's stomach cancer have been determined, this information is combined and then expressed as a stage, using Roman numerals I through IV. The process of assigning a stage number based on TNM stages is called stage grouping.

Stage 0—Tis, N0, M0: This is cancer in its earliest stage. It has not grown beyond the layer of cells that line the stomach (epithelium). This stage is also known as carcinoma in situ, which means the cancer cells are in the innermost layer, where they started. The five-year survival rate is 89 percent.

Stage IA—T1, N0, M0: The cancer has grown under the epithelium into the next layers (the lamina propria or the submucosa). However, it has not grown into the main muscle layer of the stomach (the muscularis), nor has it spread to any lymph nodes or anywhere else. The five-year survival rate for this stage is 78 percent.

Stage IB—T1, N1, M0 or T2a/b, N0, M0: Two combinations of T and N features are assigned to this stage. In the first combination, the cancer has grown under the epithelium into submucosa but it has not grown into the muscularis, the main muscle layer of the stomach. It has spread to as many as six lymph nodes near the stomach, but not to any other tissues or organs. In the second combination the cancer has grown into the main muscle layer of the stomach wall, the muscularis, and may have grown into the subserosa (outermost layer of the stomach wall). It has not spread to any other tissues or organs and has not spread to any lymph nodes. Five-year survival rate is 58 percent.

Stage II—T1, N2, M0 or T2a/b, N1, M0 or T3, N0, M0: Three combinations of T and N features are assigned to this stage, with a five-year survival rate of 34 percent:

- The cancer has grown under the epithelium into the submucosa, but it as not grown into the muscular layer; however, it has spread to between seven and 15 lymph nodes near the stomach.

- The cancer has grown into the muscular layer and may have grown into the subserosa (outermost layer of the stomach wall) but has not spread to any nearby tissues or organs; however, it has spread to no more than six lymph nodes near the stomach.

- The cancer has grown through all the layers to the outside of the stomach but has not spread to any nearby tissues or organs, and it has not spread to any lymph nodes.

Stage IIIA—T2a/b, N2, M0 or T3, N1, M0 or T4, N0, M0: Three combinations of T and N features are assigned to this stage. The five-year survival rate is 20 percent:

- The cancer has grown into the muscular layer and may have spread into the subserosa. It has not spread to any nearby tissues or organs, but it has spread to between seven and 15 lymph nodes near the stomach.
- The cancer has grown completely through the muscular layer and the subserosa to the outside of the stomach. It has not spread to any nearby tissues or organs, but it has spread to between one and six lymph nodes near the stomach.
- The cancer has grown completely through the stomach wall into other nearby organs such as the spleen, liver, intestines, kidneys, or pancreas, but it has not spread to any lymph nodes.

Stage IIIB—T3, N2, MO: The cancer has grown completely through the muscular layer and the subserosa. It has not spread to any nearby tissues or organs, but it has spread to between seven and 15 lymph nodes near the stomach. The five-year survival rate is 8 percent.

Stage IV—T4, N1-3, M0 or T1-3, N3, M0, or AnyT or N, M1:

- This is the most advanced stage of the cancer. The cancer has grown completely through the stomach wall into other nearby organs such as the spleen, liver, intestines, kidneys, or pancreas.
- Or the cancer has spread to more than 15 lymph nodes.
- Or it has spread to other organs such as the liver, lungs, brain, or bones.

Treatment

The doctor develops a treatment plan to fit each patient's needs. Treatment for stomach cancer depends on the size, location, and extent of the tumor; the stage of the disease; the patient's general health; and other factors.

Cancer of the stomach is difficult to cure unless it is found in an early stage (before it has begun to spread). Unfortunately, because early stomach cancer causes few symptoms, the disease is usually advanced when the diagnosis is made. However, advanced stomach cancer can be treated and the symptoms can be relieved. Treatment for stomach cancer may include surgery, CHEMOTHERAPY, and/or RADIATION THERAPY. New treatment approaches such as BIOLOGICAL THERAPY and improved ways of using current methods are being studied in clinical trials. A patient may have one form of treatment or a combination of treatments.

Surgery Gastrectomy is the most common treatment for stomach cancer. In this procedure, a surgeon removes either part (subtotal or partial gastrectomy) or all (total gastrectomy) of the stomach, as well as some nearby tissue. After a subtotal gastrectomy, the remaining part of the stomach is connected to the esophagus or the small intestine. After a total gastrectomy, the esophagus is connected directly to the small intestine. Because cancer can spread through the lymphatic system, lymph nodes near the tumor are often removed as well to be checked for cancer cells.

For the first few days after surgery, the patient is fed intravenously, but within a few days most patients can drink liquids, followed by soft and then solid foods. Those who have had their entire stomach removed cannot absorb vitamin B_{12}, which is necessary for healthy blood and nerves, and require regular injections of this vitamin. Patients may have temporary or permanent difficulty digesting certain foods, and they may need to change their diet. Some gastrectomy patients will need to follow a special diet for a few weeks or months, while others will need to do so permanently.

Some gastrectomy patients have cramps, nausea, diarrhea, and dizziness shortly after eating ("dumping syndrome") because food and liquid enter the small intestine too quickly. Dumping syndrome can be treated by changing the patient's diet and frequency of meals, emphasizing protein while avoiding sugary foods. To reduce the amount of fluid that enters the small intestine, patients are usually encouraged not to drink at mealtimes. Medicine also can help control the dumping syndrome. The symptoms usually disappear in three to 12 months, but they may be permanent.

Following gastrectomy, bile in the small intestine may back up into the remaining part of the stomach or into the esophagus, causing an upset stomach. Medicine or over-the-counter products can control such symptoms.

Chemotherapy   Standard chemotherapy may be useful in the treatment of stomach cancer. Scientists are exploring the benefits of giving chemotherapy before surgery to shrink the tumor, or after surgery to destroy remaining cancer cells. Various combination treatments of chemotherapy and radiation therapy are also being studied, as is a treatment in which chemotherapy is placed directly into the abdomen (intraperitoneal chemotherapy).

The cancer drug Gleevec (imatinib mesylate) was approved in 2002 to treat gastrointestinal stromal tumor (GIST), a relatively uncommon tumor that affects about 5,000 and 10,000 people each year in the United States. It is a tumor that generally begins within the stomach or intestinal tract and then spreads within the abdomen or the pelvis.

First approved in May 2001 for treatment of chronic myeloid LEUKEMIA, Gleevec works by blocking enzymes that play a role in cancer growth. In GIST, Gleevec blocks an abnormal enzyme found on the tumor cells. As these abnormal enzymes are largely confined to cancer cells, there is relatively little damage to normal cells while cancer cells are killed.

Radiation therapy   Radiation therapy with 5-Fu is usually given after surgery if the lymph nodes are positive to destroy cancer cells that may remain in the area, and to relieve pain or blockage. Researchers are also conducting clinical trials to find out whether it is helpful to give radiation therapy during surgery (intraoperative radiation therapy).

Biological therapy   Biological therapy (also called immunotherapy) is a form of treatment that helps the body's immune system attack and destroy cancer cells; it may also help the body recover from some of the side effects of treatment. In clinical trials, doctors are studying a combination of biological therapy and other treatments to try to prevent a recurrence of stomach cancer. In another use of biological therapy, patients who have low blood cell counts during or after chemotherapy may receive COLONY-STIMULATING FACTORS to help restore higher blood cell levels.

Patients may need to be hospitalized while receiving some types of biological therapy.

stomatitis   Inflammation of the soft tissues of the mouth that often occurs as a side effect of chemotherapy, radiation therapy, and some types of BIOLOGICAL THERAPY drugs, such as interleukin-2. Stomatitis can cause dry mouth, soreness, burning feelings, swelling, redness, and taste changes. In a cancer patient, this can lead to serious problems of malnutrition, which can lead to infections.

Patients can take medication to ease symptoms; they should avoid

- hot, spicy food
- highly acidic fruits and juices such as tomato or orange
- carbonated drinks
- salty food
- toothpaste or mouthwash containing salt or alcohol

Instead, patients should eat soft, unseasoned food; rinse mouth and teeth with warm water or a rinse of baking soda and warm water; and use lip balm.

stress   The complex relationship between physical and psychological health is not completely understood. Scientists do know that many types of stress activate the body's endocrine system, which can affect the immune system, although it has not been shown that stress-induced changes in the immune system directly cause cancer.

Some studies have indicated an increased incidence of early cancer death among people who have experienced the recent loss of a spouse or other loved one. However, most cancers develop for many years and are diagnosed only after they have been growing in the body for a long time. This suggests there cannot always be a link between the death of a loved one and the onset of cancer.

The relationship between BREAST CANCER and stress has received particular attention, since some studies have shown significantly higher rates of this disease among women who experienced traumatic life events and losses within several years before their diagnosis. Although studies have shown that stress factors (such as death of a spouse, social isolation, and medical school examinations) alter the way the immune system functions, they have not provided scientific evidence of a direct cause-and-effect relationship between these immune system changes and the development of cancer.

One area currently being studied is the effect of stress on women already diagnosed with breast cancer. The idea is to discover whether stress reduction can improve the immune response and possibly slow cancer progression. Researchers are trying to answer this question by investigating whether women with breast cancer who are in support groups have better survival rates than those not in support groups.

sun exposure Direct exposure to the ultraviolet rays of the Sun causes SKIN CANCER in 900,000 Americans each year. It is responsible for almost all cases of BASAL CELL CARCINOMA and squamous cell carcinoma and is a major underlying cause of malignant MELANOMA.

Ultraviolet radiation is made up of wavelengths shorter than those found in the visible spectrum. This means that even when the Sun's rays are not particularly bright (such as on a hazy day), ultraviolet radiation is still capable of burning the skin. Two types of ultraviolet radiation bands increase the risk of cancer: ultraviolet A (UVA), which is not absorbed by ozone, and ultraviolet B (UVB). UVB is especially damaging to cells' DNA, and that damage can lead to cancer. UVB can be absorbed by ozone, but as the ozone layer becomes depleted, the cancer risk posed by UVB rays will become greater.

Prevention

Skin cancer from sun overexposure can be prevented in the following ways:

Avoid sunlight If people must go out in the sun, they should try to avoid doing so in the middle of the day (between 10 A.M. and 3 P.M.), when the rays are the strongest.

Watch the UV index This measurement of the strength of the sun is often included in the weather report on television or in newspapers. It is a rela-tive measure of how damaging exposure to the sun will be on any particular day. The scale is listed from a low of 1 to a high of 10+; an index value below 5 means that exposure to UV will be low, 5 to 6 means exposure will be moderate, and 7 or higher indicates that the sun will include a danger-ously high level of UV rays. Experts recommend remaining indoors if the index tops 10.

Cover up It is possible to block UV rays from reaching the skin by wearing a hat to shade the face and the back of the neck, long-sleeve shirts, and long pants. The thicker the weave, the more protection.

Use sunscreen When out in the sun, everyone should use a sunscreen with a sun protection fac-tor (SPF) of at least 15 that works against both UVA and UVB rays. Sunscreen should be reapplied after sweating or swimming.

Stay out of tanning booths These booths or beds should be avoided, because they use UV rays. Recent studies have shown that they increase the risk of cancer.

Wear sunglasses When going outside, every-one should wear UV-light-filtering sunglasses to protect eyelids and the eye's lens.

Don sun badges Inexpensive badges can be worn that measure UV light exposure, issuing a warning when overexposure is imminent.

See also SUN LAMPS.

sun lamps A special lamp or tanning bed used to induce a tan without spending time in the sun. Tanning lamps and beds can double the risk of some common types of SKIN CANCER, particularly for the young, according to researchers, who believe that tanning salons should be closed to minors. In one recent study, people who used tan-ning devices were 1.5 to 2.5 times more likely to have common kinds of skin cancer than were peo-ple who did not use the devices. The studies show it is actually worse to go to the tanning parlor and get a little bit of ultraviolet-ray damage each day than it is to get an infrequent sunburn. Although both types of exposure can seriously damage the skin, the small, day-to-day exposure is worse for the skin in the long run. The risk is highest for those who first use the tanning devices before the age of 20. It appears that people who are younger when they start using tanning lamps are at greater risk.

See also MELANOMA; BASAL CELL CARCINOMA; SUN EXPOSURE.

support groups Groups that give people affected by cancer an opportunity to meet and discuss ways to cope with the illness. People diagnosed with cancer and their families face many challenges that may lead to feelings of being overwhelmed, afraid, and alone. Cancer support groups can help people affected by cancer feel less alone and can improve their ability to deal with the uncertainties and challenges that cancer brings.

People who have been diagnosed with cancer sometimes find they need help coping with the emotional as well as the practical aspects of their disease. In fact, attention to the emotional burden of cancer is sometimes part of a patient's treatment plan. Cancer support groups are designed to provide a confidential atmosphere where cancer patients or cancer survivors can discuss the challenges that accompany the illness with others who may have experienced the same challenges. Support groups have helped thousands of people cope with similar situations.

Family and friends also are affected when cancer touches someone they love, and they may need help in dealing with stresses such as family disruptions, financial worries, and changing roles. To help meet these needs, some support groups are designed just for family members of people diagnosed with cancer; other groups encourage families and friends to participate along with the cancer patient or cancer survivor.

Several kinds of support groups are available to meet the individual needs of people at all stages of cancer treatment. There are general cancer support groups, as well as more specialized groups that work with teens or young adults, family members, or people affected by a particular type of cancer.

Support groups may be led by a professional, such as a psychiatrist, psychologist, or social worker, or by cancer patients or survivors. In addition, support groups can vary in approach, size, and how often they meet. Many groups are free, but some require a fee (people can contact their health insurance companies to find out whether their plans will cover the cost).

Locating a Group

Many hospitals and medical centers run support groups for cancer patients. In addition, some disease-specific cancer organizations also run support groups.

American Cancer Society Support Groups

The ACS organizes, runs and facilitates thousands of cancer support groups through its state and local affiliates. These support groups are free and meet at various times of the day on different days of the week. Meetings are held in a variety of settings, including hospitals, clinics, civic organizations, community centers, churches, and so on.

The Cancer Survivors Network

The AMERICAN CANCER SOCIETY launched its first web-based virtual cancer support group in 2001. Called the cancer Survivors Network, the site has 9,000 registered users and offers safeguards to protect confidentiality, allowing users to design a support group that fits individual needs.

American Cancer Society Phone Network

Patients who do not have a computer or an Internet account can call toll-free (877) 333-HOPE to reach the phone version of the Cancer Survivors Network. The phone network is aimed at people who may live in remote areas, are too sick or otherwise cannot attend a support group meeting.

The Wellness Community

This organization offers support groups and related services for a broad-based population of cancer patients. The WELLNESS COMMUNITY was founded by Harold Benjamin in the 1980s in Santa Anna, California, as a way to help his wife, who had been diagnosed with breast cancer but was unable to find the kind of psychological support she needed for herself and her family.

Today, The Wellness Community has grown into a network of 19 facilities in 25 locations across the country with a diverse menu of weekly cancer support group meetings—as well as other services and education programs—to complement standard medical and experimental cancer treatment.

Cancer support groups can range in membership from several people to a dozen or more per group. Groups are often are based on a common denominator, such as the following:

Type of cancer Some support groups are cancer-specific, focusing on only one type of cancer, such as LUNG CANCER or BLADDER CANCER. This may mean that some groups are gender-specific (a cervical cancer group is likely to include only women, and a prostate cancer support is aimed at men).

Stage The key criterion for some groups is whether a potential member is newly diagnosed and just starting treatment, recovering from treatment, recently deemed cancer-free, or terminally ill.

Age In some cancer support groups, the age of the group members is as important as the cancer that each member has. Some support groups specialize in children and teens (with or without their parents or other family members); others are for adults and the elderly.

How Support Groups Are Structured

The structure of cancer support groups varies in terms of group leadership, longevity, and meeting schedules.

Self-help cancer support groups Also called mutual help support groups, some of these groups have no leader; others may include veteran cancer patients. Some leaders simply evolve, gradually taking on a leadership role. Self-help cancer support groups may form around a common interest beyond cancer, such as books or golfing. Membership is typically free, although voluntary donations (for refreshments) may be requested at times.

Professionally led cancer support groups In these groups members may decide on specific goals and "group work" and be led by a health-care professional who usually is experienced in cancer, mental health, or group dynamics. There may be a fee to join a group like this; financial aid may be available to cover costs. Some health insurance plans may cover the costs of groups such as these.

Ongoing support groups These ongoing groups meet at an established time on certain days, and members may join or leave the group as they wish. This may make it hard for a new member to feel part of the group, especially if there is a core of veteran participants.

Time-limited groups These groups typically start and end over a relatively short period of time, such as from one full day or for six weeks. Some groups may only convene occasionally, while others may be held periodically throughout the year. Health-care professionals usually lead these types of groups, and there is usually a fee.

Surveillance, Epidemiology, and End Results (SEER) A program of the NATIONAL CANCER INSTITUTE (NCI) that is the most authoritative source of information on cancer incidence and survival in the United States. NCI's SEER cancer registry program has been expanded to cover more racial, ethnic, and socioeconomic groups in the United States, allowing for better description and tracking of trends in health disparities. Methodological studies are seeking better ways to measure socioeconomic factors and determine their relationship to cancer incidence, survival, and mortality.

Additionally, NCI supports a growing body of research into the environmental, sociocultural, behavioral, and genetic causes of cancer in different populations. The agency seeks to apply this research through interventions in clinical and community settings. Among these interventions are tobacco control, dietary modification, and adherence to screening practices.

Susan G. Komen Breast Cancer Foundation A leader in the field of BREAST CANCER education, screening, and treatment, and the largest private funding source for breast cancer research and community outreach programs in the world.

The foundation was started in 1982 by Nancy Goodman Brinker, two years after her sister Susan Goodman Komen died from breast cancer. By the end of 2000, the Komen Foundation and its affiliates had raised more than $300 million since its inception. Key to its success is the Komen Race for the Cure, the largest series of 5-K runs/fitness walks in the world. This event, created by Nancy, has grown from one local race with 800 participants to a national series of more than 100 races with more than one million participants.

Nancy Brinker has served under three U.S. presidents on the National Cancer Advisory Board, and testified before the Congressional Subcommittee on Labor, Health and Human Services, Education and Related Agencies in 2000. She has also testified before the Democratic Policy Committee's Congressional Breast Cancer Forum, participated in the International Women's Forum, and is a collaborating partner for the National Dialogue on Cancer. For contact information, see Appendix I.

Tarceva A novel cancer drug that significantly improved survival for certain LUNG CANCER patients who failed to respond to standard chemotherapy, according to research results released in spring 2004. The drug is the first of its kind to show in a major study that the approach can extend survival in patients in non-small-cell lung cancer. This is the most common form of lung cancer, accounting for almost 80 percent of all lung cancer, a disease that results in 1.1 million deaths a year.

Tarceva is one of a new generation of cancer medications designed to directly attack cancer cells. It blocks a protein called EPIDERMAL GROWTH FACTOR RECEPTOR (EGFR), which is common in cancer cells and which experts believe may play a key role in helping them divide uncontrollably. The drug is similar in many respects to Iressa, which was launched in 2002.

Traditional chemotherapy drugs are toxins that kill many normal cells as well as tumors, one reason they often result in serious side effects, such as nausea, hair loss, and susceptibility to infection.

Tarceva is the first EGFR inhibitor that has been shown to extend survival in patients with relapsed non-small-cell lung cancer, for whom there are very limited treatments possible. It is the fifth cancer medicine with a proven survival benefit (the others include breast cancer drugs Herceptin and Xeloda, the blood cancer treatment Mabthera, and colorectal cancer drug Avastin).

The study results surprised researchers, since Tarceva in earlier studies failed to prolong survival in patients whose lung cancer had spread, when used as the first treatment tried. At the time, two studies in which Tarceva was used with traditional chemotherapy showed no sign of helping lung-cancer patients live longer. However, the most recent study of more than 700 patients looked at the benefits of using Tarceva by itself, without chemotherapy, in patients who had already had chemotherapy treatment. The drug improved overall survival, with patients on Tarceva living longer than those on placebo.

The drug is expected to be launched in late 2005 or early 2006.

taxanes A group of drugs, including paclitaxel (Taxol) and docetaxel (Taxotere), that are used in the treatment of cancer. Taxanes have a unique way of preventing the growth of cancer cells: they affect cell structures called microtubules, which play an important role in cell functions.

In normal cell growth, microtubules are formed when a cell starts dividing. Once the cell stops dividing, the microtubules are broken down or destroyed. Taxanes stop the microtubules from breaking down; cancer cells become so clogged with microtubules that they cannot grow and divide.

tea Tea drinking is an ancient tradition dating back 5,000 years in China and India, where it has long been regarded as an aid to good health. Researchers now are studying tea for possible use in the prevention and treatment of a variety of cancers.

Investigators are especially interested in the antioxidants found in tea, called catechins. These may selectively inhibit the growth of cancer. In animal studies, catechins scavenged oxidants before cell damage occurred, reduced the number and size of tumors, and inhibited the growth of cancer cells. However, human studies have proved to be more contradictory, perhaps due to such factors as variations in DIET, environments, and populations. Some studies comparing tea drinkers to non–tea drinkers support the claim that drinking tea prevents cancer; others do not.

The human body constantly produces unstable molecules called oxidants (also known as "FREE RADICALS"). To become stable, oxidants steal electrons from other molecules and, in the process, damage cell proteins and genetic material. This damage may leave the cell vulnerable to cancer. ANTIOXIDANTS are substances that allow the human body to scavenge and seize oxidants. Like other antioxidants, the catechins found in tea selectively interfere with specific enzyme activities that lead to cancer. They may also target and repair DNA aberrations caused by oxidants.

All varieties of tea come from the leaves of a single evergreen plant (*Camellia sinensis*). All tea leaves are picked, rolled, dried, and heated; black tea leaves are also allowed to ferment and oxidize. Possibly because it is less processed, green tea contains higher levels of antioxidants than black tea.

Although tea is drunk in different ways and varies in its chemical makeup, one study showed steeping either green or black tea for about five minutes released more than 80 percent of its catechins. Instant iced tea, on the other hand, contains negligible amounts of catechins.

In one Chinese study involving more than 18,000 men, tea drinkers were about half as likely to develop stomach or ESOPHAGEAL CANCER, even after adjusting for smoking and other health and diet factors. A second study at the Beijing Dental Hospital found that drinking about two cups of tea a day, along with the application of a tea extract, reduced the size and proliferation of a precancerous oral plaque called leukoplakia.

However, a study in the Netherlands did not support these findings. It investigated the link between black tea consumption and the subsequent risk of stomach, colorectal, lung, and BREAST CANCERS among 58,279 men and 62,573 women aged 55 to 69 and found no link between tea consumption and protection against cancer.

NATIONAL CANCER INSTITUTE (NCI) researchers who are investigating the therapeutic use of green tea have concluded that the beverage has limited antitumor benefit for PROSTATE CANCER patients. Other ongoing NCI studies are testing green tea as a preventive agent against SKIN CANCER. For example,

one is investigating the protective effects of a pill form of green tea against sun-induced skin damage while another explores the topical application of green tea in shrinking precancerous skin changes.

teratocarcinoma   A MIXED GERM CELL TUMOR made up of EMBRYONAL CELL CANCER and TERATOMA.

teratoma   A benign tumor composed of a number of different normal types of tissue, growing in abnormal places. Although it is technically benign, it can act like a malignant tumor and spread; eventually, it can become malignant. Because a teratoma is made up of normal cells, CHEMOTHERAPY does not affect it.

testicular cancer   A disease in which cells become malignant in one or both testicles. About 7,400 men in the United States are diagnosed with testicular cancer each year. Although testicular cancer accounts for only one percent of all cancers in men, it is the most common form of cancer in men between the ages of 15 and 35. Although any man can get testicular cancer, it is more common in Caucasians than in African Americans.

More than 95 percent of men with stage I or stage II testicular cancer are successfully treated. Stage III testicular cancer has about a 75 percent recovery rate.

Types of Testicular Cancer

About 95 percent of all testicular tumors are GERM CELL tumors. Germ cell (or sex cell) tumors in men are classified as either seminomas or nonseminomas. Each type grows and spreads differently; treatment and prognosis also vary according to type.

About half of all testicular cancers are seminomas, which begin in germ cells at a very early stage in their development. Seminomas are the most common testicular germ cell tumor, accounting for between 30 and 45 percent of all such tumors. A pure seminoma is very sensitive to radiation treatment, and almost all men recover from this type of cancer if it is treated early.

Nonseminomas   include   CHORIOCARCINOMA, embryonal carcinoma, TERATOMA, and YOLK SAC TUMORS. Most nonseminomas have more than one cell type and are known as MIXED GERM CELL

TUMORS. Knowing the cell type of these tumors is important for estimating the risk of spreading and response to chemotherapy. These cancers often develop earlier in life than seminomas, usually occurring in men in their 20s.

A testicular cancer may have a combination of both seminoma and nonseminoma types.

Risk Factors

Although the causes of testicular cancer are not known, studies show that several factors increase a man's chance of developing testicular cancer.

Undescended testicle (cryptorchidism) Normally, the testicles descend into the scrotum before birth. Men who have had a testicle that did not move down into the scrotum are at greater risk for developing the disease, even if surgery is performed to place the testicle in the scrotum. (However, most men who develop testicular cancer do not have a history of undescended testicles).

Abnormal testicular development Men whose testicles did not develop normally are at increased risk.

Klinefelter's syndrome This sex chromosome disorder characterized by low levels of male hormones, sterility, breast enlargement, and small testes has been linked to a greater risk of developing testicular cancer.

Personal history Men who have previously had cancer in one testicle are at increased risk of developing cancer in the other one.

Age Testicular cancer affects younger men, particularly those between ages 15 and 35; it is uncommon in children and in men over age 40.

Symptoms

The following symptoms can be caused by testicular cancer or by other conditions:

- painless lump or swelling in either testicle
- enlargement of a testicle or change in the way it feels
- heavy feeling in the scrotum
- dull ache in the lower abdomen, lower back, or groin
- sudden appearance of fluid buildup in the scrotum
- pain or discomfort in a testicle or the scrotum

Occasionally, men with germ cell cancer notice breast tenderness or enlarged breasts, because certain types of germ cell tumors secrete high levels of a hormone called human chorionic gonadotropin (HCG), which stimulates breast development. Because blood tests can measure HCG levels, these tests are important in diagnosis, staging, and follow-up of some testicular cancers.

Some men with testicular cancer have no symptoms at all; instead, their cancer is found during medical testing for other conditions. Sometimes imaging tests or biopsies to find the cause of infertility can uncover a small testicular cancer.

Self-Exams

Because the earlier that testicular cancer is found, the better the chance for cure, experts recommend that men of all ages, starting in the mid-teenage years, should examine their testicles regularly. The best time to do this is during or after a bath or shower, when the skin of the scrotum is relaxed.

To perform a testicular self-exam:

1. Stand in front of a mirror, looking for any swelling on the skin of the scrotum.

2. Hold the penis out of the way and examine each testicle separately.

3. Place the index and middle fingers under the testicle while placing your thumbs on the top, and roll the testicle gently between the fingers.

4. Look and feel for any hard lumps or smooth round masses, or any change in the size, shape, or consistency of the testes. Each normal testis has an epididymis, which feels like a small bump on the upper or middle outer side of the testis. Normal testicles also contain blood vessels, supporting tissues, and tubes that conduct sperm.

5. It is normal for one testicle to be a bit bigger than the other. Sometimes, a testicle can be enlarged because fluid has collected around it. This is called a hydrocele. Or the veins in the testicle can dilate and cause enlargement and lumpiness around the testicle; this is called a varicocele. A doctor may need to examine these conditions to make sure cancer is not present.

Diagnosis

Men find most testicular cancers themselves, although a doctor usually examines the testicles during routine physical exams. When testicular cancer is found early, the treatment can often be less aggressive and may cause fewer side effects.

Blood tests   Certain blood tests are sometimes helpful in diagnosing testicular tumors. Many testicular cancers (not including Sertoli or Leydig cell tumors) secrete high levels of certain proteins such as alpha-fetoprotein (AFP) and HCG. Tumors also may boost the levels of enzymes such as lactate dehydrogenase (LDH). These proteins are important because their presence in the blood suggests that a testicular tumor is present. However, they can also be found in conditions other than cancer.

Nonseminomas often raise AFP and HCG levels; seminomas sometimes raise HCG levels but never AFP levels. A high LDH often indicates widespread disease. Because levels of these proteins are not usually high if the tumor is small, blood tests can also be helpful in estimating how large the cancer is, and in evaluating the response to therapy to make sure the tumor has not returned.

Imaging tests   Ultrasound of the scrotum can reveal the presence and size of a mass in the testicle, or rule out other conditions, such as swelling due to infection. An ultrasound can help doctors tell if a mass is solid or fluid filled, which can help distinguish some types of benign and malignant tumors from one another. If the mass is solid, it is probably either a benign tumor or cancer, but since it could also be some form of infection, it is essential to follow up with further tests.

Biopsy   If a tumor is suspected, the doctor will probably suggest a BIOPSY, which involves surgery to remove the testicle. In nearly all cases of suspected cancer, the entire affected testicle is removed through an incision in the groin. This procedure is called inguinal orchiectomy. The surgeon will try to remove the entire tumor together with the testicle and spermatic cord. The spermatic cord contains blood and lymph vessels that may act as a pathway for testicular cancer to spread to the rest of the body. To minimize the risk that cancer cells will spread, these vessels are tied off early in the operation. This is best done by performing the operation through an incision in the groin (inguinal) area.

In rare cases (for example, when a man has only one testicle, or if cancer is not certain), the surgeon performs an inguinal biopsy before removing the testicle; in this case, only a sample of tissue from the testicle is removed through an incision in the groin. During this operation, the surgeon makes a cut in the groin, withdraws the testicle from the scrotum, and examines it without cutting the spermatic cord. If the mass is not cancerous, the testicle can often be returned to the scrotum. The testicle would be removed only if the pathologist finds cancer cells. (The surgeon does not cut through the scrotum to remove tissue, because if there were cancer, this procedure could cause the disease to spread.)

Staging

If testicular cancer is found, more tests are needed to classify the cancer according to its stage (whether or not it has spread from the testicle to other parts of the body). A chest X-ray can determine if cancer has spread to the lungs or lymph nodes. Computerized tomography (CT) scans are helpful in detecting if it has spread into the liver, other organs, or lymph nodes. Magnetic resonance imaging (MRI) scans are particularly helpful in examining the brain and spinal cord. Position-emission tomography (PET) scans are very useful for spotting cancer that has spread beyond the testes, and for checking enlarged lymph nodes to reveal if they contain scar tissue or active tumor.

The stages of testicular cancer include

Stage I: Testicular cancer is found only in the testicle.

Stage II: Testicular cancer has spread to the lymph nodes in the abdomen.

Stage III: Testicular cancer has spread beyond the lymph nodes to other areas, such as the lungs or liver.

Treatment

Most men with testicular cancer can be cured with surgery, RADIATION THERAPY, or CHEMOTHERAPY. Because seminomas and nonseminomas grow in different ways, each type may need different treatment. Treatment also depends on the stage of the cancer, the patient's age and general health, and other factors.

Men with testicular cancer should discuss their concerns about sexual function and fertility with a doctor. If both testicles are removed, the man will be infertile. However, male hormones can be administered to ensure that sexual function remains essentially normal. Testosterone can be replaced by intramuscular injection, usually given every two weeks; patches, applied to the skin daily; or testosterone gel, rubbed into the skin daily.

If a particular treatment might cause infertility, sperm can be frozen for future use. This procedure can allow some men to father children after loss of fertility.

Surgery Surgery to remove the testicle through an incision in the groin is called a radical inguinal orchiectomy; as long as a man has one remaining healthy testicle, he can still have a normal erection and produce sperm. An artificial testicle can be placed in the scrotum, providing the weight and feel of a normal testicle, if a man wishes.

Some of the lymph nodes located deep in the abdomen also may be removed. This type of surgery does not change a man's ability to have an erection or an orgasm, but it can cause sterility because it interferes with ejaculation. If this is a concern, the doctor may be able to remove the lymph nodes using a special nerve-sparing surgical technique that may protect the ability to ejaculate normally.

Surgery may be combined with radiation therapy or chemotherapy or both.

Radiation therapy Radiation alone is often used for seminoma; chemotherapy is added if it is advanced or if there is a recurrence. Radiation therapy for testicular cancer is external and is usually aimed at lymph nodes in the abdomen. Seminomas are highly sensitive to radiation; however, because nonseminomas are less sensitive to radiation, men with this type of cancer usually do not undergo radiation. Radiation therapy interferes with sperm production, but most patients regain their fertility within a few months after treatment ends. Just in case fertility does not return, many men store sperm at a special facility or "bank" before treatment, where it can be preserved for later use.

Chemotherapy Chemotherapy alone (cisplatin, etoposide or Bleomycin) is used primarily in patients with nonseminoma. Chemotherapy may be the first treatment if the cancer has spread outside the testicle. Some anticancer drugs interfere with sperm production, which may result in permanent sterility for some patients but only a temporary condition in others. Chemotherapy has made the biggest difference in reducing deaths from testicular cancer.

Bone marrow transplant In this procedure, bone marrow is removed from the patient, treated with drugs to kill the cancer cells, and then frozen. The patient then is given chemotherapy, with or without radiation, to destroy the remaining cancer cells (the chemotherapy also destroys the remaining bone marrow). The frozen marrow is then thawed and injected back into the patient. This relatively new treatment for testicular cancer has shown some promising initial results, but it is not routinely recommended by doctors since traditional chemotherapy is typically very successful.

Follow-up Care

Men who have had cancer in one testicle have a higher risk of developing cancer in the remaining testicle, as well as certain types of LEUKEMIA and other types of cancers. For this reason, regular follow-up is extremely important. It usually involves frequent exams and regular blood tests to measure tumor marker levels. X-rays and CT scans are usually performed at regular intervals.

thalidomide Drug that once was prescribed as a sedative but that caused severe birth defects in pregnant women and was withdrawn from the market. New research, however, is finding evidence that this much-maligned drug may be a powerful cancer treatment and possibly could help people with bone marrow cancer live longer.

Recent Mayo Clinic studies tested 32 people with advanced MULTIPLE MYELOMA whose treatments with standard CHEMOTHERAPY or STEM CELL transplantation had failed. Almost a third of those in the study responded to thalidomide for an average of about a year. This confirmed findings from an earlier University of Arkansas study. Multiple myeloma is an incurable cancer of the

BONE MARROW. About 14,600 people in the United States are diagnosed each year, and about 10,800 people die. The average survival time from diagnosis is three to four years for people treated with conventional chemotherapy. Thalidomide is not approved by the U.S. Food and Drug Administration for the treatment of myeloma, but it is widely used together with the steroid dexamethasone.

thermal imaging   A new way of diagnosing breast problems, by measuring and mapping the heat from the breast with the use of a special camera. A computer looks for "hot spots" or differences in heat, then analyzes the images. The theory is that if an area of increased heat is found, it may indicate an increase in blood vessel formation due to cancer. However, studies have not proven this to be an effective screening tool for early diagnosis of BREAST CANCER, and it is not a replacement for mammograms.

While thermography has been approved by the U.S. Food and Drug Administration as safe, it is not approved as a stand-alone screening test for breast cancer. It is not a reliable diagnostic test since it can miss some cancers and has a high false-positive rate.

See also MAMMOGRAPHY, DUCTOGRAM, and DIGITAL MAMMOGRAPHY.

thoracentesis   A diagnostic procedure in which a small amount of fluid is removed from the space between the lungs and the chest wall. The fluid is examined in the lab for cancer cells.

thoracotomy   The surgical opening of the chest in order to remove a piece of lung as a last resort in an attempt to diagnose LUNG CANCER when other diagnostic methods have failed. Performed under general anesthesia, it is considered to be major surgery.

throat cancer   See LARYNGEAL CANCER.

thrombocytopenia   A drop in the number of platelets (blood cells responsible for clotting), which is often a side effect of RADIATION THERAPY or CHEMOTHERAPY. Certain types of cancer also may directly destroy platelets in the blood. Severe cases of thrombocytopenia can have grave consequences if minor injuries result in serious blood loss.

The condition can be treated with transfusions of platelets, intravenous gamma globulin, removal of the spleen, and medications to boost the platelet count. When radiation or chemotherapy is stopped, the platelet count should return to normal.

thyroid cancer   Tiny and usually insignificant carcinomas can be found in 5 to 10 percent or more of all thyroid glands that are carefully examined under the microscope at autopsy, but relatively few thyroid tumors grow or spread to produce symptoms that lead to their detection during a person's lifetime.

The thyroid cancers that are diagnosed each year represent about 1 percent of all cancers in the U.S. population. Each year in the United States, thyroid cancer is diagnosed in 14,900 women and 4,600 men. Most types of thyroid cancer are easily treated and allow long-term survival, although some rare subtypes may have a poor prognosis.

If thyroid cancer spreads outside the thyroid, cancer cells are often found in nearby LYMPH NODES, nerves, or blood vessels. If the cancer reaches these lymph nodes, it indicates that cancer cells may have also spread to other lymph nodes or to other organs, such as the lungs or bones.

Types of Thyroid Cancer

Many types of tumors can develop in the thyroid gland, most of which (95 percent) are benign. Harmless thyroid nodules can develop at any age, but they appear most often in adults (one-third of adults have them), and can be found in normal-sized thyroid glands and goiters. A few types are malignant and can spread into nearby tissues and to other parts of the body. The following are the major types of thyroid cancer:

Papillary and follicular thyroid cancers   These account for 80 to 90 percent of all thyroid cancers. Both types begin in the follicular cells of the thyroid. Most papillary and follicular thyroid cancers grow slowly. If they are detected early, most can be treated successfully.

The most common type of thyroid cancer is papillary carcinoma (also called papillary cancer or papillary adenocarcinoma). Papillary cancers usually occur in only one lobe of the thyroid gland, although about 10 to 20 percent of the time both lobes are involved. Even though papillary cancer grows slowly, it often spreads early to the lymph nodes in the neck. Fortunately, few people with papillary cancer die of this thyroid cancer.

The next most common type of thyroid cancer is called follicular cancer, follicular carcinoma, or follicular ADENOCARCINOMA. Follicular cancer is much less common than papillary thyroid cancer. These cancers usually remain in the thyroid gland but can spread to other parts of the body, such as lungs and bone. Unlike papillary carcinoma, follicular carcinomas less often spread to lymph nodes. The prognosis for patients with follicular thyroid cancer is somewhat worse than for those with papillary cancer, but most patients with follicular thyroid cancer do not die from it.

Hürthle cell carcinoma is a subtype of follicular cancer and follows a similar course in patients. Papillary and Hürthle cell cancers have the same prognosis and are treated the same. The other variants tend to spread more quickly and have a worse prognosis.

Medullary thyroid cancer This type of cancer accounts for about 10 percent of thyroid cancer cases. Medullary thyroid cancer is easier to control if it is found and treated before it spreads to other parts of the body; however, sometimes this cancer can spread to lymph nodes, the lungs, or liver even before a thyroid nodule has been discovered.

There are two types of medullary thyroid carcinoma: sporadic and inherited. The sporadic type is far more common, occurring in 80 percent of cases, usually in one thyroid lobe in older adults. The inherited form can occur in each generation.

Anaplastic thyroid cancer It is the least common type of thyroid cancer (it occurs in only 1 to 2 percent of cases). Experts believe it may develop from an existing papillary or follicular cancer. The cancer cells are highly abnormal and difficult to recognize, and hard to control because they may grow and spread very quickly. This very aggressive cancer is usually fatal.

Thyroid lymphoma Occasionally LYMPHOMA can develop in the thyroid gland from lymphocytes, the main cell type of the immune system. Most thyroid lymphomas occur in people who have a disease called chronic lymphocytic thyroidi-

tis (also known as Hashimoto's thyroiditis), in which the immune system attacks the patient's own thyroid gland. In this disease, many lymphocytes are found in the thyroid gland. If a thyroid lymphoma has not spread beyond the gland, it is usually treated by surgical removal or radiation therapy. If it has spread, chemotherapy, with or without radiation therapy, is used.

Risk Factors

There are a number of risk factors that can be linked to thyroid cancer. These include:

Gender The highest incidence of thyroid cancer occurs in women, particularly in the Pacific Island and Southeast Asian populations living in California and Hawaii. The rates are highest among Filipino women (14.6 per 100,000), Vietnamese women (10.5), and Hawaiian women (9.1), and lowest among African-American women (3.3). Within each racial/ethnic group, incidence in women consistently exceeds incidence in men by a factor of about three.

Radiation Many studies report an association between thyroid cancer and radiation exposure. In the 1930s and 1940s, X-rays were often used to treat skin diseases and enlarged tonsils. Increased risks have been described in Japanese atomic bomb survivors and in persons exposed to fallout from atomic testing in the Marshall Islands. Goiter and other thyroid diseases, as well as diets high or low in iodine, have been suspected risk factors. Medullary carcinomas of the thyroid, which account for about 10 percent of cases, are often a part of an inherited disease complex called the multiple endocrine neoplasia syndrome.

Heredity A single genetic mistake—a mutation of the BRAF gene—causes about two-thirds of papillary thyroid cancers. These tumors account for about 75 percent of all thyroid cancer and occur mostly in women.

Diagnosis

Fine-needle aspiration biopsy The simplest way to test whether a thyroid nodule is cancerous is with a FINE-NEEDLE ASPIRATION (FNA), which can be performed in a doctor's office. Between 60 and 80 percent of FNA tests clearly show that the nodule is benign.

Blood tests Blood tests cannot tell whether a thyroid nodule is cancerous or not, but a thyroid-stimulating hormone blood test may help check the overall condition of the thyroid gland.

Thyroid scan For this test, the patient swallows a small amount of radioactive iodine or technetium, and the body concentrates these radioactive chemicals in the thyroid gland. A special camera is placed in front of the neck to measure the amount of radiation in the gland. Abnormal areas of the thyroid that contain less radioactivity are called cold nodules, while nodules that take up more radiation are called hot nodules. Most malignant thyroid nodules appear as cold nodules on thyroid scans, but since both benign and cancerous nodules can appear cold, this test is usually not very helpful in diagnosing thyroid cancer.

Ultrasound Normal thyroid tissue and most thyroid nodules make different echo patterns detectable on ultrasound, which are then processed by a computer to create a picture of the thyroid gland. This test can be used to check the number and size of thyroid nodules.

Treatment

There are a number of treatments, depending on the age and health of the patient and the stage of the disease, including surgery, radiation therapy, hormone therapy, or chemotherapy.

Surgery is the most common treatment for cancer of the thyroid, and may include:

- Lobectomy removes only the side of the thyroid where the cancer is found. Lymph nodes in the area may be taken out to see if they contain cancer.
- Near-total thyroidectomy removes most of the thyroid.
- Total thyroidectomy removes the entire thyroid.
- Lymph node dissection removes lymph nodes in the neck that contain cancer.

Chemotherapy, hormone therapy, and radiation therapy all may be used to treat thyroid cancer.

toxins See CARCINOGENS.

TRAM flap See BREAST RECONSTRUCTION.

transverse rectus abdominus myocutaneous flap See BREAST RECONSTRUCTION.

tubular carcinoma A special type of infiltrating ductal BREAST CANCER that makes up only about 2 percent of all breast cancers. These tumors have a slightly better prognosis and a slightly lower chance of spreading than invasive lobular or invasive ductal cancers of the same size.

tumor lysis syndrome A complication of CHEMOTHERAPY that is most common when treating high-grade LYMPHOMA or acute LEUKEMIA. As the cancer cells die, they release chemicals into the blood that alter the normal balance of substances circulating in the blood, such as potassium, sodium, phosphates, and urea. Abnormal levels of these chemicals can upset the heart rhythm and kidneys. The best way of dealing with this complication is to prevent it in the first place; patients at risk should be given extra fluids before the start of chemotherapy to flush out extra chemicals.

tyrosine kinase (TK) genes Genes that encode an enzyme that play key roles in controlling cell growth, differentiation, motility, and nearby tissue invasion. A few TK genes have been shown to be mutated in specific cancers, and in the spring of 2003 a new study at Johns Hopkins revealed how many or how often members of the TK gene family are altered in COLORECTAL CANCER. Investigators completed what is believed to be the first systematic analysis of a disease-related gene family, uncovering gene mutations linked to more than 30 percent of colon cancers.

TKs are "activating proteins" that, when damaged, signal cells to continually divide and take other actions that can lead to cancer. Drugs such as Gleevec, Herceptin, and other inhibitor-class compounds that block the proteins made by mutated TK genes have been shown in both human clinical trials and animal studies to halt the cancer process.

Scientists hope that this new research might pave the way for personalized treatment designed to match the mutated TK pathways present in each patient's particular tumor DNA.

To conduct this research, the investigators focused on the 138 normal TK genes that all humans have. They were able to identify mutations in 14 of these genes only after sifting through more than 4 million base pairs of DNA. The researchers are now looking more closely at the TK genes most commonly mutated in the colon cancers they studied in hopes of developing new drugs to target them.

ultrasound scan   Also called sonography, this is a diagnostic technique that uses high-frequency sound waves (above the range of human hearing) to produce images of structures inside the body.

United Ostomy Association (UOA)   A nonprofit association of ostomy chapters dedicated to complete rehabilitation of all ostomates. It provides information, education, support, and advocacy for those who already have or may soon need bowel or bladder diversions. There are more than 440 chapters and 77 satellites meeting in 47 U.S. states, Washington, D.C., and Puerto Rico. UOA and its chapters offer the only direct national person-to-person support group assistance on this issue. They have helped thousands of people to adjust to normal life after surgery.

UOA has national networks to meet the needs of parents of children with an ostomy, gay and lesbian ostomates, young adults, and those with continent diversions. For contact information, see Appendix I.

ureterostomy   A surgical procedure in which an opening is created in the abdominal wall so that urine can be excreted.

urethral cancer   A rare type of cancer in which malignant cells are found in the urethra (the tube that empties urine from the bladder). Cancer of the urethra affects women more often than men and is often associated with BLADDER CANCER. It has often spread to nearby soft tissue before it is diagnosed.

Urethral cancer is more common in women. Although it can occur at any age, it appears most often in patients in their 60s. In men 80 percent of cases are squamous cell carcinomas, most of which occur in the urethra at the base of the penis. In women 60 percent of cases are squamous cell carcinomas.

Symptoms

There may be no symptoms of early cancer of the urethra. If symptoms do appear, they may include

- lump or growth on the urethra
- diminished urine stream
- straining to void
- frequent urination and increased nighttime urination
- hardening of tissue in the perineum, labia, or penis
- itching
- incontinence
- pain during or after sex
- painful urination
- urinary tract infections
- urethral discharge and swelling
- swollen LYMPH NODES in the groin

Types of Urethral Cancer

Different types of urethral cancer develop in different types of cells in different areas of the urethra. In women the urethra is lined with transitional cells near the urethral opening and in squamous cells near the bladder. In men transitional cells line the portion of the urethra and squamous cells line the urethra at the base of and within the penis.

Squamous cell carcinoma   The most common type of urethral cancer, this develops in flat, scaly surface cells.

Transitional cell carcinoma This type of cancer appears in the surface cells of the urethra.

Adenocarcinoma A type of cancer that develops in glands located near the urethra.

Melanoma This type of urethral cancer is extremely rare; it develops in the pigment-producing skin cells.

Sarcoma Another extremely rare type of cancer, this develops in blood vessels, smooth muscle, and connective tissue.

Risk Factors

The cause of urethral cancer is unknown, but there are a number of risk factors, including:

Bladder cancer The primary risk factor for urethral cancer is a history of bladder cancer.

HPV Infection with HUMAN PAPILLOMAVIRUS (HPV) or other sexually transmitted diseases is also a risk factor. HPV is a group of more than 70 viruses that are transmitted sexually and cause genital warts. Two types of HPV are associated with warts that appear on the urethra. Having unprotected sexual intercourse with multiple partners increases the risk for HPV infection.

Age People over age 60 are at higher risk.

Chronic irritation Irritation of the urethra, as a result of childbirth, sexual intercourse, chronic urinary tract infection, and so on.

Smoking This increases the risk for bladder cancer, which is a risk factor for urethral cancer.

Diagnosis

If there are urethral cancer symptoms, a doctor will examine the patient to feel for lumps in the urethra. In men a thin lighted tube called a cystoscope may be inserted into the penis so the doctor can see inside the urethra. If the doctor finds cells or other signs that are not normal, the doctor may perform a biopsy, removing a piece of tissue to check for cancer cells.

Staging

If malignant cells are found, imaging tests are performed to find out if cancer cells have spread to other parts of the body. These tests include X-ray, ultrasound, computed tomography scan, and magnetic resonance imaging (MRI). MRI is the preferred method to evaluate urethral cancer. Patients are grouped into the following stages, depending on where the tumor is and whether it has spread to other places:

Anterior urethral cancer The anterior urethra is the part of the urethra that is closest to the outside of the body. Urethral cancer that is superficial and located toward the urethral opening often can be treated successfully.

Posterior urethral cancer The posterior urethra is the part of the urethra that connects to the bladder. Cancers that start here are more likely to be invasive, to grow through the inner lining of the urethra and affect nearby tissues. They are rarely curable. In women urethral cancer often spreads to the labia, vagina, and bladder neck. In men the condition may spread to the tissues of the penis and perineum, the prostate gland, the ligament that surrounds the urethra, the regional lymph nodes, and the penile and scrotal skin.

Recurrent urethral cancer The cancer has returned after it has been treated, either in the same place or in another part of the body.

Treatment

Treatment for cancer of the urethra depends on the stage and location of the disease, and the patient's age, sex, and overall health. It includes surgery, radiation therapy, and chemotherapy.

Surgery This is the most common treatment of cancer of the urethra. A doctor may remove the cancer using one of the following operations:

Electrofulguration In this method, electric current is used to burn away the tumor and the area around it.

Laser therapy This method uses a narrow beam of intense light to kill cancer cells.

Cystourethrectomy The removal of the bladder and the urethra.

Partial penectomy This type of surgery removes the part of the penis containing the urethra that has cancer.

Total penectomy Sometimes the entire penis is removed; plastic surgery is then used to create a new penis.

Cystoprostatectomy The removal of the bladder and prostate along with the seminal vesicles. Lymph nodes in the pelvis also may be removed.

Anterior exenteration In women, surgery to remove the urethra, the bladder, and the vagina, along with lymph node removal. Plastic surgery may be needed to create a new vagina.

If the urethra is removed, the doctor will need to fashion a new way for the urine to pass from the body; if the bladder is removed, a new way to store and pass urine must be devised. Sometimes part of the small intestine can be used to make a tube through which urine can pass out of the body through an opening (stoma) on the outside of the body. (This is sometimes called an OSTOMY or UROSTOMY.)

Urethral cancer and invasive bladder cancer Because people with bladder cancer sometimes also have cancer of the urethra, the urethra may be removed at the same time that the bladder is taken out. If the urethra is not removed during surgery for bladder cancer, the doctor may follow the patient closely so treatment can be started if cancer of the urethra develops.

Radiation therapy Radiation may combined with surgery in advanced urethral cancer, or as primary treatment for early urethral cancer that has not spread. Radiation can be applied using external sources, or by surgically implanting radioactive seeds or pellets (BRACHYTHERAPY) to destroy cancer cells. External radiation and brachytherapy are sometimes used together. External beam radiation usually involves treatment five days a week for about six weeks. Brachytherapy involves surgical implantation of the seeds, which become inactive over time and remain in place.

Chemotherapy A number of different drugs can be used in combination to destroy urethral cancer that has spread. Commonly used drugs include cisplatin (Platinol), vincristine (Oncovin), and methotrexate (Trexall).

Prognosis
The chance of recovery depends on the stage of the cancer and the patient's general state of health. Five-year survival rates for noninvasive urethral cancer treated surgically or with radiation are about 60 percent. Recurrence rates for invasive urethral cancer treated with a combination of surgery, chemotherapy, and radiation are higher than 50 percent. Early diagnosis and treatment offers the best chance for cure.

urostomy   A surgically created opening in the abdominal wall through which urine passes, as part of the treatment for BLADDER CANCER. A section either at the end of the small bowel (ileum) or at the beginning of the large intestine (cecum) is surgically removed and relocated as a passageway (conduit) for urine to pass from the kidneys to the outside of the body through a stoma. The procedure may include removal of the diseased bladder. An odor-free pouch system collects the urine.

With a securely attached pouch, a patient can swim, camp out, and play baseball and most other sports. Doctors advise caution with heavy body-contact sports, but travel is not restricted. Patients may bathe and shower with or without the pouch in place.

Usually there are no dietary restrictions, although it is important to drink between eight and 10 glasses of fluid a day to help decrease the chance of kidney infection.

US TOO! International   The world's largest independent charitable network of education and support groups for men with PROSTATE CANCER and their families. Us Too! International and hundreds of local affiliated support group chapters offer education, publications, fellowship, peer counseling, treatment option information, and discussion of medical alternatives. The group's goals include education, advocacy, patient and family support, and public awareness of prostate cancer and prostate disease. For contact information, see Appendix I.

uterine cancer   The most common cancer of the female reproductive system in the United States, accounting for 6 percent of all cancers in American women. The most common type of cancer of the uterus begins in the lining (endometrium) and is called ENDOMETRIAL CANCER. Uterine sarcoma, a different type of cancer, develops in the muscle of the uterus (myometrium). Cancer that begins in the cervix is also called CERVICAL CANCER and is a different type of cancer.

Uterine cancer is usually curable when detected early. It is the third most common cancer in women, affecting more than 40,000 each year.

Risk Factors

Experts do not know the exact cause of uterine cancer, but women who get this disease are more likely than other women to have certain risk factors. However, most women who have known risk factors do not get uterine cancer, and many who do get this disease have none of these factors. Doctors can seldom explain why one woman gets uterine cancer and another does not.

Risk factors include:

Age   Cancer of the uterus occurs mostly in women over age 50.

Hormone replacement therapy (HRT)   Until recently, menopausal women experiencing unpleasant side effects were often prescribed replacement hormones to ease these symptoms. In the past, women who had no uterus could take ESTROGEN alone as a form of hormone replacement therapy; in other women, estrogen use alone (called "unopposed estrogen") had been linked to an increase in uterine cancer. Women whose uterus was still intact used a combination of PROGESTIN and estrogen as hormone replacement therapy; adding the progestin to the estrogen reduced the risk of uterine cancer.

For a long time, doctors had thought that using estrogen together with progestin as hormone replacement therapy would keep women healthier after menopause by reducing heart attacks and keeping the brain sharp. However, millions of women abandoned the estrogen-progestin combination in 2002, when a major federal study concluded that those pills raised the risk of BREAST CANCER, strokes and heart attacks. At that time, the scientists were not sure whether estrogen alone was as risky. Women abandoned estrogen-alone HRT in 2004, when studies also revealed serious stroke risks and lack of any heart benefits with this type of treatment.

Obesity   Because fatty tissue produces estrogen, obese women are more likely than thin women to have high levels of estrogen in their bodies, which may be why obese women have an increased risk of developing uterine cancer (and breast cancer). The risk of this disease is also higher in women with diabetes or high blood pressure (conditions that occur in many obese women).

Tamoxifen   Women who take the drug tamoxifen to prevent or treat breast cancer increase their risk for uterine cancer, which appears to be related to the estrogen-like effect of this drug on the uterus. Because of this, doctors monitor women taking tamoxifen for possible signs or symptoms of uterine cancer. The benefits of taking tamoxifen to treat breast cancer outweigh the risk that it will result in other cancers.

Race   Caucasian women are more likely than African-American women to get uterine cancer.

Colorectal cancer   Women who have had an inherited form of COLORECTAL CANCER have a higher risk of developing uterine cancer than other women.

Estrogen   Other risk factors are related to how long a woman's body is exposed to estrogen. Women who have no children, begin menstruation at a very young age, or enter menopause late in life are exposed to estrogen longer and have a higher risk.

Symptoms

Uterine cancer usually occurs around the time menopause begins or after. Abnormal vaginal bleeding with a watery flow that gradually worsens is the most common symptom. Women should not assume that abnormal vaginal bleeding is part of menopause. Symptoms include

- unusual vaginal discharge
- difficult or painful urination
- painful intercourse
- pelvic pain

Diagnosis

In the presence of symptoms, a doctor may do a physical exam and order blood and urine tests, or perform any of the following:

Pelvic exam   A pelvic exam can reveal the health of the vagina, uterus, bladder, and rectum.

Pap test   This test is typically used to detect cervical cancer, and cells from inside the uterus usually do not show up on a PAP TEST. This is why a BIOPSY is a better way to diagnose uterine cancer.

Transvaginal ultrasound   An ultrasound of the uterus uses an instrument inserted into the vagina.

If the endometrium looks too thick, a biopsy should be performed.

Biopsy A procedure that can be performed in a doctor's office to remove a sample of uterine lining tissue. In some cases, however, a woman may need to have a dilation and curettage (D & C), which can be done as same-day surgery with anesthesia in a hospital. A pathologist examines the tissue to check for cancer cells, hyperplasia, and other conditions. For a short time after the biopsy, some women have cramps and vaginal bleeding.

Staging

If uterine cancer is diagnosed, the doctor needs to know the stage of the disease to plan the best treatment. To find out whether the cancer has spread, the doctor may order blood and urine tests, chest X-rays, scans, or colonoscopy.

Usually, the most reliable way to stage this disease is to remove and examine the uterus during a HYSTERECTOMY and check the lymph nodes and other organs in the pelvic area.

Stage I: The cancer is only in the body of the uterus and is not in the cervix.

Stage II: The cancer has spread from the body of the uterus to the cervix.

Stage III: The cancer has spread outside the uterus, but not outside the pelvis, nor to the bladder or rectum. Lymph nodes in the pelvis may contain cancer cells.

Stage IV: The cancer has spread into the bladder or rectum, or beyond the pelvis to other body parts.

Treatment

There are many different treatment options for uterine cancer, but surgery is usually the first choice. Some patients also have RADIATION THERAPY or HORMONAL THERAPY, and others have a combination of therapies.

Surgery The most common surgery is a HYSTERECTOMY with an abdominal incision and removal of both fallopian tubes and both ovaries (bilateral SALPINGO-OOPHORECTOMY). The LYMPH NODES near the tumor may be removed for lab inspection; if cancer cells have reached the lymph nodes, it may

mean that the disease has spread to other parts of the body. If cancer cells have not spread beyond the endometrium, the woman may not need to have any other treatment. The length of the hospital stay may vary from several days to a week.

Some doctors are experimenting with less extensive ways of removing the uterus. For instance, they may use a lighted tube called a laparoscope to help remove the uterus through the vagina. The doctor also can use the laparoscope to help remove the ovaries and lymph nodes and to inspect the abdomen for signs of cancer.

Radiation therapy Some women with stage I, II, or III uterine cancer need both radiation therapy and surgery. Radiation may be given to shrink the tumor before surgical removal, or after surgery to destroy any remaining cancer cells. Radiation treatments may also be given to those women who cannot have surgery. Radiation therapy may be given either externally, five days a week for several weeks, or internally. Internal radiation involves the use of small radioactive tubes inserted through the vagina and left in place for a few days. The woman stays in the hospital during this treatment. To protect others from radiation exposure, the patient may not be able to have visitors or may have visitors only for a short period of time while the implant is in place. Once the implant is removed, the woman has no radioactive material in her body.

Hormonal therapy Sometimes medications can be administered to prevent cancer cells from getting or using the hormones they need to grow. If lab tests indicate that the cancer cells have estrogen and progesterone receptors, the woman is more likely to respond to hormonal therapy. Usually, hormonal therapy involves a type of progesterone taken as a pill.

The doctor may use hormonal therapy for women with uterine cancer who are unable to have surgery or radiation therapy, or if the uterine cancer has spread to the lungs or other distant sites. It is also given to women with recurrent uterine cancer.

vaccine   A form of BIOLOGICAL THERAPY that would encourage a cancer patient's IMMUNE SYSTEM to recognize and destroy cancer cells. The immune system is constantly scanning the body for foreign invaders, but because cancer cells originate in the body, they are usually not detected by the immune system.

In cancer vaccine technology, tumor cells would be removed, marked as "foreign" by adding a special gene, and then injected beneath the skin along with an immunostimulant (such as interleukin-2). This stimulates the immune system into thinking it has just been newly infected with cancer, so that it destroys this "new" antigen. Scientists hope such a vaccine would help the body recognize cancer and reject tumors, preventing cancer from recurring.

Unlike vaccines against infectious diseases, cancer vaccines are designed to be injected after the disease is diagnosed, rather than before it develops. Cancer vaccines given when a tumor is small may be able to eradicate the cancer.

Early cancer vaccine studies primarily involved patients with MELANOMA, but scientists are also testing vaccines for many other types of cancer, including LYMPHOMA and cancers of the kidney, breast, ovary, prostate, colon, and rectum.

In one study of vaccines against PROSTATE CANCER that had spread to the bone, patients were given 13 shots of the vaccine for four months: 41 percent who got a low dose and 70 percent who got a high dose were alive two years later, prompting researchers to schedule larger trials for late in 2003. The vaccine, known as GVAX, is also being tested for lung, pancreas, and colon cancers.

In a slightly different attack, scientists in California and Germany have successfully used an oral vaccine to stop cancerous tumor growth in animals by choking off the tumor's blood supply.

Researchers first targeted a protein produced in new blood vessels (VEGF receptor 2), one of several substances that trigger new blood vessel growth (a process called ANGIOGENESIS). New blood vessel growth is critical for cancerous tumors to grow and spread. When researchers administered genetically engineered bacteria that contained a gene to express the VEGF receptor 2 protein, it triggered the animals' immune system to fight off the mild infection from the bacteria— and in the process, killed the protein that spurs new blood vessel growth to the tumors. The vaccine worked against melanoma, colon cancer, and lung cancer in the animals. The immune response triggered by the vaccine destroys the blood vessels that nourish the tumor. Researchers estimate that studies in humans may not begin until at least 2010.

vaginal cancer   A rare kind of cancer in women that affects the tissues of the vagina. There are two main types of cancer of the vagina: squamous cell carcinoma and ADENOCARCINOMA.

Women of any age can have cancer of the vagina, but typically, squamous carcinoma usually occurs in women between the ages of 60 and 80 and accounts for between 85 and 90 percent of all vaginal cancers. Adenocarcinoma is more often found in women between the ages of 12 and 30, and accounts for between 5 and 10 percent of all vaginal cancers.

Young women whose mothers took DES (DIETHYLSTILBESTROL) to prevent miscarriage are at risk for getting tumors in their vaginas, including a rare form of adenocarcinoma called CLEAR CELL ADENOCARCINOMA.

Other types of vaginal cancer include malignant MELANOMA, LEIOMYOSARCOMA, and RHABDOMYOSARCOMA.

Risk Factors

The following risk factors have been linked to the development of vaginal cancer:

- *Age:* Half of the women affected are older than 60, with most between ages 50 and 70.
- *Fetal DES exposure*
- *History of cervical cancer or cervical precancerous conditions*
- *HUMAN PAPILLOMAVIRUS (HPV) infection*
- *Vaginal adenosis*
- *Vaginal irritation*
- *Uterine prolapse*
- *Smoking*

Although these factors can increase a woman's risk, they do not necessarily cause the disease. Some women with one or more risk factors never develop cancer, while others develop cancer and have no known risk factors.

Symptoms

The most common symptom of cancer of the vagina is bleeding after having sex. Other symptoms include

- bleeding or discharge not related to menstrual periods
- difficult or painful urination
- pain during intercourse in the vagina or pelvic area

Diagnosis

If abnormal cells are discovered during a pelvic exam, a biopsy of the vagina will be performed to check for cancer cells. The doctor should look not only at the vagina but also at the other organs in the pelvis to see where the cancer started and where it may have spread. The doctor may take an X-ray of the chest to make sure the cancer has not spread to the lungs.

The prognosis and choice of treatment depend on how far the cancer has progressed and the patient's general state of health.

Staging

The following stages are used for cancer of the vagina.

Stage 0 (carcinoma in situ): This very early cancer is found inside the vagina only, in only a few layers of cells.

Stage I: Cancer has occurred in the vagina, but has not spread beyond it.

Stage II: Cancer has spread to the tissues just outside the vagina, but has not moved into the pelvic bones.

Stage III: Cancer has spread to the bones of the pelvis and may also have spread to other organs and the lymph nodes in the pelvis.

Stage IVA: Cancer has spread into the bladder or rectum.

Stage IVB: Cancer has spread to other parts of the body, such as the lungs.

Recurrent: The cancer has recurred after it has been treated, either in the vagina or in another part of the body.

Treatment

Treatments are available for all patients with cancer of the vagina. In most cases, radiation therapy is used to treat cancer of the vagina. Surgery may be performed only for small tumors confined to the vaginal mucosa only. Chemotherapy rarely is used in treating vaginal cancer.

Surgery The most common treatment of all stages of vaginal cancer is surgical removal of the tumor. Laser surgery uses a narrow beam of light to kill cancer cells and is useful for stage 0 cancer. Wide local excision can remove the tumor and some of the tissue around it, but the patient may need to have skin grafts to repair the vagina after the surgery. In some cases, surgical removal of the vagina (vaginectomy) may be recommended. When the cancer has spread outside the vagina, the surgeon may remove not just the vagina but also the uterus, ovaries, and fallopian tubes. During these operations, LYMPH NODES in the pelvis also may be removed.

If the cancer has spread outside the vagina and the other reproductive organs, the doctor also may remove the lower colon, rectum, or bladder (depending on where the cancer has spread). A woman may need skin grafts and plastic surgery to create an artificial vagina after these operations.

vasectomy and cancer About one out of every six American men over age 35 has had a vasectomy, and some studies have suggested there might be a relationship between vasectomy and cancer (especially PROSTATE CANCER or TESTICULAR CANCER).

To this point, scientists who have carefully reviewed all of the data, including results from published and unpublished studies, believe that there is no consistent link between vasectomy and prostate cancer. Nor could experts find a convincing biological explanation for a link between vasectomy and an increased risk of prostate cancer.

Although most studies find no connection, a few have reported a link between vasectomy and prostate cancer. It is possible that other factors, including chance, may be responsible for the increased prostate cancer risk seen in these studies. Scientists expect that additional research will clarify this issue.

Several studies looking at a possible connection between vasectomy and prostate cancer are currently under way. The largest of these studies is the NATIONAL CANCER INSTITUTE's Prostate, Lung, Colorectal, and Ovarian (PLCO) Cancer Screening Trial, which began in 1992 and will end by 2015. The PLCO Trial is evaluating screening procedures for prostate cancer and will prospectively examine potential risk factors, including vasectomy, associated with prostate cancer.

Testicular cancer is much less common than prostate cancer, accounting for only 1 percent of cancers in American men. A few studies have suggested a link between vasectomy and an increased risk of testicular cancer, but it is possible that this increase may be due to factors other than vasectomy. It is also possible that the vasectomy procedure increases the rate at which an existing, but undetected, testicular cancer progresses. At this time, experts believe there is either no association, or only a weak link, between vasectomy and testicular cancer.

vesicant An intravenous CHEMOTHERAPY drug capable of damaging tissue and causing pain and swelling if it leaks into the skin. Many chemotherapy drugs will cause local tissue damage if they leak out of the vein. They include

- anthracyclines (daunorubicin, adriamycin [doxorubicin], epirubicin, idarubicin)
- antibiotics (bleomycin, mitomycin, actinomycin)

- mustards (mustine)
- vinca alkaloids (vincristine, vinblastine, vindesine)
- other (etoposide, tenoposide, amsacrine, mitozantrone)

virtual colonoscopy An experimental method that would allow doctors to examine the colon by taking a series of computerized tomography scans and then using a high-powered computer to reconstruct 2-D and 3-D pictures of the interior surfaces of the colon from these X-rays. The pictures can be saved, manipulated to better viewing angles, and reviewed after the procedure, even years later.

von Hippel-Lindau's disease (VHL) An inherited cancer syndrome that causes multiple tumors, including cancers of the kidney, eye, brain, spinal cord, and adrenal gland. This genetic condition involves the abnormal growth of blood vessels in some parts of the body, forming tangles of capillaries called angiomas or hemangioblastomas.

The disease can be different in every patient, even among members of the same family. Since it is impossible to predict which symptoms of VHL each person will have, it is important to check for all the possibilities.

The syndrome was named for Dr. Eugen von Hippel, who described the angiomas in the eye in 1904. Dr. Arvid Lindau described angiomas of the cerebellum and spine in 1926; his name is usually associated with occurrence of VHL in the central nervous system.

As the angioma grows, the walls of the blood vessels may weaken and some blood may leak out, damaging surrounding tissues. Blood leakage from angiomas in the retina can interfere with vision. Early detection and careful monitoring of the eye are very important to maintain healthy vision.

Some male patients experience tumors in the scrotal sacs. These are almost always benign but should be examined by a urologist because some could be malignant. Early detection and careful monitoring are particularly important for these organ systems.

Cause

Von Hippel-Lindau is a genetically transmitted condition caused by a dominant gene, although patients differ in age at onset, the organ system in which the problem occurs, and the severity.

Symptoms

There is no consistent set of symptoms from person to person. Angiomas in the brain or spinal cord may press on nerve or brain tissue and cause symptoms such as headaches. Cysts may grow around angiomas, which can exert pressure or create blockages that can cause symptoms. Cysts and tumors may also occur in the kidney, pancreas, or liver. If they affect the adrenal glands, high blood pressure may result.

Diagnosis

Anyone with a family history of VHL should be screened early in life before symptoms occur, usually by age six or younger. One clear screening does not necessarily mean there is no VHL present.

DNA testing is the best way to diagnose VHL. Using DNA testing, people with no symptoms have been found to have a change in the VHL gene even in old age. Although they themselves had no symptoms, their children were still at risk for VHL.

Once VHL has been diagnosed in any one part of the body, it is important to undergo a full screening for other possible evidences of the disease in other parts of the body, and to return for additional screening on the schedule recommended by the medical team.

vulvar cancer Cancer of the vulva (the outer part of the vagina) is a rare malignancy that can occur on any part of the female external reproductive system, but most often affects the inner edges of the labia majora or the labia minora. Less often, cancer occurs on the clitoris or the Bartholin's glands (small mucus-producing glands on either side of the vaginal opening). Most women with cancer of the vulva are over age 50, but it is becoming more common in women under age 40. In the United States, vulvar cancer accounts for about 4 percent of cancers in the female reproductive organs and 0.6 percent of all cancers in women. In 2003 about 4,000 cancers of the vulva were diagnosed, with about 800 deaths.

When vulvar cancer is detected early, it is highly curable. If the LYMPH NODES are not involved, the overall five-year survival rate is 90 percent. The survival rate drops to 30 to 55 percent when cancer has spread to the lymph nodes, and outlook for survival is influenced by the number of lymph nodes involved.

Types of Vulvar Cancer

About 90 percent of vulvar cancers are squamous cell carcinomas. Next most common are MELANOMAS, usually in the labia minora or clitoris. Other types of vulvar cancer include ADENOCARCINOMA, Paget's disease, SARCOMAS, verrucous carcinoma, and BASAL CELL CARCINOMA.

Squamous cell carcinoma Squamous cell carcinomas begin in the outermost skin layer. This type of cancer usually forms slowly over many years and is usually preceded by precancerous changes called "vulvar intraepithelial neoplasia" (VIN) (or "DYSPLASIA"). VIN is often divided into three categories—VIN1, VIN2, and VIN3—with the last closest to a true cancer. Alternatively, the precancerous cell changes may be called mild dysplasia, moderate dysplasia, severe dysplasia, or finally, carcinoma in situ. Not all women with VIN or dysplasia will develop vulvar cancer. However, because it is impossible to predict which women will, treatment of every woman with VIN is very important.

Verrucous carcinoma resembles a large wart and requires a biopsy to distinguish it from an actual wart. This form of vulvar cancer is a slow-growing subtype of squamous cell carcinoma and usually has a good prognosis.

Melanoma The second most common type of vulvar cancer (about 4 percent) is melanoma, which begins in the pigment-producing cells that determine the skin's color. About 5 to 8 percent of melanomas in women occur on the vulva, usually on the labia minora and clitoris.

Adenocarcinomas A small percentage of vulvar cancers develop from glands and are called adenocarcinomas. Some develop from the Bartholin's glands, which are found at the opening of the vagina and which produce a mucuslike lubricating fluid. Although most Bartholin's gland cancers are adenocarcinomas, some (particularly those developing from the ducts of the gland) may be different types, either transitional cell carcinomas or squamous cell carcinomas. Adenocarcinomas can also form in the sweat glands of the vulvar skin, although this is quite rare. Paget's disease of the vulva is a condition in which adenocarcinoma cells are found in the vulvar skin. Between 20 and 25 percent of patients with vulvar Paget's disease also have an invasive adenocarcinoma of a Bartholin's gland or sweat gland. The remaining 75 to 80 percent of cases have malignant cells only in the skin's top layer. Since a tumor in the Bartholin's gland is easily mistaken for a cyst, delay in accurate diagnosis is common.

Sarcomas   Less than 2 percent of vulvar cancers are sarcomas (tumors of the connective tissues under the skin), which tend to grow rapidly. Unlike other cancers of the vulva, vulvar sarcomas can occur at any age, including in childhood.

Basal cell carcinoma   Basal cell carcinoma, the most common cancer of sun-exposed areas of the skin, occurs very rarely on the vulva.

Symptoms

The most common symptom of vulvar cancer is itching. Other symptoms include burning or discomfort, a sore on the vulva, or changes in skin color. However, nearly 20 percent of women with vulvar cancer have no symptoms.

Cause

Recent studies suggest that squamous cell vulvar cancer can develop in at least two ways. In a third to half of all cases, infection with the HUMAN PAPILLOMAVIRUS (HPV) appears to play an important role. Two proteins produced by certain high-risk HPV varieties can interfere with the functioning of tumor suppressor gene products (called p53 and Rb). Vulvar cancers associated with HPV infection seem to have certain distinctive features. Women with these cancers often have multiple areas of VIN elsewhere on their vulvas, are usually smokers, and tend to be younger (aged 35 to 55) than typical vulvar cancer patients.

The second process by which vulvar cancers develop does not involve HPV infection. Vulvar cancers not associated with HPV infection usually are diagnosed in older women (aged 55 to 85) who rarely have VIN. DNA tests from vulvar cancers in older women not infected by HPV often show mutations of the p53 tumor suppressor gene; younger patients with HPV infection and vulvar cancer rarely have p53 mutations.

Because of their rarity, much less is known about how vulvar melanomas and adenocarcinomas develop.

Risk Factors

There are several risk factors that increase the odds of developing vulvar cancer; however, most women with these risk factors do not develop cancer, while other women without any apparent risk factors do. When a woman develops vulvar cancer or precancerous changes, it is usually not possible to say with certainty that a particular risk factor was the cause.

Age   Three-fourths of women with vulvar cancer are over age 50, and two-thirds are over age 70 at the time their cancer is first diagnosed. However, 15 percent of new patients are under age 40, and the number of vulvar cancer patients in this age group is increasing. The average age of women diagnosed with invasive cancer is 65 to 70, while women diagnosed with noninvasive vulvar cancer average about 20 years younger.

Human papillomavirus (HPV) infection   Human papillomavirus infection is thought to be responsible for between 30 percent and 50 percent of vulvar cancers. HPVs are a group of more than 70 types of viruses that are called papillomaviruses because they can cause "papillomas" (warts). Different HPVs cause different types of warts in different parts of the body; some cause common warts on the hands and feet, while others cause warts on the lips or tongue. Certain HPV types can infect the genital organs and the anal area. These HPV types are passed from one person to another during sexual contact. Sexual contact at a young age increases the likelihood of HPV infection and increases the time during which HPV infection may progress to cancer. Having a large number of sexual partners or having sex with persons who have had many sexual partners increases the risk of exposure to HPV. When HPVs infect the skin of the external genital organs and anal area, they often cause raised, bumpy warts. These may be barely visible or they may be several inches across.

Most genital warts are caused by two HPV types, HPV 6 and HPV 11. These rarely develop into cancer and are called "low-risk" viruses. However, other sexually transmitted HPVs have been linked with genital or anal cancers in both men and women. These are considered "high-risk" types of HPV and include HPV 16, HPV 18, HPV 31, and some others. Infection with high-risk HPVs often produces no visible signs until precancerous changes or cancer develop.

Smoking SMOKING exposes the body to many cancer-causing chemicals, which can be absorbed into the lining of the lungs and spread throughout the body. Among women who have a history of genital warts, smoking further increases the risk of developing vulvar cancer.

HIV infection Because HIV (the AIDS virus) damages the body's immune system, it makes women more susceptible to persistent HPV infections, which may, in turn, increase the risk of precancerous vulvar changes and vulvar cancer. Scientists also believe that the immune system plays a role in destroying cancer cells and slowing their growth and spread.

Low income Many people with low incomes do not have easy access to good health care, including routine gynecologic examinations. This may be an important factor in explaining the link between low income and increased vulvar cancer risk.

Vulvar intraepithelial neoplasia (VIN) Women with a condition known as VIN have an increased risk of progression to invasive vulvar cancer. Although most cases of VIN never progress to cancer, it is not possible to tell which will, so treatment and/or close medical follow-up is needed.

Lichen sclerosus This disorder, sometimes called lichen sclerosus et atrophicus, makes the vulvar skin very thin and itchy. This condition has been linked to a 4 percent increased risk of vulvar cancer.

Inflammation Some experts believe that chronic irritation of the vulvar skin by infections and poor hygiene may be a vulvar cancer risk factor.

Other genital cancers Experts estimate that up to 15 percent of women with vulvar cancer also have CERVICAL CANCER. The likely reason for this association is the role of HPV infection in causing both of these cancers.

Melanoma or atypical moles Women with a family history of melanoma or atypical moles elsewhere on the body are at risk for developing a melanoma on the vulva.

Diagnosis

A doctor may discover vulvar cancer during a routine pelvic examination. If there is a suspicion of cancer, the doctor may perform a biopsy of the vulva and check for malignant cells. This test is often done in a doctor's office.

Stages

Once cancer of the vulva is diagnosed, more tests will be done to find out if the cancer has spread from the vulva to other parts of the body. A doctor needs to know the stage of the disease to plan treatment. The following stages are used for cancer of the vulva.

Stage 0 (carcinoma in situ): A very early cancer in which the malignancy is found in the vulva only and is only in the surface of the skin.

Stage I: Cancer is found only in the vulva or the perineum, and the tumor is 2 centimeters or less in size.

Stage II: Cancer is found only in the vulva or perineum, and the tumor is larger than 2 centimeters.

Stage III: Cancer is found in the vulva or perineum and has spread to nearby tissues such as the lower part of the urethra, the vagina, the anus, or has spread to nearby lymph nodes.

Stage IV: Cancer has spread beyond the urethra, vagina, and anus into the lining of the bladder and the bowel; or it may have spread to the lymph nodes in the pelvis or to other parts of the body.

Recurrent: The cancer has recurred after it has been treated, either in its original location or elsewhere in the body.

Treatment

Treatment of cancer of the vulva depends on the stage of the disease, the type of disease, and the patient's age and overall condition, but surgery is the most common treatment.

Surgery A doctor may remove the cancer using one of the following operations:

- *Wide local excision* to remove the cancer and some of the normal neighboring tissue
- *Radical local excision* to remove the cancer and a larger portion of normal tissue around the cancer.
- *Laser surgery*
- *Skinning vulvectomy* to remove only the skin of the vulva that contains the cancer
- *Partial vulvectomy* to remove less than the entire vulva
- *Radical vulvectomy* to remove the entire vulva

If the cancer has spread outside the vulva and the other female organs, the surgeon may also remove the lower colon, rectum, or bladder (depending on where the cancer has spread) along with the cervix, uterus, and vagina. A patient may need to have skin grafts and plastic surgery to create an artificial vulva after these operations.

Radiation therapy Either external or internal radiation may be used to kill cancer cells. Radiation may be used alone, or may be used either before or after surgery.

Prevention

There are two ways to prevent vulvar cancer: avoid any controllable risk factors and treat precancerous conditions before an invasive cancer develops. These steps cannot guarantee prevention, but they can greatly reduce the chances of developing vulvar cancer.

HPV infection is a vulvar cancer risk factor that can be reduced by avoiding certain sexual practices, or by delaying onset of sexual activity. Recent research shows that condoms cannot protect against infection with HPV because HPV can be passed from one person to another via skin-to-skin contact involving any HPV-infected area of the body, such as skin of the genital or anal area not covered by the condom. (However, it is still important to use condoms to protect against HIV/AIDS and other sexually transmitted diseases.)

The earlier that sexual contact begins, and the more sexual partners a person has, the more likely it is that she will become infected with HPV, and the more time any HPV infection will have to progress to cancer. For these reasons, postponing the beginning of sexual activity and limiting the number of sexual partners are two ways to reduce the risk of developing HPV infection and vulvar cancer. Not smoking is another way to lower vulvar cancer risk.

Precancerous vulvar conditions can be identified by having regular reproductive system checkups and by having a doctor evaluate any persistent vulvar rashes, moles, lumps, or other abnormalities. Treatment of VIN can prevent many cases of invasive squamous cell vulvar cancer. Some vulvar melanomas can be prevented by removal of atypical moles.

Screening

A doctor routinely examines the vulva during a PAP TEST and pelvic examination. The AMERICAN CANCER SOCIETY recommends that:

- All women should begin cervical cancer screening about three years after they begin having sex, but no later than age 21.

- Screening should be done every year with a regular Pap test or every two years using the newer liquid-based Pap test.

- Beginning at age 30, women who have had three normal Pap test results in a row may get screened every two to three years with either the conventional (regular) or liquid-based Pap test. Or women over 30 may be screened every three years (but not more frequently) with either the conventional or liquid-based Pap test, plus the HPV DNA test.

- Annual screenings are recommended for women with certain risk factors, such as diethylstilbestrol (DES) exposure before birth, HIV infection, or a weakened immune system due to organ transplant, chemotherapy, or chronic steroid use.

- Women 70 years of age or older who have had three or more normal Pap tests in a row and no abnormal Pap test results in the previous 10 years may choose to stop having cervical cancer screening. Women with a history of cervical cancer, HIV infection or a weakened immune system should continue to have screening as long as they are in good health.

- Women who have had a total hysterectomy (removal of the uterus and cervix) may also choose to stop having cervical cancer screening, unless the surgery was done as a treatment for cervical cancer or precancer. Women who have had a hysterectomy without removal of the cervix should continue to follow the guidelines above.

Self-examination

Some doctors recommend that women examine their own vulvas for early detection of vulvar cancer and other disorders. A woman can become aware of any changes in the skin of her vulva by examining herself monthly. Using a mirror, she can look for any areas that are red and irritated, white, or darkly pigmented. Any abnormal growths, nodules, bumps, or ulcers should also be noted. These should be reported to a physician, since they may indicate vulvar cancers or precancerous conditions.

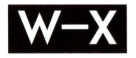

Wellness Community A national nonprofit organization dedicated to providing free emotional support, education, and hope for people with cancer and their loved ones. Through participation in professionally led support groups, educational workshops, and mind/body programs, people affected by cancer can learn vital skills to regain control, reduce feelings of isolation, and restore hope—regardless of the stage of disease.

With 21 facilities nationwide, the Virtual Wellness Community on the Internet, and international centers in Tel Aviv and Tokyo, the Wellness Community provides a free, homelike setting for people living with cancer and their loved ones to connect with and learn from each other. Services include counseling, support groups, networking groups, educational information, nutritional information, volunteer services, and addressing survivor concerns.

The Wellness Community was founded by Dr. Harold Benjamin in Santa Monica, California, in 1982 after his wife experienced BREAST CANCER. After subsequent years of study on the psychological and social impact of cancer, Dr. Benjamin formulated the Patient Active concept, which was recognized years later at the Walt Disney World Epcot Metropolitan Life exhibit as one of the most significant developments in the evolution of modern health care.

The Patient Active concept is based on Dr. Benjamin's belief that people with cancer who participate in their fight for recovery—who see themselves as partners with their physicians and health-care team—will improve the quality of their life and may enhance the possibility of their recovery.

From Dr. Benjamin's first program in a little yellow house in Santa Monica, the Wellness Community has grown to 22 facilities throughout the country with four additional facilities cur-

rently in development. For contact information, see Appendix I.

Wilms' tumor A type of solid tumor of the kidneys that is the most common KIDNEY CANCER among children. It is currently curable about 90 percent of the time, but patients sometimes relapse; if this happens, the disease can be fatal. This rapidly developing tumor most often appears in children between the ages of two and four and, unlike kidney cancer in adults, often spreads to the lungs. In the past, the death rate from this cancer was extremely high. However, treatment combining surgery, RADIATION THERAPY, and CHEMOTHERAPY have been very effective in controlling the disease. As a result, cure rates for Wilms' tumor have improved.

Diagnosis

If a child has symptoms, the doctor will assess the abdomen for lumps, perform blood and urine tests, and may order a special X-ray called an intravenous pyelogram. During this test, a dye is injected that helps the kidney appear more clearly on X-ray. An ultrasound, CT, or MRI scan may be ordered to better visualize the kidney. Chest and bone X-rays may also be taken.

If abnormal tissue is found, the doctor will need to perform a biopsy of the kidney to check the tissue for cancer cells. In Wilms' tumor, the appearance of cancer cells is very important. The child's prognosis and choice of treatment depend on whether the cancer has spread, how the cancer cells look under a microscope, tumor size, and the child's age and general health.

Staging

If Wilms' tumor has been found, more tests will pinpoint whether cancer cells have spread from the kidney to other parts of the body. The following stages are used for Wilms' tumor:

Stage I: Cancer is found only in the kidney and can be completely removed by surgery.

Stage II: Cancer has spread beyond the kidney to areas of fat, soft tissue, or blood vessels, but the cancer can be completely removed by surgery.

Stage III: Cancer has spread within the abdomen and cannot be completely removed by surgery. The cancer may have spread to the lymph nodes near the kidney, blood vessels, or the peritoneum.

Stage IV: Cancer has spread to other parts of the body, such as the lungs, liver, bone, or brain.

Stage V: Cancer cells are found in both kidneys when the disease is first diagnosed.

Recurrent: Cancer has recurred after it has been treated, either in its original location or in another part of the body.

Treatment

Wilms' tumor is treated with surgery, chemotherapy, or radiation. After several years, some children develop another form of cancer as a result of their treatment with chemotherapy and radiation. Clinical trials are ongoing to determine if lower doses of chemotherapy and radiation can be used.

Surgery This is a common treatment for Wilms' tumor and may involve one of three different types of operations:

- *Partial nephrectomy* removes the cancer and part of the kidney around the cancer and is usually used only in special cases, such as when the other kidney is damaged or has already been removed.

- *Simple nephrectomy* removes the entire affected kidney; the healthy kidney on the other side of the body can take over filtering blood.

- *Radical nephrectomy* removes the entire affected kidney with the tissues around it. Some lymph nodes in the area may also be removed.

Chemotherapy Chemotherapy drugs may be given either before surgery, to help shrink the tumor before removal, or after surgery, to kill any remaining cancerous cells.

A new genetic test may help better identify those children with Wilms' tumor who need more intensive treatment and those who can be treated with less. Researchers found a difference in the genetic makeup of Wilms' tumor that is present at first diagnosis and that seems to predict the child's chance of having a relapse in the future. The new test may also help scientists design drugs for more effective treatment of the genetic variant of the disease that is not now curable and may help some children avoid toxic treatment.

Doctors now look at the microscopic appearance of a patient's Wilms' tumor cells to separate cases into anaplastic tumors, which have a poor prognosis, and non-anaplastic, which have a good prognosis and are likely to be cured. But even within the good-prognosis group, a very small percent of children relapse. Scientists know that genes control almost all cell functions and that cancer usually begins with change in a gene. Scientists found that in all the tumors from patients who had relapsed, the genes on a certain part of chromosome 1q were activated and affecting the cells' growth. If they were not very active, then the tumors did not relapse.

Radiation Radiation may be used either before surgery, or after surgery and chemotherapy.

wine and cancer There are many biologically active plant-based chemicals in wine. Some scientists believe that particular compounds called polyphenols found in red wine (such as catechins and RESVERATROL) may have antioxidant or anticancer properties.

Polyphenols are ANTIOXIDANT compounds found in the skin and seeds of grapes, which are dissolved by alcohol produced by the fermentation process. Red wine contains more polyphenols than white wine because when white wine is made, the skins are removed after the grapes are crushed. The phenols in red wine include catechin, gallic acid, and epicatechin.

Polyphenols have been found to possess antioxidant properties, which means they can protect cells from damage caused by molecules called "FREE RADICALS." These free radicals can damage important parts of cells, including proteins, membranes, and DNA, which may lead to cancer.

Research on the antioxidants found in red wine has shown that they may help inhibit the development of certain cancers.

Resveratrol is a type of polyphenol that is produced as part of a plant's defense system in response to an invading fungus, stress, injury, infection, or ultraviolet irradiation. Red wine contains high levels of the antioxidant resveratrol, as do grapes, raspberries, peanuts, and other plants. Resveratrol has been shown to reduce tumor incidence in animals by affecting one or more stages of cancer development and has been shown to inhibit growth of many types of cancer cells in culture. It also appears to reduce inflammation and activation of a protein produced by the body's immune system when it is under attack. This protein affects cancer cell growth and metastasis.

However, it is still too early to make conclusions about the association between red wine consumption and cancer in humans. Although consumption of large amounts of alcoholic beverages may increase the risk of some cancers, there is growing evidence that the health benefits of red wine are related to its nonalcoholic components.

Xcytrin (motexafin gadolinium) A drug that makes certain tumors more sensitive to radiation, thereby allowing RADIATION THERAPY to kill off more cancer cells. A study of 30 patients with a kind of brain tumor called glioblastoma multiforme showed an increase in survival among those given the drug from 10 months up to 17 months. Possible side effects of the drug include skin discoloration, NAUSEA, and diarrhea.

Y-ME National Breast Cancer Organization

National nonprofit BREAST CANCER organization founded in 1978 by two breast cancer patients dedicated to providing information, empowerment, and peer support, so that no one faces breast cancer alone.

The group operates a 24-hour breast cancer hotline (800-221-2141), the only hotline in the United States staffed by trained peer counselors who are breast cancer survivors. It is a convenient, anonymous resource for breast cancer and breast health information, as well as support for anyone touched by or concerned about this disease. Callers can be matched with a survivor, patient, or supporter who has had a similar experience with breast cancer. The group also offers a monthly one-hour teleconference featuring a breast-cancer-related presentation by a medical professional followed by a question-and-answer session. Participants are divided into small groups for discussions, which are moderated by volunteers who match the profile of the participants.

Publications include a national quarterly newsletter providing the latest information on breast cancer issues, research, and concerns surrounding breast cancer, and *Latina News,* a bilingual quarterly newsletter distributed nationwide to address breast cancer issues, research, and concerns specific to the Latina community. Y-ME also offers a program to help men who are supporting a wife, mother, daughter, or friend through breast cancer.

The group's Web site (http://www.y-me.org) offers information and resources for the public and for medical professionals. Guests can submit questions concerning breast health or breast cancer and have them answered by breast cancer survivors within 48 hours. The site is available in both English and Spanish.

The organization also offers free wigs and prostheses to women with limited resources, monitors federal breast-cancer-related legislation and regulations, and works with several patient advocacy groups to impact breast cancer policy as it develops. For contact information, see Appendix I.

yolk sac carcinoma   A malignant tumor that produces ALPHA-FETOPROTEIN and is thought to be derived from primitive endodermal cells. The yolk sac tumor is the most common testicular tumor among infants and children up to age three. A pure yolk sac tumor is extremely rare in adults, but it is seen as a component in a MIXED GERM CELL TUMOR in about 30 percent of cases. It is also known as an endodermal sinus tumor or infantile embryonal carcinoma.

See also TESTICULAR CANCER.

APPENDIXES

APPENDIX I
ASSOCIATIONS

ADENOID CYSTIC CARCINOMA

Adenoid Cystic Carcinoma Organization
P.O. Box 15482
San Diego, CA 92175
http://www.orgsites.com/ca/acco/

ADVOCACY

Breast Cancer Resource Committee (BCRC)
2005 Belmont Street, NW
Washington, DC 2009
(202) 463-8040
http://www.bcresource.org

The BCRC is a nonprofit organization based in Washington, D.C. The goal of the BCRC is to reduce the incidence and mortality rates from breast cancer among African-American women.

Children's Cause, Inc.
1010 Wayne Street
Suite 770
Silver Spring, MD 20910
(301) 562-2765
http://www.childrenscause.org

The Children's Cause is dedicated to accelerating the discovery of and access to innovative, safer, and more effective treatments for childhood cancer via advocacy.

National Breast Cancer Coalition
1707 L Street, NW
Suite 1060
Washington, DC 20036
(202) 296-7477
(800) 622-2838
http://www.natlbcc.org

NBCC is a grassroots advocacy group of more than 300 member organizations fighting breast cancer through action, advocacy, and public education. Ser-

vices: referrals, education and training, advocacy, volunteer services.

National Childhood Cancer Foundation
440 East Huntington Drive
P.O. Box 60012
Arcadia, CA 91066
(626) 447-1674 (The Foundation)
(626) 447-0064 (Children's Oncology Group)
(800) 458-6223
http://www.nccf.org

NCCF funds research and treatment of children with cancer through the Children's Oncology Group (CCG), a network of 2,500 pediatric cancer specialists. Services: advocacy, public education, referrals to CCG treatment centers, and clinical trial information.

National Children's Cancer Society
1015 Locust Street
Suite 600
St. Louis, MO 63101
(800) 532-6459
http://www.children-cancer.com

A nonprofit organization that provides children (from birth to 18 years) who have cancer, and their families, with emotional support and direct financial support for cancer-related expenses. Services: financial and in-kind assistance, advocacy, support services, education and prevention programs.

National Latina Health Organization
P.O. Box 7567
Oakland, CA 94601
(510) 534-1362

An organization committed to working toward bilingual access to quality health care and self-empowerment of Latinas, through health education, health advocacy, and public policy. All Latinas as well as women of color are welcome.

National Patient Advocate Foundation
753 Thimble Shoals Boulevard
Suite A
Newport News, VA 23606
(757) 873-0438
(800) 532-5274
http://www.npaf.org

A national network for health-care reform which supports legislation to enable cancer survivors to obtain insurance funding for medical care and participation in clinical trials. Services: referrals, information education, advocacy, benefits and health insurance.

National Prostate Cancer Coalition (NPCC)
1158 15th Street, NW
Washington, DC 20005
(202) 463-9455
(888) 245-9455 (toll free)
http://www.pcacoalition.org

NPCC, a grassroots awareness and advocacy group, is interested in the outreach and advocacy of prostate cancer. Services: advocacy, public education, referrals, education information.

Ovarian Cancer National Alliance
910 17th Street, NW
Suite 413
Washington, DC 20006
(202) 331-1332
http://www.ovariancancer.org

The Ovarian Cancer National Alliance is a patient-led, umbrella organization uniting ovarian cancer activists, women's health advocates, and health-care professionals in an effort to increase public and professional understanding of ovarian cancer and to work toward more effective diagnostics, treatments, and a cure. Services: advocacy, referrals, education information.

AFRICAN-AMERICAN ISSUES

See RACIAL ISSUES IN CANCER.

AIRLINE TRANSPORTATION (FREE)

Air Care Alliance
1515 East 71st Street
Suite 312
Tulsa, OK 74136
(918) 745-0384
(888) 260-9707 (toll-free)
http://www.aircareall.org/

The Air Care Alliance is a nationwide league of humanitarian flying organizations dedicated to community service. The ACA has member groups whose activities involve health care, patient transport, and related kinds of public benefit flying.

Angel Flight America
50 Fullerton Court
Suite 200
Sacramento, CA 95825
(877) 858-7788 (toll-free)
http://www.angelflightamerica.org

Provides transportation to and from medical destinations for patients in financial need, 1,000 air miles from any departure point in the United States.

Corporate Angel Network
Building 1
Westchester County Airport
White Plains, NY 10604
(914) 328-1313
(866) 328-1313 (toll-free)
http://www.corpangelneetwork.org

CAN finds free air transportation (on corporate planes) for cancer patients who need medical attention. Patients must be able to walk.

National Patient Air Transport Hotline (NPATH)
P.O. Box 1940
Manassas, VA 22110-0804
(800) 296-1217
http://www.npath.org

NPATH is a clearinghouse for patients who cannot afford travel for medical care.

National Patient Travel Center (NPTC)
4620 Haygood Road
Suite 1
Virginia Beach, VA 23455
(800) 296-1217
http://www.patienttravel.org

The NPTC provides the National Patient Travel Helpline, a telephone service that facilitates patient access to charitable medical air transportation resources in the United States. The NPTC also offers information about discounted airline ticket programs for patients and patient escorts, operates Special-Lift and Child-Lift programs, and brings ambulatory outpatients to the United States from many overseas locations.

ALOPECIA

See HAIR LOSS.

ALVEOLAR SOFT PART SARCOMA

Alliance Against Soft Part Sarcoma
http://www.alveolarspsarcoma.net

AMPUTATION

American Amputee Foundation, Inc.
P.O. Box 250218
Hillcrest Station
Little Rock, AR 72225
(501) 666-9540
http://www.arcat.com

Provides information and referrals to amputees and their families and prints a National Resource Directory every two years as a source for amputees and professionals in the amputee related field. Services: people without financial means are given prosthesis devices. The agency makes referrals to different support groups and publishes a biannual newsletter. The Give-A-Limb program is unique (a person can apply for this program but must be approved by the board of directors). For those who have been denied SSI, for whom rehabilitation is not working, or for those too old or not old enough.

APPEARANCE

Let's Face It
P.O. Box 29972
Bellingham, WA 98228
(360) 676-2972
http://www.faceit.org

A nonprofit support network that links disfigured people and all who care for them to resources that can enrich their lives. Services: an annual resource directory and "self-help network" book, and phone consultations.

Look Good . . . Feel Better (LGFB)
CTFA Foundation
1101 17th Street, NW
Washington, DC 20036
(800) 395-5665
(202) 331-1770
http://www.lookgoodfeelbetter.org

A program that helps cancer patients improve their appearance during cancer treatment. LGFB offers workshops across the country, often in conjunction with the local American Cancer Society chapters. Services: makeup kits; free program materials; patient education; counseling; hair care, skin care, and makeup tips; voluntary services.

National Foundation for Facial Reconstruction (NFFR)
317 East 34th Street
Suite 901
New York, NY 10016
(212) 263-6656
http://www.nffr.org

NFFR is a voluntary organization aiding the rehabilitation of people suffering from facial disfigurement. Services: physician, hospital, or clinic referrals to those unable to afford private reconstructive surgical care.

ASIAN ISSUES

See RACIAL ISSUES IN CANCER.

ATAXIA TELANGIECTASIA

A-T Children's Project
668 South Military Trail
Deerfield Beach, FL 33442
(800) 5-HELP-A-T
http://www.atcp.org

BLADDER CANCER

American Foundation for Urologic Disease (AFUD)
1128 North Charles Street
Baltimore, MD 21201
(410) 468-1800
(800) 242-2383
http://www.afud.org

BONE MARROW TRANSPLANT

Blood & Marrow Transplant Information Network
2900 Skokie Valley Road
Suite B
Highland Park, IL 60035
(847) 433-3313
(888) 597-7674 (toll-free)
http://www.marrow.org

A nonprofit organization that provides publications and support services to bone marrow, peripheral blood stem cell, and cord blood transplant patients and survivors. Services: publishes a quarterly newsletter (*Blood & Marrow Transplant Newsletter*) for bone marrow, peripheral stem cell, and cord blood transplant patients; a resource directory; a "patient-to-survivor" telephone link; and a 157-page book describing physical and emotional aspects of marrow and stem cell transplantation. Another book, *Mira's Month* ($5), helps prepare young children for their parent's transplant. A directory of transplant centers, which includes information on types and number of transplants performed and diseases treated, and an attorney list, to help resolve insurance problems, are additional resources for the public.

Bone Marrow Foundation
70 East 55th Street
20th Floor
New York, NY 10022
(212) 838-3029
(800) 365-1336
http://www.bonemarrow.org

Provides eligible transplant candidates with financial assistance limited to help defray the cost of ancillary services needed to ensure proper care during the transplant procedure, as well as in pre- and post-transplant treatment phases.

**Bone Marrow Transplant Family Support
  Network**
P.O. Box 845
Avon, CT 06001
(800) 826-9376

A national telephone support network for patients and their families. Services include referrals, bone marrow transplant information, counseling, children's services, health insurance information. The network answers questions raised by the person calling and connects newly diagnosed patients with a recovered BMT patient who is the same age, has the same diagnosis, stage of disease, and so on.

National Bone Marrow Transplant (BMT) Link
20411 West 12 Mile Road
Suite 108
Southfield, MI 48076
(800) LINK-BMT or (800) 546-5268
http://www.comnet.org

BMT Link is a national clearinghouse on a variety of bone marrow transplant issues. Services: patient advocacy, referrals, and an excellent resource guide on BMT. BMT Link also funds research.

National Marrow Donor Program (NMDP)
3001 Broadway Street, NE
Suite 500
Minneapolis, MN 55413-1753
(800) MARROW2 or (800) 627-7692
(888) 999-6743 (Office of Patient Advocacy)
http://www.marrow-donor.org

NMDP maintains a registry of bone marrow donors, provides information on how to become a donor, and organizes donor recruitment drives. The program, which is funded by the federal government, was created to improve the effectiveness of the search for bone marrow donors. It keeps a registry of potential bone marrow donors and provides free information on bone marrow transplantation, peripheral blood stem cell transplant, and unrelated donor stem cell transplant, including the use of umbilical cord blood. The NMDP's Office of Patient Advocacy assists transplant patients and their physicians through the donor search and transplant process by providing information, referrals, support, and advocacy.

BRACHYTHERAPY

American Brachytherapy Society
11250 Roger Bacon Drive
Suite 8
Reston, VA 20190-5202
(703) 234-4078
http://www.americanbrachytherapy.org

BRAIN TUMORS

American Brain Tumor Association (ABTA)
2720 River Road
Suite 146
Des Plaines, IL 60018
(847) 827-9910
(800) 886-2282 (patient line)
http://www.abta.org

A national organization founded in 1973 that offers more than 20 publications about brain tumors, treatment, and coping with the disease; free social service consultations; a mentorship program for new support group leaders; and a resource listing of physicians. Services are provided free of charge to patients and to their families. ABTA also funds research.

Brain Tumor Foundation for Children, Inc. (BTFC)

1835 Savoy Drive
Suite 316
Atlanta, GA 30341
(770) 458-5554
http://www.btfcgainc.org

A nonprofit organization that provides information and patient services for children with brain tumors. Services: family support and education programs, public awareness and information activities, a telephone support network, and regular meetings and recreational events for children and their families. BTFC also funds research.

Brain Tumor Society (BTS)

124 Watertown Street
Suite 3-H
Watertown, MA 02472
(800) 770-8287
(617) 924-9998
http://www.tbts.org

The Brain Tumor Society exists to find a cure for brain tumors and strives to improve the quality of life of brain tumor patients and their families. It also raises funds to advance selected scientific research projects, improve clinical care, and find a cure. Services: BTS provides educational material for patients and physicians, and a resource guide, "Color Me Hope." Also offered are a support and information hotline (staffed by social workers), a newsletter, "Head Up," and a Brain Tumor Booklist, as well as funding for professional conferences and research.

Children's Brain Tumor Foundation

274 Madison Avenue
Suite 1301
New York, NY 10016
(212) 448-9494
http://www.cbtf.org

Group that seeks to improve treatment and outlook for children with brain and spinal cord tumors through research and treatment, education and support. Services: a monthly support group for parents who have a child with a brain or spinal cord tumor, a resource guide, and a newsletter.

Dana Alliance for Brain Initiatives

745 Fifth Avenue
Suite 700
New York, NY 10151
http://www.dana.org

The Dana Alliance, a nonprofit organization of 150 neuroscientists, was formed to help provide information about the personal and public benefits of brain research.

National Brain Tumor Foundation (NBTF)

414 Thirteenth Street
Suite 700
Oakland, CA 94612
(510) 839-9777
(800) 934-CURE
http://www.braintumor.org

NBTF provides information, counseling, and support services to brain tumor patients and their families. Services: a newsletter, a patient-to-patient telephone support line, a free resource guide, a list of support groups, and training for caregivers of brain tumor patients. NBTF also funds research.

National Institute of Neurological Disorders and Stroke

NIH Neurological Institute
P.O. Box 5801
Bethesda, MD 20824
(800) 352-9424

This federal institute conducts and supports research on many serious diseases affecting the brain.

BREAST CANCER

Breast Cancer Resource Committee

2005 Belmont Street, NW
Washington, DC 20009
(202) 463-8040

The BCRC is a nonprofit organization based in Washington, D.C. The goal of the BCRC is to reduce the incidence and mortality rates from breast cancer among African-American women.

ENCOREplus

YWCA of the USA
1015 18th Street, NW
Suite 700
Washington, DC 20036

(202) 467-0801
(800) 95-EPLUS
http://www.ywca.org

Encore Plus is for women over 50 years of age who need early detection information, breast and cervical cancer screening, or support services. Services: counseling, information, diagnostic screenings, rehabilitation, advocacy, transportation, housing, children's services, financial assistance. Call for local Encore Plus programs.

Judges and Lawyers Breast Cancer Alert (JALBCA)

369 Madison Avenue
PMB 424
New York, NY 10128
(212) 683-6630
http://www.jalbca.org

A confidential hotline for judges, lawyers, and law students who have been diagnosed with breast cancer.

Living Beyond Breast Cancer (LBBC)

10 East Athens Avenue
Suite 204
Ardmore, PA 19003
(610) 645-4567
(888) 735-5222
http://www.lbbc.org

An educational organization that aims to empower women with breast cancer to live as long as possible with the best quality of life. The LBBC offers an interactive message board and information about upcoming conferences and teleconf\erences on its Web site. In addition, the organization has a toll-free Survivors' Helpline, a Young Survivors Network for women diagnosed with breast cancer who are age 45 or younger, and outreach programs for medically underserved communities. The LBBC also offers a quarterly educational newsletter and a book for African-American women living with breast cancer.

Mothers Supporting Daughters with Breast Cancer (MSDBC)

21710 Bayshore Road
Chestertown, MD 21620-4401
(410) 778-1982
http://www.mothersdaughter.org

MSDBC helps women whose daughters have breast cancer, so they can better help their daughters cope with the disease and treatment. Call for information

and handbook. Services: referrals, counseling, support groups.

National Alliance of Breast Cancer Associations (NABCO)

9 East 37th Street
10th Floor
New York, NY 10016
(888) 80-NABCO
(212) 719-0154
(212) 889-0606
http://www.nabco.org

NABCO, a network of breast cancer organizations, provides information, assistance, and referrals to anyone with questions about breast cancer and acts as a voice for the interests and concerns of breast cancer survivors and women at risk. Services: information referrals, job discrimination-related advocacy, and professional education.

National Asian Women's Health Organization (NAWHO): Breast and Cervical Cancer

250 Montgomery Street
Suite 900
San Francisco, CA 94104
(415) 989-9747
http://www.nawho.org

NAWHO created Communicating Across Boundaries: the Asian American Women's Breast and Cervical Cancer Program to eliminate the threat of these diseases in Asian American communities nationwide by increasing provider awareness of and responsiveness to the health needs of Asian American women. Services: early detection screening, educational programs, health promotion activities, advocacy, raises awareness through community health forums and training sessions.

National Breast and Cervical Cancer Early Detection Program (NBCCEDP)

Centers for Disease Control and Prevention
4770 Buford Highway, NE
MS K64
Atlanta, GA 30341
(888) 842-6355 (toll-free)
http://www.cdc.gov/cancer/nbccedp

A government program that provides screening services, including clinical breast examinations, mammograms, pelvic examinations, and Pap tests to underserved women. The program also funds postscreening diagnostic services, such as surgical consultation and biopsy, to ensure that all women with abnormal results receive timely and adequate referrals. Services: breast and cervical cancer screening, referrals, public information and education programs, appropriate surveillance and epidemiological systems.

National Breast Cancer Coalition (NBCC)
1707 L Street, NW
Suite 1060
Washington, DC 20036
(202) 296-7477
(800) 622-2838
http://www.natlbcc.org

NBCC is a grassroots advocacy group of more than 600 member organizations fighting breast cancer through action, advocacy, and public education. Services: referrals, education and training, advocacy, volunteer services.

National Lymphedema Network
Latham Square, 1611 Telegraph Avenue
Suite 1111
Oakland, CA 94612-2138
(800) 541-3259
(510) 208-3200
http://www.lymphnet.org

NLN provides support, education, and information on lymphedema. Services: a toll-free information line, professional education, counseling, referrals, and a newsletter (membership fee required for newsletter).

Susan B. Komen Breast Cancer Foundation (SBKCF)
5005 LBJ Freeway
Suite 250
P.O. Box 650309
Dallas, TX 75244
(972) 855-1600
(800) 462-9273
http://www.komen.org

SBKCF is dedicated to eradicating breast cancer as a life-threatening disease through research, education, screening, and treatment. Services: a toll-free "Helpline" (1-800-IM-AWARE) staffed by trained volunteers, referrals, screening. SKBFC also funds research and other cancer-related programs.

Women's Healthcare Educational Network, Inc. (WHEN)
P.O. Box 5061
Tiffin, OH 44883

(800) 991-8877
http://www.whenusa.org

WHEN is an organization of independent businesses that specialize in serving women who have had breast surgery. Services: information and referrals to physicians, nurses, and managed care providers, specialty items like wigs, maternity and nursing products, compression therapy products, prostheses, etc.

Women's Information Network (WIN) Against Breast Cancer
536 South Second Avenue
Suite K
Covina, California 91723-3043
(866) 294-6222 (toll-free)
(626) 332-2255
http://www.winabc.org

A national nonprofit organization that offers information, resources, peer support and referral sources for breast cancer patients and their families through telephone counseling, mail support, and community outreach.

Y-Me National Breast Cancer Organization
212 West Van Buren
Suite 500
Chicago, IL 60607
(312) 986-8338
(800) 986-9505 (Spanish)
(800) 221-2141 (24-hr)
http://www.y-me.org

A nonprofit consumer-oriented organization that provides information, referral, and emotional support to individuals concerned about or diagnosed with breast cancer. Hotline is staffed by trained counselors and volunteers who have experienced breast cancer and can offer peer support. Services: referrals, educational programs, counseling, rehabilitation, advocacy, health insurance information. Y-ME Men's Support Line Monday through Friday 9 a.m. to 5 p.m. CST. Men can call the Y-ME 800 number and request to speak to a male counselor. The counselor most closely matched in experience to the caller will return the call within 24 hours.

Young Survival Coalition
Box 528
52A Carmine Street
New York, NY 10014
(212) 916-7667
http://www.youngsurvival.org

Organization that focuses on the issues and challenges faced by women aged 40 and under who are diagnosed with breast cancer.

CAMPS

See also CHILDREN.

Camp Adventure American Cancer Society
75 Davids Drive
Hauppauge, NY 11788
(631) 436-7070
http://www.bravekids.org

Camp Adventure is a one-week sleepaway camp program for children with cancer and their brothers and sisters, age six to 18.

Children's Oncology Camps of America
Children's Center for Cancer and Blood Disorders
7 Richland Medical Park
Suite 203
Columbia, SC 29203
(803) 434-3503

Hole in the Wall Gang Camp
565 Ashford Center Road
Ashford, CT 06278
(860) 429-3444
http://www.holeinthewallgang.org

Started and funded by actor Paul Newman, this summer camp is designed for children with cancer and/or serious blood diseases. The camp provides year-round activities for campers and other seriously ill children and their siblings at camp and in their own communities.

CANCER

AMC Cancer Research Center–Cancer Information and Counseling Line
1600 Pierce Street
Denver, CO 80214
(303) 233-6501
(800) 525-3777
(800) 321-1557
http://www.amc.org

A nonprofit research institute dedicated to the prevention of cancer. Services: provides up-to-date facts about all aspects of cancer as well as personal assistance from counselors trained and experienced in dealing with the fear, confusion, conflicts, and other problems often associated with the disease. All staff are paid professionals with degrees in counseling or related health areas. Through the CICL, members of the general public have access to the latest information on cancer prevention, detection, diagnosis, treatment, and rehabilitation, including the Physicians' Data Query (PDQ), a database of research studies and treatment protocols from the nation's cancer centers. The service mails out thousands of free brochures and other literature every year and helps put callers in touch with cancer-related resources in their communities. In addition, AMC-CRC funds research.

American Cancer Society (ACS)
1599 Clifton Road, NE
Atlanta, GA 30329-4251
(800) 227-2345
http://www.cancer.org

Dedicated to eliminating cancer as a major health problem through research, education, and service. ACS is a nationwide, community-based organization with chartered divisions in every state plus Washington, D.C., and Puerto Rico. Services: the variety of programs include but are not limited to "Reach to Recovery," "Cansurmount," "I Can Cope," "Road to Recovery," "Man to Man," "International Association of Laryngectomees," "Look Good . . . Feel Better," and "Resources, Information, and Guidance" (RIG). ACS also operates "Hope Lodges" (temporary housing) in selected areas.

American Joint Committee on Cancer
633 North Saint Clair
Chicago, IL 60611
(312) 202-5290

Cancer Care
275 Seventh Avenue
New York, NY 10001
(212) 712-8080
(800) 813-HOPE (4673)
http://www.cancercare.org

A national nonprofit agency offering a range of free support services to cancer patients and their families. Services: professional individual and group counseling, bereavement counseling, online support and counseling, educational programs, workshops, teleconferences, financial assistance, and referrals. Services are offered at all stages of the disease, to patients and to their families. Supplementary financial assistance is awarded for home care, transportation, and pain medication. The funds are limited to cancer treatment in the NY, NJ, and CT regions only. There are African-American and Hispanic Outreach programs, as well. Review the Web site for detailed program information and online services; Cancer Care has offices in New Jersey, Connecticut, and Long Island.

Cancer Hope Network
Two North Road
Suite A
Chester, NJ 07930
(877) 467-3638
(877) HOPENET
http://www.cancerhopenetwork.org

Cancer Hope Network is a nonprofit organization that provides free and confidential one-on-one support to cancer patients and their families. Services: volunteer training programs, peer support for individuals and families, and a toll-free information number. It matches cancer patients and/or family members with trained volunteers who have themselves undergone and recovered from a similar cancer experience. Through the matching process, Cancer Hope Network strives to provide support and hope.

Cancer Information and Counseling Line
1600 Pierce Street
Denver, CO 80214
(800) 525-3777
http://www.amc.org

Cancer Information Service
Building 31, Room 101A16
9000 Rockville Pike
Bethesda, MD 20892
(301) 402-5874
(800) 4 CANCER
http://www.icic.nci.nih.gov

Nationwide network founded by the National Cancer Institute (NCI). Calls are routed to local CIS offices where trained cancer information specialists answer virtually any question on cancer. More than 100 free pamphlets are available. In addition to answering callers' questions, the CIS is committed to increasing the public's awareness through outreach. The CIS Outreach Coordinator is available to groups and can help them set up their own education programs.

Cancer Net
Building 31, Room 10A03
31 Center Drive, MSC 2580
Bethesda, MD 20892-2580
(301) 435-3848
http://cancernet.nci.nih.gov/index.html

Cancer Research Institute
681 Fifth Avenue
New York, NY 10022-4209
(212) 688-7515
(800) 99-CANCER
http://www.cancerresearch.org

A nonprofit organization that funds research projects and scientists across the country. Services: *The Cancer Research Institute Help Book* and information on clinical trials using immunological treatments.

Cancer Survivors Network
American Cancer Society (ACS)
1599 Clifton Road, NE
Atlanta, GA 30329-4251
(877) 333-4673
http://www.cancer.org

Cancervive
11636 Chayote Street
Suite 500
Los Angeles, CA 90049
(310) 203-9232
(800) 4 TO-CURE

Assists cancer survivors to face and overcome the challenges of "life after cancer." Services: support groups, educational materials, insurance information and assistance, and advocacy for cancer survivors.

CanSurmount
(800) ACS-2345

Exceptional Cancer Patient, Inc. (EcaP)
522 Jackson Park Drive
Meadville, PA 16335
(814) 337-8192
http://www.ecap-online.org

EcaP offers programs and services to cancer patients, people with terminal illness, and health professionals. Services are based in Connecticut only; referrals are national.

I Can Cope
American Cancer Society (ACS)
1599 Clifton Road, NE
Atlanta, GA 30329-4251
(800) 227-2345
http://www.cancer.org

Information and Referral Network
http://www.ir-net.com/index.html

Provides a place where people who need help can find information about information and referral services and other community resources. A kind of "one-stop" shopping center for human services.

International Union Against Cancer
3 rue du Conseil General
1205 Geneva
Switzerland
http://www.uicc.org

National Comprehensive Cancer Network
50 Huntingdon Pike
Suite 200
Rockledge, PA 19046
(215) 728-4788
(888) 909-6226
http://www.nccn.org

A nonprofit alliance of the world's leading cancer centers established in 1995 to enhance the leadership role of member institutions in the evolving managed care environment. The NCCN seeks to support and strengthen the mission of member institutions by providing state-of-the-art cancer care, advance cancer prevention, screening, diagnosis, and treatment through excellence in basic and clinical research, and also seeks to enhance the effectiveness and efficiency of cancer care delivery.

CARCINOID CANCER

Carcinoid Cancer Foundation, Inc.
333 Mamaroneck Avenue # 492
White Plains, NY 10605
(914) 968-1001
(888) 722-3132
http://www.carcinoid.org

The foundation was formed to encourage research and education about carcinoid cancer.

CAREGIVERS

National Family Caregivers Association (NFCA)
10400 Connecticut Avenue
Suite 500
Kensington, MD 20895-3944
(301) 942-6430
(800) 896-3650 (toll-free)
http://www.nfcacares.org

NFCA provides educational and emotional support for family caregivers. Services: advocacy; individual, family, group, peer, and bereavement counseling; information education.

Well Spouse Foundation
P.O. Box 30093
Elkins Park, PA 19027
(800) 838-0879
http://www.wellspouse.org

A membership organization providing emotional support and information to the "well spouse" or the caregiver of the chronically ill. Services: a newsletter, local support groups, "round-robin" letter writing, an annual weekend conference, and bereavement counseling.

CERVICAL CANCER

See also DES.

Center for Cervical Health
54 Sunrise Boulevard
Toms River, NJ 08753
(732) 255-1132
http://www.cervicalhealth.org

The Center for Cervical Health is a nonprofit organization based in New Jersey. Its goals are to provide emotional support for women and their families touched by cervical disease and to provide information to the public and professionals on cervical health issues through education and advocacy.

ENCOREplus
YWCA of the USA
726 Broadway
New York, NY 10003
(212) 614-2827
http://www.ywca.org/html/B4d1.asp

National Asian Women's Health Organization (NAWHO): Breast and Cervical Cancer
250 Montgomery Street
Suite 900
San Francisco, CA 94104
(415) 989-9747
http://www.nawho.org

NAWHO created Communicating Across Boundaries: the Asian American Women's Breast and Cervical Cancer Program to eliminate the threat of these diseases in Asian American communities nationwide by increasing provider awareness of and responsiveness to the health needs of Asian American women. Services: early detection screening, educational programs, health promotion activities, advocacy, raises awareness through community health forums and training sessions.

National Breast and Cervical Cancer Early Detection Program (NBCCEDP)
Centers for Disease Control and Prevention
4770 Buford Highway, NE
MS K64
Atlanta, GA 30341
(888) 842-6355 (toll-free)
http://www.cdc.gov/cancer/nbccedp

A CDC program that provides screening services, including clinical breast examinations, mammograms, pelvic examinations, and Pap tests to underserved women. The program also funds post-screening diagnostic services, such as surgical consultation and biopsy, to ensure that all women with abnormal results receive timely and adequate referrals. Services: breast and cervical cancer screening, referrals, public information and education programs, appropriate surveillance and epidemiological systems.

National Cervical Cancer Coalition (NCCC)
16501 Sherman Way
Suite 110
Van Nuys, CA 91406
(818) 909-3849
(800) 685-5531
http://www.nccc-online.org

A grassroots advocacy group whose goal is to educate the public and legislators about the issues facing cervical cancer patients, including Pap smear reimbursement, access to testing for all women, and treatment and research in the field of cervical cancer.

CHEMOTHERAPY

CHEMOcare
231 N. Avenue
Westfield, NJ 07090
(800) 552-4366
(908) 233-1103

Chemotherapy Foundation
183 Madison Avenue
Suite 302
New York, NY 10016
(212) 213-9292
http://www.neoplastics.mssm.edu/sympbrochure.html

CHILDREN

See also CAMPS; HOSPICE.

Brain Tumor Foundation for Children, Inc. (BTFC)
1835 Savoy Drive
Suite 316
Atlanta, GA 30341
(770) 458-5554
http://www.btfcgainc.org

A nonprofit organization that provides information and patient services for children with brain tumors. Services: family support and education programs, public awareness and information activities, a telephone support network, and regular meetings and recreational events for children and their families. BTFC also funds research.

Candlelighters Childhood Cancer Foundation
P.O. Box 498
Kensington, MD 20895-0498
(301) 962-3520
(800) 366-2223
http://www.candlelighters.org

The foundation provides support, information, and advocacy to those whose lives are touched by childhood cancer. Services: a network of peer-support groups for parents, a "Youth Newsletter," a bibliography of cancer-related materials, an Ombudsman Program on insurance concerns, a long-term survivors' network, bereavement counseling, pain management, a speaker's bureau, and a toll-free phone number.

Children's Brain Tumor Foundation
274 Madison Avenue
Suite 1301
New York, NY 10016
(212) 448-9494
http://www.cbtf.org

Group that seeks to improve treatment and outlook for children with brain and spinal cord tumors through research and treatment, education and support. Services: a monthly support group for parents who have a child with a brain or spinal cord tumor; a resource guide; and a newsletter.

Children's Cancer Association
7524 S.W. Macadam Avenue
Suite B
Portland, OR 97219

(503) 244-3141
http://www.childrenscancerassociation.org

The Alexandra Ellis Memorial Children's Cancer Association is dedicated to improving the care and quality of children with cancer and life-threatening illnesses, and to easing the burdens of their families. Services: emphasis and direct hospital programs in Oregon only. Kids' Cart Tune hospital music program, Pediatric Chemo Pal Program; Alexandra Ellis Family Resource Center; Kids Cancer Pages—national resource on childhood cancer; Dream Catcher Wishing Program; and "Our Children, Your Patients" medical presentations.

Children's Cause, Inc.
1010 Wayne Street
Suite 770
Silver Spring, MD 20910
(301) 562-2765
http://www.childrenscause.org

The Children's Cause is dedicated to accelerating the discovery and access to innovative, safer, and more effective treatments for childhood cancer. Services: advocacy, counseling for children with cancer and long-term survivors, training workshops, educational programs, referrals, information on clinical trials.

Children's Hopes & Dreams Foundation Inc.
280 Route 46
Dover, NJ 07801
(973) 361-7366
http://www.childrenswishes.org

Offers pen-pal program for children five through 17 and siblings who have been diagnosed with a life-threatening and chronic illness or crisis situation. Services: housing/lodging and children's services.

Children's Hospice International
901 North Pitt Street
Suite 230
Alexandria, VA 22314
(703) 684-0330
(800) 24-CHILD
http://www.chionline.org

Nonprofit organization to promote hospice support through pediatric care facilities, to encourage the inclusion of children in existing and developing hospice/home care programs, and to include the hospice perspectives in all areas of pediatric care, education, and the public arena. Asks a fee for membership. Is currently expanding to reach out to professionals. Publishes a newsletter. Services: information and referral service for child care, counseling, support groups, and pain management. Also funds research and education.

Children's Organ Transplant Association, Inc.
2501 COTA Drive
Bloomington, IN 47403
(812) 336-8872
(800) 366-2682
http://www.cota.org

COTA provides support and financial assistance to the families of children who need organ transplants; educates the public about the need for organ donors; promotes and contributes to medical research to develop new antirejection drugs for transplant recipients; and builds a network of COTA organizations to coordinate services nationwide. Services: a speaker's bureau, cancer information, and a toll-free information line.

Kids Cancer Network
P.O. Box 4545
Santa Barbara, CA 93140
http://www.kidscancernetwork.org

A national nonprofit organization that offers a national cancer activities newsletter (The Funletter) to help children with cancer.

Locks of Love
2925 10th Avenue North
Suite 102
Lake Worth, FL 33461
(561) 963-1677
(888) 896-1588 (toll-free)
http://www.locksoflove.org

Locks of Love is a nonprofit organization that provides hairpieces to financially disadvantaged children across the United States under age 18 who are suffering from hair loss. Services: provides hair prosthetics, resources, volunteer services, a newsletter. Also, Locks of Love accepts tax-deductible financial contributions and donations of human hair. Hair donations must meet the following criteria: 10″ or longer, clean and dry, bundled in a ponytail or braid, and not overly gray.

Make-A-Wish Foundation (MAWF)
2600 North Central Avenue
Suite 936
Phoenix, AZ 85013

(800) 722-9474
(602) 279-9474
http://www.wish.org

MAWF is a foundation that grants "special wishes" to children (up to age 18) who have a life-threatening illness. Services: devoted to fulfilling dreams; wish requests are granted; volunteer services.

National Childhood Cancer Foundation

440 East Huntington Drive
P.O. Box 60012
Arcadia, CA 91066
(626) 447-1674 (The Foundation)
(626) 447-0064 (Children's Oncology Group)
(800) 458-6223
http://www.nccf.org

NCCF funds research and treatment of children with cancer through the Children's Cancer Group (CCG), a network of 2,500 pediatric cancer specialists. Services: advocacy, public education, referrals to CCG treatment centers, and clinical trial information.

National Children's Cancer Society

1015 Locust
Suite 600
St. Louis, MO 63101
(800) 532-6459
http://www.children-cancer.com

National Children's Leukemia Foundation (NCLF)

172 Madison Avenue
New York, NY 10016
(212) 686-2722
(800) GIVE-HOPE (out of state)
http://www.leukemiafoundation.org

One of the leading nonprofit organizations in the fight against leukemia and cancer for children and adults. The NCLF is established to support the unfortunate in various programs, to provide the cure for children and adults, and to ease the family's burden during their hospital stay. The 24-hour hotline (800) GIVE HOPE (800-448-3467) offers comprehensive information to any caller, and provides referrals for initial testing, physicians, hospital admissions, and treatment options.

Planet CANCER

1804 East 39th Street
Austin, TX 78722
(512) 481-9010
http://www.planetcancer.org

Planet Cancer is an international network of young adults (between ages 18 and 35) with cancer who support each other in communities online and face-to-face. Services: peer support, a "Planet Cancer Forum" where patients communicate directly with each other, advocacy, and "Adventure Therapy"—a type of outdoor expedition for young adults.

Ronald McDonald House (RMH) Charities

One Kroc Drive
Oak Brook, IL 60523
(630) 623-7048
http://www.rmhc.com

RMH is a national network of temporary housing facilities for families of children hospitalized with lifethreatening illnesses. Many states and major cities have Ronald McDonald Houses. Call for locations, service information, and eligibility. Services: housing/ lodging, referrals, and children's services.

STARBRIGHT Foundation

11835 West Olympic Boulevard
Suite 500
Los Angeles, CA 90064
(310) 479-1212
http://www.starbright.org

The STARBRIGHT Foundation creates projects that are designed to help seriously ill children and adolescents cope with the psychosocial and medical challenges they face. The STARBRIGHT Foundation produces materials such as interactive educational CD-ROMs and videos about medical conditions and procedures, advice on talking with a health professional, and other issues related to children and adolescents who have serious medical conditions. All materials are available to children, adolescents, and their families free of charge. Staff can respond to calls in Spanish.

Starlight Children's Foundation (SCF)

5900 Wilshire Boulevard
Suite 2530
Los Angeles, CA 90036
(323) 634-0080
(800) 274-7827
http://www.starlight.org

SCF grants the "special wishes" of critically, chronically, and/or terminally ill children aged 4–18. Services: provides in-hospital entertainment, grants wishes to ill children, and plans family outings.

Sunshine Foundation
1041 Mill Creek Drive
Feaster Ville, PA 19053
(215) 396-4770
(800) 767-1976
http://www.sunshinefoundation.org

This foundation grants the "special wishes" of critically, chronically, and/or terminally ill children, ages 3–21, whose families are under financial strain due to the child's illness. It is the original dream-granting organization.

CLINICAL TRIALS

Cancer Liaison Program (CLP)
Food and Drug Administration
FDA Room 9-49CFH-12
5600 Fishers Lane
Rockville, MD 20857
(888) INFO-FDA (toll-free)
http://www.fda.gov

As a division of the FDA, the Cancer Liaison Program works directly with cancer patients and advocacy programs. They provide information and education on the FDA drug approval process, cancer clinical trials, and access to investigational therapies when entering into an existing clinical trial is not possible. Services: provides information and education on the FDA drug approval process, cancer clinical trials, and access to investigational therapies.

Coalition of National Cancer Cooperative Groups, Inc.
1818 Market Street
#1100
Philadelphia, PA 19103
(877) 520-4457
http://www.ca-coalition.org

The Coalition of National Cancer Cooperative Groups, Inc., is the nation's premier network of cancer clinical trials specialists. Services: a variety of programs and information for physicians, payers, patient advocate groups, and patients, designed to improve the clinical trials process.

COLORECTAL CANCER

American Gastroenterological Association
7910 Woodmont Avenue
7th Floor
Bethesda, MD 20814

(301) 654-2055
http://www.gastro.org

Colon Cancer Alliance
175 Ninth Avenue
New York, NY 10011
(212) 627-7451
(877) 422-2030 (toll free)
http://www.ccalliance.org

An organization of colon and rectal cancer survivors, caregivers, people with a genetic predisposition to the disease, and other individuals touched by colorectal cancer. Services: information, quarterly newsletter, support program, and advocacy.

Colorectal Cancer Network (CCNetwork)
P.O. Box 182
Kensington, MD 20895-0182
(301) 879-1500
http://www.colorectal-cancer.net

CCNetwork offers support to colorectal patients, as well as to their family and friends. Services: advocacy; family, individual, and peer to peer counseling, information on clinical trials; referrals.

United Ostomy Association, Inc. (UOA)
19772 MacArthur Boulevard
Suite 200
Irvine, CA 92612-2405
(949) 660-8624
(800) 826-0826
http://www.uoa.org

UOA is an association of ostomy chapters dedicated to complete rehabilitation of all ostomates. Call for a listing of local chapters. Services: publication, OQ (quarterly newsletter), peer groups, and educational material.

CUTANEOUS LYMPHOMA

See LYMPHOMA.

DEATH AND DYING

See also HOSPICE.

Candlelighters Childhood Cancer Foundation
7910 Woodmont Avenue
Suite 460
Bethesda, MD 20814
(301) 657-8401
(800) 366-2223

Compassionate Friends

P.O. Box 3696
Oak Brook, IL 60522-3696
(630) 990-0010
(877) 969-0010 (toll-free)
http://www.compassionatefriends.org/

A national nonprofit, self-help support organization that offers friendship and understanding to bereaved families, following the death of a child of any age. Services: online support groups, a chat room, monthly meetings, monthly newsletters, literature, and a quarterly magazine.

Partnership for Caring

1620 Eye Street, NW
Suite 202
Washington, DC 20006
(202) 296-8071
(800) 989-9455
http://www.partnershipforcaring.org

Partnership for Caring is an advocacy and research organization protecting the rights of dying patients that provides information to help people prepare for end-of-life decisions. Services: referrals; guest speakers; counseling; legal assistance; patient advocacy; pain management; volunteer services; hospice care; distributes advance directives, including living wills, durable power of attorney, and explanatory guidelines appropriate to state of residence. Additionally, various publications, videos, and audios that deal with advance care planning and end-of-life issues are provided.

Widowed Persons Service

NY Service Program for the Older People, Inc. (SPOP)
188 West 88th Street
New York, NY 10024
(212) 787-7120 (ext 139)
(212) 721-6279
http://www.spop.org

SPOP's Widowed Persons Service, cosponsored by the American Association of Retired Persons, serves widows, men and women of all ages, offering peer support and information to the newly widowed.

DES

DES Action USA

610 16th Street
Suite 301
Oakland, CA 94612

(510) 465-4011
http://www.desaction.org

A nonprofit consumer group for professionals and the public concerned with Diethylstilbestrol (DES) exposure. Services: referrals for medical care, peer counseling, and newsletter (available with membership at $35).

DES Cancer Network (DCN)

514 10th Street, NW
Suite 400
Washington DC, 20004
(800) 337-6384
(202) 628-6330
http://www.descancer.org

DCN is a national organization for DES-exposed men and women who also have cancer. Services: advocacy and patient-to-patient support. DCN also funds research.

EYE CANCER

American Society of Ophthalmic Plastic and Reconstructive Surgery

1133 West Morse Boulevard, #201
Winter Park, FL 32789
(407) 647-8839
http://www.asoprs.org

A nonprofit organization founded in 1969 to advance training, education, research, and the quality of clinical practice in the fields of aesthetic, plastic, and reconstructive surgery specializing in the face, eyelids, orbits, and lacrimal system.

National Eye Institute (NEI)

2020 Vision Place
Bethesda, MD 20892-3655
(301) 496-5248
http://www.nei.nih.gov

One of the federal government's National Institutes of Health (NIH), the NEI conducts and supports research that helps prevent and treat eye diseases and other disorders of vision. This research leads to sight-saving treatments, reduces visual impairment and blindness, and improves the quality of life for people of all ages.

FERTILITY

Fertile Hope

P.O. Box 624
New York, NY 10014

(888) 994-HOPE
http://www.fertilehope.org

Fertile Hope is a national nonprofit organization addressing the reproductive needs of cancer patients and survivors. Services: awareness, education, financial assistance, research, and support.

FINANCIAL AID

American Amputee Foundation, Inc.
P.O. Box 250218
Hillcrest Station
Little Rock, AR 72225
(501) 666-9540
http://www.arcat.com

People without financial means can receive prosthesis devices. The agency makes referrals to different support groups and publishes a biannual newsletter. Foundation helps patients who have been denied SSI, or whose rehabilitation is not working.

American Kidney Fund (AKF)
6110 Executive Boulevard
Suite 1010
Rockville, MD 20852
(301) 881-3052
(800) 638-8299
http://www.kidneyfund.org

A national voluntary health organization dedicated to relieving the staggering financial burden associated with chronic kidney failure through patient aid programs and by offering direct financial assistance.

Bone Marrow Foundation
70 East 55th Street
20th Floor
New York, NY 10022
(212) 838-3029
(800) 365-1336
http://www.bonemarrow.org

Provides eligible transplant candidates with financial assistance limited to helping defray the cost of ancillary services needed to ensure proper care during the transplant procedure, as well as in pre- and post-transplant treatment phases.

Cancer Fund of America (CFA)
2901 Breezewood Lane
Knoxville, TN 37921-1009

(865) 938-5281
http://www.cfoa.org

CFA is dedicated to providing direct aid to financially indigent patients in the form of goods.

Corporate Angel Network (CAN)
Westchester County Airport
Building 1
White Plains, NY 10604
(914) 328-1313
http://www.corpangelneetwork.org

CAN finds free air transportation (on corporate planes) for cancer patients who need medical attention. Patients must be ambulatory.

Ensure Health Connection
P.O. Box 29139
Shawnee, KS 66201
(800) 986-8501
http://www.ensure.com

Provides coupons and valuable information to people in need of the nutritional supplement Ensure. Ensure donates their product to food banks, where a person in need may be able to receive a free supply when available.

Hill-Burton Free Hospital Care
5600 Fishers Lane
Rockville, MD 20857
(800) 638-0742
(301) 443-5656
Email: dfcrcomm@hrsa.gov
http://www.hrsa.gov/osp.dfcr/

Hill-Burton is a program run by the U.S. government that can arrange for certain medical facilities or hospitals to provide free or low-cost care. For information, call hotline or access through Web site (click on "Obtaining Free Care").

Medicine Program
P.O. Box 520
Doniphan, AL 63935
(573) 996-7300
http://www.themedicineprogram.com

Provides free prescription medicine to those who qualify. Services: assistance for medicine. The Medicine Program requires a $5 processing fee for each medication requested.

Mission of Hope Cancer Fund

802 First Street
Jackson, MI 49023
(517) 782-4643
(888) 544-6423
http://www.cancerfund.org

A nonprofit organization established by a cancer survivor to help cancer patients and their families with special financial needs. Our goal is to help relieve some of the extra financial burdens of cancer patients and their families while dealing with cancer treatment and recovery. Services: information education, counseling, housing, financial assistance, assistance for medications.

National Association of Hospital Hospitality Houses

4915 Auburn Avenue
Bethesda, MD 20814
(800) 542-9730
http://www.nahhh.org/

A nonprofit corporation serving facilities that provide lodging and other supportive services to patients and their families when confronted with medical emergencies: Services: referrals; housing/lodging facilities.

National Patient Air Transport Hotline (NPATH)

P.O. Box 1940
Manassas, VA 22110-0804
(800) 296-1217
http://www.npath.org

NPATH is a clearinghouse for patients who cannot afford travel for medical care.

Patient Advocate Foundation (PAF)

753 Thimble Shoals Boulevard
Suite B
Newport News, VA 23606
(757) 873-6668
(800) 532-5274
http://www.patientadvocate.org

PAF helps cancer patients deal with insurance coverage, paying for managed care treatment, and understanding managed care. Services: specializing in mediation, negotiation, and education on behalf of patients experiencing the following issues: preauthorization, coding and billing, insurance appeal process, expedited appeal process, debt crisis, job retention, access to pharmaceutical agents, access to chemotherapy, access to medical devices, access to surgical procedures, and expedited applications for Social Security Medicare, Medicaid, and other agencies.

Ronald McDonald House (RMH) Charities

One Kroc Drive
Oak Brook, IL 60523
(630) 623-7048
http://www.rmhc.com

RMH is a national network of temporary housing facilities for families of children hospitalized with life-threatening illnesses. Many states and major cities have "Ronald McDonald Houses." Call for locations, service information, and eligibility. Services: housing/lodging, referrals, and children's services.

FOOD ASSISTANCE

Ensure Health Connection

P.O. Box 29139
Shawnee, KS 66201
(800) 986-8501
http://www.ensure.com

Provides coupons and valuable information to people in need of the nutritional supplement Ensure. Ensure donates their product to food banks, where a person in need may be able to receive a free supply when available.

GENETICS INFORMATION

Hereditary Cancer Institute

Creighton University School of Medicine
California at 24th
Omaha, NE 68178
(800) 648-8133
(402) 280-2942
http://www.medicine.Creighton.edu/medschool/
    prevmd/hc.jtml

National Society of Genetic Counselors (NSGC)

233 Canterbury Drive
Wallingford, PA 19086-6617
(610) 872-7608
http://www.nsgc.org/

NSGC will promote the genetic counseling profession as a recognized and integral part of health-care delivery, education, research and public policy. Services: referrals, educational programs, genetic screening.

GOVERNMENT AGENCIES

Cancer Liaison Program (CLP)
Food and Drug Administration
FDA Room 9-49CFH-12
5600 Fishers Lane
Rockville, MD 20857
(888) INFO-FDA (toll-free)
http://www.fda.gov

As a division of the FDA, the Cancer Liaison Program works directly with cancer patients and advocacy programs. They provide information and education of the FDA drug approval process, cancer clinical trials, and access to investigational therapies when entering into an existing clinical trial is not possible. Services: provides information and education on the FDA drug approval process, cancer clinical trials, and access to investigational therapies.

Centers for Disease Control and Prevention Division of Cancer Prevention and Control (DCPC)
4770 Buford Highway, NE
MS K-64
Atlanta, GA 30341-3717
(770) 488-4751
(800) 311-3435
http://www.cdc.gov/cancer

The Division of Cancer Prevention and Control of the Centers for Disease Control serves as a leader for nationwide cancer prevention and control and as a partner with state health agencies and other key groups.

National Breast and Cervical Cancer Early Detection Program (NBCCEDP)
Centers for Disease Control and Prevention (CDC)
4770 Buford Highway, NE
MS K64
Atlanta, GA 30341
(888) 842-6355 (toll-free)
http://www.cdc.gov/cancer/nbccedp

A CDC program that provides screening services, including clinical breast examinations, mammograms, pelvic examinations, and Pap tests, to underserved women. The program also funds post-screening diagnostic services, such as surgical consultation and biopsy, to ensure that all women with abnormal results receive timely and adequate referrals. Services: breast and cervical cancer screening, referrals, public information and education programs, appropriate surveillance and epidemiological systems.

National Cancer Institute (NCI)
Building 31, Room 10A03
31 Center Drive, MSC 2580
Bethesda, MD 20892-2580
(301) 435-3848
(800) 422-6237
http://www.cancer.gov

NCI is the federal government's principal agency for cancer research. Services: NCI's comprehensive database, PDQ, contains: peer-reviewed summaries and the most current information on cancer treatment, screening, prevention, genetics, and supportive care; a registry of cancer clinical trials being conducted worldwide; directories of physicians, professionals who provide genetic services, and organizations that provide care to people with cancer.

National Center for Complementary and Alternative Medicine (NCCAM)
NCCAM Clearinghouse
P.O. Box 7923
Gaithersburg, MD 20893-7923
(301) 519-3153
(866) 464-3615 (TTY)
(888) 644-6226 (toll-free)
http://www.nccam.nih.gov

The NCCAM supports rigorous research on complementary and alternative medicine (CAM), trains researchers in CAM, and disseminates information to the public and professionals on which CAM modalities work, which do not, and why. Services: a toll-free telephone line, information packages, fact sheets, a newsletter, referrals, meetings and workshops, treatment information.

Social Security Administration (SSA)
Office of Public Inquiries
Room 4-C-5 Annex
6401 Security Boulevard
Baltimore, MD 21235
(800) 772-1213
http://www.ssa.gov

The SSA is the U.S. government agency that runs the Social Security program. It also provides information about retirement and disability benefits, Supplemental Security Income (SSI), and Medicare (the government program that pays for the medical care of the elderly). Services: a toll-free number, referrals, financial assistance, education information.

GYNECOLOGIC CANCERS

See also specific types of cancer.

Gynecologic Cancer Foundation (GCF)
401 North Michigan Avenue
Chicago, IL 60611
(312) 644-6610
(800) 444-4441 (toll-free)
http://www.wcn.org/gcf/

The Gynecologic Cancer Foundation is a nonprofit organization that supports programs designed to benefit women who have, or are at risk for developing, a gynecologic cancer. Services: information hotline, referrals, educational booklet, interactive Internet Web site.

HAIR LOSS

Locks of Love
2925 10th Avenue North
Suite 102
Lake Worth, FL 33461
(561) 963-1677
(888) 896-1588 (toll-free)
http://www.locksoflove.org

Locks of Love is a nonprofit organization that provides hairpieces to financially disadvantaged children across the United States under age 18 who are suffering from hair loss. Services: provides hair prosthetics, resources, volunteer services, a newsletter. Also, Locks of Love accepts tax-deductible financial contributions and donations of human hair. Hair donations must meet the following criteria: 10″ or longer, clean and dry, bundled in a ponytail or braid, and not overly gray.

Studio International
2100 18th Street
San Francisco, CA 94107
(415) 626-5583
http://www.studiosf.com

Salon based in San Francisco that specializes in working with those suffering from hair loss due to medical treatments. There is also a full service online salon.

HEAD AND NECK CANCER

International Association of Laryngectomees
8900 Thornton Road
Box 99311
Stockton, CA 95209
(866) IAL-FORU or 425-3678 (toll-free)
http://www.larynxlink.com

National Oral Health Information Clearinghouse (NOHIC)
1 NOHIC Way
Bethesda, MD 20892-3500
(301) 402-7364
http://www.aerie.com/nohicweb/

NOHIC, a service of the National Institute of Dental and Craniofacial Research, one of the National Institutes of Health, provides information for both patients and professionals regarding special care topics in oral health, including oral complications of cancer treatments.

Support for People with Oral and Head and Neck Cancer (SPOHNC)
P.O. Box 53
Locust Valley, NY 11560
(516) 759-5333
(800) 377-0928
http://www.spohnc.org

SPOHNC is a patient-run support group for people who have or have had oral, head, and neck cancer. Services: small group meetings, patient networking, a nationwide newsletter ($20/year), survivor-to-survivor network, and 18 chapters nationwide.

HELICOBACTER PYLORI

Helicobacter Foundation
P.O. Box 7965
Charlottesville, VA 22906-7965
http://www.helico.com

International Research Foundation for Helicobacter and Intestinal Immunology
P.O. Box 7965
Charlottesville VA 22906
(804) 977-1594
http://www.helico.com

HISPANIC ISSUES

See RACIAL ISSUES IN CANCER.

HOME CARE

See also HOSPICE.

Visiting Nurse Association of America (VNAA)
11 Beacon Street
Suite 910
Boston, MA 02108
(617) 523-4042g

(800) 426-2547
http://www.vnaa.org

VNAA provides information on all aspects of home health care, including general nursing; physical, occupational, and speech therapy; medical social service; home health aide and homemaker services; nutritional counseling and hospice care. Callers will be referred to a local VNS service. Services: educational information, referrals, home care/hospice care.

HOSPICE

Children's Hospice International
2202 Mt. Vernon Avenue
Suite 3C
Alexandria, VA 22301
(800) 242-4453
http://www.chionline.org

Hospice Education Institute
3 Unity Square
P.O. Box 98
Machiasport, Maine 04655-0098
(207) 255-8800
(800) 331-1620
http://www.hospiceworld.org

An independent, nonprofit organization serving the public and health-care professionals with information and education about the many facets of caring for the dying and the bereaved. Services: a toll-free information and referral service (HospiceLink), regional seminars, professional education, advice, and assistance.

HospiceLink
Hospice Education Institute
190 Westbrook Road
Essex, CT 06426
(800) 331-1620
(203) 767-1620
http://www.hospiceworld.org

National Hospice and Palliative Care Organization, The (NHPCO)
1700 Diagonal Road
Suite 625
Alexandria, VA 22314
(703) 837-1500
(800) 658-8898
http://www.nhpco.org

NHPCO provides information and referrals to nationwide hospice programs via a toll-free phone number.

Services: referrals, patient advocacy, research, public engagement, and professional education.

National Hospice Foundation
1700 Diagonal Road
Suite 625
Alexandria, VA 22314
(703) 516-4928
http://www.nhpco.org

Visiting Nurse Association of America (VNAA)
11 Beacon Street
Suite 910
Boston, MA 02108
(617) 523-4042
(800) 426-2547
http://www.vnaa.org

VNAA provides information on all aspects of home health care, including general nursing; physical occupational, and speech therapy; medical social service; home health aide and homemaker services; nutritional counseling and hospice care. Callers will be referred to a local VNS service. Services: educational information, referrals, home care/hospice care.

HOUSING (TEMPORARY)

American Cancer Society (ACS)
1599 Clifton Road, NE
Atlanta, GA 30329-4251
(800) 227-2345
http://www.cancer.org

ACS operates "Hope Lodges" (temporary housing) in selected areas.

National Association of Hospital Hospitality Houses, Inc.
P.O. Box 18087
Asheville, NC 28814-0087
(828) 253-1188
(800) 542-9730
http://www.nahhh.org

A nonprofit corporation serving facilities that provide lodging and other supportive services to patients and their families when confronted with medical emergencies. Services: referrals, housing/lodging facilities.

Ronald McDonald House (RMH) Charities
One Kroc Drive
Oak Brook, IL 60523
(630) 623-7048
http://www.rmhc.com

RMH is a national network of temporary housing facilities for families of children hospitalized with life-threatening illnesses. Many states and major cities have "Ronald McDonald Houses." Call for locations, service information, and eligibility. Services: housing/lodging, referrals, and children's services.

KIDNEY CANCER

American Association of Kidney Patients
3505 East Frontage Road
Suite 315
Tampa, FL 33607
(800) 749-2257
http://www.aakp.org

American Foundation for Urologic Disease (AFUD)
1120 North Charles Street
Baltimore, MD 21201
(410) 468-1800
(800) 242-2383
http://www.afud.org

The mission of the American Foundation for Urologic Disease is the prevention and cure of urologic disease, through the expansion of patient education, public awareness, research, and advocacy. Provides support groups for people with prostate cancer. Services: a toll-free phone line, a resource guide on prostate cancer, support group listings, referrals for incontinence and erectile dysfunctions. There is a Spanish-speaking operator available.

American Kidney Fund (AKF)
6110 Executive Boulevard
Suite 1010
Rockville, MD 20852
(301) 881-3052
(800) 638-8299
http://www.kidneyfund.org

A national voluntary health organization dedicated to improving the daily lives of people with chronic kidney disease. The AKF's primary goal is to relieve the often staggering financial burden associated with chronic kidney failure through patient aid programs by offering direct financial assistance.

Kidney Cancer Association (KCA)
1234 Sherman Avenue
Suite 203
Evanston, IL 60202
(847) 332-1051
(800) 850-9132
http://www.kidneycancerassociation.org

KCA is a membership organization providing information to professionals and the public and advocating on behalf of kidney cancer patients. Services: information and referrals, advocacy, professional education, and a speaker's bureau. KCA also funds research.

National Kidney Foundation
30 East 33rd Street
New York, NY 10016
(800) 622-9010
http://www.kidney.org

National Kidney and Urologic Diseases
Information Clearinghouse
3 Information Way
Bethesda, MD 20892
(301) 654-4415

KLINEFELTER'S SYNDROME

Klinefelter Syndrome Associates
P.O. Box 119
Roseville, CA 95678-0119
(916) 773-2999
http://www.genetic.org/ks

LATINO ISSUES

See RACIAL ISSUES IN CANCER.

LEGAL ISSUES

Cancer Legal Resource Center
919 South Albany Street
Los Angeles, CA 90019-0015
(213) 736-1455
http://www.lls.edu/community/clrc.htm

LESBIAN/GAY GROUPS

Mary-Helen Mautner Project for Lesbians with Cancer (MHMPLC)
1707 L Street, NW
Washington, DC 20036
(202) 332-5536
http://www.mautnerproject.org

MHMPLC provides services and support to lesbians who have cancer, their partners, and their caregivers.

Services: advocating for benefits, volunteer services (home care, etc.), transportation to and from treatment, legal assistance, bereavement counseling, support groups, library, and a smoking cessation program.

LEUKEMIA

Leukemia & Lymphoma Society
1311 Mamaroneck Avenue
White Plains, NY 10605
(914) 949-5213
(800) 955-4572
http://www.leukemia-lymphoma.org

The Leukemia and Lymphoma Society's mission is to cure leukemia, lymphoma, Hodgkin's disease, and myeloma, and to improve the quality of life of patients and their families. The Society has dedicated itself to being one of the top-rated voluntary health agencies in terms of dollars that directly fund our mission. Services: counseling, referrals, survivor concerns, volunteer services, financial assistance. Each of the 59 chapters offers: First Connection, a peer-to-peer support program for patients and survivors; a Family Support Group; patient education programs; Trish Greene Back to School program for children with cancer; the Information Resource Center.

Leukemia Society of America
733 Third Avenue
New York, NY 10017
(800) 955-4572
(812) 573-8484

National Children's Leukemia Foundation (NCLF)
172 Madison Avenue
New York, NY 10016
(212) 686-2722
(800) GIVE-HOPE (out of state)
http://www.leukemiafoundation.org

One of the leading nonprofit organizations in the fight against leukemia and cancer for children and adults. The NCLF is established to support the unfortunate in various programs, to provide the cure for children and adults, and to ease the family's burden during their hospital stay. The 24-hour hotline (800) GIVE HOPE (800-448-3467) offers comprehensive information to any caller and provides referrals for initial testing, physicians, hospital admissions, and treatment options.

LIVER CANCER

American Liver Foundation
75 Maiden Lane
Suite 603
New York, NY 10038
(800) 465-4837 (toll-free)
(888) 4HEP-USA
http://www.liverfoundation.org

A national, voluntary nonprofit organization dedicated to the prevention, treatment, and cure of hepatitis and other liver diseases through research, education, and legal or patient advocacy assistance. Services: referrals, a newsletter, provides guest speakers, advocacy. The Foundation also provides funding for research and educational programs.

LUNG CANCER

Alliance for Lung Cancer Advocacy, Support, and Education (ALCASE)
P.O. Box 849
Vancouver, WA 98666
(360) 696-2436
(800) 298-2436
http://www.alcase.org

ALCASE is an advocacy, support, and education organization that helps people with lung cancer and their families. Services: a toll-free telephone support and information line, a quarterly newsletter "Spirit and Breath," customized information, and a resource list.

American Lung Association (ALA)
61 Broadway
6th Floor
New York, NY 10006
(212) 315-8700
(800) LUNG-USA
http://www.lungusa.org

ALA is a national nonprofit organization dedicated to conquering lung disease and promoting lung health. Services: provides cancer information, professional education, smoking cessation programs, and a speakers bureau.

Lung Cancer.org
(877) 646-LUNG or (877) 646-5864
http://www.lungcancer.org

LYMPHEDEMA

National Lymphedema Network
2211 Post Street
Suite 404
San Francisco, CA 94115-3427
(800) 541-3259
http://www.lymphnet.org

LYMPHOMA

Cure for Lymphoma Foundation
215 Lexington Avenue
New York, NY 10016
(212) 213-9595
(800) CFL-6848
http://www.cfl.org

A nonprofit organization established to raise money for lymphoma research, support, and education for those whose lives have been touched by lymphoma.

Cutaneous Lymphoma Network
c/o Department of Dermatology
234 Goodman Street
Cincinnati, OH 45267-0523
http://www.med.uc.edu/departme/dermatol/
    dermatol.htm

Provides a newsletter distributed quarterly to 1,800 physicians and patients. Working on producing a videotape to educate about the disease and treatment.

Leukemia & Lymphoma Society
1311 Mamaroneck Avenue
White Plains, NY 10605
(914) 949-5213
http://www.leukemia.org

The world's largest voluntary health organization dedicated to funding blood cancer research, education, and patient services. The society's mission is to cure leukemia, lymphoma, Hodgkin's disease, and myeloma, and to improve the quality of life of patients and their families. Since its founding in 1949, the society has provided more than $280 million for research specifically targeting blood-related cancers.

Lymphoma Foundation of America
P.O. Box 15335
Chevy Chase, MD 20825
(202) 223-6181

Lymphoma Foundation of American is a nonprofit charitable organization devoted to helping lymphoma patients and their families.

Lymphoma Research Foundation (LRF)
111 Broadway
19th Floor
New York, NY 10006
(212) 348-2810
(800) 235-6848
http://www.lymphoma.org

LRF raises money for lymphoma medical research and provides support and education for lymphoma patients and families. Services: "patient-to-patient" telephone network, a Buddy Program, library, newsletter, counseling, advocacy, and financial assistance.

MOUTH CANCER

See ORAL CANCER.

MULTIPLE MYELOMA

International Myeloma Foundation (IMF)
12650 Riverside Drive
Suite 206
North Hollywood, CA 91607-3421
(818) 487-7455
(800) 452-2873 (United States and Canada)
http://www.myeloma.org

IMF provides up-to-date information and services for the treatment and management of multiple myeloma. Services: a toll-free hotline, patient and family seminars, clinical conferences, and a bimonthly newsletter, Myeloma Today. IMF also funds research.

Multiple Myeloma Research Foundation (MMRF)
3 Forest Street
New Canaan, CT 06840
(203) 972-1250
http://www.multiplemyeloma.org

The MMRF provides research funding in the field of multiple myeloma, and information to people with cancer and their family members. Services: a quarterly newsletter, research roundtables, seminars, advocacy, fund-raising events, referrals to support groups and financial assistance.

NASOPHARYNGEAL CANCER

International Association of Laryngectomees
8900 Thornton Road
Box 99311
Stockton, CA 95209
(866) IAL-FORU or 425-3678
http://www.larynxlink.com

ORAL CANCER

**National Oral Health Information
  Clearinghouse (NOHIC)**
1 NOHIC Way
Bethesda, MD 20892-3500
(301) 402-7364
http://www.aerie.com/nohicweb/

NOHIC, a service of the National Institute of Dental and Craniofacial Research, one of the National Institutes of Health, provides information for both patients and professionals regarding special care topics in oral health, including oral complications of cancer treatments.

Oral Cancer Foundation
3419 Via Lido #205
Newport Beach, CA 92663
(949) 646-8000
http://www.oralcancerfoundation.org

A nonprofit organization dedicated to saving lives through education, research, prevention, advocacy, and support for persons with oral cancer. The Foundation provides an online Oral Cancer Forum, which includes a message board and chat room that connect newly diagnosed patients, family members, and the public.

**Support for People with Oral and Head and
  Neck Cancer (SPOHNC)**
P.O. Box 53
Locust Valley, Ny 11560
(516) 759-5333
(800) 377-0928
http://www.spohnc.org

SPOHNC is a patient-run support group for people who have or have had oral, head, and neck cancer. Services: small group meetings, patient networking, a nationwide newsletter ($20/year), survivor-to-survivor network, and 18 chapters nationwide.

ORGAN TRANSPLANTS

**Children's Organ Transplant Association, Inc.
  (COTA)**
2501 COTA Drive
Bloomington, IN 47403
(812) 336-8872
(800) 366-2682
http://www.cota.org

COTA provides support and financial assistance to the families of children who need organ transplants; educates the public about the need for organ donors; promotes and contributes to medical research to develop new antirejection drugs for transplant recipients; and builds a network of COTA organizations to coordinate services nationwide. Services: a speaker's bureau, cancer information, and a toll-free information line.

OSTOMY PATIENTS

See also COLORECTAL CANCER.

United Ostomy Association, Inc. (UOA)
19772 MacArthur Boulevard
Suite 200
Irvine, CA 92612-2405
(949) 660-8624
(800) 826-0826
http://www.uoa.org

UOA is an association of ostomy chapters dedicated to complete rehabilitation of all ostomates. Call for a listing of local chapters. Services: publication, OQ (quarterly newsletter), peer groups, and educational material.

OVARIAN CANCER

**Gilda Radner Familial Ovarian Cancer Registry
  (FOCR)**
Roswell Park Cancer Institute
Elm and Carlton Streets
Buffalo, NY 14263
(800) 682-7426
(716) 845-3110
http://www.ovariancancer.com

A project collecting data on the link between heredity and ovarian cancer. Services: genetic counseling, support groups, referrals, and assistance with genetic screening. (FOCR is not a treatment center.)

National Ovarian Cancer Coalition (NOCC)
500 NE Spanish River Boulevard
Suite 14
Boca Raton, FL 33431
(561) 393-0005
(888) OVARIAN
http://www.ovarian.org

NOCC's mission is to raise awareness about ovarian cancer and to promote education about the disease. NOCC has chapters throughout the country. Services: patient advocacy, toll-free phone line, information education, referrals.

Ovarian Cancer National Alliance
910 17th Street, NW
Suite 413
Washington, DC 20006
(202) 331-1332
http://www.ovariancancer.org

The Ovarian Cancer National Alliance is a patient-led, umbrella organization uniting ovarian cancer activists, women's health advocates, and health-care professionals in an effort to increase public and professional understanding of ovarian cancer and to work toward more effective diagnostics, treatments, and a cure. Services: advocacy, referrals, education information.

Yale University—Ovarian Screening Program
Yale Comprehensive Cancer Center—OB/GYN
P.O. Box 208063
New Haven, CT 06520-8063
(203) 785-4014

University offers information and screening (nationwide) to anyone at "high risk" for ovarian cancer (e.g., a mother, sister, grandmother, or aunt who has had ovarian cancer). Clinical trials are also available. Services: referrals, and genetic and diagnostic screenings.

PAIN

American Chronic Pain Association (ACPA)
P.O. Box 850
Rocklin, CA 95677
(800) 533-3231
http://www.theacpa.org

A self-help organization that offers educational material and peer support to help people combat chronic pain. Services: refers to pain control facilities. Has publications on managing daily pain. Organizes support groups; call for a referral. Publishes a quarterly newsletter and a book on coping with pain for which a donation is requested. Provides no direct physician referral, or for biofeedback, hypnosis, etc.

American Pain Society
4700 West Lake Avenue
Glenview, IL 60025
(847) 375-4715
http://www.ampainsoc.org

A multidisciplinary educational and scientific organization dedicated to serving people in pain. Members research and treat pain and advocate for patients with pain. Services: the "Pain Facilities Directory" has information on more than 500 "specialized pain treatment centers" across the country (these are usually a part or a program of a hospital, clinic, or medical care complex); counseling for pain; referrals; education programs.

**National Chronic Pain Outreach
   Association, Inc.**
P.O. Box 274
Millboro, VA 24460
(540) 862-9437
http://www.chronicpain.org

A nonprofit organization whose purpose is to lessen the suffering of people with chronic pain by educating pain sufferers, health-care professionals, and the public about chronic pain and its management.

PANCREATIC CANCER

Hirshberg Foundation for Pancreatic Cancer
375 Homewood Road
Los Angeles, CA 90049
(310) 472-6310
Email: agirsh@aol.com
http://www.pancreatic.org

National nonprofit organization, supported by donations, serves as a help line for patients with pancreatic cancer. Primary function is to fund research for early detection of this cancer. Services: referrals, counseling, home care/hospice. Two research laboratories at UCLA Medical Center are the major recipients of the research grants. Patient financial aid is offered.

National Pancreas Foundation
P.O. Box 15333
Boston, MA 02215
http://www.pancreasfoundation.org/

Nonprofit foundation that supports research into diseases of the pancreas and provides information and humanitarian services to those people who are suffering from such illnesses.

Pancreatic Cancer Action Network (PANCAN)
2221 Rosecrans Avenue
Suite 131
El Segundo, CA 90245
(877) 2-PANCAN
(310) 725-0025
http://www.pancan.org

A nonprofit advocacy organization that educates health professionals and the general public about pancreatic cancer to increase awareness of the disease. PanCan also advocates for increased funding of pancreatic cancer research and promotes access to and awareness of the latest medical advances, support networks, clinical trials, and reimbursement for care.

PARENTS' ISSUES

Candlelighters Childhood Cancer Foundation
7910 Woodmont Avenue
Suite 460
Bethesda, MD 20814
(301) 657-8401
(800) 366-2223
http://www.candlelighters.org

Compassionate Friends
P.O. Box 3696
Oak Brook, IL 60522-3696
(630) 990-0010
(877) 969-0010 (toll-free)
http://www.compassionatefriends.org/

A national nonprofit, self-help support organization that offers friendship and understanding to bereaved families, following the death of a child of any age. Services: online support groups, a chat room, monthly meetings, monthly newsletters, literature, and a quarterly magazine.

PITUITARY TUMOR

Pituitary Network Association
P.O. Box 1958
Thousand Oaks, CA 91358
(805) 499-9973
http://www.pituitary.org

PREGNANCY AND CANCER

Pregnant With Cancer Support Group
P.O. Box 1243
Buffalo, NY 14220
(800) 743-6724 (ext 308)
http://pregnantwithcancer.org

A national organization created to offer hope and support to women who are diagnosed with cancer while pregnant. Services: education information, peer counseling, medical referrals, a free quarterly newsletter, survivor concerns.

PROFESSIONAL GROUPS

American College of Radiology
1891 Preston White Drive
Reston, VA 20191
(703) 648-8912
(703) 648-8900
(800) 227-5463
http://www.acr.org

A medical professional organization designed to advance the science of radiology, improve radiologic service to the patient, study the economic aspects of the practice of radiology, and encourage improved and continuing education for radiologists and allied professional fields.

American Society of Clinical Oncology
1900 Duke Street
Suite 200
Alexandria, VA 22314
(703) 299-0150
http://www.asco.org

An organization that represents more than 10,000 cancer professionals worldwide and offers scientific and educational programs and other initiatives intended to foster the exchange of information about cancer. Services: "ASCO OnLine" offers services for both professionals and people with cancer, including extensive information on its patient page.

Association of Community Cancer Centers
11600 Nebel Street
Suite 201
Rockville, MD 20852-2557
(301) 984-9496 (ext 200)
http://www.accc-cancer.org

National Society of Genetic Counselors (NSGC)
233 Canterbury Drive
Wallingford, PA 19086-6617
(610) 872-7608
http://www.nsgc.org/

NSGC will promote the genetic counseling profession as a recognized and integral part of health-care delivery, education, research, and public policy. Services: referrals, educational programs, genetic screening.

Society of Gynecologic Oncologists (SGO)
401 North Michigan Avenue
Chicago, IL 60611-4267
(312) 644-6610
(800) 444-4441 (referral)
http://www.sgo.org

The SGO is a nonprofit, international organization made up of obstetricians and gynecologists specializing in gynecologic oncology. Its purpose is to improve the care of women with gynecologic cancer, to raise standards of practice in gynecologic oncology, and to encourage ongoing research.

PROSTATE CANCER

American Foundation for Urologic Disease (AFUD)
1128 North Charles Street
Baltimore, MD 21201
(410) 468-1800
(800) 242-2383
http://www.afud.org

The AFUD supports research; provides education to patients, the general public, and health professionals; and offers patient support services for those who have or may be at risk for a urologic disease or disorder. They provide information on urologic disease and dysfunctions, including prostate cancer treatment options, bladder health, and sexual function. They also offer prostate cancer support groups (Prostate Cancer Network). Some Spanish-language publications are available.

American Prostate Society
P.O. Box 870
Hanover, MD 21076
(800) 308-1106
Email: ameripros@mindspring.com
http://www.ameripros.org

CaP CURE (Association for the Cure of Cancer of the Prostate)
1250 Fourth Street
Suite 360
Santa Monica, CA 90401
(310) 458-2873
(800) 757-2873 or (800) 757-CURE
http://www.capcure.org

Cap CURE is dedicated to finding a cure for prostate cancer through support of research, education, and prevention. Services: advocacy; identify and support prostate cancer research; referrals; information on clinical trials.

Man to Man
American Cancer Society
1599 Clifton Road, NE
Atlanta, GA 30329
(800) 227-2345
(404) 320-3333
http://www.cancer.org

Support group that includes an educational presentation by a health-care professional. Offers support, one-on-one visitation, and telephone support from specially trained prostate cancer survivors.

Men's Cancer Resource Group
1001 South MacDill Avenue
Tampa, FL 33629
(800) 227-2345

Organized by prostate cancer survivors and concerned professionals, the MCRG offers a support network as well as an education clearinghouse for current information on research and treatment. The groups offers support group meetings and community outreach in the Tampa Bay area. Callers from anywhere can discuss concerns with another man by calling the 24-hour information line at 1-800-309-6467.

National Prostate Cancer Coalition (NPCC)
1158 15th Street, NW
Washington, DC 20005
(202) 463-9455

(888) 245-9455 (toll-free)
http://www.pcacoalition.org

NPCC, a grassroots awareness and advocacy group, is interested in both outreach and advocacy for people with prostate cancer. Services: advocacy, public education, referrals, education information.

Patient Advocates for Advanced Cancer Treatments (PAACT)

1143 Parmelee, NW
Grand Rapids, MI
(616) 453-1477
http://www.paactusa.org

A nonprofit prostate cancer advocacy organization that provides prostate cancer patients with the most advanced methods of detection, diagnostic procedures, evaluations, and treatments. The legal action committee can help patients with insurance problems. Services: referrals, public library, education information, a quarterly "Cancer Communication" newsletter, counseling, sex therapy, advocacy, volunteer services, medical assistance, alternative therapies; support group information, elderly services, health insurance information.

US TOO International, Inc.

5003 Fairview Avenue
Downers Grove, IL 60515-5286
(630) 795-1002
(800) 80-USTOO
http://www.ustoo.com

US TOO is an international network of chapters providing support and services to prostate cancer survivors. Services: support groups, referrals for clinical trials, educational information, advocacy. US TOO also provides professional education.

RACIAL ISSUES IN CANCER

Intercultural Cancer Council (ICC)

6655 Travis Street
Suite 322
Houston, TX 77030
(713) 798-4617
http://www.icc.bcm.tmc.edu

While cancer rates are declining nationwide, racial and ethnic minorities and medically underserved populations have higher incidence and lower survival rates from this disease. The mission of the ICC is to develop and promote policies and programs to redress this tragic imbalance.

National Asian Women's Health Organization (NAWHO): Breast and Cervical Cancer

250 Montgomery Street
Suite 900
San Francisco, CA 94104
(415) 989-9747
http://www.nawho.org

NAWHO created Communicating Across Boundaries: the Asian American Women's Breast and Cervical Cancer Program to eliminate the threat of these diseases in Asian American communities nationwide by increasing provider awareness of and responsiveness to the health needs to Asian American women. Services: early detection screening, educational programs, health promotion activities, advocacy, raises awareness through community health forums and training sessions.

National Latina Health Organization

P.O. Box 7567
Oakland, CA 94601
(510) 534-1362

An organization committed to working toward bilingual access to quality health care and self-empowerment of Latinas, through health education, health advocacy, and public policy. All Latinas as well as women of color are welcome.

Native American Cancer Survivors Network

St. Joseph Hospital Foundation/Attn: NAWWA
1835 Franklin St.
Denver, CO 80218
http://natamcancer.org/community.html

An educational community-based research study to help improve the quality of cancer care and the quality of life for all American Indian, Alaska Native, and First Nations cancer patients and their loved ones.

Sisters Network (SN)

8787 Woodway Drive
Suite 4206
Houston, TX 77063
(713) 781-0255
http://www.sistersnetworkinc.org

SN is the first national breast cancer survivors support group organized for African-American women. Services: community education and awareness programs, person-to-person support, a speakers' bureau, and national newsletter. Call for local chapters' information.

RESEARCH

American Institute for Cancer Research (AICR)
1759 R Street, NW
Washington, DC 20009
(202) 328-7744
(800) 843-8114
http://www.aicr.org

A national cancer organization focusing exclusively on the relationship between nutrition and cancer. The Institute supports research in the area of nutrition and cancer treatment and cancer prevention. Through its extensive education programs the Institute builds awareness and knowledge of diet, nutrition, and cancer. Services: AICR offers a wide array of education materials for consumers to help them lower their cancer risk through diet. The AICR Nutrition toll-free hotline allows consumers to speak personally with a registered dietitian about dietary concerns.

Brain Tumor Society (BTS)
124 Watertown Street
Suite 3-H
Watertown, MA 02472
(800) 770-8287
(617) 924-9998
http://www.tbts.org

The Brain Tumor Society exists to find a cure for brain tumors, raising funds to advance selected scientific research projects, improve clinical care, and find a cure. Services: BTS provides educational material for patients and physicians, as well as funding professional conferences and research.

Cancer Research Foundation of America (CRFA)
1600 Duke Street
Suite 110
Alexandria, VA 22314
(703) 836-4412
(800) 227-2732 or (800) 227-CRFA)
http://www.preventcancer.org

CRFA is a nonprofit organization dedicated to cancer prevention through research and education. Services: CRFA funds peer-reviewed research grants and fellowships and develops educational programs

that focus on prevention and early detection, including free newsletters, brochures, videos, PSAs and CD-ROMS.

Cancer Research Institute
681 Fifth Avenue
New York, NY 10022-4209
(212) 688-7515
http://www.cancerresearch.org

DES Cancer Network
514 10th Street, NW
Suite 400
Washington, DC 20004
(800) 337-6384
(202) 628-6330
http://www.descancer.org

DCN is a national organization that funds research into DES and cancer.

European Organisation for Research and Treatment of Cancer
Central Office/Data Center
Avenue E. Mounier, 83/11
B-1200 Brussels, Belgium
+32 2 774 16 11
http://www.eortc.be

International Myeloma Foundation (IMF)
12650 Riverside Drive
Suite 206
North Hollywood, CA 91607-3421
(818) 487-7455
(800) 452-2873 (United States and Canada)
http://www.myeloma.org

IMF funds research into multiple myeloma.

International Research Foundation for Helicobacter and Intestinal Immunology
P.O. Box 7965
Charlottesville, VA 22906
(804) 977-1594
http://www.helico.com

National Childhood Cancer Foundation (NCCF)
400 East Huntington Drive
P.O. Box 60012
Arcadia, CA 91066
(626) 447-1674 (The Foundation)
(626) 447-0064 (Children's Oncology Group)
(800) 458-6223
http://www.nccf.org

NCCF funds research and treatment of children with cancer through the Children's Cancer Group (CCG), a network of 2,500 pediatric cancer specialists. Services: advocacy, public education, referrals to CCG treatment centers, and clinical trial information.

Susan B. Komen Breast Cancer Foundation (SBKBCF)
5005 LBJ Freeway
Suite 250
P.O. Box 650309
Dallas, TX 75244
(972) 855-1600
(800) 462-9273
http://www.komen.org

SBKBCF funds research and other cancer-related programs.

SKIN CANCER

Skin Cancer Foundation
245 Fifth Avenue
Suite 1403
New York, NY 10016
(800) SKIN-490
http://www.skincancer.org

Major goals of the Skin Cancer Foundation are to increase public awareness of the importance of taking protective measures against the damaging rays of the sun and to teach people how to recognize the early signs of skin cancer. They conduct public and medical education programs to help reduce skin cancer.

SUPPORT (GENERAL)

Cancer Care Connection (CCC)
3 Innovation Way
Suite 210
Newark, DE 19711
(302) 266-8050
(866) 266-7008 (toll-free)
http://www.cancercareconnection.org

A nonprofit agency that provides information, referrals, and compassionate listening to people affected by cancer through a free phone service. CCC specializes in providing referrals for services ranging from local solutions to global cancer information via a specially designed searchable database. CCC also provides referrals to physician locator services and to clinical trial principal investigators. Services offered in Delaware,

Southern Pennsylvania, Southern New Jersey, and Northern Maryland.

Center for Attitudinal Healing (CAH)
33 Buchanan Drive
Sausalito, CA 94965
(415) 331-6161
http://www.healingcenter.org

CAH is an agency providing nonsectarian spiritual and emotional support.

Comfort Connection
269 East Main Street
Newark, DE 19711
(302) 455-1501

The Comfort Connection is committed to improving overall well-being and making life a little more peaceful through new services aimed at supporting the mind, body, and soul. Services: massage therapy; relaxation for stress management (including muscle relaxation, guided imagery, meditation, and problem-solving tactics); counseling; nutrition support; cosmetic services; volunteer services. Gift certificates are available.

Gilda's Club Worldwide
322 Eighth Avenue
Suite 1402
New York, NY 10001
(800) GILDA-4-U
http://www.gildasclub.org

The headquarters organization for the Gilda's Club network works with communities around the world to start and sustain Gilda's Clubs. In addition, it is a leading global advocate for the principle that emotional and social support are as essential as medical care when cancer is in the family. There are 12 Gilda's Clubs nationwide. Services: referrals, counseling, support systems, advocacy, nutrition services, and volunteer services.

Group Room Radio Talk Show
Vital Options TeleSupport Cancer Network
15821 Ventura Boulevard
Suite 645
Encino, CA 91436
(818) 788-5225
(800) GRP-ROOM
http://www.vitaloptions.org

A weekly syndicated call-in cancer talk show linking patients, survivors, and health-care professionals. Call

1-800-GRP-ROOM for a station in your area. Services: using communication technology, counseling, and support for patients and their families and friends; referrals.

National Association of Hospital Hospitality Houses, Inc.
P.O. Box 18087
Asheville, NC 28814-0087
(828) 253-1188
(800) 542-9730

A nonprofit corporation serving facilities that provide lodging and other supportive services to patients and their families when confronted with medical emergencies. Services: referrals, housing/lodging facilities, volunteer services.

R. A. Bloch Cancer Foundation
4435 Main Street
Kansas City, MO 64111
(816) 932-8453
(800) 433-0464
http://www.blochcancer.org

The Foundation provides a toll-free hotline that matches newly diagnosed patients with someone who has survived the same cancer. It also offers free information lists of multidisciplinary second-opinion centers. Services: Cancer Hotline, home volunteers with similar diagnosis to clients, support groups, educational and special interest presentations, and a list of medical multidisciplinary second opinion boards.

Wellness Community
National Office
35 East Seventh Street
Cincinnati, OH 45202
(513) 421-7111
(888) 793-WELL (toll-free)
http://www.wellness-community.org

The Wellness Community provides free psychosocial support to people fighting to recover from cancer. There are 21 Wellness Community facilities nationwide. Services include: counseling, support groups, networking groups, educational information, nutritional information, volunteer services, and survivor concerns.

Well Spouse Foundation
P.O. Box 30093
Elkins Park, Pa 19027
(800) 838-0879
http://www.wellspouse.org

A membership organization providing emotional support and information to the "well spouse" or the caregiver of the chronically ill. Services: a newsletter, local support groups, "round-robin" letter writing, an annual weekend conference, and bereavement counseling.

SURVIVORS

National Coalition for Cancer Survivorship (NCCS)
1010 Wayne Avenue
Suite 770
Silver Spring, MD 20910
(301) 650-9127
(877) NCCS-YES (toll-free)
http://www.canceradvocacy.org

NCCS is a survivor-led organization working on behalf of all cancer survivors. NCCS's mission is to ensure quality cancer care for all Americans. Services: referrals, information education, advocacy.

TEENS/YOUNG ADULTS

Planet CANCER
1804 East 39th Street
Austin, TX 78722
(512) 481-9010
http://www.planetcancer.org

Planet Cancer is an international network of young adults (between ages 18 and 35) with cancer who support each other in communities online and face-to-face. Services: peer support; a "Planet Cancer Forum" where patients communicate directly with each other; advocacy; "Adventure Therapy," which is a type of outdoor expedition for young adults.

Ulman Cancer Fund for Young Adults
4725 Dorsey Hall Drive
Suite A, PMB #505
Ellicott City, MD 21042
(410) 964-0202
(888) 393-FUND (toll-free)
http://www.ulmanfund.org

The Ulman Cancer Fund for Young Adults was founded to provide support programs, education, and resources, free of charge, to benefit young adults, their families and friends, who are affected by cancer, and to promote awareness and prevention. Services: support groups; a guidebook ("No Way, It Can't Be": A Young Adult Faces Cancer); a nationwide skin protection campaign; and scholarship program.

TESTICULAR CANCER

Klinefelter Syndrome and Associates
P.O. Box 119
Roseville, CA 95678-0119
(916) 773-2999
http://www.genetic.org/ks/

Lance Armstrong Foundation (LAF)
P.O. Box 161150
Austin, TX 78716-1150
(512) 236-8820
http://www.laf.org

A nonprofit organization founded by cancer survivor and cyclist Lance Armstrong that provides resources and support to people diagnosed with cancer and their families. The LAF's services include Cycle of Hope, a national cancer education campaign for people with cancer and those at risk for developing the disease, and the Cancer Profiler, a free interactive treatment decision support tool. The LAF also provides scientific and research grants for the better understanding of cancer and cancer survivorship.

THYROID CANCER

American Thyroid Association
6066 Leesburg Pike
Suite 650
Falls Church, VA 22041
(703) 998-8890
http://www.thyroid.org

ThyCa: Thyroid Cancer Survivors' Association, Inc.
P.O. Box 1545
New York, NY 10159-1545
(877) 588-7904
http://www.thyca.org

A nonprofit organization providing information about thyroid cancer and support for thyroid cancer survivors.

Thyroid Foundation of America
350 Ruth Sleeper Hall, RSL 350
40 Parkman Street
Boston, MA 02114
(800) 832-8321

(617) 726-8500
http://www.tsh.org

TRANSPLANTS

National Foundation for Transplants (NFT)
1102 Brookfield
Suite 200
Memphis, TN 38119
(901) 684-1697
(800) 489-3863
http://www.transplants.org

NFT assists transplant candidates, recipients, and their families. Services: financial assistance, patient advocacy, insurance information, and help locating housing during treatment.

URINARY TRACT CANCERS

American Foundation for Urologic Disease (AFUD)
1128 North Charles Street
Baltimore, MD 21201
(410) 468-1800
(800) 242-2383
http://www.afud.org

VON HIPPEL-LINDAU

Von Hippel-Lindau Family Alliance (VHLFA)
171 Clinton Road
Brookline, MA 02445
(617) 232-5946
(617) 277-5667
(800) 767-4VHL
http://www.vhl.org

VHLFA works to improve the diagnosis, treatment, and quality of life of individuals with VHL, one of the family of diseases known as hereditary cancer syndromes. Services: referrals, counseling, support groups.

VULVAR CANCER

Vulvar Pain Foundation (VPF)
Post Office Drawer 177
Graham, NC 27253
(336) 226-0704
http://www.vulvarpainfoundation.org

The Vulvar Pain Foundation is a nonprofit organization established to end the isolation of women suffering from vulvar pain, and to give them hope, support, and reliable information in their quest for freedom from pain. The Network support is manned by volunteers. There is a patient-to-patient network established by the VPF either through telephone, correspondence, or support groups. The Network membership is at a yearly cost of $40.

WALDENSTROM'S MACROGLOBULINEMIA

International Waldenstrom's Macroglobulinemia Foundation (IWMF)
2300 Bee Ridge Road
Suite 301
Sarasota, FL 34239-6226
(941) 927-4963
http://www.iwmf.com

Nonprofit foundation that provides encouragement and support to people with WM and their families. The IWMF also supports increased research toward finding more effective treatments and ultimately a cure. The IWMF offers publications, regional support groups, and telephone Lifeline Project.

WISH FULFILLMENT GROUPS

Dream Foundation
621 Chapala Street
Suite D
Santa Barbara, CA 93101-7011
(805) 564-2131
http://www.dreamfoundation.org

The Dream Foundation tries to fulfill last wishes of terminal adults (aged 18–65) when life expectancy is less than one year.

Make-A-Wish Foundation (MAWF)
2600 North Central Avenue
Suite 936
Phoenix, AZ 85013
(800) 722-9474
(602) 279-9474
http://www.wish.org

MAWF is a foundation that grants "special wishes" to children (up to age 18) who have a life-threatening illness. Services: devoted to fulfilling dreams; wish requests are granted; volunteer services.

STARBRIGHT Foundation
11835 West Olympic Boulevard
Suite 500
Los Angeles, CA 90064
(310) 479-1212
http://www.starbright.org

The STARBRIGHT Foundation creates projects that are designed to help seriously ill children and adolescents cope with the psychosocial and medical challenges they face. The STARBRIGHT Foundation produces materials such as interactive educational CD-ROMs and videos about medical conditions and procedures, advice on talking with a health professional, and other issues related to children and adolescents who have serious medical conditions. All materials are available to children, adolescents, and their families free of charge. Staff can respond to calls in Spanish.

Starlight Children's Foundation
5900 Wilshire Boulevard
Suite 2530
Los Angeles, CA 90036
(323) 634-0080
(800) 274-7827
http://www.starlight.org

SCF grants the "special wishes" of critically, chronically, and/or terminally ill children aged 4–18. Services: provides in-hospital entertainment, grants wishes to ill children, and plans family outings.

Sunshine Foundation (SFO)
1041 Mill Creek Drive
Feaster Ville, PA 19053
(215) 396-4770
(800) 767-1976
http://www.sunshinefoundation.org

SFO grants the "special wishes" of critically, chronically, and/or terminally ill children, aged three to 21, whose families are under financial strain due to the child's illness. It is the original dream-granting organization.

WOMEN'S ISSUES

National Asian Women's Health Organization
250 Montgomery Street
Suite 900
San Francisco, CA 94104
(415) 989-9747
http://www.nawho.org

National Women's Health Information Center (NWHIC)
8550 Arlington Boulevard
Suite 300
Fairfax, VA 22031
(800) 994-9662
http://www.4woman.org

Women's Cancer Resource Center (WCRC)
3023 Shattuck Avenue
Berkeley, CA 94705
(510) 548-WCRC
http://www.wcrc.org

WCRC's mission is to empower women with cancer to be active and informed consumers and survivors, provide community for women with cancer and their supporters, and educate the general community about cancer.

Women's Healthcare Educational Network, Inc. (WHEN)
P.O. Box 5061
Tiffin, OH 44883
(800) 991-8877
http://www.whenusa.org

WHEN is an organization of independent businesses that specialize in serving women who have had breast surgery. Services: information and referrals to physicians, nurses, and managed care providers; specialty items like wigs, maternity and nursing products, compression therapy products, prostheses, etc.

APPENDIX II
CANCER CENTERS

ALABAMA

University of Alabama at Birmingham Comprehensive Cancer Center*
1824 Sixth Avenue South
Birmingham, AL 35294
(205) 975-8222
(800) 822-0933 or (800) UAB-0933
http://www.ccc.uab.edu/

ARIZONA

Arizona Cancer Center*
The University of Arizona
1515 North Campbell Avenue
P.O. Box 245024
Tucson, AZ 85724
(520) 626-2900 (new patient registration line)
(800) 622-COPE (2673)
http://www.azcc.arizona.edu/

CALIFORNIA

Chao Family Comprehensive Cancer Center*
University of California at Irvine
Building 23, Route 81
101 The City Drive
Orange, CA 92868
(714) 456-8200
http://www.ucihs.uci.edu/cancer/

City of Hope*
Cancer Center and Beckman Research Institute
1500 East Duarte Road
Duarte, CA 91010
(626) 359-8111
(800) 826-4673
E-mail: becomingapatient@coh.org
http://www.cityofhope.org/

*Comprehensive cancer centers
**Clinical cancer centers

Jonsson Comprehensive Cancer Center at UCLA*
8-684 Factor Building
UCLA Box 951781
Los Angeles, CA 90095
(310) 825-5268
E-mail: jcccinfo@mednet.ucla.edu
http://www.cancer.mednet.ucla.edu/

University of California, San Diego Cancer Center*
9500 Gilman Drive
La Jolla, CA 92093
(858) 534-7600
http://cancer.ucsd.edu/

University of California, San Francisco Comprehensive Cancer Center*
Box 0128, UCSF
2340 Sutter Street
San Francisco, CA 94143
(415) 476-2201 (general information)
(800) 888-8664 (cancer referral line)
E-mail: cceditor@cc.ucsf.edu
http://cc.ucsf.edu/

USC/Norris Comprehensive Cancer Center and Hospital*
1441 Eastlake Avenue
Los Angeles, CA 90033
(323) 865-3000
(800) 872-2273 or (800) USC-CARE
E-mail: cainfo@ccnt.hsc.usc.edu
http://ccnt.hsc.usc.edu/

COLORADO

University of Colorado Cancer Center*
Box F-704
1665 North Ursula Street
Aurora, CO 80010
(720) 848-0300

(800) 473-2288 (cancer referral line)
http://uch.uchsc.edu/uccc/

CONNECTICUT

Yale Cancer Center*
Yale University School of Medicine
333 Cedar Street
P.O. Box 208028
New Haven, CT 06520
(203) 785-4095
http://www.info.med.yale.edu/ycc/

DISTRICT OF COLUMBIA

Lombardi Cancer Center*
Georgetown University Medical Center
3800 Reservoir Road, NW
Washington, DC 20007
(202) 784-4000
http://lombardi.georgetown.edu/

FLORIDA

**H. Lee Moffitt Cancer Center & Research
   Institute at the University of South Florida***
12902 Magnolia Drive
Tampa, FL 33612
(813) 972-4673
http://www.moffitt.usf.edu/

HAWAII

Cancer Research Center of Hawaii**
1236 Lauhala Street
Honolulu, HI 96813
(808) 586-3010
http://www.hawaii.edu/crch/

ILLINOIS

Robert H. Lurie Comprehensive Cancer Center*
Northwestern University
Olson Pavilion 8250
710 North Fairbanks Court
Chicago, IL 60611
(312) 908-5250
E-mail: s-markman@northwestern.edu
http://www.lurie.nwu.edu/

University of Chicago Cancer Research Center*
Mail Code 9015
5758 South Maryland Avenue
Chicago, IL 60637

(773) 702-9200
(888) 824-0200 (new patients)
E-mail: aholub@mcis.bsd.uchicago.edu
http://www.uccrc.uchicago.edu/

INDIANA

Indiana University Cancer Center**
535 Barnhill Drive
Indianapolis, IN 46202
(317) 278-4822
(888) 600-4822
http://iucc.iu.edu/

IOWA

**Holden Comprehensive Cancer Center at the
   University of Iowa***
5970-Z JPP
200 Hawkins Drive
Iowa City, IA 52242
(800) 237-1225 (general information)
(800) 777-8442 (patient referral)
E-mail: Cancer-Center@uiowa.edu
http://www.uihealthcare.com/DeptsClinicalServices/
   CancerCenter

MARYLAND

Johns Hopkins Oncology Center*
401 North Broadway
Weinberg Building
Baltimore, MD 21231
(410) 502-1033
http://www.hopkinskimmelcancercenter.org

MASSACHUSETTS

Dana-Farber Cancer Institute*
44 Binney Street
Boston, MA 02115
(617) 632-3000
http://www.dana-farber.org/

MICHIGAN

Barbara Ann Karmanos Cancer Institute*
Operating the Meyer L. Prentis Comprehensive
   Cancer Center of Metropolitan Detroit
Wertz Clinical Center
4100 John R Street
Detroit, MI 48201
(800) 527-6266
E-mail: info@karmanos.org
http://www.karmanos.org/

University of Michigan Comprehensive Cancer Center*
1500 East Medical Center Drive
Ann Arbor, MI 48109
(800) 865-1125
E-mail: wwwcancer@umich.edu
http://www.cancer.med.umich.edu/

MINNESOTA

Mayo Clinic Cancer Center*
200 First Street, SW
Rochester, MN 55905
(507) 284-2111
http://www.mayo.edu/cancercenter/

University of Minnesota Cancer Center*
420 Delaware Street, SE
Mayo Mail Code Box 806
Minneapolis, MN 55455
(612) 624-8484
http://www.cancer.umn.edu/

MISSOURI

Siteman Cancer Center**
Barnes-Jewish Hospital and
   Washington University School of Medicine
660 South Euclid
Box 8100
St. Louis, MO 63110
(314) 747-7222
(800) 600-3606
E-mail: info@ccadmin.wustl.edu
http://www.siteman.wustl.edu/

NEBRASKA

UNMC Eppley Cancer Center**
University of Nebraska Medical Center
986805 Nebraska Medical Center
Omaha, NE 68198
(402) 559-4238
http://www.unmc.edu/cancercenter/

NEW HAMPSHIRE

Norris Cotton Cancer Center*
Dartmouth-Hitchcock Medical Center
One Medical Center Drive
Lebanon, NH 03756
(603) 650-6300 (administration)
(800) 639-6918 (cancer help line)
E-mail: cancerhelp@dartmouth.edu
http://www.dartmouth.edu/dms/nccc

NEW JERSEY

Cancer Institute of New Jersey**
Robert Wood Johnson Medical School
195 Little Albany Street
New Brunswick, NJ 08901
(732) 235-2465
http://cinj.umdnj.edu

NEW YORK

Albert Einstein Comprehensive Cancer Center*
Albert Einstein College of Medicine
1300 Morris Park Avenue
Bronx, NY 10461
(718) 430-2302
E-mail: aeccc@aecom.yu.edu
http://www.aecom.yu.edu/cancer

Herbert Irving Comprehensive Cancer Center*
Columbia Presbyterian Center
New York-Presbyterian Hospital
PH 18, Room 200
622 West 168th Street
New York, NY 10032
(212) 305-9327 (office of administration)
http://www.ccc.columbia.edu/

Kaplan Comprehensive Cancer Center*
New York University School of Medicine
550 First Avenue
New York, NY 10016
(212) 263-6485
http://www.nyucancerinstitute.org/

Memorial Sloan-Kettering Cancer Center*
1275 York Avenue
New York, NY 10021
(800) 525-2225
http://www.mskcc.org/

Roswell Park Cancer Institute*
Elm and Carlton Streets
Buffalo, NY 14263
(800) 767-9355
http://www.roswellpark.org/

NORTH CAROLINA

Comprehensive Cancer Center of Wake Forest University*
Wake Forest University Baptist Medical Center
Medical Center Boulevard
Winston-Salem, NC 27157

(336) 716-4464
http://www.bgsm.edu/cancer/

Duke Comprehensive Cancer Center*
Duke University Medical Center
Box 3843
301 MSRB
Durham, NC 27710
(919) 684-3377
http://www.cancer.duke.edu

**UNC Lineberger Comprehensive Cancer
   Center***
School of Medicine
University of North Carolina at Chapel Hill
Campus Box 7295
Chapel Hill, NC 27599
(919) 966-3036
E-mail: dgs@med.unc.edu
http://cancer.med.unc.edu/

OHIO

Ireland Cancer Center*
University Hospitals of Cleveland
11100 Euclid Avenue
Cleveland, OH 44106
(216) 844-5432
(800) 641-2422
E-mail: info@irelandcancercenter.org
http://www.irelandcancercenter.org

**Ohio State University Comprehensive Cancer
   Center***
The Arthur G. James Cancer Hospital and
   Richard J. Solove Research Institute
300 West 10th Avenue
Suite 519
Columbus, OH 43210
(800) 293-5066
E-mail: cancerinfo@jamesline.com
http://www.jamesline.com

OREGON

Oregon Cancer Center**
The Oregon Health Sciences University
CR145
3181 Southwest Sam Jackson Park Road
Portland, OR 97201
(503) 494-1617
http://www.ohsu.edu/oci/

PENNSYLVANIA

Fox Chase Cancer Center*
7701 Burholme Avenue
Philadelphia, PA 19111
(215) 728-2570 (to schedule an appointment) or
(888) 369-2427
E-mail: info@fccc.edu
http://www.fccc.edu/

Kimmel Cancer Center**
Thomas Jefferson University
233 South 10th Street
Bluemle Life Sciences Building
Philadelphia, PA 19107
(215) 503-4500
(800) 533-3669 (Jefferson Cancer Network)
(800) 654-5984 (TDD)
http://www.kcc.tju.edu/

University of Pennsylvania Cancer Center*
3400 Spruce Street
15th Floor, Penn Tower
Philadelphia, PA 19104
(215) 662-4000 (main)
(800) 789-7366 (referral/schedule an appointment)
http://www.oncolink.upenn.edu/

University of Pittsburgh Cancer Institute*
Iroquois Building
3600 Forbes Avenue
Suite 206
Pittsburgh, PA 15213
(800) 237-4724
E-mail: PCI-INFO@msx.upmc.edu
http://www.upci.upmc.edu/

TENNESSEE

St. Jude Children's Research Hospital**
332 North Lauderdale Street
Memphis, TN 38105
(901) 495-3300
http://www2.stjude.org

Vanderbilt-Ingram Cancer Center*
Vanderbilt University
649 The Preston Building
Nashville, TN 37232
(615) 936-1782
(615) 936-5847
(800) 811-8480 (clinical trial or treatment option
   information)

(888) 488-4089 (all other calls)
http://www.vicc.org/

TEXAS

San Antonio Cancer Institute*
8122 Datapoint Drive
San Antonio, TX 78229
(210) 616-5590
http://www.ccc.saci.org/

**University of Texas M. D. Anderson
Cancer Center***
1515 Holcombe Boulevard
Houston, TX 77030
(713) 792-6161
(800) 392-1611
http://www.mdanderson.org/

UTAH

Huntsman Cancer Institute**
University of Utah
2000 Circle of Hope
Salt Lake City, UT 84112
(801) 585-0303
(877) 585-0303
http://www.hci.utah.edu/

VERMONT

Vermont Cancer Center*
University of Vermont
Medical Alumni Building
Burlington, VT 05401
(802) 656-4414
E-mail: vcc@uvm.edu
http://www.vermontcancer.org

VIRGINIA

Cancer Center at the University of Virginia**
University of Virginia Health System
Box 800334
Charlottesville, VA 22908

(804) 924-9333
(800) 223-9173
http://www.med.virginia.edu/medcntr/cancer/
home.html

Massey Cancer Center**
Virginia Commonwealth University
401 College Street
P.O. Box 980037
Richmond, VA 23298
(804) 828-0450
http://www.vcu.edu/mcc/

WASHINGTON

Fred Hutchinson Cancer Research Center*
LA-205
1100 Fairview Avenue North
P.O. Box 19024
Seattle, WA 98109
(206) 288-1024
(800) 804-8824 (appointments and medical
referral—Seattle Cancer Care Alliance)
E-mail: hutchdoc@seattlecca.org
(patient information)
http://www.fhcrc.org/

WISCONSIN

**University of Wisconsin Comprehensive
Cancer Center***
600 Highland Avenue, K5/601
Madison, WI 53792
(608) 263-8600
(608) 262-5223 (Cancer Connect)
(800) 622-8922
E-mail: uwccc@uwcc.wisc.edu/
http://www.cancer.wisc.edu

APPENDIX III
CARCINOGENS

A. KNOWN TO BE A HUMAN CARCINOGEN

Aflatoxins
Alcoholic Beverage Consumption
4-Aminobiphenyl
Analgesic Mixtures Containing Phenacetin
Arsenic Compounds, Inorganic
Asbestos
Azathioprine
Benzene
Benzidine
Beryllium and Beryllium Compounds
1,3-Butadiene
1,4-Butanediol Dimethylsulfonate (Myleran)
Cadmium and Cadmium Compounds
Chlorambucil
1-(2-Chloroethyl)-3-(4-methylcyclohexyl)-1-nitrosourea (MeCCNU)
bis(Chloromethyl) Ether and Technical-Grade Chloromethyl Methyl Ether
Chromium Hexavalent Compounds
Coal Tar Pitches
Coal Tars
Coke Oven Emissions
Cyclophosphamide
Cyclosporin A (Ciclosporin)
Diethylstilbestrol
Dyes Metabolized to Benzidine
Environmental Tobacco Smoke
Erionite
Estrogens
Ethylene Oxide
Melphalan
Methoxsalen with Ultraviolet A Therapy (PUVA)
Mineral Oils (Untreated and Mildly Treated)
Mustard Gas
2-Naphthylamine
Nickel Compounds

Radon
Silica, Crystalline (Respirable Size)
Smokeless Tobacco
Solar Radiation
Soots
Strong Inorganic Acid Mists Containing Sulfuric Acid
Sunlamps or Sunbeds, Exposure to
Tamoxifen
2,3,7,8-Tetrachlorodibenzo-p-dioxin (TCDD); "Dioxin"
Thiotepa
Thorium Dioxide
Tobacco Smoking
Ultraviolet Radiation, Broad Spectrum UV Radiation
Vinyl Chloride
Wood Dust

B. REASONABLY ANTICIPATED TO BE A HUMAN CARCINOGEN

Acetaldehyde
2-Acetylaminofluorene
Acrylamide
Acrylonitrile
Adriamycin (Doxorubicin Hydrochloride)
2-Aminoanthraquinone
o-Aminoazotoluene
1-Amino-2-methylanthraquinone
2-Amino-3-methylimidazo[4,5-f]quinoline (IQ)
Amitrole
o-Anisidine Hydrochloride
Azacitidine (5-Azacytidine, 5-AzaC)
Benz[a]anthracene
Benzo[b]fluoranthene
Benzo[j]fluoranthene
Benzo[k]fluoranthene

Benzo[a]pyrene
Benzotrichloride
Bromodichloromethane
2,2-bis-(Bromoethyl)-1,3-propanediol (Technical
    Grade)
Butylated Hydroxyanisole (BHA)
Carbon Tetrachloride
Ceramic Fibers (Respirable Size)
Chloramphenicol
Chlorendic Acid
Chlorinated Paraffins (C12, 60% Chlorine)
1-(2-Chloroethyl)-3-cyclohexyl-1-nitrosourea
bis(Chloroethyl) nitrosourea
Chloform
3-Chloro-2-methylpropene
4-Chloro-o-phenylenediamine
Chloroprene
p-Chloro-o-toluidine and p-Chloro-o-toluidine
    Hydrochloride
Chlozotocin
C.I. Basic Red 9 Monohydrochloride
Cisplatin
p-Cresidine
Cupferron
Dacarbazine
Danthron (1,8-Dihydroxyanthraquinone)
2,4-Diaminoanisole Sulfate
2,4-Diaminotoluene
Dibenz[a,h]acridine
Dibenz[a,j]acridine
Dibenz[a,h]anthracene
7H-Dibenzo[c,g]carbazole
Dibenzo[a,e]pyrene
Dibenzo[a,h]pyrene
Dibenzo[a,i]pyrene
Dibenzo[a,l]pyrene
1,2-Dibromo-3-chloropropane
1,2-Dibromoethane (Ethylene Dibromide)
2,3-Dibromo-1-propanol
tris(2,3-Dibromopropyl) Phosphate
1,4-Dichlorobenzene
3,3'-Dichlorobenzidine and 3,3'-
    Dichlorobenzidine Dihydrochloride
Dichlorodiphenyltrichloroethane (DDT)
1,2-Dichloroethane (Ethylene Dichloride)
Dichloromethane (Methylene Chloride)
1,3-Dichloropropene (Technical Grade)
Diepoxybutane

Diesel Exhaust Particulates
Diethyl Sulfate
Diglycidyl Resorcinol Ether
3,3'-Dimethoxybenzidine
4-Dimethylaminoazobenzene
3,3'-Dimethylbenzidine
Dimethylcarbamoyl Chloride
1,1-Dimethylhydrazine
Dimethyl Sulfate
(Continued)Dimethylvinyl Chloride
1,6-Dinitropyrene
1,8-Dinitropyrene
1,4-Dioxane
Disperse Blue 1
Dyes Metabolized to 3,3'-Dimethoxybenzidine
Dyes Metabolized to 3,3'-Dimethylbenzidine
Epichlorohydrin
Ethylene Thiourea
di(2-Ethylhexyl) Phthalate
Ethyl Methanesulfonate
Formaldehyde (Gas)
Furan
Glasswool (Respirable Size)
Glycidol
Hexachlorobenzene
Hexachlorocyclohexane Isomoers
Hexachloroethane
Hexamethylphosphoramide
Hydrazine and Hydrazine Sulfate
Hydrazobenzene
Indeno[1,2,3-cd]pyrene
Iron Dextran Complex
Isoprene
Kepone (Chlordecone)
Lead Acetate
Lead Phosphate
Lindane and Other Hexachlorocyclohexane
    Isomers
2-Methylaziridine (Propylenimine)
5-Methylchrysene
4,4'-Methylenebis(2-chloroaniline)
4-4'-Methylenebis(N,N-dimethyl)benzenamine
4,4'-Methylenedianiline and 4,4'-
    Methylenedianiline Dihydrochloride
Methyleugenol
Methyl Methanesulfonate
N-Methyl-N'-nitro-N-nitrosoguanidine
Metronidazole

Michler's Ketone [4,4'-
(Dimethylamino)benzophenone]
Mirex
Nickel (Metallic)
Nitrilotriacetic Acid
o-Nitroanisole
6-Nitrochrysene (see Nitroarenes [selected])
Nitrofen (2,4-Dichlorophenyl-p-nitrophenyl
ether)
Nitrogen Mustard Hydrochloride
2-Nitropropane
1-Nitropyrene
4-Nitropyrene
N-Nitrosodi-n-butylamine
N-Nitrosodiethanolamine
N-Nitrosodiethylamine
N-Nitrosodimethylamine
N-Nitrosodi-n-propylamine
N-Nitroso-N-ethylurea
4-(N-Nitrosomethylamino)-1-(3-pyridyl)-1-
butanone
N-Nitroso-N-methylurea
N-Nitrosomethylvinylamine
N-Nitrosomorpholine
N-Nitrosonornicotine
N-Nitrosopiperidine
N-Nitrosopyrrolidine
N-Nitrososarcosine
Norethisterone
Ochratoxin A
4,4'-Oxydianiline
Oxymetholone
Phenacetin
Phenazopyridine Hydrochloride

Phenolphthalein
Phenoxybenzamine Hydrochloride
Phenytoin
Polybrominated Biphenyls (PBBs)
Polychlorinated Biphenyls (PCBs)
Polycyclic Aromatic Hydrocarbons (PAHs)
Procarbazine Hydrochloride
Progesterone
1,3-Propane Sultone
â-Propiolactone
Propylene Oxide
Propylthiouracil
Reserpine
Safrole
Selenium Sulfide
Streptozotocin
Styrene-7,8-oxide
Sulfallate
Tetrachloroethylene (Perchloroethylene)
Tetrafluoroethylene
Tetranitromethane
Thioacetamide
Thiourea
Toluene Diisocyanate
o-Toluidine and o-Toluidine Hydrochloride
Toxaphene
Trichloroethylene
2,4,6-Trichlorophenol
1,2,3-Trichloropropane
Ultraviolet A, B and C radiation
Urethane
Vinyl Bromide
4-Vinyl-1-cyclohexene Diepoxide
Vinyl Fluoride

GLOSSARY

adrenal glands A pair of small glands, one located on top of each kidney, that produce steroid hormones, adrenaline and noradrenaline to help control heart rate, blood pressure, and other important body functions.

agonists Drugs that trigger an action from a cell or another drug.

agranulocyte A type of white blood cell that includes monocytes and lymphocytes.

anaplastic A term used to describe cancer cells that divide rapidly and bear little or no resemblance to normal cells.

autologous Taken from an individual's own tissues, cells, or DNA.

axilla The underarm or armpit.

B cell White blood cells that make antibodies and are an important part of the immune system. B cells come from bone marrow and are also called B lymphocytes.

blood-brain barrier A network of blood vessels with closely spaced cells that makes it difficult for potentially toxic substances (such as chemotherapy drugs) to enter the brain.

B lymphocytes See **B cell.**

central nervous system The brain and spinal cord.

cerebellum The largest part of the hind brain, responsible for maintaining muscle tone, balance, and muscle activity.

cerebrum The largest, most highly developed part of the brain composed of two hemispheres. Each hemisphere has an outer layer of gray matter (the cerebral cortex) below which lies white matter containing the basal ganglia. The cortex is the seat of all intelligent behavior.

cervix The lower, narrow end of the uterus that forms a canal between the uterus and vagina.

chromosome Part of a cell that contains genetic information. Except for sperm and eggs, all human cells contain 46 chromosomes.

coenzyme A substance needed for the proper functioning of an enzyme.

colon The long, tubelike organ that is connected to the small intestine and rectum. The colon removes water and some nutrients and electrolytes from digested food. The remaining solid waste moves through the colon to the rectum and leaves the body through the anus.

cytokines A class of substances produced by immune system cells that affect the immune response. Cytokines can also be produced in the laboratory and given to people to affect their immune response.

cytopenia A reduction in the number of blood cells.

cytotoxic Cell-killing.

diuretic A drug that increases the volume of urine.

endocrine glands Glands that manufacture and secretes hormones into the blood. Endocrine glands include the pituitary, thyroid, parathyroid, adrenal glands, ovary and testis, placenta and part of the pancreas.

endometrium The lining of the uterus.

enzyme A protein that speeds up the rate at which chemical reactions take place in the body.

eosinophil A type of white blood cell.

epithelium Tissue that covers the external surface of the body and that lines hollow structures.

granulocyte A type of white blood cell that fights bacterial infection. Neutrophils, eosinophils, and basophils are granulocytes.

islets of Langerhans Cells in the pancreas that produce hormones (including insulin).

killer cells White blood cells that attack tumor cells and body cells that have been invaded by foreign substances.

larynx Also called the "voice box," this is the part of the throat containing the vocal cords.

leukocytes   A white blood cell that does not contain hemoglobin. White blood cells include lymphocytes, neutrophils, eosinophils, macrophages, and mast cells, all of which are produced by bone marrow and help the body fight infection.

lymph   The clear fluid of the lymphatic system through which cells travel as they fight infection and disease.

lymph gland   Also known as a lymph node, this tissue mass contains lymphocytes that filter the lymphatic fluid.

lymphocyte   A type of white blood cell that helps produce antibodies and other substances that fight infection and diseases.

mast cell   A type of white blood cell.

meninges   The membranes that cover and protect the brain and spinal cord.

monoclonal antibodies   A substance produced in the lab that can locate and bind to cancer cells wherever they are in the body. Many monoclonal antibodies are used in cancer diagnosis or treatment. Each one recognizes a different protein on certain cancer cells. Monoclonal antibodies can be used alone, or they can be used to deliver drugs, toxins, or radioactive material directly to a tumor.

monocyte   A type of white blood cell.

myeloid   Derived from or pertaining to bone marrow.

myometrium   The muscular outer layer of the uterus.

nasopharynx   The upper part of the throat behind the nose.

natural killer cells (NK cells)   A type of white blood cell that can kill tumor cells.

neutrophil   A type of white blood cell.

oropharynx   The middle part of the throat that includes the soft palate, the base of the tongue, and the tonsils.

parathyroid glands   Four pea-sized glands found on the thyroid that produce parathyroid hormone, which increases the calcium level in the blood.

peptide   Any compound consisting of two or more amino acids, the building blocks of proteins.

pharynx   The throat area that starts behind the nose and ends at the top of the trachea (windpipe) and esophagus.

pineal gland   A tiny organ located in the brain that produces melatonin, a hormone that plays an important role in the sleep-wake cycle.

plasma   The clear, yellowish, fluid part of the blood that carries the blood cells.

platelets   A type of blood cell that helps prevent bleeding by causing blood clots to form.

polyp   A growth that protrudes from a mucous membrane.

protein   A molecule made up of amino acid chains that the body needs for proper function. Proteins form the structure of skin, hair, enzymes, cytokines, and antibodies.

radioisotope   An unstable element that releases radiation as it breaks down. Radioisotopes can be used in imaging tests or as a treatment for cancer.

receptor   A molecule inside or on the surface of a cell that binds to a specific substance.

red blood cell   A cell (also called an erythrocyte) that carries oxygen to all parts of the body.

serum   The clear liquid part of the blood that remains after blood cells and clotting proteins have been removed.

stem cells   Cells from which other types of cells can develop.

T cell   A type of white blood cell that attacks invaders such as cancer cells, and that produces substances that regulate the immune response.

thyroid gland   A gland located beneath the larynx that produces thyroid hormone and that helps regulate growth and metabolism.

white blood cell   A blood cell that does not contain hemoglobin, including lymphocytes, neutrophils, eosinophils, macrophages, and mast cells. These cells are made by bone marrow and help the body fight infection and other diseases.

BIBLIOGRAPHY

Abramova, L., Parekh, J., Irvin, W. P., Jr., et al. "Sentinel Node Biopsy in Vulvar and Vaginal Melanoma: Presentation of Six Cases and a Literature Review," *Annals of Surgical Oncology* 9/9 (November 2002): 840–846.

Adami, H. O., Bergstrom, R., Lund, E., and Meirik, O. "Absence of Association between Reproductive Variables and the Risk of Breast Cancer in Young Women in Sweden and Norway," *British Journal of Cancer* 62 (1990): 122–126.

Adjetey, V., Ganesan, R., Downey, G. P. "Primary Vaginal Endometrioid Carcinoma following Unopposed Estrogen Administration," *Journal of Obstetrics and Gynecology* 23/3 (May 2003): 316–317.

Adlercreutz H., Goldin, B. R., Gorbach, S. I., et al. "Estrogen Excretion Patterns and Plasma Levels in Vegetarian and Omniverous Women," *New England Journal of Medicine* 307 (1982): 1,542–1,547.

Adlercreutz, H. "Evolution, Nutrition, Intestinal Microflora, and Prevention of Cancer: a Hypothesis," *Proceedings of the Society for Experimental Biology and Medicine* 217 (1998): 241–246.

Adlercreutz, H. "Evolution, Nutrition, Intestinal Microflora, and Prevention of Cancer: a Hypothesis," *Proceedings of the Society for Experimental Biology and Medicine* 217 (1998): 241–246.

Ah Lee S., Kang D., Soo Seo S., et al. "Multiple HPV Infection in Cervical Cancer Screened by HPVDNA Chip," *Cancer Letter* 198/2 (August 2003): 187–192.

Albanes, D., Blair, A., and Taylor, P. R. "Physical Activity and Risk of Cancer in the NHANES I Population," *American Journal of Public Health* 79 (1989): 744–750.

Albertazzi, P., et al. "Dietary Soy Supplementation and Phytoestrogen Levels," *Obstetrics and Gynecology* 94 (1999): 229–231.

Altman, Roberta, and Sarg, Michael J. *The Cancer Dictionary, Revised Edition.* New York: Facts On File, 2000.

Ambrosone, C. B., et al. "Breast Cancer Risk, Meat Consumption, and N-acetyltransferase Genetic Polymorphisms," *International Journal of Cancer* 75 (1998): 30.

American Cancer Society. "Unproven Methods of Cancer Management: Laetrile," *CA: A Cancer Journal for Clinicians* 41/3 (1991): 187–192.

———. "American Cancer Society Updates Prostate Cancer Screening Guidelines," available online at: http://www.cancer.org.

Anderson, J. J. B., and Garner, S. C. "Phytoestrogens and Human Function," *Nutrition Today* 32 (1997): 39.

Ardies, C. M., and Dee, C. "Xenoestrogens Significantly Enhance Risk for Breast Cancer during Growth and Adolescence," *Medical Hypotheses* 50 (1998): 457–464.

Armstrong B. K., Brown J. B., Clarke H. T., et al. "Diet and Reproductive Hormones: A Study of Vegetarian and Nonvegetarian Postmenopausal Women," *Journal of the National Cancer Institute* 67 (1981): 761–767.

Armstrong, C., Stern, C., and Corn, B. "Memory Performance Used to Detect Radiation Effects on Cognitive Functioning," *Applied Neuropsychology* 8 (2001): 129–139.

Atallah, D., Chahine, G., Voutsadakis, I. A. "Brain Metastasis from Ovarian Cancer," *Journal of Clinical Oncology* 21/15 (Aug. 1, 2003): 2,996–2,998.

Austin, H, Drews, C., Partridge, E. E., "A Case-control Study of Endometrial Cancer in Relation to Cigarette Smoking, Serum Estrogen Levels, and Alcohol Use," *American Journal of Obstetrics and Gynecology* 169 (1993): 1,086–1,091.

Bal, D. G., and Forester, S. B. "Dietary Strategies for Cancer Prevention," *Cancer* 72 (1992): 1,005–1,010.

Barger-Lux, M. J., and Heaney, R. P. "The Role of Calcium Intake in Preventing Bone Fragility, Hypertension, and Certain Cancers," *Journal of Nutrition* 124 (1994): 1,406S–1,411S.

Barnes, M. N., Grizzle, W. E., Grubbs, C. J., Partridge, E. E. "Paradigms for Primary Prevention of Ovarian Carcinoma," *CA: Cancer Journal for Clinicians*. 52 (2002): 216–225.

Barnholtz-Sloan, J. S., Sloan, A. E., Schwartz, A. G. "Racial Differences in Survival after Diagnosis with Primary Malignant Brain Tumor," *Cancer* 98/3 (Aug. 1, 2003): 603–609.

Beaty, O., Hudson, M., Greenwald, C., et al. "Subsequent Malignancies in Children and Adolescents after Treatment for Hodgkin's Disease," *Journal of Clinical Oncology* 13 (1995): 603–609.

Beecher, C. W. W. "Cancer Preventive Properties of Varieties of *Brassica oleracea*: a Review," *American Journal of Clinical Nutrition* 59 (1994): 166S–1,170S.

Beeson W. L., Fraser G. E., Mills P. K, et al. "Cancer Incidence among California Seventh-Day Adventists 1976–1982," *American Journal of Clinical Nutrition* 59 (1994): 1,136S–1,142S.

Berman, M. L., Brinton, L. A., Mortel, R., et al. "Reproductive, Menstrual and Medical Risk Factors for Endometrial Cancer: Results from a Case-Control Study," *American Journal of Obstetrics and Gynecology* 167 (1993): 1,317–1,325.

Bessho, F. "Effects of Mass Screening on Age-Specific Incidence of Neuroblastoma," *International Journal of Cancer* 67 (1996): 520–522.

Bhatia, S., Robison, L. L., Oberlin, O., et al. "Breast Cancer and Other Second Neoplasms after Childhood Hodgkin's Disease," *New England Journal of Medicine* 334 (1996): 745–751.

Bingham, S. A. "Meat or Wheat for the Next Millennium? High-Meat Diets and Cancer Risk," *Proceedings of the Nutrition Society* 58 (1999): 243–248.

Bingham, S. A., Atkinson, C., Liggins, J., et al. "Phyto-oestrogens: Where Are We Now?" *British Journal of Nutrition* 79 (1998): 393–406.

Blot, W., Henderson, B., and Boice, J. J. "Childhood Cancer in Relation to Cured Meat Intake: Review of the Epidemiological Evidence," *Nutrition and Cancer* 34 (1999): 111–118.

Bocciolone L., La Vecchia C., Parazzini F., et al. "The Epidemiology of Endometrial Cancer," *Gynecologic Oncology* 41 (1991): 1–16.

Boran, N., Kayikcioglu, F., Kir, M. "Sentinel Lymph Node Procedure in Early Vulvar Cancer," *Gynecologic Oncology* 90/2 (August 2003): 492–493.

Bouker, K. B., and Hilakivi-Clarke, L. "Genistein: Does It Prevent or Promote Breast Cancer?" *Environmental Health Perspectives* 108 (2000): 701–708.

Bowlin, S. J., Leske, M. C., Varma, A., et al. "Breast Cancer Risk and Alcohol Consumption: Results from a Large Case-Control Study," *International Journal of Epidemiology* 26 (1997): 915–923.

Bradlow, H. L., Sepkovic, D. W., Telang, N. T., et al. "Indole-3-carbinol: A Novel Approach to Breast Cancer Prevention," *Annals of the New York Academy of Science* 768 (1995): 180–200.

Braga, C., La Vecchia, C., Negri, E., et al. "Intake of Selected Foods and Nutrients and Breast Cancer Risk: an Age- and Menopause-Specific Analysis," *Nutrition and Cancer* 28 (1997): 258–263.

Brekelmans, C. T., Seynaeve, C., Bartels, C. C., et al. "Rotterdam Committee for Medical and Genetic Counselling: Effectiveness of Breast Cancer Surveillance in *BRCA* 1/2 Gene Mutation Carriers and Women with High Familial Risk," *Journal of Clinical Oncology* 19/4 (2001): 924–930.

Brenner, A. V. "Polio Vaccination and Risk of Brain Tumors in Adults: No Apparent Association," *Cancer. Epidemiology, Biomarkers, and Prevention* Cancer Epidemiol Biomarkers Prev. 12 (2003): 177–178.

Brinton, L. A., Potischman, N. A., Swanson, C. A., et al. "Breastfeeding and Breast Cancer Risk," *Cancer Causes and Control* 6 (1995): 199–208.

Brinton, L. A. "Breast Cancer Following Augmentation Mammoplasty (United States)," *Cancer Causes and Control* 11/9 (2000): 819–827.

Brinton, L. A., Daling, J. R., Liff, J. M., et al. "Oral Contraceptives and Breast Cancer Risk among Younger Women," *Journal of the National Cancer Institute* 87/13 (1995): 827–835.

Brown, S., and Degner, L. "Delirium in the Terminally Ill Cancer Patient: Aetiology, Symptoms and Management," *International Journal of Palliative Nursing* 7 (2001): 266–272.

Bruera, E. "Current Pharmacological Management of Anorexia in Cancer Patients," *Oncology* 6/1 (1992): 125–130.

Burke, G. L., Vitolins, M. Z., and Bland, D. "Soybean Isoflavones as an Alternative to Traditional Hormone Replacement Therapy: Are We There Yet?" *Journal of Nutrition* 130 (2000): 664S–665S.

Burke, W., Daly, M., Garber, J., et al. "Recommendations for Follow-up Care of Individuals with an Inherited Predisposition to Cancer. II. *BRCA1* and *BRCA2*." Cancer Genetics Studies Consortium. *Journal of the American Medical Association* 277/12 (1997): 997–1,003.

Byers, T., and Guerrero, N. "Epidemiologic Evidence for Vitamin C and Vitamin E in Cancer Prevention," *American Journal of Clinical Nutrition* 62 (1995): 1,385S–1,392S.

Byrne, C., Sinha, R., Platz, E., et al. "Predictors of Dietary Heterocyclic Amine Intake in Three Prospective Cohorts," *Cancer Epidemiology, Biomarkers and Prevention* 7 (1998): 523–529.

Byrne, C., Ursin, G., and Ziegler, R. "A Comparison of Food Habit and Food Frequency Data as Predictors of Breast Cancer in the NHANES I / NHEFS Cohort," *Journal of Nutrition* 126 (1996): 2,757–2,764.

"California Seventh-Day Adventists 1976–1982," *American Journal of Clinical Nutrition* 59 (1994): 1,136S–1,142S.

Calle, E. E., Murphy, T. K., Rodriguez, C., et al. "Occupation and Breast Cancer Mortality in a Prospective Cohort of U.S. Women," *American Journal of Epidemiology* 148 (1998): 191–197.

Calle, E. E., Patel, A. V., Rodriguez, C., et al. "Estrogen Replacement Therapy and Ovarian Cancer Mortality in a Large Prospective Study of U.S. Women," *Journal of the American Medical Association* 185/11 (March 2001): 1,460S–1,465.

Cantor, K. "Drinking Water and Cancer," *Cancer Causes and Control* 8 (1997): 292–308.

Caygill, C., Charlett, A., and Hill, M. "Fat, Fish, Fish Oil, and Cancer," *British Journal of Cancer* 74 (1996): 159–164.

Cedars-Sinai Medical Center. "Possible Effects of Plant Compounds on Uterus," *Media Advisory* (July 31, 1999).

Chang, Hsueh-Wei. "Assessment of Plasma DNA Levels, Allelic Imbalance, and CA125 as Diagnostic Tests for Cancer," *Journal of the National Cancer Institute* 94/22 (Nov. 20, 2002).

Chang, S., and Risch, H. A. "Perineal Talc Exposure and Risk of Ovarian Carcinoma," *Cancer* 79/12 (June 15, 1997): 2,396–2,401.

Chlebowski, R. T., Bulcavage, L., Grosvenor, M., et al. "Hydrazine Sulfate Influence on Nutritional Status and Survival in Non-Small-Cell Lung Cancer," *Journal of Clinical Oncology* 8/1 (1990): 9–15.

Clinical Evidence editors: "Pancreatic Cancer," *Clinical Evidence* 9 (June 2003): 528–533.

Cohen, S. M. "Cell Proliferation in the Bladder and Implications for Cancer Risk Assessment," *Toxicology* 102/1–2 (1995): 149–159.

Coley, C. M., Barry, M. J., Fleming, C. M., et al. "Early Detection of Prostate Cancer. Part II: Estimating the Risks, Benefits, and Costs," *Annals of Internal Medicine* 126 (1997): 468–479.

Collaborative Group on Hormonal Factors in Breast Cancer. "Breast Cancer and Hormonal Contraceptives: Collaborative Reanalysis of Individual Data on 53,297 Women with Breast Cancer and 100,239 Women without Breast Cancer from 54 Epidemiological Studies," *Lancet* 347 (1996): 1,713–1,727.

Cox, J. T. "The Clinician's View: Role of Human Papillomavirus Testing in the American Society for Colposcopy and Cervical Pathology Guidelines for the Management of Abnormal Cervical Cytology and Cervical Cancer Precursors," *Archives of Pathology and Laboratory Medicine* 127/8 (August 2003): 950–958.

Cramer, D. W., Liberman, R. F., Titus-Ernstoff, L., et al. "Genital Talc Exposure and Risk of Ovarian Cancer," *International Journal of Cancer* 81/3 (May 5, 1999): 351–356.

Cryns, P., Roofthooft, N. J., and Tjalma, W. A. "Ovarian Sex Cord-Stromal Tumors in Children and Adolescents," *Journal of Clinical Oncology* 15/21 (June 12, 2003): 2,357–2,363.

Daling, J. R., Madeleine, M. M., McKnight, B., et al. "The Relationship of Human Papillomavirus-Related Cervical Tumors to Cigarette Smoking, Oral Contraceptive Use, and Prior Herpes Simplex Virus Type 2 Infection," *Cancer Epidemiology, Biomarkers, and Prevention* 5/7 (1996): 541–548.

D'Avanzo, B., La Vechia, C., Parazzini, F., et al. "Alcohol and Endometrial Cancer Risk: Findings from an Italian Case-control Study," *Nutritional Cancer* 23 (1995): 55–62.

Davidson, E. J., Sehr, P., Faulkner, R. L., et al. "Human Papillomavirus Type 16 E2- and L1-Specific Serological and T-cell Responses in Women with Vulval Intraepithelial Neoplasia," *Journal of General Virology* 84/Pt 8 (August 2003): 2,089–2,097.

Dearnaley, D. P., Sydes, M. R., Mason, M. D., et al. "A Double-Blind, Placebo-Controlled, Randomized Trial of Oral Sodium Clodronate for Metastatic Prostate Cancer (MRC PR05 Trial)," *Journal of the National Cancer Institute* 95/17 (Sept. 3, 2003): 1,300–1,311.

Decarli, A., Fasoli, M., La Vecchia, C., et al. "Nutrition and Diet in the Etiology of Endometrial Cancer," *Cancer* 57 (1986): 1,248–1,253.

Decker, E. A. "The Role of Phenolics, Conjugated Linoleic Acid, Carnosine, and Pyrroloquinoline Quinone as Nonessential Dietary Antioxidants," *Nutrition Review* 53 (1995): 49–58.

Department of Health, Education, and Welfare. "FDA and NCI Announce Plans to Conduct a Nationwide Study on the Possible Role of Saccharin in Causing Bladder Cancer in Humans," (*press release*) January 25, 1978.

Dibble, S. L., Chapman, J., Mack, K. A., et al. "Acupressure for Nausea: Results of a Pilot Study," *Oncology Nursing Forum* 27/1 (February 2000): 41–47.

Djuric, Z., Depper, J. B., Uhley, V., et al. "Oxidative DNA Damage Levels in Blood from Women at High Risk for Breast Cancer Are Associated with Dietary Intake of Meats, Vegetables, and Fruits," *Journal of the American Dietetic Association* 98 (1998): 524–528.

Domchek, S. M. "The Utility of Ductal Lavage in Breast Cancer Detection and Risk Assessment," *Breast Cancer Research* 4/2 (2002): 51–53.

Downing, S. R., Russell, P. J., Jackson, P. "Alterations of p53 Are Common in Early Stage Prostate Cancer," *Canadian Journal of Urology* 10/4 (August 2003): 1,924–1,933.

Duenas-Gonzales, A., Cetina, L., Mariscal, I., et al. "Modern Management of Locally Advanced Cervical Carcinoma," *Cancer Treatment Review* 29/5 (October 2003): 389–399.

Dufresne, C. J., and Farnworth, E. R. "A Review of Latest Research Findings on the Health Promotion Properties of Tea," *Journal of Nutritional Biochemistry* 12/7 (2001): 404–421.

Elit, L. "Familial Ovarian Cancer," *Canadian Family Physician* 47 (April 2001): 778–784.

Ellison, N. M., Byar, D. P., Newell, G. R. "Special Report on Laetrile: the NCI Laetrile Review: Results of the National Cancer Institute's Retrospective Laetrile Analysis," *New England Journal of Medicine* 299/10 (1978): 549–552.

Engels, E. A. "Cancer Incidence in Denmark Following Exposure to Poliovirus Vaccine Contaminated with Simian Virus 40," *Journal of the National Cancer Institute* 95 (2003): 24.

Environmental Health Information Service, U.S. Department of Health and Human Services, Public Health Service, National Toxicology Program. "Ninth Report on Carcinogens, Revised January 2001," available online at http://ehis.niehs.nih.gov/roc/t oc9.html.

Fiorica, J. V. "The Role of Topotecan in the Treatment of Advanced Cervical Cancer," *Gynecologic Oncology* 90/3 Pt. 2 (September 2003): S16–21.

Fisher, B., Constantino, J. P., Wickerham, D. L., et al. "Tamoxifen for Prevention of Breast Cancer: Report of the National Surgical Adjuvant Breast and Bowel Project P-1 Study," *Journal of the National Cancer Institute* 90/18 (1998): 1,371–1,388.

Fleischer, A. C., Cullinan, J. A., Peery, C. V., et al. "Early Detection of Ovarian Carcinoma with Transvaginal Color Doppler Ultrasonography," *American Journal of Obstetrics and Gynecology* 174/1 Pt. 1 (1996): 101–106.

Folsom, A. R., Kaye, S. A., Potter, J. D., et al. "Association of Incident Carcinoma of the Endometrium with Body Weight and Fat Distribution in Older Women: Early Findings of the Iowa Women's Health Study," *Cancer Research* 49 (1989): 6,828–6,831.

Foster, R. D., Esserman, L. J., Anthony, J. P., et al. "Skin-Sparing Mastectomy and Immediate Breast Reconstruction: A Prospective Cohort Study for the Treatment of Advanced Stages of Breast Carcinoma," *Annals of Surgical Oncology* 9/8 (October 2002): 820–821.

Foth, D., and Cline, M. J. "Effects of Mammalian and Plant Estrogens on Mammary Glands and

Uteri of Macaques," *American Journal of Clinical Nutrition* 68 (1998): 1,413S–1,417S.

Frank, S. J., Jhingran, A., Levenback, C., et al. "Definitive Treatment of Vaginal Cancer with Radiation Therapy," *International Journal of Radiation Oncology and Biological Physics* 57 (2 Suppl.); (October 2003): S194.

Frank, T. S. "Testing for Hereditary Risk of Ovarian Cancer," *Cancer Control* 6/4 (July 1999): 327–334.

Freeman, Harold P., and Alshafie, T. A. "Colorectal Carcinoma in Poor Blacks," *Cancer* 94:9 (May 1, 2002): 2,327–2,332.

Freudenheim, J. L., Marshall, J. R., Vena, J. E., et al. "Premenopausal Breast Cancer Risk and Intake of Vegetables, Fruits, and Related Nutrients," *Journal of National Cancer Institute* 88 (1996): 340–348.

Friedenreich, C. M., and Courneya, K. S. "Exercise as Rehabilitation for Cancer Patients," *Clinical Journal of Sport Medicine* 6 (1996): 237–244.

Friess, H., Beger, H. G., Kunz, J., et al. "Treatment of Advanced Pancreatic Cancer with Mistletoe: Results of a Pilot Trial," *Anticancer Research* 16/2 (March–April 1996): 915–920.

Frydenberg, M., Stricker, P. D., Kaye, K. W. "Prostate Cancer Diagnosis and Management," *The Lancet* 349 (1997): 1,681–1,687.

Gammon, M. D., John, E. M., and Britton, J. A. "Recreation and Occupational Physical Activities and Risk of Breast Cancer," *Journal of the National Cancer Institute* 90 (1998): 100–117.

Gapstur, S. M., Potter, J. D., Sellers, T. A., et al. "Alcohol Consumption and Postmenopausal Endometrial Cancer: Results from the Iowa Women's Health Study," *Cancer Control* 4 (1993): 323–329.

Garland, M., Hunter, D. J., Colditz, G. A., et al. "Alcohol Consumption in Relation to Breast Cancer Risk in a Large Cohort of United States Women 25–42 Years of Age," *Cancer Epidemiology, Biomarkers, and Prevention* 8 (1999): 1,017–1,021.

Garro, A. J., and Lieber, C. S. "Alcohol and Cancer," *Annual Review of Pharmacology and Toxicology* 30 (1990): 219–249.

Gavaler, J. S. "Protective Effect of Alcohol Against Endometrial Cancer," *Lancet* 2/983 (1983): 627.

Geller, A. C., Colditz, G., Oliveria, S., et al. "Use of Sunscreen, Sunburning Rates, and Tanning Bed Use among More than 10,000 U.S. Children and Adolescents," *Pediatrics* 109/6 (2002): 1,009–1,014.

Gertig, D. M., Hankinson, S. E., Hough, H., et al. "N-Acetyl Transferase 2 Genotypes, Meat Intake and Breast Cancer Risk," *International Journal of Cancer* 80 (1999): 13–17.

Gill, W. B., Schumacher, G. F. B., and Bibbo, M. "Structural and Functional Abnormalities in the Sex Organs of Male Offspring of Mothers Treated with Diethylstilbestrol (DES)," *Journal of Reproductive Medicine* 16 (1976): 147–153.

Ginsberg, J., and Prelevic, G. M. "Lack of Significant Hormonal Effects and Controlled Trials of Phyto-oestrogens," *Lancet* 355 (2000): 163–164.

Giovannucci, E. "An Updated Review of the Epidemiological Evidence that Cigarette Smoking Increases Risk of Colorectal Cancer," *Cancer Epidemiology, Biomarkers, and Prevention* 10 (2001): 725–731.

Giovannucci, E., Pollak, M., Platz, E. A., et al. "Insulin-like Growth Factor I (IGF-I), IGF-Binding Protein-3 and the Risk of Colorectal Adenoma and Cancer in the Nurses' Health Study," *Growth Hormone IGF Research* 10/Suppl. A (2000): S30–31.

Giuliano, A. R., Papenfuss, M., Schneider, A., et al. "Risk Factors for High-Risk Type Human Papillomavirus Infection among Mexican-American Women," *Cancer Epidemiology, Biomarkers, and Prevention* 8/7 (1999): 615–620.

Godard, B., Foulkes, W. D., Provencher, D., et al. "Risk Factors for Familial and Sporadic Ovarian Cancer among French Canadians: a Case-Control Study. *American Journal of Obstetrics and Gynecology* 179/2 (1998): 403–410.

Gold, J. "Use of Hydrazine Sulfate in Terminal and Preterminal Cancer Patients: Results of Investigational New Drug (IND) Study in 84 Valuable Patients," *Oncology* 32/1 (1975): 1–10.

Goldacre, M. J. "Abortion and Breast Cancer: A Case-Control Record Linkage Study," *Journal of Epidemiology and Community Health* 55 (2001): 336–337.

Goldbohm, R. A., Hertog, M. G., Brants, H. A., et al. "Consumption of Black Tea and Cancer Risk: A Prospective Cohort Study," *Journal of the National Cancer Institute* 88/2 (1996): 93–100.

Goldin, B., Gorbach, S., Longcope, C., et al. "The Effect of a Low Fat Diet on Estrogen Metabolism," *Journal of Clinical Endocrinology and Metabolism* 64 (1987): 1,246–1,250.

Goldsmith, J. D., "Cystic Neoplasms of the Pancreas," *American Journal of Clinical Pathology* 119 Suppl (June 2003): S3–16.

Goodman, M. T., Wilkins, L. R., Hankin, J. H., et al. "Association of Soy and Fiber Consumption with the Risk of Endometrial Cancer," *American Journal of Epidemiology* 146 (1997): 294–306.

Gowen, L. C., Avrutskaya, A. V., Latour, A. M., et al. "*BRCA1* Required for Transcription-Coupled Repair of Oxidative DNA Damage," *Science* 281/5379 (1998): 1,009–1,012.

Grady, D., Herrington, D., Blumenthal, R., et al. "Cardiovascular Disease Outcomes during 6.8 Years of Hormone Therapy: Heart and Estrogen/Progestin Replacement Study Follow-up (HERS II)," *Journal of the American Medical Association* 288 (2002): 49–57.

Grant, W. B. "An Estimate of Premature Cancer Mortality in the United States due to Inadequate Doses of Solar Ultraviolet-B Radiation, a Source of Vitamin D," *Cancer,* 94/6 (March 15, 2002): 1,867–1,875.

Gray, S., and Olopade, O. I. "Direct-to-Consumer Marketing of Genetic Tests for Cancer: Buyer Beware," *Journal of Clinical Oncology* 21 (2003): 3,191–3,193.

Greenlee, R. T., Hill-Harmon, M. B., Murray, T., et al. "Cancer Statistics, 2001," *CA: A Cancer Journal for Clinicians* 56 (2001): 15–36.

Greenwald, P. "The Potential of Dietary Modification to Prevent Cancer," *Preventive Medicine* 25 (1996): 41–43.

Grodstein, F., Newcomb, P. A., and Stampfer, M. J. "Postmenopausal Hormone Therapy and the Risk of Colorectal Cancer: A Review and Meta-analysis," *American Journal of Medicine* 106 (1999): 574–582.

Grossarth-Maticek, R., Kiene, H., Baumgartner, S. M., et al. "Use of Iscador, an Extract of European Mistletoe (*Viscum album*), in Cancer Treatment: Prospective Nonrandomized and Randomized Matched-Pair Studies Nested within a Cohort Study," *Alternative Therapies in Health and Medicine* 7/3 (May–June 2001): 57–66, 68–72, 74–76.

Guillette, L. H., Jr. "Endocrine Disrupting Environmental Contaminants and Developmental Abnormalities in Embryos," *Human and Ecological Risk Assessment* 1/2 (1995): 25–36.

Guillette, L. H., Jr., Gross, T. S., Masson, G. R., et al. "Developmental Abnormalities of the Gonad and Abnormal Sex Hormone Concentrations in Juvenile Alligators from Contaminated and Control Lakes in Florida," *Environmental Health Perspectives* 102/8 (1994): 680–688.

Gurney, J. G., Ross, J. A., Wall, D. A., et al. "Infant Cancer in the US: Histology-Specific Incidence and Trends, 1973 to 1992," *Journal of Pediatrics, Hematology and Oncology* 19 (1997): 428–432.

Hahn, N. I. "Are Phytoestrogens Nature's Cure for What Ails Us? A Look at the Research," *Journal of the American Dietetic Association* 98 (1998): 974–976.

Hainer, M. I., Tsai, N., Komura, S. T., et al. "Fatal Hepatorenal Failure Associated with Hydrazine Sulfate," *Annals of Internal Medicine* 133/11 (2000): 877–880.

Hall, A. H., Spoerke, D. G., Rumack, B. H. "Assessing Mistletoe Toxicity," *Annals of Emergency Medicine* 15/11 (1986): 1,320–1,323.

Hamdy, R. C. "Hormonal Replacement Therapy," *Southern Medical Journal* 94 (2001): 1,141–1,142.

Hammar, M., Frisk, J., Grimas, O., et al. "Acupuncture Treatment of Vasomotor Symptoms in Men with Prostatic Carcinoma: A Pilot Study," *Journal of Urology* 161 (1999): 853–856.

Hammes, B., and Laitman, C. J., "Diethylstilbestrol (DES) Update: Recommendations for the Identification and Management of DES-Exposed Individuals," *Journal of Midwifery and Women's Health* 48/1 (January–February 2003): 19–29.

Hankinson, S. E., Colditz, G. A., Hunter, D. J., et al. "A Prospective Study of Reproductive Factors and Risk of Epithelial Ovarian Cancer," *Cancer* 76/2 (1995): 284–290.

Hankinson, S. E., Colditz, G. A., Manson, J. E., et al. *Healthy Women, Healthy Lives: A Guide to Preventing Disease, from the Landmark Nurses' Health Study.* New York: Simon & Schuster, Inc., 2001.

Hartge, P., Itnyre, J., Whittemore, A. S., et al. "Rates and Risks of Ovarian Cancer in Subgroups of White Women in the United States," The Collaborative Ovarian Cancer Group. *Obstetrics and Gynecology* 84/5 (November 1994): 760–764.

Hartmann, L. C., Sellers, T. A., Schaid, D. J., et al. "Efficacy of Bilateral Prophylactic Mastectomy in *BRCA1* and *BRCA2* Gene Mutations Carriers," *Journal of the National Cancer Institute* 93/21 (2001): 1,633–1,637.

He, J. P., Friedrich, M., Ertan, A. K., et al. "Pain-Relief and Movement Improvement by Acupuncture after Ablation and Axillary Lymphadenectomy in Patients with Mammary Cancer," *Clinical and Experimental Obstetrics and Gynecology* 26 (1999): 81–84.

Herbert, J. R., and Rosen, A. "Nutritional Socioeconomic, and Reproductive Factors in Relation to Female Breast Cancer Mortality: Findings from a Cross-National Study," *Cancer Detection and Prevention* 20 (1996): 234–244.

Herman, C., Adlercreutz, T., Golin, B. R., et al. "Soybean Phytoestrogen Intake and Cancer Risk," *Journal of Nutrition* 125 (1995): 757S–770S.

Herndon, J. E., Fleishman, S., Kosty, M. P., et al. "A Longitudinal Study of Quality of Life in Advanced Non-Small Cell Lung Cancer: Cancer and Leukemia Group B (CALGB) 8931," *Controlled Clinical Trials* 18/4 (1997): 286–300.

Hertel, H., Kohler, C., Michels, W., et al. "Laparoscopic-Assisted Radical Vaginal Hysterectomy (LARVH): Prospective Evaluation of 200 Patients with Cervical Cancer," *Gynecologic Oncology* 90/3 (September 2003): 505–511.

Herzog, T. J. "New Approaches for the Management of Cervical Cancer," *Gynecologic Oncology* 90/3 Pt. 2 (September 2003): S22–27.

Hoffman-Goetz, L., Apter, D., Denmark-Wahnefried, W., et al. "Possible Mechanisms Mediating an Association between Physical Activity and Breast Cancer," *Cancer* 83 (1998): 621–628.

Holmes, M. D., Stampfer, M. J., Colditz, G. A., et al. "Dietary Factors and the Survival of Women with Breast Carcinoma," *Cancer* 86 (1999): 826–835.

Holschneider, C. H., and Berek, J. S. "Ovarian Cancer: Epidemiology, Biology, and Prognostic Factors," *Seminar in Surgical Oncology* 19/1 (July–August 2000): 3–10.

Horsman, M. R., Alsner, J., Overgaard, J. "The Effect of Shark Cartilage Extracts on the Growth and Metastatic Spread of the SCVII Carcinoma," *Acta Oncologica* 37 (1998): 441–445.

Hulley, S., Furberg, C., Barrett-Connor, E., et al. "Noncardiovascular Disease Outcomes during 6.8 Years of Hormone Therapy. Heart and Estrogen/Progestin Replacement Study Follow-up (HERS II)," *Journal of the American Medical Association* 288 (2002): 58–66.

Hunter, D. J., and Willet, W. C. "Nutrition and Breast Cancer," *Cancer Causes and Control* 7 (1996): 56–68.

Hunter, D. J., Manson, J. E., Colditz, G. A., et al. "A Prospective Study of the Intake of Vitamins C, E, and A and the Risk of Breast Cancer," *The New England Journal of Medicine* 329 (1993): 234–240.

Inskip, P. D. "Multiple Primary Tumors Involving Cancer of the Brain and Central Nervous System as the First or Subsequent Cancer," *Cancer* 98/3 (August 1, 2003): 562–570.

Institute of Medicine (US) Committee on the Early Detection of Breast Cancer. *Mammography and Beyond: Developing Technologies for the Early Detection of Breast Cancer.* Washington, D.C.: National Academy Press, 2001.

International Journal of Gynecologic Cancer 13/4 (July–August 2003): 466–471.

Jain, M. "Dairy Foods, Dairy Fats and Cancer: A Review of Epidemiological Evidence," *Nutrition Research* 18 (1998): 905–937.

Jobling, J. S., and Sumpter, J. P. "Detergent Component in Sewage Effluent Are Weakly Oestrogenic to Fish: An Invitro Study Using Rainbow Trout (*Oncorhynchus mykiss*) Hepatocyctes," *Aquatic Toxicology* 27 (1993): 361–372.

Kaegi, E. "Unconventional Therapies for Cancer," *Canadian Medical Association Journal* 158/9 (1998): 1,157–1,159.

Kalandidi, A., Lipworth, L., Tzonou, A., et al. "Case-control Study of Endometrial Cancer in Relation to Reproductive, Omatometric, and Life-style Variables," *Oncology* 53 (1996): 354–359.

Kaminski, J. M., Anderson, P. R., Han, A. C., et al. "Primary Small Cell Carcinoma of the Vagina," *Gynecologic Oncology* 88/3 (March 2003): 451–455.

Kamradt, J. M., and Pienta, K. J. "The Effect of Hydrazine Sulfate on Prostate Cancer Growth," *Oncology Reports* 5 (1998): 919–921.

Karlan, B. Y., and Platt, L. D. "Ovarian Cancer Screening. The Role of Ultrasound in Early Detection," *Cancer* 76/10 Suppl. (1995): 2,011–2,015.

Kattlove, H., and Winn, R. J. "Ongoing Care of Patients after Primary Treatment for Their Cancer," *CA: A Cancer Journal for Clinicians* 53 (2003): 172–196.

Kauff, Noah D., Satagopan, J. M., Robson, M. E., et al. "Risk-Reducing Salpingo-Oophorectomy in Women with a *BRCA1* or *BRCA2* Mutation," *New England Journal of Medicine* 346/21 (May 23, 2002): 1,609–1,615.

Kennedy, E., Bowman, S., and Powell, R. "Dietary-Fat Intake in the U.S. Population," *Journal of the American College of Nutrition* 18 (1999): 207–212.

Kerber, R. A., and Slattery, M. L. "The Impact of Family History on Ovarian Cancer Risk: The Utah Population Database," *Archives of Internal Medicine* 155/9 (1995): 905–912.

King, C. "On Pharmacologic Management of Chemotherapy-Induced Nausea and Vomiting," *Oncology Nursing Forum* 24 (1997) (suppl. 7): 41–48.

King M. C., Wieand, S., Hale, K., et al. "National Surgical Adjuvant Breast and Bowel Project: Tamoxifen and Breast Cancer Incidence among Women with Inherited Mutations in *BRCA1* and *BRCA2*: National Surgical Adjuvant Breast and Bowel Project (NSABP-P1) Breast Cancer Prevention Trial," *Journal of the American Medical Association* 286/18 (2001): 2,251–2,256.

Kjellberg, L., Hallmans, G., Ahren, A. M., et al. "Smoking, Diet, Pregnancy, and Oral Contraceptive Use as Risk Factors for Cervical Intra-Epithelial Neoplasia in Relation to Human Papillomavirus Infection," *British Journal of Cancer* 82 (2000): 1,332–1,338.

Kopp, P. "Resveratrol, a Phytoestrogen Found in Red Wine. A Possible Explanation for the Conundrum of the 'French paradox'?" *European Journal Endocrinology* 138 (1998): 619–620.

Kramer, B. S., Gohagan, J., Prorok, P. C., et al. "A National Cancer Institute Sponsored Screening Trial for Prostatic, Lung, Colorectal, and Ovarian Cancers," *Cancer* 71 (2 Suppl.) (1993): 589–593.

Krzyzanowska, M. K., Weeks, J. C., Earle, C. C. "Treatment of Locally Advanced Pancreatic Cancer in the Real World: Population-Based Practices and Effectiveness," *Journal of Clinical Oncology* 21/18 (September 23, 2003): 3,409–3,414.

Kuhl, C. K., Schmutzler, R. K., Leutner, C. C., et al. "Breast MR Imaging Screening in 192 Women Proved or Suspected to be Carriers of a Breast Cancer Susceptibility Gene: Preliminary Results," *Radiology* 215/1 (2000): 267–279.

Kurzer, M. S. "Hormonal Effect of Soy Isoflavones: Studies in Premenopausal and Postmenopausal Women," *Journal of Nutrition* 130 (2000): 6,60S–6,661S.

Lacey, J. V., Mink, P. J., Lubin, J. H., et al. "Menopausal Hormone Replacement Therapy and Risk of Ovarian Cancer," *Journal of the American Medical Association* 288 (2002): 334–341.

Laing, A. E., Demenais, F. M., Williams, R., et al. "Breast Cancer Risk Factors in African-American Women: the Howard University Tumor Registry Experience," *Journal of the National Medical Association* 85 (1993): 931–939.

Lamartiniere, C. A. "Protection against Breast Cancer with Genistein: A Component of Soy," *American Journal of Clinical Nutrition* 71 (2000): 1,705S–1,707S.

Lantz, P., Orians, C., Liebow, E., et al. "Implementing Women's Cancer Screening Programs in American Indian and Alaska Native Populations," *Health Care Women International* 24/8 (September 2003): 674–696.

Lawlor, P. "The Panorama of Opioid-Related Cognitive Dysfunction in Patients with Cancer: A Critical Literature Appraisal," *Cancer* 94 (2002): 1,836–1,863.

Lazovich, D. "Induced Abortion and Breast Cancer Risk," *Epidemiology* 11 (2000): 76–80.

Leiserowitz, G. S., Gumbs, J. L., Oi, R., et al. "Endometriosis-Related Malignancies," *International Journal of Gynecological Cancer* 13/4 (July–August 2003): 466–471.

Leiss, J. K., and Savitz, D. A. "Home Pesticide Use and Childhood Cancer: a Case-Control Study," *American Journal of Public Health* 85 (1995): 249–252.

Lenartz, D., Dott, U., Menzel, J., et al. "Survival of Glioma Patients after Complementary Treatment with Galactoside-Specific Lectin from Mistletoe," *Anticancer Research* 20/3B (May–June 2000): 2,073–2,076.

Lerman, C., Hughes, C., Croyle, R. T., et al. "Prophylactic Surgery Decisions and Surveillance

Practices One Year Following *BRCA1/2* Testing," *Preventive Medicine* 31/1 (2000): 75–80.

Lerner, I. J. "Laetrile: a Lesson in Cancer Quackery," *CA: A Cancer Journal for Clinicians* 31/2 (1981): 91–95.

Levi, F., Franceschi, S., Negri, E., et al. "Dietary Factors and the Risk of Endometrial Cancer," *Cancer* 71 (1983): 3,575–3,581.

Lewin, J. M., D'Orsi, C. J., Hendrick, R. E., et al. "Clinical Comparison of Full-Field Digital Mammography and Screen-Film Mammography for Detection of Breast Cancer," *American Journal of Roentgenology* 179/3 (2002): 671–677.

Lewin, J. M., Hendrick, R. E., D'Orsi, C. J., et al. "Comparison of Full-Field Digital Mammography with Screen-Film Mammography for Cancer Detection: Results of 4,945 Paired Examinations," *Radiology* 218/3 (2001): 873–880.

Lipkin, M., and Newmark, H. L. "Vitamin D, Calcium, and Prevention of Breast Cancer: a Review," *Journal of the American College of Nutrition* 18 (1999): 392S–397S.

Long, H. J., Rayson, S., Podratz, K. C., et al. "Long-term Survival of Patients with Advanced/Recurrent Carcinoma of Cervix and Vagina after Neoadjuvant Treatment with Methotrexate, Vinblastine, Doxorubicin, and Cisplatin with or without the Addition of Molgramostim, and Review of the Literature," *American Journal of Clinical Oncology* 25/6 (December 2002): 547–551.

Longnecker, M. P., Newcomb, P. A., Mittendorf, R., et al. "Intake of Carrots, Spinach, and Supplements Containing Vitamin A in Relation to Risk of Breast Cancer," *Cancer Epidemiology, Biomarkers, and Prevention* 6 (1997): 887–892.

Lynch, H. T., Watson, P., Bewtra, C., et al. "Hereditary Ovarian Cancer. Heterogeneity in Age at Diagnosis," *Cancer* 67/5 (1991): 1,460–1,466.

Lynch, H. T., Ens, J. A., and Lynch, J. F. "The Lynch Syndrome II and Urological Malignancies," *Journal of Urology* 143/1 (January 1990): 24–28.

Marchbanks, P. A., McDonald, J. A., Wilson, H. G., et al. "Oral Contraceptives and the Risk of Breast Cancer," *The New England Journal of Medicine* 346 (2002): 2,025–2,032.

Martin, A. M., Blackwood, M. A., Antin-Ozerkis, D., et al. "Germline Mutation in *BRCA1* and *BRCA2* in Breast-Ovarian Families from a Breast Cancer Risk Evaluation Clinic," *Journal Of Clinical Oncology* 19/8 (April 15, 2001); 2,247–2,253.

McGinn, Kerry A., and Haylock, Pamela J. *Women's Cancers: How to Prevent Them, How to Treat Them, How to Beat Them.* Alameda, Calif.: Hunter House, 1998.

Mcleod, D. G., and Kolvenbag, G. J. "Defining the Role of Antiandrogens in the Treatment of Prostate Cancer," *Urology* 47 (suppl. 1A) (1996): 85–89.

Meijers-Heijboer, E. J., Verhoog, L. C., Brekelmans, C. T., et al. "Presymptomatic DNA Testing and Prophylactic Surgery in Families with a *BRCA1* or *BRCA2* Mutation," *Lancet* 355/9220 (2000): 2,015–2,020.

Meijers-Heijboer, H., Brekelmans, C. T., Menke-Pluymers, M. "Use of Genetic Testing and Prophylactic Mastectomy and Oophorectomy in Women with Breast or Ovarian Cancer from Families with a *BRCA1* or *BRCA2* Mutation," *Journal of Clinical Oncology* 21 (2003): 1,675–1,681.

Menczer, J., Chetrit, A., Barda, G., et al. "Frequency of *BRCA* Mutations in Primary Peritoneal Carcinoma in Israeli Jewish Women," *Gynecologic Oncology* 88/1 (January 2003): 58–61.

Michels, K. B., Trichopoulos, D., Rosner, B. A., et al. "Being Breastfed in Infancy and Breast Cancer Incidence in Adult Life: Results from the Two Nurses' Health Studies," *American Journal of Epidemiology* 153/3 (2001): 275–283.

Miller, A. B., To, T., Baines, C. J., et al. "Canadian National Breast Screening Study-2: 13-Year Results of a Randomized Trial in Women Aged 50–59 Years," *Journal of the National Cancer Institute* 92/18 (2000): 1,490–1,499.

Miller, R. W. "Special Susceptibility of the Child to Certain Radiation-Induced Cancers," *Environmental Health Perspectives* 103 (1995): 41–44.

Milner, J. A. "A Historical Perspective on Garlic and Cancer," *Journal of Nutrition* 131 (2001): 1,027S–1,031S.

Mirhashemi, R., Ganjei-Azar, P., Nadji, M., et al. "Papillary Squamous Cell Carcinoma of the Uterine Cervix: An Immunophenotypic Appraisal of 12 Cases," *Gynecologic Oncology* 90/3 (September 2003): 657–661.

Modan, B., Hartge, P., Hirsh-Yechezkel, G., et al. "Oral Contraceptives, and the Risk of Ovarian Cancer among Carriers and Noncarriers of a

BRCA1 or *BRCA2* Mutation," *New England Journal of Medicine* 345/4 (July 26, 2001): 235–240.

———. "National Israel Ovarian Cancer Study Group: Parity, Oral Contraceptives, and the Risk of Ovarian Cancer among Carriers and Noncarriers of a *BRCA1* or *BRCA2* Mutation," *New England Journal of Medicine* 345/4 (2001): 235–240.

Mohamed, A. A., and Sharma, S. D. "Fallopian Tube Hydatidiform Mole," *Journal of Obstetrics and Gynecology* 23/3 (May 2003): 330–331.

Moreno, V., Bosch, F. X., Munoz, N., et al. "Effect of Oral Contraceptives on Risk of Cervical Cancer in Women with Human Papillomavirus Infection: The IARC Multicentric Case-Control Study," *Lancet* 359/9312 (2002): 1,085–1,092.

Moslehi, R., Narod, S. A., Risch, H., et al. "Oral Contraceptives and Hereditary Ovarian Cancer," *New England Journal of Medicine* 340/1 (January 7, 1999): 59.

Mullineaux, L., Rahm, A. K., Wood, et al. "Impact of *BRCA1* Testing on Women with Cancer: A Pilot Study," *Genetic Testing* 4/3 (2000): 265–272.

Narod, S. A. "Oral Contraceptives and the Risk of Ovarian Cancer," *New England Journal of Medicine* 339 (1998): 424–428.

Narod, S. A., Dubé, M. P., Klijn, J., et al. "Oral Contraceptives and the Risk of Breast Cancer in *BRCA1* and *BRCA2* Mutation Carriers," *Journal of the National Cancer Institute* 94/23 (2002): 1,773–1,779.

Narod, S. A., Risch, H., Moslehi, R., et al. "Oral Contraceptives and the Risk of Hereditary Ovarian Cancer. Hereditary Ovarian Cancer Clinical Study Group," *New England Journal of Medicine* 339/7 (1998): 424–428.

Narod, S. A., Sun, P., Ghadirian, P., et al. "Tubal Ligation and Risk of Ovarian Cancer in Carriers of *BRCA1* or *BRCA2* Mutations: A Case-Control Study," *Lancet* 357/9267 (2001): 1,467–1,470.

Neto, A. G., Deavers, M. T., Silva, E. G., et al. "Metastatic Tumors of the Vulva: A Clinicopathologic Study of 66 Cases," *American Journal of Surgical Pathology* 27/6 (June 2003): 799–804.

Newcomb, P. A., Storer, B. E., Trentham, Dietz, A. "Alcohol Consumption in Relation to Endometrial Cancer Risk," *Cancer Epidemiology, Biomarkers, and Prevention* 6 (1997): 773–778.

NIH consensus conference. Ovarian cancer. Screening, treatment, and follow-up. NIH Consensus Development Panel on Ovarian Cancer. *Journal of the American Medical Association* 273/6 (1995): 491–497.

NIH editors (*press release*). "NHLBI Stops Trial of Estrogen plus Progestin due to Increased Breast Cancer Risk, Lack of Overall Benefit," Bethesda, Md.: National Institutes of Health (July 9, 2002).

Ohgaki, H. "Cell and Molecular Biology of Simian Virus 40: Implications for Human Infections and Disease," *Journal of the National Cancer Institute* 92 (2000): 495–496.

Olin, P., and Giesecke, J. "Potential Exposure to SV40 in Polio Vaccines Used in Sweden during 1957—No Impact on Cancer Incidence Rates 1960 to 1993," *Developments in Biological Standards* 94 (1997): 227–233.

Olney, John. "Increasing Brain Tumor Rates: Is There a Link to Aspartame?" *Journal of Neuropathology and Experimental Neurology* 55 (1996): 1,115–1,123.

Paley, P. J., Swisher, E. M., Garcia, R. L., et al. "Occult Cancer of the Fallopian Tube in *BRCA-1* Germline Mutation Carriers at Prophylactic Oophorectomy: A Case for Recommending Hysterectomy as Surgical Prophylaxis," *Gynecologic Oncology* 80/2 (2001): 176–180.

Park, K. S., Kim, M., Park, S. H., et al. "Nervous System Involvement by Pancreatic Cancer," *Journal of Neurooncology* 63/3 (July 2003): 313–316.

Parnes, H. L., and Aisner, J. "Protein Calorie Malnutrition and Cancer Therapy," *Drug Safety* 7/6 (1992): 404–416.

Parodi, P. W. "Conjugated Linoleic Acid and Other Anticarcinogenic Agents of Bovine Milk Fat," *Journal of Dairy Science* 82 (1999): 1,339–1,349.

Paul, C., Skegg, D. C. G., Spears, G. F. S. "Oral Contraceptives and Risk of Breast Cancer," *International Journal of Cancer* 46 (1990): 366–373.

Perera, F. P. "Molecular Epidemiology: Insights into Cancer Susceptibility, Risk Assessment, and Prevention," *Journal of the National Cancer Institute* 88 (1996): 496–509.

Peterson, E. P. "Endometrial Carcinoma in Young Women," *Obstetrics and Gynecology* 31 (1968): 702–707.

Pichert, G., Bolliger, B., Busek, K., et al. "Evidence-based Management Options for Women at Increased Breast/Ovarian Cancer Risk," *Annals of Oncology* 14 (2003): 9–19.

Piek, J. M., Verheijen, R. H., Kenemans, P., et al. "*BRCA1/2*-Related Ovarian Cancers Are of Tubal Origin: A Hypothesis," *Gynecologic Oncology* 90/2 (August 2003): 491.

Pinilla, L., Barreiro, M. L., Gonzales, L. C., et al. "Comparative Effects of Testosterone Propionate, Oestradiol Benzoate, ICI 182,780, Tamoxifen and Raloxifene on Hypothalamic Differentiation in the Female Rat," *Journal of Endocrinology* 172/3 (2002): 441–448.

Pivers, M. S., Jishi, M. F., Tsukada, Y., et al. "Primary Peritoneal Carcinoma after Prophylactic Oophorectomy in Women with a Family History of Ovarian Cancer: A report of the Gilda Radner Familial Ovarian Cancer Registry," *Cancer* 71/9 (May 1, 1993): 2,751–2,755.

Piver, M. S., Baker, T. R., Jish, M. F., et al. "Familial Ovarian Cancer. A Report of 658 Families from the Gilda Radner Familial Ovarian Cancer Registry 1981–1991," *Cancer* 71/2 Suppl (1993): 582–528.

Pizzo, P., and Poplack, D., eds. *Principles and Practices of Pediatric Oncology.* 3rd ed. Philadelphia, Pa.: Lippincott-Raven, 1997.

Pongprasobchai, S., and Chari, S. T. "Management of Patients at High Risk for Pancreatic Cancer," *Current Treatment Options in Gastroenterology* 6/5 (October 2003): 349–358.

Powell, J. L. "Extrammary Paget's Disease," *Journal of the American College of Surgeons* 196/5 (May 2003): 824.

Puskin, J. S., and Nelson, C. B. "Estimates of Radiogenic Cancer Risks," *Health Physics* 69 (1995): 93–101.

Rebbeck, T. R. "Prophylactic Oophorectomy in *BRCA1* and *BRCA2* Mutation Carriers," *Journal of Clinical Oncology* 18/21 Suppl. (November 1, 2002): 100S–103S.

Riggs, B. L., and Hartmann, L. C. "Selective Estrogen-Receptor Modulators—Mechanisms of Action and Application to Clinical Practice," *New England Journal of Medicine* 348 (2003): 618–629.

Rockhill, B., Willett, W. C., Hunter, D. J., et al. "Physical Activity and Breast Cancer Risk in a Cohort of Young Women," *Journal of the National Cancer Institute* 90 (1998): 1,155–1,160.

Rodriguez, C., Patel, A. V., Calle, E. E., et al. "Estrogen Replacement Therapy and Ovarian Cancer Mortality in a Large Prospective Study of U.S. Women," *Journal of the American Medical Association* 285/11 (March 2001): 1,460–1,465.

Rosenberg, L., Slone, D., Shapiro, S., et al. "Breast Cancer and Alcoholic Beverage Consumption," *Lancet* 1 (1982): 267–271.

Ross, L., Johansen, C., Dalton, S. O., et al. "Psychiatric Hospitalizations among Survivors of Cancer in Childhood or Adolescence," *New England Journal of Medicine* 349/7 (August 14, 2003): 650–657.

Roukos, D. H., Kappas, A. M., Tsianos, E. "Role of Surgery in the Prophylaxis of Hereditary Cancer Syndromes," *Annals of Surgical Oncology* 9 (2002): 607–609.

Rozario, D., Brown, I., Fung, M. F., et al. "Is Incidental Prophylactic Oophorectomy an Acceptable Means to Reduce the Incidence of Ovarian Cancer?" *American Journal of Surgery* 173/6 (June 1997): 495–498.

Ruffin, M. T., 4th. "Family Physicians' Knowledge of Risk Factors for Cervical Cancer," *Journal of Women's Health* 12/6 (July–August 2003): 561–567.

Rutter, J. L., Wacholder, S., Chetrit, A., et al. "Gynecologic Surgeries and Risk of Ovarian Cancer in Women with *BRCA1* and *BRCA2* Ashkenazi Founder Mutations: An Israeli Population-Based Case-Control Study." *Journal of the National Cancer Institute* 95 (2003): 1,072–1,078.

Sahmoun, A. E., D'Agostino, R. A., Jr., Bell, R. A., et al. "International Variation in Pancreatic Cancer Mortality for the Period 1955–1998," *European Journal of Epidemiology* 18/8 (2003): 801–816.

Satagopan, J. M., Boyd, J., Kauff, N. D., et al. "Ovarian Cancer Risk in Ashkenazi Jewish Carriers of *BRCA1* and *BRCA2* Mutations," *Clinical Cancer Research* 8 (2002): 3,776–3,781.

Schaefermeyer, G., and Schaefermeyer, H. "Treatment of Pancreatic Cancer with *Viscum album* (Iscador): A Retrospective Study of 292 Patients 1986–1996," *Complementary Therapies in Medicine* 6 (1998): 172–177.

Schagen, S., Hamburger, H., Muller, M., et al. "Neurophysiological Evaluation of Late Effects of Adjuvant High-Dose Chemotherapy on Cognitive Function," *Journal of Neurooncology* 51 (2001): 159–162.

Schellhammer, P. F., Sharifi, R., Block, N. I., et al. "Clinical Benefits of Bicalutamide Compared with Flutamide Capsules in Combined Androgen Blockade for Patients with Advanced Prostatic Carcinoma: Final Report of a Double-blind, Randomized, Multicenter Trial, " *Urology* 50 (1997): 330–336.

Schneider, D. T., Calaminus, G., Wessalowksi, R., et al. "A Population Based Case-Control Study of Endometrial Cancer in Shanghai, China," *International Journal of Cancer* 49 (1991): 38–43.

Schwingl, P. J., and Guess, H. A. "Safety and Effectiveness of Vasectomy," *Fertility and Sterility 2000* 73 (5): 923–936.

Serra-Majem, L., La Vecchia, C., Ribas-Barba, L., et al. "Changes in Diet and Mortality from Selected Cancers in Southern Mediterranean Countries," *European Journal of Clinical Nutrition* 47 (1993): S25–S34.

Sigurdsson, S., Thorlacius, S., Tomasson, J., et al. "*BRCA2* Mutation in Icelandic Prostate Cancer Patients," *Journal of Molecular Medicine* 75 (1997): 758–761.

Simcox, N. J., Fenske, R. A., Wolz, S. A., Lee, I.-C., and Kalman, D. A. "Pesticides in Household Dust and Soil: Exposure Pathways for Children of Agricultural Families," *Environmental Health Perspectives* 103 (1995): 1,126–1,134.

Simone, C. B., Simone, N. L., Simone, C. B.; 2nd "Shark Cartilage for Cancer," *Lancet* 351 (1998): 9,113.

Simone, J. V. "Childhood Leukemia—Successes and Challenges for Survivors," *New England Journal of Medicine* 349/7 (August 14, 2003): 627–628.

Snijders, P. J., Van Den Brule, A. J., Meijer, C. J. "The Clinical Relevance of Human Papillomavirus Testing: Relationship Between Analytical and Clinical Sensitivity," *Journal of Pathology* 201/1 (September 23, 2003): 1–6.

Spremulli, E., Wampler, G. L., Regelson, W. "Clinical Study of Hydrazine Sulfate in Advanced Cancer Patients," *Cancer Chemotheraphy and Pharmacology* 3/2 (1979): 121–124.

Stanford, J. L., Brinton, L. A., Berman, M. L., et al. "Oral Contraceptives and Endometrial Cancer: Do Other Risk Factors Modify the Association?" *International Journal of Cancer* 54/2 (1993): 243–248.

Steuer-Vogt, M. K., Bonkowsky, V., Ambrosch, P., et al. "The Effect of an Adjuvant Mistletoe Treatment Programme in Resected Head and Neck Cancer Patients: A Randomised Controlled Clinical Trial," *European Journal of Cancer* 37/1 (2001): 23–31.

Strickler, H. D. "Trends in U.S. Pleural Medothelioma Incidence Rates Following Simian Virus 40 Contamination of Early Polio Virus Vaccines," *Journal of the National Cancer Institute* 95 (2003): 38–45.

Strickler, H. D., Rosenberg, P. S., Devesa, S. S., et al. "Contamination of Poliovirus Vaccines with Simian Virus 40 (1955–1963) and Subsequent Cancer Rates," *Journal of the American Medical Association* 279 (1998): 292–295.

Struewing, J. P., Watson, P., Easton, D. F., et al. "Prophylactic Oophorectomy in Inherited Breast/Ovarian Cancer Families," *Journal of the National Cancer Institute* Monographs 17 (1995): 33–35.

Struewing, J. P., Hartge, P., Wacholder, S., et al. "The Risk of Cancer Associated with Specific Mutations of *BRCA1* and *BRCA2* among Ashkenazi Jews," *New England Journal of Medicine* 336 (1997): 1,401–1,408.

Sun, C. L., Yuan, J. M., Lee, M. J., et al. "Urinary Tea Polyphenols in Relation to Gastric and Esophageal Cancers: a Prospective Study of Men in Shanghai, China," *Carcin* 23 (2002): 1,497–1,503.

Suzuki, F. "Cartilage-derived Growth Factor and Antitumor Factor: Past, Present, and Future Studies," *Biochemical and Biophysical Research Communications* 259 (1999): 1–7.

Swanson, C. A., Wilbanks, G. D., Twiggs, L. B., et al. "Moderate Alcohol Consumption and the Risk of Endometrial Cancer," *Epidemiology* 4 (1993): 530–536.

Tao, L. C. "Oral Contraceptive-Associated Liver Cell Adenoma and Hepatocellular Carcinoma," *Cancer* 68 (1991): 341–347.

Tayek, J. A., Sutter, L., Manglik, S., et al. "Altered Metabolism and Mortality in Patients with

Colon Cancer Receiving Chemotherapy," *American Journal of Medical Sciences* 310/2 (1995): 48–55.

Teeley, Peter, and Bashe, Philip. *The Complete Cancer Survival Guide.* New York: Doubleday, 2000.

Thorgeirsson, U. P. "Tumor Incidence in a Chemical Carcinogenesis Study of Nonhuman Primates," *Regulatory Toxicology and Pharmacology* 19/2 (1994): 130–151.

Tobacman, J. K., Greene, M. H., Tucker, M. A., et al. "Intra-abdominal Carcinomatosis after Prophylactic Oophorectomy in Ovarian-Cancer-Prone Families," *Lancet* 2/8302 (1982): 795–797.

Toth, B. "A Review of the Antineoplastic Action of Certain Hydrazines and Hydrazine-Containing Natural Products," *In Vivo* 10/1 (1996): 65–96.

Vachon, C. M., Mink, P. J., Janney, C. A., et al. "Association of Parity and Ovarian Cancer Risk by Family History of Breast or Ovarian Cancer in a Population-Based Study of Postmenopausal Women," *Epidemiology* 13/1 (2002): 66–71.

Volpert, Olga V. "Id1 Regulates Angiogenesis Through Transcriptional Repression of Thrombospondin-1," *Cancer Cell* 2 (December 2002).

Weiderpass, E., Baron, J. A., Adami, H. O., et al. "Low-Potency Estrogen and Risk of Endometrial Cancer: A Case-Control Study," *Lancet* 353 (199): 1,824–1,828.

Weiner, Z., Beck, D., Shteiner, M., et al. "Screening for Ovarian Cancer in Women with Breast Cancer with Transvaginal Sonography and Color Flow Imaging," *Journal of Ultrasound Medicine* 12/7 (1993): 387–393.

Wideroff, L., Freedman, A. N., Olson, L. "Physician Use of Genetic Testing for Cancer Susceptibility: Results of a National Survey. *Cancer Epidemiology, Biomarkers, and Prevention* 12 (2003): 295–303.

Wilkes, Gail M., Ades, Terri B., and Krakoff, Irwin. *American Cancer Society's Consumers Guide to Cancer Drugs.* Sudbury, Mass.: Jones and Bartlett Publishers, 2000.

Willett, W. C. "Diet and Cancer," *Oncologist* 5/5 (2000): 393–404.

Willett, W. C., Colditz, G. A., Stampfer, M. J. "Postmenopausal Estrogens—Opposed, Unopposed, or None of the Above" (editorial), *Journal of the American Medical Association* 283/4 (2000): 534–535.

Writing Group for the Women's Health Initiative Investigators. "Risks and Benefits of Estrogen plus Progestin in Healthy Postmenopausal Women: Principal Results from the Women's Health Initiative Randomized Controlled Trial," *Journal of the American Medical Association* 28 (2002): 321–333.

Zhuang, S. H., Leonard, G. D., Swain, S. M. "Oophorectomy in Carriers of *BRCA* Mutations," *New England Journal of Medicine* 47 (2002): 1,037–1,040.

INDEX

Boldface page numbers indicate major treatment of a subject. (Numerals are ignored in alphabetization.)

A

ABCD **1**
abdominal cancer **1**
abdominoperineal resection **1,** 15–16
ABNOBAviscum 239
acesulfame potassium 24
acetaminophen 270
achlorhydria **1**
acinar cell carcinoma. *See* pancreatic cancer
acoustic neuroma 54–55
acquired immunodeficiency syndrome. *See* AIDS
acral lentiginous melanoma 235
acrylamide **1–2,** 85, 122, 211
ACS. *See* American Cancer Society
actinic cheilitis 3
actinic keratosis **2–3,** 51, 311
acupressure **3**
acupuncture **3–4,** 271
acute lymphocytic leukemia (ALL) 100, 128, 208–210
acute myeloid leukemia (AML) 10, 22, 208, 242–243, 245, 292
acute promyelocytic leukemia (APL) 22
adenocarcinoma(s) **4**
  anal 15
  bladder 45

clear cell **103–104,** 339
duodenal 126
esophageal 136
fallopian tube 145
follicular 331
gastric 316. *See also* stomach cancer
lung 218, 222
pancreatic 272
papillary 330–331
penile 275
sinus and nasal cavity 165
urethral 335
vaginal 339
vulvar 342–343
adenoid cystic carcinoma (ACC) **4–5**
Adenoid Cystic Carcinoma Organization 353
adenoma(s) **5,** 58
adenomatoid tumor **5**
adenomatous hyperplasia **5,** 132
adenomatous polyps **5**
adenovirus **5,** 110–111
adjuvant therapy **5,** 71, 95
adrenal cancer **5–6,** 6–7, 32
adrenalectomy 7
adrenal glands 395
adrenocortical cancer 5–6, **6–7**
advance directives **7,** 124
advocacy groups 12, 251, 275, 353–354
aflatoxins **7–8,** 214
AFP. *See* alpha-fetoprotein

African American(s) 380–381
  cancer in **8–9,** 78
    bladder 45
    breast 8–9, 305, 380–381
    causes of 8
    colorectal 8–9, 107
    education on 9
    endometrial 130
    kidney 8, 196
    laryngeal 201
    leukemia 208
    liver 214
    lung 8–9, 218–219
    oral 260
    prevention of 9
    prostate 8–9, 285–286, 313
    stomach 8–9, 316
  men 8
  women 9, 78
after loading **9,** 52
age
  and benign prostatic hyperplasia 33
  and cancer **9–10,** 78. *See also specific cancers*
  and myelodysplasia 242, 245
  and ovarian cysts 268
  and support groups 323
Agent Orange **10–11**
agonists 395
agranulocyte 395
agranulocytosis. *See* neutropenia